SECONDARY SOURCES IN THE HISTORY OF CANADIAN MEDICINE

A Bibliography

SECONDARY SOURCES IN THE HISTORY OF CANADIAN MEDICINE
A Bibliography

Compiled by **Charles G. Roland**, M.D.

THE HANNAH INSTITUTE FOR THE HISTORY OF MEDICINE

Canadian Cataloguing in Publication Data

Roland, Charles G., 1933-
    Secondary sources in the history of Canadian
medicine : a bibliography

ISBN 0-88920-182-X

1. Medicine — Canada — History — Bibliography.
2. Medicine — Canada — Bibliography.   I. Hannah
Institute for the History of Medicine.   II. Title.

Z6661.C2R64 1984   016.61′0971   C85-098066-6

Published 1984 for the Hannah Institute for the History of Medicine
          by Wilfrid Laurier University Press, Waterloo, Ontario   N2L 3C5

ISBN 0-88920-182-X

This book was phototypeset from an electronic file provided by the compiler.

Printed in Canada

Dedicated to my parents
Leona (Roland) Steel
and
John Sanford Roland (1910-1960)

———————————

Among their unwitting gifts to me
was an appreciation
of
intellectual order and organization,
attributes that are, I hope, reflected in this volume

Contents

Page

Introduction ix

Using the Bibliography xiii

Searching the McMaster University Data Base xv

List of Journals Examined xvii

Table 1.   Subject Classification Codes xix

Table 2.   "Diseases & Injuries" Subclassification xxi

Table 3.   Era and Place Divisions xxiii

Biographical Listing 1

Subject Listing 47

Author Listing 117

Introduction

Medical-historical bibliography has made great progress since the 1960s, thanks substantially, although by no means entirely, to the availability of the digital computer. Excellent reference works such as Garrison and Morton[1] and Genevieve Miller's bibliography[2] remain standards, but for the latter, at least, the task of supplementing or revising manually would become increasingly arduous. (The work has, to a significant degree, been continued by the National Library of Medicine's efforts.) The Wellcome Library has issued a splendid quarterly bibliography since 1965, a work that unfortunately is more and more weakened by the lack of a cumulative index. We entered the Computer Age in that year, when the National Library of Medicine, in Bethesda, Maryland, began to produce its annual bibliographies, cumulated quinquennially.

Readers will be well aware of the merits and weaknesses of these various tools. Canadian readers will also know that our medical-historical literature has had little bibliographic attention, with two general exceptions. First, the major reference tools mentioned above do carry citations of Canadian material. However, such citations are far from comprehensive, even within the differing scopes of these bibliographies; local publications rarely are cited and none of the tools except Garrison and Morton is retrospective. Secondly, there have been some bibliographic efforts carried out in specialized fields. In the 1930s, MacDermot compiled a useful bibliography of Canadian medical periodicals[3] that recently was brought up-to-date and expanded.[4] A little-known but very useful bibliography has been prepared on the history of Indian and Inuit health.[5] And a few individuals have received bibliographic attention, most particularly William Osler.[6] Beyond these kinds of works, there has been little of specific assistance to historians of Canadian medicine. It is that gap that this volume is intended to fill.

Thirty years ago I began to collect material for my personal bibliography of Canadian medical history, little suspecting the scope this personal project would attain. This book represents the attainment of the first goal of three that were defined formally some years ago in seeking support for a project to enlarge Canadian medical-historical bibliographic resources. The three goals were:
• to publish a bibliography categorized by biographical and subject entries;
• to maintain an expanded data file that could be searched by any scholar seeking greater depth of information;
• to keep that file up-to-date for the indefinite future.
The data files do exist at McMaster University and are available to scholars. That option will be described later. The intention is to pursue the third goal, although to some degree success here is in the laps of the gods.

Scope and Definitions

This work is presented as a *bibliography* of *secondary sources* in *Canadian medical history*. Each of these words deserves some explanation and definition.

Bibliography: This is an enumerative bibliography without annotations. Since the material is in general not rare or difficult to find, no effort has been made to describe locations. Nor is it an elitist document in any way; the compiler has made no attempt to exclude "bad" history (whatever that may be), nor badly written history. The spectrum will be found to be extremely broad, accurately reflecting the historical and contemporary state of the discipline. The work is avowedly retrospective, every reasonable effort having been made to find older material, especially that pre-dating the existing bibliographic tools—i.e. pre-1939.

Secondary Sources: These are *published* sources that are written *about* an event or person. To be published, a work must be available to the public; included are books, book chapters, journal and magazine articles, pamphlets, brochures, and theses. Primary sources, both published and unpublished, are excluded. For example, the original papers by Banting *et al* on their researches into insulin do not appear within these pages, although later retrospective considerations of these times and events, both by Banting and by Best, are included.

Canadian: Here the intent has been to encompass everything that fits all the other criteria and that took place in what is now Canada, or what was once Canada, including New France, British North America, and the territories of the Hudson's Bay Company (but expressly excluding the now U.S.A., a huge subject in its own right). In addition, activities of Canadians outside the country have been included where these activities are identifiably "Canadian": for example, military medical work in Europe in World War I, and the medical-missionary efforts of numerous individuals in Asia and Africa.

Medical: The broadest scope has been used in defining this word, as should be evident in scanning the list of subject categories. However, some specific exclusions should be noted: a few general works on the history of dentistry, pharmacy, and nursing are cited, but these fields have not been tilled systematically. The same is true of related fields such as physiotherapy. On the other hand, the history of medical topics that are not medical-scientific, but rather "social," is included, as shown by the entries on subjects such as poor relief and famine.

History: This criterion also has been defined as having a wide spectrum. The result is perhaps most evident in the large number of obituaries that are included, some of them quite short and most of them uncritical; the rationale has been, first, that the obituary is a deliberate attempt to create an historical record, no matter how biased the eulogist may be, and second, that obituaries often are the sole published record of a life or the only accessible entree to a life. Thus obituaries have been entered in generous numbers.

If any simple statement can synopsize the editorial intention in compiling this bibliography, it might be this: where decisions to include/exclude have had to be made, I have tried to be inclusive rather than exclusive. Data presented in this bibliography need not be used, but data not presented might be lost or ignored.

There will be numerous omissions in this bibliography (without, I hope, many errors). I accept full responsibility for both, but I hope readers will see their occurrence as providing an opportunity to contribute to the increased usefullness of the work, and will notify me promptly. I also accept total responsibility for some discrepancies of style that continue to exist in the present work despite much effort to eliminate these; in a project pursued over many years, such inconsistencies seem as inevitable as they are frustrating. Ultimately, in the interests of getting the volume into the hands of historians, the time came when a halt had to be called to further resetting of type. One final apology is in order: although every effort was made to design the computer programmes to include them, and though they were all entered into the computer, nevertheless, it has proved impossible to print the proper accents for any of the items published in French. This inconsistency will be corrected in future editions.

Acknowledgements

Scholars throughout the field and in many parts of the world have suggested entries and assisted in many other ways. Although they are too numerous to mention by name, I hope they will accept this blanket note of appreciation as well as my warm invitation to continue to make recommendations. This book is only one stage in a continuing project.

Two secretaries, Sue Glover and, for a few months, Cora Miszuk, have had the unenviable task of typing thousands of entry-cards. They have done so with good humour as well as skill. Khursh Ahmed and Kim Clark, of the Computation Services Unit, Health Sciences Centre, McMaster University, provided valuable guidance in setting up the program, and Clark designed the necessary software.

The Hannah Institute for the History of Medicine, and Associated Medical Services, Inc., through two grants-in-aid, provided the necessary financial nourishment without which there would have been no bibliography. From this same source came the funding that enables this publication. Additional financial support came from the John P. McGovern Research Foundation of Houston, Texas.

* * * *

Finally, may I offer the traditional, and totally deserved, tribute: an expression of appreciation to my wife, Connie Rankin Roland. She has indeed put up with lonely hours while I have laboured on this project; she has endured, patiently and with good humour, fully aware that when this responsibility has been completed, its place will be taken by another.

C.G.R.

References

1. Leslie T. Morton, *A Medical Bibliography (Garrison and Morton): An Annotated Check-List of Texts Illustrating the History of Medicine*, (4th ed.; London: A Grafton Book, 1983).

2. Genevieve Miller, editor, *Bibliography of the History of Medicine of the United States and Canada, 1939-1960* (Baltimore: The Johns Hopkins Press, 1964).

3. H. Ernest MacDermot, *A Bibliography of Canadian Medical Periodicals With Annotations* (Montreal: Renouf Publishing Co. Ltd., 1934).

4. Charles G. Roland and Paul Potter, *An Annotated Bibliography of Canadian Medical Periodicals, 1826-1975* (Toronto: The Hannah Institute for the History of Medicine, 1979).

5. Bennett McCardle, *Bibliography of the History of Canadian Indian and Inuit Health* (Edmonton: Treaty and Aboriginal Rights Research of the Indian Association of Alberta, 1981).

6. Bibliographies exist both of Osler's writings and of writings about him. See, respectively, Maude E. Abbott, *Classified and Annotated Bibliography of Sir William Osler's Publications* (Montreal: The Medical Museum, McGill University, 1939), and Earl F. Nation, Charles G. Roland, and John P. McGovern, *An Annotated Checklist of Osleriana* (Kent: The Kent State University Press, 1976).

Using the Bibliography

The format derives in large measure from the annual bibliographies issued by the National Library of Medicine in the U.S.A. There are three sections, Biographical, Subject, and Author.

The Biographical section lists biographical accounts, obituaries, etc., alphabetically by the name of the biographee. Wherever possible, birth and death dates are listed after each individual's name, not only for general information but also to assist the user in distinguishing the various McLeods and Smiths and Johnsons.

The table of subject-classification codes (Table 1, pages xix-xx) will assist the user in accessing material in the Subject section. These codes are based on those used by the N.L.M. but with some deletions, additions, and expansions. The category "Diseases and Injuries" is further subdivided as shown in Table 2 (pages xxi-xxii).

It will be obvious to the reader that many of the categories are such that the opportunity for overlap with other categories exists. Thus anyone interested in *Psychiatry* would wish to examine the entries in that category as well as *Mental Health* and *Hospitals, Psychiatric*. Similarly, one might look for material related to diabetes and the discovery of insulin under *Endocrinology* in the main subject section, but should also remember that there is a specific category *Diabetes* in the secondary codes under *Diseases and Injuries*. All entries in each category of the Subject section are grouped into time periods (roughly corresponding to significant political events in Canadian history) and into geographical areas. Both of these divisions are described and itemized in Table 3.

The author section is just that—a listing of the entries in the book, alphabetically by the name of the author. There is one major omission from this section, however. All entries by that most prolific of authors, Anonymous, are deleted, on the principle that the list is long and a reader is highly unlikely to seek a reference for which he has no subject information but which he knows to be written anonymously.

Abbreviations

In general, names of journals and magazines are spelled out fully. The exceptions, a handfull of titles that recur with high frequency, are listed here:

BHM   Bulletin of the History of Medicine
CACHB   Calgary Associate Clinic Historical Bulletin
CAMSI   Canadian Association of Medical Students and Interns
CHR   Canadian Historical Review
CMAJ   Canadian Medical Association Journal
DCB   Dictionary of Canadian Biography
JAMA   Journal of the American Medical Association
JHMAS   Journal of the History of Medicine and Allied Sciences
L'UMC   L'Union Medicale du Canada
PTRSC   Proceedings and Transactions of the Royal Society of Canada (includes all variants of this organization's name)

Searching the McMaster University Data Base

The data base is available for access by any interested scholar. Although it is assumed that the published bibliography will provide sufficient material for most users, nevertheless, searching the data base carries two advantages. First, that base will be maintained continuously, and thus after a period of time will be significantly more up-to-date than the book. (When sufficient time has passed, the desirability of publishing a second volume or a revised edition will be considered.)

Secondly, data are available from the computer that are not so readily available from the published bibliography. This is so because articles that cover more than one general subject category were assigned one primary area—the one under which the item appears in the book—and up to four additional secondary areas in the data base.

For example, the article by Hilda Neatby on "The Medical Profession in the North-West Territories" (*Saskatchewan History* 2(2): 1-15, 1949) is found in this volume under the category of *Professionalization*. But the article deals as well with *Medical Licencing*, *Frontier Medicine*, and *Economics, Medical*. A scholar not familiar with Neatby's article but interested in medical economics could miss the reference unless the data base was searched for that category, at which time all primary citations in this category (those cited in the published bibliography) plus all secondary citations (such as to the Neatby article) will be located. So using this source can expand the number of relevant citations found.

Anyone who wishes to access the data base may do so by writing the appropriate office:

> History of Medicine Datasearch
> 3N10-HSC, McMaster University
> Hamilton, Ontario L8N 3Z5

A check-list/order-form can be obtained by writing or calling (area 416 525-9140, ext. 2751); however, orders for searches will *not* be accepted on the telephone. You must specify on the appropriate form what search you wish to have made. Full details are available from the same address. A nominal charge of $10 will be made for each search made; the Hannah Institute for the History of Medicine has agreed to underwrite this programme, at least for the first few years, so that this charge can remain nominal and uniform.

Searching the McMaster University Data Base

List of Journals Examined

Acadiensis (1901-1908)
Acadiensis (1971-)
Alberta Historical Review
American Indian Quarterly
Anthropological Journal of Canada
Atlantis
BC Studies
Beaver
Boreal (Journal of Northern Ontario Studies)
British Columbia Historical Quarterly
Bulletin des Recherches Historiques
Bulletin of the History of Medicine
Cahiers des Dix
Cahiers d'Histoire
Calgary Associate Clinic Historical Bulletin
Canada: An Historical Magazine
Canadian Antiquarian and Numismatic Journal
Canadian Church Historical Society Journal
Canadian Ethnic Studies
Canadian Frontier
Canadian Geographer
Canadian Historical Review
Canadian Jewish Historical Society Journal
Canadian Journal of Archeology
Canadian Journal of History/Annales Canadienne
 d'Histoire
Canadian Journal of Public Health
Canadian Journal of Surgery
Canadian Journal of the History of Sport and Physical
 Education
Canadian Medical Association Journal
Canadian Psychiatric Association Journal
Canadian Review of Social Anthropology
Canadian Review of Sociology and Anthropology
Canadian Studies in Population
Collections of the New Brunswick Historical Society
Collections of the Nova Scotia Historical Society
Culture
Dalhousie Review
Dan Brock's Historical Almanack of London
Etudes/Inuit/Studies

Grand Manan Historian
Histoire Sociale/Social History
Historical and Scientific Society of Manitoba: Papers
Journal of Canadian Art History
Journal of Canadian Fiction
Journal of Canadian Studies
Journal of Social History
Journal of the History of Medicine and Allied Sciences
Journal of the Society for Army Historical Research
Lakehead University Review
Laurentian University Review/Revue de L'Universite
 Laurentienne
Le Canada Francais
L'Union Medicale du Canada
Manitoba History
Medical Anthropology
Medical History
Medical Services Journal of Canada
Nova Scotia Historical Quarterly
Okanagan Historical Society Annual Report
Ontario Historical Society Papers and Records
Ontario History
Proceedings and Transactions of the Royal Society of
 Canada
Proceedings of the Canadian Institute
Queen's Quarterly
Recherches Sociographiques
Revue d'Histoire de l'Amerique Francais
Revue Trimestrielle Canadienne
Saskatchewan History
Scarlet and Gold [R.C.M.P.]
Societe Historique Acadienne. Cahier
Studies in Religion/Science Religieuses
Transactions of the Literary and Historical Society of
 Quebec
University of Toronto Quarterly
Wentworth Bygones
Western Canadian Journal of Anthropology
Women's Canadian Historical Society of Toronto:
 Annual Report
York Pioneer

All of these journals have been searched systematically and retrospectively for articles suitable for inclusion in this bibliography. In addition, many articles are included from journals not on this list but which have been found to contain single or sporadic items that fit the criteria for inclusion.

Table 1
Subject Classification Codes

Acupuncture *see* Therapeutics
1 Aerospace Medicine
2 Alchemy
3 Anatomy
4 Anesthesiology
5 Animals
Anthropology *see* Anatomy; Evolution; Science;
6 Art & Medicine
7 Awards & Prizes
Bacteriology, *see* Microbiology
8 Balneology, Hydrotherapy, & Health Resorts
9 Biology
10 Biophysics
11 Birth Control
12 Blood Transfusion
13 Botany
14 Cardiology & Circulatory System
15 Chemistry & Biochemistry
16 Child Health
17 Climate
18 Cold
19 Communicable Disease Control
20 Congresses
21 Cytology
22 Death
Demography *see* Statistics
23 Dentistry
24 Dermatology
25 Diagnosis
26 Diseases & Injuries (Listing pp. xxi-xxii)
27 Drugs & Chemicals
28 Ecology
29 Economics, incl. Health Insurance
30 Education, Medical
31 Embryology
32 Emergency Care
33 Endocrinology
Engineering *see* Instruments & Equipment
Environmental Health *see* Ecology; Sanitation
34 Epidemiology
35 Ethics, Medical
36 Evolution
37 Exhibits
38 Famous Persons
Fertility *see* Generation & Reproduction;
39 Folk & Popular Medicine

40 Foods & Food Supply
41 Forensic Medicine & Legal Medicine
42 Gastroenterology & Digestive System
43 General Practice & Family Medicine
44 Generation & Reproduction
45 Genetics, incl. Eugenics
46 Gerontology & Geriatrics
47 Gynecology
48 Health Education
49 Health Occupations & Professions
Health Resorts *see* Balneology
50 Hematology
51 Herbals
52 Histology
53 Historiography & History of Medicine
54 Homeopathy
55 Hospitals
56 Hospitals, Psychiatric
57 Human Development & Growth
58 Hygiene
59 Hypnosis
60 Immunology
Industrial Medicine *see* Occupational Medicine
155 Incarceration, incl. POW & Concentration Camps
62 Instruments
Insurance *see* Economics; Statistics
62 International Health
63 Jews
Journalism *see* Periodicals
64 Laboratories & Research Institutes
65 Libraries & Archives
66 Licensure & Regulation
67 Literature & Medicine
68 Magic, Occult & Mystic
69 Manuscripts
70 Maternal Health
71 Mathematics
72 Medical Illustration
Medical Theory *see* Philosophy
73 Medicine, General History & Collective Biography
74 Mental Health
Meteorology *see* Climate
75 Microbiology
76 Microscopy
77 Military Medicine, incl. NWMP/RCMP
78 Molecular Biology

Table 1. Subject Classification Codes

Table 1. **Subject Classification Codes**—*Continued*

79 Mortuary Practices
80 Musculoskeletal System
81 Museums
82 Music & Medicine
83 Naval Medicine
84 Negroes
85 Neurology & Neurosurgery
  Nosology *see* Terminology
86 Numismatics
87 Nursing
88 Nutrition & Diet
89 Obstetrics
90 Occupational Medicine
91 Ophthalmology
92 Optics
93 Orthopedics
94 Osteopathy
95 Otorhinolaryngology
96 Paleopathology
97 Parasitology
98 Pathology
99 Pediatrics
100 Periodicals
101 Pharmacology
102 Pharmacy
103 Philately
104 Philosophy
105 Photography
106 Physical Medicine & Rehabilitation
107 Physiognomy
108 Physiology
153 Plastic Surgery
109 Podiatry
110 Politics
111 Portraits
112 Preventive Medicine
113 Primitive American & Inuit Medicine
114 Printing & Bibliography
  Proctology *see* Gastroenterology

154 Professionalization
115 Psychiatry
116 Psychology
117 Psychosomatic Medicine
118 Public Health
119 Quackery
120 Race
121 Radiology
122 Red Cross
123 Religion & Medicine
124 Research
125 Respiratory System
126 Resuscitation
127 Rural Health & Pioneer Practice
128 Sanitation
129 Science
130 Sex Behaviour
131 Social Medicine
132 Social Welfare
133 Societies, Academies, & Foundations
134 Specialization & Practice Organization
135 Sport Medicine
136 State Medicine & Medical Legislation
137 Statistics & Demography
138 Surgery
139 Symbolism & Heraldry
140 Terminology & Nomenclature
141 Therapeutic Cults excl. Homeopathy
142 Therapeutics
143 Toxicology
144 Transport of Sick & Wounded
145 Travel & Exploration
146 Tropical Medicine
147 Urology & Nephrology
148 Veterinary Medicine
149 War
150 Witchcraft
151 Women in Medicine
  Zoology *see* Animals; Biology; Parasitology

Table 2
"Diseases & Injuries" Subclassification

 1 Abdominal
 2 Abnormalities
 3 Abscess
 4 Adrenal Gland
 5 Alcoholism
 6 Altitude Sickness
 7 Anemia
 8 Anthrax
 9 Appendicitis
10 Arthritis & Rheumatism
11 Asphyxia
12 Asthma
13 Avitaminosis
14 Beriberi
15 Biliary Tract
16 Bites & Stings
17 Blood
18 Bone
19 Botulism
20 Brucellosis
21 Burns
   Cancer *see* Neoplasms
22 Cataract
23 Cerebrovascular
24 Chest
25 Chickenpox
26 Cholera
27 Cleft Palate
28 Clubfoot
167 Congenital Malformations
29 Cretinism
30 Cystic Fibrosis
31 Cysts
32 Decompression Sickness
33 Dengue
34 Diabetes
35 Diarrhea
36 Digestive System
37 Diphtheria
38 Dislocations
165 Drowning
39 Drug Addiction
40 Dwarfism
41 Dysentery
42 Ear
43 Edema

44 Encephalitis
45 Endocrine
46 Epilepsy
47 Ergotism
48 Erysipelas
49 Eye
50 Fatigue
51 Favism
52 Fever
53 Filariasis
54 Food Poisoning
55 Foot-and-Mouth
56 Fractures
57 Gangrene
58 Gigantism
59 Goiter
60 Gonorrhea
61 Gout
62 Gynecologic
63 Hay Fever
64 Headache
65 Hearing Disorders
66 Heart
67 Helminthiasis
68 Hemophilia
69 Hemorrhage
70 Hernia
71 Herpes
72 Hookworm Infection
73 Hypersensitivity
74 Iatrogenic
75 Infections
76 Infectious Mononucleosis
77 Influenza
78 Jaundice
79 Kidney
80 Laurence-Moon-Biedl Syndrome
81 Leishmaniasis
82 Leprosy
83 Leptospirosis
84 Leukemia
85 Liver
86 Lymphatic
87 Malaria
88 Marfan's Syndrome
89 Measles

Table 2.   "Diseases & Injuries" Subclassification

Table 2.   **"Diseases & Injuries" Subclassification**—*Continued*

90 Meningitis
91 Mental Disorders
92 Mental Retardation
93 Metabolic
94 Metabolism, Inborn Errors
95 Milk Sickness
96 Motion Sickness
97 Mumps
98 Musculoskeletal
99 Neoplasms
100 Nervous System
101 Obesity
102 Oral
103 Ornithosis
104 Parasitic
105 Pellagra
106 Plague
107 Plant Poisoning
108 Pneumoconiosis
109 Pneumonia
110 Poisoning
111 Poliomyelitis
112 Polyps
113 Porphyria
114 Puerperal Infection
115 Rabies
116 Radiation Injury
117 Rat-Bite Fever
118 Reiter's Disease
119 Relapsing Fever
120 Respiratory Tract
121 Rheumatic Fever
122 Rickets
123 Rocky Mountain Spotted Fever
124 Rubella
125 Salmonella Infections
126 Sarcoidosis
127 Scabies

128 Scarlet Fever
129 Schistosomiasis
130 Scrofula
131 Scurvy
132 Sex Deviation
133 Sex Disorders
134 Shock
135 Sjogren's Syndrome
136 Skin
137 Smallpox
138 Speech Disorders
139 Splenic
140 Spontaneous Combustion
166 Suicide
141 Sweating Sickness
142 Syphilis
143 Tetanus
144 Thymus
145 Thyroid
146 Tonsillitis
147 Toxoplasmosis
148 Treponemal Infection
149 Trichinosis
150 Trypanosomiasis
151 Tuberculosis
152 Tularemia
153 Typhoid
154 Typhus
155 Urinary Calculi
156 Urogenital System
157 Vascular
158 Venereal, General
159 Vision Disorders
160 Waterhouse-Friderichsen Syndrome
161 Whooping Cough
162 Wound Infection
162 Wounds & Injuries
164 Yellow Fever

Table 3
Era and Place Divisions

Era: Divisions are as follows:

Pre-1500	1500-1699	1700-1759	1760-1815
1816-1867	1868-1918	1919-1945	1946-1979
1980-1989	All-embracing		

Place: Divisions are as follows:

Canada	Alberta	British Columbia	Manitoba
New Brunswick	Newfoundland	Northwest Territories	Nova Scotia
Ontario	Prince Edward Island	Quebec	Saskatchewan
Yukon	United Kingdom	USA	Others

BIOGRAPHICAL LISTING

A

Abbott, A.C. (1898-1983)

Beamish, R.E.: Dr. Albert Clifford Abbott: Pioneer Surgeon of Western Canada. CMAJ 128:862, 864, 1983 ⟨I-05072⟩

Beamish, R.E.: Dr. Albert Clifford Abbott: Pioneer Experimental Surgeon of Western Canada. University of Manitoba Medical Journal 53:84-88, 1983 ⟨I-05288⟩

Abbott, M.E.S. (1869-1940)

MacDermot, H.E.: Maude Abbott: A Memoir. Toronto, Macmillan Co. of Canada Ltd., 1941. 264 p. ⟨I-00024⟩

MacDermot, H.E.: Nora Livingston and Maude Abbott. CACHB 22:228-235, 1958 ⟨I-00023⟩

Roland, C.G.: Maude Abbott and J.B. MacCallum: Canadian Cardiac Pioneers. Chest 57:371-377, 1970 ⟨I-03565⟩

Smith, K.: Maude Abbott: Pathologist and Historian. CMAJ 127:774-776, 1982 ⟨I-04976⟩

Abbott, W.O. (-1943)

E.R.: Dr. William Osler Abbott. CMAJ 49:447, 1943 ⟨I-04264⟩

Abramson, H.L. (1886-1934)

Roberts, W.F.: Dr. H.L. Abramson. CMAJ 30:696, 1934 ⟨I-03541⟩

Adami, J.G. (1862-1926)

Adami, J.G.: An Epizootic of Rabies; and a Personal Experience of M. Pasteur's Treatment. British Medical Journal 2:808-810, 1889 ⟨I-03413⟩

Adami, M.: J. George Adami: A Memoir. London, Constable and Co., Ltd., 1930. 179 p. ⟨I-00028⟩

Fulton, J.F.: John George Adami (1862-1926). In Kelly HW, Burrage WL: Dictionary of American Medical Biography. New York and London, D. Appleton and Co., 1928. p.3. ⟨I-00022⟩

Martin, C.F.: Dr. J.G. Adami. CMAJ 16:1281-1282, 1926 ⟨I-01616⟩

Nicholls, A.G.: Dr. J.G. Adami. CMAJ 16:1282, 1926 ⟨I-01615⟩

Oertel, H.: Dr. J.G. Adami. CMAJ 16:1282, 1926 ⟨I-01955⟩

Power, D'Arcy: John George Adami. In: Plarr's Lives of the Fellows of the Royal College of Surgeons of England. Bristol and London, The Royal College of Surgeons, 1930. Vol. I, pp 2-3 ⟨I-02760⟩

Adamson, J.D. (1890-1964)

Thompson, I.M.: Dr. Adamson as a medical historian. Manitoba Medical Review 44:564-565, 1964 ⟨I-00018⟩

Addison, W.L.T. (-1930)

Gwyn, N.B.: Dr. William Lockwood T. Addison. CMAJ 23:727, 1930 ⟨I-03025⟩

Addy, G.A.B. (1869-1945)

Kirkland, A.S.: Dr. George Arthur Beldon Addy. CMAJ, 52:312, 1945 ⟨I-04368⟩

Ahern, G. (1887-1927)

Vallee, A.: Dr. Georges Ahern. CMAJ 17:1233, 1927 ⟨I-03423⟩

Ahern, M.J. (1844-1914)

Kelly, H.A.: Michael Joseph Ahern (1844-1914). In Kelly HW, Burrage WL: Dictionary of American Medical Biography. New York, London, D. Appleton and Co., 1928. p. 10. ⟨I-00027⟩

Vallee, A.: Feu Dr. Ahern. In: Annuaire de l'Universite Laval pour l'annee 1914-15. Quebec 1914 ⟨I-05214⟩

Aikenhead, A.E. (1882-1954)

Scarlett, E.P.: Ave Atque Vale: Albert Earl Aikenhead 1882-1954. CACHB 19:84-85, 1954 ⟨I-00021⟩

Aikins, W.T. (1827-1895)

Cameron, M.H.V.: William Thomas Aikins (1827-1895). CMAJ 64:161-163, 1951 ⟨I-01068⟩

Harris, C.W.: William Thomas Aikins, M.D., LL.D.,. Canadian Journal of Surgery 5:131-137, 1962 ⟨I-04243⟩

Alavoine, C. (ca1695-1764)

Douville, R.: Charles Alavoine. DCB 3:7-8, 1974 ⟨I-00032⟩

Alcorn, D.E. (1906-1968)

Margetts, E.L.: Dr. Douglas Earle Alcorn. CMAJ 100:42, 1969 ⟨I-05040⟩

Alexander, H.E. (1884-1942)

Valens, J.A.: Dr. Harold Egbert Alexander. CMAJ 47:599, 1942 ⟨I-04278⟩

Alleyn, R.E. (1895-1931)

Mitchell, R.: Dr. R.E. Alleyn. CMAJ 24:474, 1931 ⟨I-03065⟩

Allin, A.E. (1906-1966)

Hogarth, W.P.: Dr. Albert E. Allin. CMAJ 96:61-62, 1967 ⟨I-03910⟩

Allin, E.W. (1875-1933)

Whitelaw, T.H.: Dr. Edgar W. Allin. CMAJ 29:338, 1933 ⟨I-03070⟩

Almon, W.J. (1755-1817)

Kernaghan, L.K.: William James Almon. DCB 5:23-24, 1983 ⟨I-05318⟩

Almon, W.J. (1816-1901)

Campbell, D.A.: William Johnston Almon (1816-1901). In Kelly HW, Burrage WL: Dictionary of American Medical Biography. New York, London, D. Appleton and Co., 1928. p. 22. ⟨I-00029⟩

Amyot, G.F. (1897-1967)

Taylor, J.A.: Dr. Gregoire F. Amyot. CMAJ 98:795, 1968 ⟨I-03908⟩

Amyot, J.A. (1868-1940)

Heagerty, J.J.: The retirement of Lt.-Col. John Andrew Amyot, CMG, MB, Deputy Minister of Pensions and National Health, Canada. CMAJ 27:544-545, 1933 ⟨I-03909⟩

Anderson, F. U. (1859-1929)
Walker, S.L.: Fitzgerald Uniacke Anderson. CMAJ 20:681, 1929 ⟨I-03500⟩

Anderson, G. L. (1908-1981)
Duncan, L.M.C.: Gordon L. Anderson. CMAJ 125:1059, 1981 ⟨I-04650⟩

Anderson, W. J. (1812-1873)
Waterson, E.: William James Anderson. DCB 10:13-14, 1972 ⟨I-00026⟩

Antle, J. (-1949)
Kidd, H.M.: John Antle. CMAJ 65:484-489, 1951 ⟨I-03875⟩

Archer, A. E. (1879-1949)
Young, M.A.R.: A.E. Archer, M.D. CMAJ 61:193-4, 1949 ⟨I-04488⟩

Archibald, E. W. (1872-1945)
Gallie, W.E.: Dr. Edward Archibald. CMAJ 54:197, 1946 ⟨I-04348⟩
Graham, E.A.: Dr. Edward Archibald. CMAJ 54: 197-8, 1946 ⟨I-04347⟩
Howell, W.B.: Dr. Edward Archibald. CMAJ 54:317, 1946 ⟨I-04349⟩
MacDermot, H.E.: Dr. Edward Archibald, 1872-1945. McGill News, Spring 1946, 4p. ⟨I-04389⟩
Meakins, J.C.: Edward William Archibald, B.A., M.D., C.M. (McGill); Hon. F.R.C.S. (Eng.); F.R.C.S. [C].; Hon. F.R.C.S. (Australasia); F.A.C.S. CMAJ 54:194-7, 1946 ⟨I-04346⟩
Penfield, W.: Edward Archibald :1872-1945. Canadian Journal of Surgery 1:167-174, 1958 ⟨I-01576⟩
Robertson, H.R.: Edward Archibald, the "New Medical Science" and Norman Bethune. In: Shephard, D.A.E.; Levesque, A. (edit): Norman Bethune; His Times and His Legacy. Ottawa, Canadian Public Health Assoc., 1982 pp 71-78 ⟨I-04895⟩

Argue, A. W. (1862-1945)
Valens, J.A.: Dr. Andrew William Argue. CMAJ 52:530-1, 1945 ⟨I-04370⟩

Argue, J. F. (1871-1956)
F., T.L.: Dr. John Fenton Argue, an appreciation. CMAJ 75:456, 1956 ⟨I-04736⟩

Armitage, A. H. (-1942)
Valens, J.A.: Dr. Alexander Howard Armitage. CMAJ 48:279, 1943 ⟨I-04270⟩

Armstrong, G. E. (1855-1933)
Archibald, E.: Dr. George Eli Armstrong. CMAJ 29:103-104, 1933 ⟨I-03075⟩
Barlow, W.L.: Dr. George Eli Armstrong, an appreciation. CMAJ 29:104, 1933 ⟨I-01487⟩
MacLaren, M.: Dr. George Eli Armstrong. CMAJ 29:103, 1933 ⟨I-03074⟩

Armstrong, J. W. (1860-1928)
Thornton, R.S.: Hon. J.W. Armstrong, an appreciation. CMAJ 18:475, 1928 ⟨I-03904⟩

Arnoldi, D. (1774-1849)
Gauvreau, J.: Dr. Daniel Arnoldi (1774-1849). CMAJ 27:79-82, 1932 ⟨I-03040⟩

Arnoldi, F. C. T. (-1862)
Gauvreau, J.: L'Ecole de Medecine et de Chirurgie de Montreal Fondee en 1843: Le Docteur Thomas Arnoldi, son Premier President. L'UMC 60:818-827, 1931 ⟨I-01773⟩

Arnoux, A. (1720-1760)
Douville, R.: Andre Arnoux. DCB 3:18-20, 1974 ⟨I-00031⟩

Arthur, E. C. (1856-1932)
Bastin, C.H.: Dr. Edward Charles Arthur. CMAJ 27:332, 1932 ⟨I-03057⟩

Arthur, R. H. (1861-1941)
Lockwood, A.L.: Dr. Robert Hugh Arthur. CMAJ 46:198-9, 1942 ⟨I-04252⟩

Ash, J. (1821-1886)
Jones, O.M.: John Ash (1821-1886) [sic]. In Kelly HW, Burrage WL: Dictionary of American Medical Biography. New York and London, D. Appleton and Co., 1928. pp. 38-39. ⟨I-00030⟩
Teece, W.K.: John Ash. DCB 11:32-33, 1982 ⟨I-04839⟩

Atkin, G. M.
Stanley, G.D.: Dr. G.M. Atkin. CACHB 12(1):18-20, 1947 ⟨I-00019⟩

Atlee, H. B. (1890-1978)
Fishman, N.: Harold Benge Atlee. CMAJ 121:1439, 1441, 1979 ⟨I-00017⟩
Oxorn, H.: Harold Benge Atlee, M.D.: A Biography. Hantsport, N.S., Lancelot Press, 1983. pp 352. ⟨I-05164⟩

Austin, L. J. (1880-1945)
Austin, L.J.: My Experiences as a German Prisoner. London: Andrew Melrose Ltd., 1915, pp.158 ⟨I-04399⟩
Jones, W.A.: Lorimer John Austin, M.A., M.B., M.Ch., F.R.C.S. [C] F.A.C.S. 1880-1945. Canadian Journal of Surgery 1-5, 1962 ⟨I-04244⟩
Miller, J.: The Late Dr. L.J. Austin. CMAJ 52:644-5, 1945 ⟨I-04334⟩

B

Bacstrom, S.
Cole, D.: Sigismund Bacstrom's northwest coast drawings and an account of his curious career. British Columbia Studies, 46:61-86, 1980 ⟨I-03166⟩

Badelard, P-L-F. (1728-1802)
Bernier, J.: Philippe-Louis-Francois Badelard. DCB 5:46-47, 1983 ⟨I-05317⟩

Badgley, F. (1807-1863)
Desjardins, E.: Francis Badgley. DCB 9:16-17, 1976 ⟨I-00986⟩

Bagnall, A.W. (1881-1944)

M., J.H.: Dr. A.W. Bagnall. CMAJ 52:313, 1945 ⟨I-04369⟩

Bagshaw, E.C. (1881-1982)

Gray, C.: Elizabeth Catharine Bagshaw. CMAJ 124:211, 1981 ⟨I-03241⟩

Hellstedt, L.McG. (edit): Elizabeth Catherine Bagshaw. In: Women Physicians of the World: Autobiographies of Medical Pioneers New York, McGraw-Hill Book Co., 1978. pp 8-9 ⟨I-03942⟩

Bailey, A.A. (1910-1967)

McKerracher, D.G.: Dr. Allan A. Bailey. CMAJ 97:1428, 1967 ⟨I-01489⟩

Moore, D.F.: Dr. Allan A. Bailey, an appreciation. CMAJ 97:1429, 1967 ⟨I-01490⟩

Bain, H. (1921-)

Gray, C.: Harry Bain. CMAJ 129-614, 1983 ⟨I-05184⟩

Bajusz, E. (1926-1973)

Abelmann, W.H.: In Memoriam -- Elors Bajusz 1926-1973. Recent Advances in Studies in Cardiac Structure and Metabolism 6:5-20, 1975 ⟨I-05381⟩

Baldwin, W.W. (1774-1844)

Baldwin, R.M., Baldwin, J.: The Baldwins and The Great Experiment. Longmans, 1969, 269 p. ⟨I-04516⟩

Phelan, J.: A Duel on the Island. Ontario History 69:235-238, 1977 ⟨I-01666⟩

Balfour, D.C. (1882-1963)

Bailey, A.A.: Dr. Donald C. Balfour, an appreciation. CMAJ 89:831-382, 1963 ⟨I-03903⟩

Bowman, F.B.: Donald C. Balfour. CMAJ 89:361, 1963 ⟨I-03901⟩

Wangensteen, O.H.: Dr. Donald Church Balfour: Builder of the University Name. University of Minnesota, 1950 ⟨I-00933⟩

Ball, F.J. (1865-1928)

Moore, S.E.: Dr. F.J. Ball. CMAJ 19:628-629, 1928 ⟨I-03489⟩

Ballem, J.C. (1881-1963)

P., V.H.T.: Dr. John C. Ballem. CMAJ 90:1138, 1964 ⟨I-05225⟩

Banting, F.G. (1891-1941)

Berry, J.N.: Sir Frederick Banting's Dream. Canadian Notes and Queries 23:7, 1980 ⟨I-00961⟩

Best, C.H.: Sir Frederick Banting. University of Toronto Quarterly 10:249-254, 1940-41 ⟨I-04367⟩

Casson, A.J.: The doctor as an artist. Northward Journal No.'s 14 and 15:21-24, 1979 ⟨I-03188⟩

Greenaway, R: Banting and Medical News. In: The News Game. Toronto/Vancouver, Clarke, Irwin and Co. Ltd., 1966, pp 59-71 ⟨I-03880⟩

Harris, S.: Banting's Miracle: The Story of the Discoverer of Insulin. Toronto/Vancouver, J.M. Dent and Sons (Canada) Ltd., 1946. 245 p. ⟨I-00964⟩

Henderson, V.E.: Sir Frederick Grant Banting. CMAJ 44:429-430, 1941 ⟨I-03348⟩

Hunter, G.: Sir Frederick Banting. CMAJ 44:431, 1941 ⟨I-03349⟩

Jackson, A.Y.: Banting As an Artist. Toronto, Ryerson Press, 1943. 37 p. ⟨I-00965⟩

Jackson, A.Y.: Memories of a Fellow Artist, Frederick Grant Banting. CMAJ 92:1077-1084, 1965 ⟨I-04951⟩

Katz, S.: A new, informal glimpse of Dr. Frederick Banting. CMAJ 129:1229-1232, 1983 ⟨I-05300⟩

Lajoie, G.: A la Memoire de Sir Frederick Banting. L'UMC 71:1331-1332, 1942 ⟨I-00960⟩

Levine, I.E.: The discoverer of insulin: Dr. Frederick G. Banting. Toronto, The Copp Clark Publishing Co. Ltd., 1959. pp. 192 ⟨I-00962⟩

Rowntree, L.G.: Banting's "Miracle". In: Amid Masters of Twentieth Century Medicine. Springfield, Charles C. Thomas Publisher, 1958. pp 339-354 ⟨I-02593⟩

Shaw, M.M.: He Conquered Death: The Story of Frederick Grant Banting. Toronto, MacMillan Co., 1946, 111 p. ⟨I-01645⟩

Shaw, M.M.: Frederick Banting. Toronto, Fitzhenry and Whiteside Limited, 1976, p.62 ⟨I-04521⟩

Stevenson, L.G.: Sir Frederick Banting. Toronto, The Ryerson Press, 1946. 446 p. ⟨I-00963⟩

Stevenson, L.G.: Frederick Grant Banting. Dictionary of Scientific Biography 1:440-443, 1970 ⟨I-02761⟩

Vipond, M.: A Canadian Hero of the 1920's: Dr. Frederick G. Banting. Canadian Historical Review 58:461-486, 1982 ⟨I-05028⟩

Williams, J.R.: The "S.S. Frederick Banting". CMAJ 50:181, 1944 ⟨I-04260⟩

Wrenshall, G.A., Hetenyi, G., Feasby, W.R.: The Story of Insulin. Toronto, Max Reinhardt, 1962. 232 p. ⟨I-01039⟩

Banting, H. (1913-1977)

V., K: Lady Henrietta Banting: a life of service. CMAJ 116:85, 1977 ⟨I-03882⟩

Bardy, P.-M. (1797-1869)

LeBlond, S.: Pierre-Martial Bardy. Laval Medical 27(4):3-10, 1959 ⟨I-03876⟩

Savard, P.: Pierre-Martial Bardy. DCB 9:32-33, 1976 ⟨I-00977⟩

Barker, E.J. (1799-1884)

Spurr, J.W.: Edward John Barker, M.D. Editor and Citizen. Historic Kingston 27:113-126, 1979 ⟨I-00016⟩

Spurr, J.W.: Edward John Barker. DCB 11:47-49, 1982 ⟨I-04841⟩

Barnston, J. (-1859)

R., A.N.: James Barnston, M.D. Medical Chronicle 6:90-92, 1859 ⟨I-00987⟩

Barrett, M. (1816-1887)

Craig, G.M.: Michael Barrett. DCB 11:53-54, 1982 ⟨I-04842⟩

Barrett, W.T.
Barrett, W.T.: Reminiscences of Early Klondyke Days. University of Manitoba Medical Journal 49:141-146, 1979 ⟨I-01570⟩

Barry, J. (ca.1795-1865)
Humphrey, B.M.: A Medical Sphinx [James Barry]. CACHB 10:107-114. 1945 ⟨I-03926⟩
Rae, I.: The strange story of Dr. James Barry. London, Longmans, Green and Co., 1958. pp 124 ⟨I-00992⟩
Roland, C.G.: James Barry. DCB 9:33-34, 1976 ⟨I-00985⟩
Rose, J.: The Perfect Gentleman. London, England, Hutchinson and Co. (Publishers) Ltd., 1977. 160 p. ⟨I-00990⟩
Smith, K.M.: Dr. James Barry: military man -- or woman?. CMAJ 126:854-857, 1982 ⟨I-04770⟩

Bascom, H. (1863-1956)
Harshman, J.P.: Dr. Horace Bascom (1863-1956) Country Doctor, Court Officer. Ontario Medical Review 47(1):12-17, 1980 ⟨I-00934⟩

Basset du Tartre, V. (fl. 1665)
Nadeau, G.: Vincent Basset du Tartre. DCB 1:79-80, 1966 ⟨I-00995⟩

Bates, G.A. (1885-1975)
Robinson, R.R.: Bates of the Health League: An Insider's Reminiscence. Ontario Medical Review 49:305-308, 1982 ⟨I-04871⟩

Baudeau, P. (1643-1708)
Biron, H.: Pierre Baudeau. DCB 2:47-48, 1969 ⟨I-00993⟩

Baudoin, G. (1686-1752)
Paquin, M.: Gervais Baudoin. DCB 3:35, 1974 ⟨I-00994⟩

Baudouin, G. (1645-1700)
Nadeau, G.: Gervais Baudouin. DCB 1:80-81, 1966 ⟨I-00996⟩

Bayard, R. (1788-1868)
Gibbon, A.D.: Robert Bayard. DCB 9:35, 1976 ⟨I-00982⟩

Bayard, W. (1814-1907)
Atherton, A.B.: William Bayard (1814-1907). In Kelly HW, Burrage WL: Dictionary of American Medical Biography. New York and London, D. Appleton and Co., 1928. pp. 76-77 ⟨I-00980⟩
Cushing, J.E., Casey, T., Robertson, M.: A Chronicle of Irish Emigration to Saint John, New Brunswick, 1847. New Brunswick, The New Brunswick Museum, 1979. 77 p. ⟨I-00981⟩

Bazin, A.T. (1873-1958)
Shane, S.J.: Dr. Alfred Turner Bazin, appreciation. CMAJ 79:600-601, 1958 ⟨I-03893⟩

Beath, T. (-1923)
Cooke, R.: A Thumb-Nail Sketch of Dr. Thomas Beath. University of Manitoba Medical Journal 26:13, 1954 ⟨I-03891⟩

Beaubien, J-O. (1824-1877)
Vachon, C.: Joseph-Octave Beaubien. DCB 10:36-37, 1972 ⟨I-00015⟩

Beaubien, P. (1796-1881)
Bernier, J.: Pierre Beaubien. DCB 11:57-58, 1982 ⟨I-04843⟩
Desjardins, E.: Deux Medecins Montrealais du XIXe Siecle Adeptes de la Pensee Ecologique. L'UMC 99:487-492, 1970 ⟨I-02235⟩

Beaumont, W.R. (1803-1875)
Cosbie, W.G.: William Rawlins Beaumont. DCB 10:38-39, 1972 ⟨I-00014⟩
Power, D'Arcy: William Rawlins Beaumont. In: Plarr's Lives of the Fellows of the Royal College of Surgeons of England. Bristol and London, The Royal College of Surgeons 1930. Vol. 1:73-75 ⟨I-02759⟩

Beaupre, E. (1881-1904)
Blais, J.M.: Un geant canadien celebre: Edouard Beaupre (1881-1904). Neuro-Chirurgie 19(2):23-34, 1973 ⟨I-05295⟩

Beckingsale, D.L. (1847-1929)
Bastin, C.H.: Dr. D.L. Beckingsale. CMAJ 20:571, 1929 ⟨I-03499⟩

Beddome, H.S. (1830-1881)
Bredin, T.F.: Henry Septimus Beddome. DCB 11:63-64, 1982 ⟨I-04844⟩

Beemer, N.H. (1853-1934)
B, J.N.E.: Dr. Nelson Beemer. Canadian Journal of Medicine and Surgery 76:133-135, 1934 ⟨I-03887⟩

Bell, G. (1863-1923)
Bell, L.G.: My Father -- Gordon Bell. Winnipeg Clinic Quarterly 23:77-93, 1970 ⟨I-02047⟩
Mitchell, R.: Dr. Gordon Bell 1863-1923. Manitoba Medical Review 39:521 + 523, 1959 ⟨I-05057⟩
Moorhead, E.S.: The Late Dr. Gordon Bell. CMAJ 14:895-896, 1924 ⟨I-02992⟩

Bell, J. (1845-1878)
Fishman, N.: John Bell, MD - Teacher to William Osler. CMAJ: 1981, 125:1042-44 ⟨I-04766⟩

Bell, J. (1853-1911)
Archibald, A.: Master Surgeons of America: James Bell. Surgery, Gynecology and Obstetrics 37:93-96, 1923 ⟨I-04288⟩
Murphy, D.A.: James Bell's Appendicitis. Canadian Journal of Surgery 15:335-338, 1972 ⟨I-04224⟩

Bell, J.L.H. (1870-1964)
N, R.: Dr. Jane L. Heartz Bell. CMAJ 90:946, 1964 ⟨I-02046⟩

Bell, R. (1841-1917)
Swinton, W.E.: Robert Bell, the great geologist. CMAJ 115:948-50, 1976 ⟨I-04428⟩

Belleau, A.G. (1842-1905)
LeBlond, S.: Le docteur Alfred Gauvreau Belleau (1842-1905). Laval Medical 39:870-73, 1968 ⟨I-05296⟩

Bell-Irving, D. (1857-1929)

Bastin, C.H.: Dr. Duncan Bell-Irving. CMAJ 20:451, 1929 ⟨I-03509⟩

Bernstein , A. (1897-1952)

Howell, G.R.: Dr. Arnold Bernstein. CMAJ 68:299, 1953 ⟨I-04532⟩

Best, C.H. (1899-1978)

Best, C.H.: A Canadian Trail of Medical Research. Journal of Endocrinology 19:1-17, 1959 ⟨I-01038⟩

Best, C.H.: Forty Years of Interest in Insulin. British Medical Bulletin 16(3):179-182, 1960 ⟨I-01041⟩

C, A.W.: Charles Best: The Codiscoverer of Insulin. CMAJ 118:167-168, 1978 ⟨I-02048⟩

D., E.F.: The Best Biography. The Medical Post, pp 8, 24, 35 (Sept. 7); 20, 22 (Sept. 21); 22-23 (October 5), 1971 ⟨I-03886⟩

Haist, R.E.: Charles Herbert Best 1899-1978. PTRSC series 4, 16:45-47, 1978 ⟨I-04953⟩

Wrenshall, G.A., Hetenyi, G., Feasby, W.R.: The Story of Insulin. Canada, Max Reinhardt, 1962. 232 p. ⟨I-00935⟩

Bethune, H.N. (1890-1939)

Allan, T., Gordon, S.: The Scalpel, The Sword. (The Story of Dr. Norman Bethune). Boston, Little, Brown and co., 1952. 336 p. ⟨I-00969⟩

Barootes, E.W.: Dr. Norman Bethune: Inspiration for a Modern China. CMAJ 122:1176-1184, 1980 ⟨I-00953⟩

Beaton-Mamak, M.: The Lonely Legend of Norman Bethune. Dimensions in Health Service 51:14-6, 1974 ⟨I-05372⟩

Capacchione, L. (trans.), Endicott, J. (trans.), Perly, C. (trans.): Bethune: His Story in Pictures. Toronto, N.C. Press Ltd., 1975. 77 p. ⟨I-00970⟩

Chih-cheng, C. (adapted): Norman Bethune in China. Peking, Foreign Languages Press, 1975. 114 p. ⟨I-00954⟩

DuVernet, S.: The Muskoka Tree: Poems of Pride for Norman Bethune. Bracebridge, Herald-Gazette Press, 1976, 73 p. ⟨I-04440⟩

Fish, F.H.: Dr. Norman Bethune 1889-1939. CACHB 10(4):151-159, 1946 ⟨I-00946⟩

Jackson, P.: People's Doctor: Norman Bethune 1890-1939. Montreal, Red Flag Publications, 1979. 43 p. ⟨I-00955⟩

Langley, R.: Bethune. Vancouver, Talonbooks, 1975. 119 p. ⟨I-05185⟩

Lem, C.: Bethune Memorial House. Ontario Museum Association Quarterly 7(2):5-6, 1978 ⟨I-00966⟩

MacLeod, W., Park, L., Ryerson, S.: Bethune, the Montreal Years. (An informal portrait). Toronto, James Lorimer and Co., Publishers, 1978. 167 p. ⟨I-00967⟩

Mao Tse-Tung: In Memory of Norman Bethune. Chinese Medical Journal 84(11):699-700, 1965 ⟨I-00957⟩

Nadeau, G.: A T.B's Progress: The Story of Norman Bethune. BHM 8(8):1135-1171, 1940 ⟨I-00956⟩

Stewart, R.: Norman Bethune. Don Mills, Fitzhenry and Whiteside Ltd., 1974. 60 p. ⟨I-00971⟩

Stewart, R.: Bethune. Toronto, New Press, 1973. 210 p. ⟨I-00972⟩

Stewart, R.: The Mind of Norman Bethune. Toronto/Montreal/Winnipeg/Vancouver, Fitzhenry and Whiteside, 1977. 150 p. ⟨I-00973⟩

Stewart, R.J.: Dr. Bethune is a hero to the Chinese. The Medical Post, pp 32-33, Nov.16, 1971 ⟨I-03881⟩

Bier, T.H. (1873-1933)

Secord, E.R.: Thomas Henry Bier. CMAJ 29:575, 1933 ⟨I-03077⟩

Bigelow, W.A. (1879-1967)

Bigelow, W.A.: Forceps, Fin, and Feather. Manitoba, D.W. Friesen and Sons Ltd., 1969. 116 p. ⟨I-00940⟩

Mitchell, R.: Dr. Wilfred Abram Bigelow, an appreciation. CMAJ 97:874, 877, 1967 ⟨I-01492⟩

Mitchell, R.: Dr. Wilfred A. Bigelow. Manitoba Medical Review 47:421-422, 1967 ⟨I-01964⟩

Birchard, C.C. (1886-1951)

MacDermot, H.E.: Dr. Cecil C. Birchard. CMAJ 65:393, 1951 ⟨I-04545⟩

Bird, C.J. (1838-1876)

Smith, W.D.: Curtis James Bird. DCB 10:67-68, 1972 ⟨I-00984⟩

Birkett, H.S. (1864-1942)

McNally, W.J.: Herbert Stanley Birkett. CMAJ 47:280-283, 1942 ⟨I-02050⟩

Black, D. (1884-1934)

Hood, D.: Davidson Black: A Biography. Toronto, University of Toronto Press, 1964. 145 p. ⟨I-00959⟩

Kelly, A.D.: China Hands. CMAJ 97:1363-64, 1967 ⟨I-03917⟩

Swinton, W.E.: Davidson Black, our Peking man. CMAJ 115:251-3, 1976 ⟨I-04430⟩

Black, E.F.F. (1905-1982)

Andison, A.W.: Elinor Black. CMAJ 126:869, 1982 ⟨I-04769⟩

Black, E.F.E.: Thinking Back. CMAJ 105:143-144, 1971 ⟨I-03884⟩

Black, E.F.E.: Not So Long Ago. University of Manitoba Medical Journal 45:54-56, 1975 ⟨I-00941⟩

Mitchell, J.R.: Elinor F.E. Black, an appreciation. University of Manitoba Medical Journal 52:6-7, 1982 ⟨I-04972⟩

Roulston, T.M.: Elinor F.E. Black. University of Manitoba Medical Journal 52:5-6, 1982 ⟨I-04973⟩

S., O.A.: Elinor Frances Elizabeth Black. The Lancet 1:694, 1982 ⟨I-04963⟩

Black, J.B. (1842-1925)

H., W.H.: Dr. J.B. Black. CMAJ 15:104-105, 1925 ⟨I-01591⟩

Black, R.S. (1812-1893)

Campbell, D.A.: Rufus Smith Black (1812-1893). In Kelly HW, Burrage WL: Dictionary of American Medical Biography. New York and London, D. Appleton and Co., 1928. pp. 102-103 ⟨I-00979⟩

Black, V.E. (1884-1936)
D., W.A.: Dr. Vaughan Elderkin Black. CMAJ 35:698, 1936 ⟨I-02874⟩

Blackader, A.D. (1847-1932)
Macallum, A.B.: Alexander Dougall Blackader. CMAJ 26:519-524, 1932 ⟨I-02988⟩
N., A.G.: Dr. A.D. Blackader and the Journal. CMAJ 21:367, 1929 ⟨I-00947⟩
Stewart, J.: Alexander Dougall Blackader, MA, MD, LL.D, MRCS, FRCP(C). CMAJ 26:519-524, 1932 ⟨I-00948⟩

Blake, C. (1746-1810)
Janson, G.: Charles Blake. DCB 5:88-89, 1983 ⟨I-05316⟩

Blanchard, R.J. (1853-1928)
Chown, H.H.: Dr. Robert Johnstone Blanchard. CMAJ 19:500, 1928 ⟨I-03505⟩
Stewart, J.: Dr. Robert Johnstone Blanchard, an appreciation. CMAJ 19:500-501, 1928 ⟨I-03504⟩

Blanchet, F. (1776-1857)
Bernier, J.: Francois Blanchet et le Mouvement Reformiste en Medecine au Debut du XIXe Siecle. Revue d'histoire de l'amerique Francaise 34:223-244, 1980 ⟨I-04657⟩

Blanchet, J-B.
Tache, J.C.: The late Dr. Blanchet. Medical Chronicle 5:165-169, 1857-58 ⟨I-00988⟩

Blanchet, J-G (1829-1890)
Caissie, F.: Joseph-Godric Blanchet. DCB 11:85-86, 1982 ⟨I-04861⟩

Blatchford, E.C. (1900-)
Hellstedt, L. McG (edit): Ellen C. Blatchford. In: Women Physicians of the World: Autobiographies of Medical Pioneers New York, McGraw Hill Book Co., 1978. pp 223-225 ⟨I-03919⟩

Blatz, W.E.
Northway, M.L.: William Emet Blatz. CMAJ 123:15-16, 1980 ⟨I-01066⟩

Blow, T.H. (1862-1932)
Learmonth, G.E.: Dr. Thomas Henry Blow. CMAJ 28:227. 1933 ⟨I-03081⟩

Bonamour, J. de. (fl. 1670)
Nadeau, G.: Jean de Bonamour. DCB 1:106-107, 1966 ⟨I-00997⟩

Bond, J.N. (1758-1830)
Farish, G.W.T.: A medical biography of the Bond-Farish family. CMAJ 23:696-698, 1930 ⟨I-03170⟩

Bonnemere, F. (1600-1683)
Drolet, A.: Florent Bonnemere. DCB 1:107-108, 1966 ⟨I-00998⟩

Botsford, L.B. (1812-1888)
Murray, F.E.: Memoir of LeBaron Botsford, M.D. New Brunswick, J. and A. McMillan, 1892. 285 p. ⟨I-00983⟩

Bouchard, E. (1622-1676)
Nadeau, G.: Etienne Bouchard. DCB 1:108-109, 1966 ⟨I-00999⟩

Boucher de la Bruere (1808-1871)
Roby, Y.: Pierre-Claude Boucher de la Bruere. DCB 10:76-77, 1972 ⟨I-00013⟩

Bourgeois, B.G. (1877-1943)
Desjardins, E.: B.G. Bourgeois (1877-1943). Canadian Journal of Surgery 9:1-5, 1966 ⟨I-04230⟩

Bourgeois, J. (1621-1701)
Jost, A.C.: Jacques Bourgeois, Chirurgien 1621-1701. CMAJ 16:190-191, 1926 ⟨I-01603⟩

Bourgeois, J. de L.
LeSage, A.: Jacques de Lorimier Bourgeois. L'UMC 72:1-4, 1943 ⟨I-02001⟩

Bourne, W. (1886-1965)
Griffith, H.R.: Dr. Wesley Bourne, an appreciation. CMAJ 92:895-896, 1965 ⟨I-02052⟩
Griffith, H.R.: Wesley Bourne (1886-1965). Canadian Anaesthetists' Society Journal 12:315-317, 1965 ⟨I-02053⟩

Boutillier, T. (1797-1861)
Bernard, J.P.: Thomas Boutillier. DCB 9:73-74, 1976 ⟨I-00989⟩

Bovell, J. (1817-1880)
Blogg, H.: James Bovell (1817-1880). In Kelly HW, Burrage WL: Dictionary of American Medical Biography. New York and London, D. Appleton and Co., 1928. pp.126-127. ⟨I-00012⟩
Dolman, C.E.: The Reverend James Bovell, M.D. 1817-1880. In: G.F.G. Stanley(edit.): Pioneers of Canadian Science Toronto, University of Toronto Press, 1966 ⟨I-02496⟩
Dolman, C.E.: James Bovell. DCB 10:83-85, 1972 ⟨I-00011⟩
McKillop, A.B.: Dr. Bovell's Quadrilateral Mind. In: A Disciplined Intelligence. Montreal, McGill-Queen's University Press, 1979, pp 73-91. ⟨I-03189⟩
[Osler, W.]: James Bovell, M.D. The Canada Lancet 12:249-51, 1880 ⟨I-01580⟩
Roland, C.G.: James Bovell (1817-1880): The Toronto Years. CMAJ 91:812-814, 1964 ⟨I-00010⟩

Bowie, D.I. (1887-1968)
Mitchell, R.: Dr. Donald I. Bowie. CMAJ 99:509, 1968 ⟨I-01961⟩

Bowman, F.B. (1883-1976)
K[elly], A.D.: W.O. and F.B.B. CMAJ 103:231-232 ⟨I-02883⟩

Boyce, B.F. (1866-1945)
Schoenfeld, R.: Dr. B.F. Boyce. Okanagan Historical Society Annual Report 37:52-55, 1973 ⟨I-05067⟩

Boyd, W. (1885-1979)
B., H.J.: Dr. William Boyd. Bulletin Academy of Medicine, Toronto 52(8):110-115, 1979 ⟨I-00937⟩
Becker, W.J.: Biography: Dr. William Boyd. University of Manitoba Medical Journal 39:41-45, 1967 ⟨I-02057⟩

Boyd, W.: With A Field Ambulance at Ypres. Toronto, Musson Book Co. Ltd., 1916. 110 p. ⟨I-00936⟩

Duff, G.L.: William Boyd: a Biographical Sketch. Laboratory Investigation 5:389-395, 1956 ⟨I-04758⟩

Feasby, W.R.: Professor William Boyd. Medical Post, Aug 16, Aug 30, Sept 13, 1966 ⟨I-02059⟩

Boyer, G.F. (-1966)

Keith, W.S.: Dr. George F. Boyer. CMAJ 96:505-506, 1967 ⟨I-02055⟩

Boys, H. (1775-1868)

Rudkin, D.W.: Henry Boys. DCB 9:79-80, 1976 ⟨I-00009⟩

Braithwaite, E.A.

Stanley, G.D.: Medical Pioneering in Alberta (Dr. E.A. Braithwaite). CACHB 1(4):7-8, 1937 ⟨I-00975⟩

Brandson, B.J. (1874-1944)

Montgomery, E.W.: Dr. Brandur Jonsson Brandson. CMAJ 51:185-6, 1944 ⟨I-04257⟩

Thorlakson, P.H.T.: The Late Brandur Jonsson Brandson. Manitoba Medical Review 24:223, 1944 ⟨I-05029⟩

Brasset, E.A. (1907-)

Brasset, E.A.: A Doctor's Pilgrimage: an autobiography. Philadelphia, J.B. Lippincott Co., 1951. 256 p. ⟨I-04828⟩

Brett, R.G. (1851-1929)

Learmonth, G.E.: The Hon. Dr. R.G. Brett. CMAJ 21:621, 1929 ⟨I-02045⟩

Stanley, G.D.: Dr. Robert George Brett (1851-1929). CACHB 4(1):5-12, 1939 ⟨I-00976⟩

Watson, I.A.: Robert George Brett. In: Physicians and Surgeons of America. Concord, Republican Press Association, 1896. pp 753. ⟨I-02509⟩

Woods, J.H.: Hon. Dr. Robert George Brett, an appreciation. CMAJ 21: 621-622, 1929 ⟨I-02003⟩

Briault, A. (fl. 1760)

Nadeau, G.: Le dernier chirurgien du roi a Quebec, Antoine, Briault, 1742-1760. L'UMC 8:720, 1951 ⟨I-04938⟩

Britton, W. (-1915)

Hunter, J.: An appreciation of Dr. Wm. Britton. Canadian Journal of Medicine and Surgery 37:165-167, 1915 ⟨I-01554⟩

Brouse, W.H. (1824-1881)

Swainson, D.: William Henry Brouse. DCB 11:114, 1982 ⟨I-04862⟩

Brown, G.M. (1916-1977)

Wilson, D.L.: G. Malcolm Brown 1916-1977. PTRSC series 4, 16:59-60, 1978 ⟨I-04954⟩

Brown, W.G. (1902-1968)

Nicholas, W.B.: Dr. W. Gordon Brown, an appreciation. CMAJ 98:795, 1968 ⟨I-01705⟩

Bruce, H.A. (1868-1963)

Bruce, H.A.: Varied Operations. Toronto, Longmans, Green and Co., 1958. 366 p. ⟨I-00939⟩

Bruce, H.A.: Memories of a Fellow of the Royal College of Surgeons of 1896. CMAJ 84:762, 733, 1961 ⟨I-03885⟩

K(elly), A.D.: Herbert Alexander Bruce, M.D., FACS, LRCP, (Eng.). CMAJ 89:232-233, 1963 ⟨I-01483⟩

Bryce, P.H. (1853-1932)

Fitzgerald, J.G.: Doctor Peter H. Bryce. Canadian Public Health Journal 23:88-91, 1932 ⟨I-05297⟩

Watson, I.A.: Peter H. Bryce. In: Physicians and Surgeons of America. Concord, Republican Press Association, 1896. pp 268-69 ⟨I-02510⟩

Buchanan, D. (1868-1933)

Woolner, W.: Dr. Dan Buchanan. CMAJ 29:575-576, 1933 ⟨I-03078⟩

Buchanan, R.W. (1860-1895)

Scammell, H.L.: Medicine Hat. Nova Scotia Medical Bulletin 28:146-148, 1949 ⟨I-03553⟩

Buck, A. (1833-1919)

Corrigan, S.H.: Anson Buck, MD, MRCS (Eng.) 1833-1919. CMAJ 34:564-569, 1936 ⟨I-01706⟩

Bucke, R.M. (1837-1902)

Berry, E.G.: Whitman's Canadian Friend. Dalhousie Review 24:77-82, 1944-45 ⟨I-02024⟩

Coyne, J.H.: Richard Maurice Bucke--A Sketch. PTRSC Section 2, 159-196, 1906 ⟨I-00004⟩

Coyne, J.H.: Richard Maurice Bucke. Toronto, Henry S. Saunders, 1923. 77 p. ⟨I-01165⟩

Greenland, C.: Richard Maurice Bucke, M.D. Canada's Mental Health 11:6, 1963 ⟨I-04388⟩

Greenland, C.: Richard Maurice Bucke, M.D., 1837-1902 (A Pioneer of Scientific Psychiatry). CMAJ 91:385-391, 1964 ⟨I-01709⟩

Greenland, C.: Richard Maurice Bucke, 1837-1902. CMAJ 92:1136, 1965 ⟨I-01710⟩

Greenland, C.: Richard Maurice Bucke, M.D. 1837-1902: The Evolution of a Mystic. Canadian Psychiatric Association Journal 11:146-154, 1966 ⟨I-01712⟩

Greenland, C.: Three Pioneers of Canadian psychiatry. JAMA 200:833-842, 1967 ⟨I-00008⟩

Greenland, C.: The Compleat Psychiatrist: Dr. R.M. Bucke's Twenty-Five Years as Medical Superintendent, Asylum for the Insane, London, Ontario 1877-1902. Canadian Psychiatric Association Journal 17:71-77, 1972 ⟨I-03566⟩

Horne, J.: R.M. Bucke: Pioneer Psychiatrist, Practical Mystic. Ontario History 59:197-208, 1967 ⟨I-01662⟩

Jameson, M.A.: Richard Maurice Bucke: A catalogue based upon the collections of the University of Western Ontario libraries. London, The Libraries, University of Western Ontario, 1978. 126 pp. ⟨I-00003⟩

Kelly, A.D.: Richard Maurice Bucke. CMAJ 91:769, 1964 ⟨I-01550⟩

Lauder, B.: Two Radicals: Richard Maurice Bucke and Lawren Harris. Dalhousie Review 56:307-318, 1976-77 ⟨I-02580⟩

Lozynsky, A.: Richard Maurice Bucke, Medical Mystic. Detroit, Wayne State University Press, 1977. 203 p. ⟨I-00001⟩

McMullin, S.E.: Walt Whitman's Influence in Canada. Dalhousie Review 49:361-368, 1969-70 ⟨I-02022⟩

Mitchinson, W.: R.M. Bucke: A Victorian Asylum Superintendent. Ontario History 63:239-254, 1981 ⟨I-04715⟩

Shortt, S.E.D.: The Influence of French Biomedical Theory on Nineteenth-Century Canadian Neuropsychiatry: Bichat and Comte in the Work of R.M. Bucke. International Congress for the History of Medicine, Paris, 1982. Proceedings, vol. 1:309-312, 1982 ⟨I-05219⟩

Stevenson, G.H.: The Life and Work of Richard Maurice Bucke. American Journal of Psychiatry 93:1127-50, 1937 ⟨I-02305⟩

Stevenson, G.H.: Bucke and Osler: a personality study. CMAJ 44:183-188, 1941 ⟨I-03337⟩

Timothy, H.B.: Rediscovering R.M. Bucke. Western Historical Notes 21(1):34-40, 1965 ⟨I-03187⟩

Buckwold, A.E. (1918-1965)
Gerrard, J.W.: Dr. Alvin E. Buckwold. CMAJ 93:1044, 1965 ⟨I-01713⟩

Buller, F. (1844-1905)
Birkett, H.S.: Buller, the Ophthalmologist, Politzer, the Otologist, and Lefferts, the Laryngologist. Transactions of the American Academy of Ophthalmology and Oto- Laryngology, pp 24-34, 1927 ⟨I-01714⟩

Macphail, A.: Francis Buller (1844-1905). In Kelly HW, Burrage WL: Dictionary of American Medical Biography. New York and London, D. Appleton and Co., 1928. pp. 170-171 ⟨I-00978⟩

Bunn, J. (1802-1861)
Klassen, H.C.: John Bunn. DCB 9:102-103, 1976 ⟨I-00991⟩

Stubbs, R.S.: Dr. John Bunn. In: Four Recorders of Rupert's Land. Winnipeg, Peguis Publishers, 1967. pp 91-134 ⟨I-04779⟩

Burgess, J.F. (-1953)
Forsey, R.R.: J. Frederick Burgess. CMAJ 68:625, 1953 ⟨I-04529⟩

M[acDermot], H.E.: J. Frederick Burgess. CMAJ 68:625, 1953 ⟨I-04530⟩

Burgess, T.J.W. (1849-1925)
Morphy, A.G.: Thomas J.W. Burgess, M.D., F.R.C.S. CMAJ 16:203, 1926 ⟨I-01569⟩

Burnett, W.B. (1871-1964)
MacD(ermot), J.H.: Dr. William Brenton Burnett, an appreciation. CMAJ 90:1478, 1964 ⟨I-01549⟩

Burnham, F.W.E. (1872-1957)
Mitchell, R.: Dr. F.W.E. Burnham 1872-1957: A Life of Strange Adventure. Manitoba Medical Review 46:569-570, 1966 ⟨I-02130⟩

Burns, C.W. (-1967)
K(elly), A.D.: Dr. C.W. Burns, an appreciation. CMAJ 96:1542-1543, 1967 ⟨I-01493⟩

Burns, J.H. (1845-1898)
C,J.J.: Dr. James H. Burns. Canadian Journal of Medicine and Surgery 3:47-48, 1898 ⟨I-01548⟩

Burris, J.S. (1875-1953)
Murphy, H.H.: Dr. J.S. Burris 1875-1953. CMAJ, 70:479, 1954 ⟨I-04564⟩

Burton, A.C. (1904-1979)
Roach, M.R.: Alan Chadburn Burton 1904-1979. PTRSC series 4, 18: 57-59, 1980 ⟨I-04955⟩

Butters, T.L. (1890-1934)
L., A.: Dr. Thomas Lowell Butters. CMAJ 31:452-453, 1934 ⟨I-03513⟩

Byers, H.P. (1860-1933)
Rawson, N.B.: Dr. Herbert P. Byers. CMAJ 30:108-109, 1934 ⟨I-03543⟩

C

Cadham, F.T. (-1961)
Bigelow, W.A.: Dr. Frederick Todd Cadham, an appreciation. CMAJ 84:673-674, 1961 ⟨I-01481⟩

M., R.: Dr. Frederick Todd Cadham. CMAJ 84:673, 1961 ⟨I-01482⟩

Caldwell, W. (1782-1833)
Bensley, E.H.: The Caldwell - O'Sullivan Duel: A Prelude to the Founding of the Montreal General Hospital. CMAJ 100:1092-1095. 1969 ⟨I-00926⟩

Caleff, J. (1726-1812)
Condon, A.G.: John Caleff. DCB 5:134-135, 1983 ⟨I-05315⟩

Everett, H.S.: Dr. John Calef, Physician, Naval and Military Surgeon and Statesman. CMAJ 72:390-391, 1955 ⟨I-01547⟩

Cameron, A. (1830-)
Watson, I.A.: Allan Cameron. In: Physicians and Surgeons of America. Concord, Republican Press Association, 1896. pp 277 ⟨I-02511⟩

Cameron, A.T. (1882-1947)
G., A.: Alexander Thomas Cameron. CMAJ 57:504-5, 1947 ⟨I-04401⟩

Cameron, D.E. (1901-1967)
Cleghorn, R.A.: D. Ewan Cameron, M.D., F.R.C.P. (C). CMAJ 97:984-985, 1967 ⟨I-01701⟩

Silverman, B.: Dr. E. Ewan Cameron. CMAJ 97:985-986, 1967 ⟨I-01700⟩

Cameron, G.D. (-1983)
Moore, P.E.: George Donald [Don] Cameron. CMAJ 129:771, 1983 ⟨I-05162⟩

Cameron, H.M. (1882-1929)
Mitchell, R.: H.M. Cameron, M.C., B.A., M.D., LL.B. CMAJ 20:329-330, 1929 ⟨I-01568⟩

Cameron, I.H. (1855-1933)
Harris, C.W.: Irving Heward Cameron (1855-1933): Professor of Surgery, University of Toronto, 1897-1920. Canadian Journal of Surgery 8:131-136, 1965 ⟨I-01565⟩

McCrae, T.: Mr. Irving Heward Cameron. CMAJ 30:225-226, 1934 ⟨I-03550⟩

Primrose, A.: Irving Heward Cameron. CMAJ 30:224-225, 1934 ⟨I-03480⟩

Stanley, G.D.: Irving Heward Cameron: The Philosophical Surgeon. CACHB 6:1-11, 1941 ⟨I-01564⟩

Stanley, G.D.: Further notes on Irving Heward Cameron. CACHB 7:8-10, 1942 ⟨I-01566⟩

Caminetsky, S. (1920-1967)

Peikoff, S.S.: Dr. Sydney Caminetsky. CMAJ 97:1495, 1967 ⟨I-01562⟩

Campbell, F.W. (1837-1905)

Macphail, A.: Francis Wayland Campbell (1837-1905). In Kelly HW, Burrage WL: Dictionary of American Medical Biography. New York and London, D. Appleton and Co., 1928. pp. 195-196 ⟨I-00911⟩

Watson, I.A.: Francis W. Campbell. In: Physicians and Surgeons of America. Concord, Republican Press Association, 1896. pp 675 ⟨I-02512⟩

Campbell, G.W. (1810-1882)

Howard, R.P.: A Sketch of the Life of the Late G.W. Campbell A.M.,M.D.,LL. D., Late Dean of the Medical Faculty, and a Summary of the History of the Faculty; Being the Introductory Address of the Fiftieth Session of the Medical Faculty of McGill University. Montreal Gazette, 1882 ⟨I-00910⟩

Roland, C.G.: George William Campbell. DCB 11:148-149, 1982 ⟨I-04868⟩

Campbell, P.McG. (1872-1954)

Stanley, G.D.: Campbell of Lethbridge. CACHB 12:56-62, 1947 ⟨I-01563⟩

Tuttle, M.W.: Peter McGregor Campbell. CMAJ, 71:631, 1954 ⟨I-04568⟩

Campbell, W.A. (1873-1934)

Somerville, A.: Dr. William Alexander Campbell. CMAJ 31:573, 1934 ⟨I-03516⟩

Campbell, W.R. (1890-1981)

Campbell, W.R.: Walter R. Campbell 1890-1981. PTRSC series 4, 19:69-71, 1981 ⟨I-04956⟩

Cannell, D.E.

H., J.L.: Douglas Edward Cannell, M.C. LL.D., University of Toronto, Honoris Causa - B.Sc., (Med.) F.R.C.S.(C), F.A.C.O.G., F.R.S.M. (Hon.), F.R.C.O.G. Bull of the Academy of Med, Toronto 53:53-54, 1980 ⟨I-00892⟩

Caplan, H. (1920-1980)

Sarwer-Foner, G.J.: Hyman Caplan, M.D., C.M., F.R.C.P.(C). Psychiatric Journal of the University of Ottawa 5:145-146, 1980 ⟨I-01585⟩

Weiss, G.: Hyman Caplan: 1920-1980. Canadian Journal of Psychiatry 25:684, 1980 ⟨I-02879⟩

Carigouan (-1634)

Jury, E.M.: Carigouan. DCB 1:164-165, 1966 ⟨I-00931⟩

Carlisle, A.M.

Fryer, H.: Pioneer Doctor (A.M. Carlisle). Heritage 7:21-24, 1979 ⟨I-00906⟩

Carrall, R.W.W. (1837-1879)

Smith, D.B.: Robert William Weir Carrall. DCB 10:138-140, 1972 ⟨I-00924⟩

Casgrain, G. (-1966)

Desjardins, E.: Dr. Gerard Casgrain. CMAJ 95:738, 1966 ⟨I-01560⟩

Cass, E.E. (1905-)

Hellstedt, L.McG. (edit): E. Elizabeth Cass. In: Women Physicians of the World: Autobiographies of Medical Pioneers New York, McGraw-Hill Book Co., 1978. pp 306-12 ⟨I-03921⟩

Cassidy, J.J. (1843-1914)

Watson, I.A.: John J. Cassidy. In: Physicians and Surgeons of America. Concord, Republican Press Association, 1896. pp 86-87 ⟨I-02513⟩

Catellier, L. (1839-1918)

Cauvreau, J.: Le Docteur Laurent Catellier: Ex-Doyen de l'Universite-Laval, Quebec 1839-1918. L'UMC 47:86, 1918 ⟨I-00913⟩

Chapoton, J.-B. (1690-1760)

Kelsey, H.: Jean-Baptiste Chapoton. DCB 3:102-103, 1974 ⟨I-00925⟩

Charlton, M. (1858-1931)

LeBlond, S.: Margaret Charlton. CSHM Newsletter, Spring 1983, pp 15-16 ⟨I-05063⟩

Chartier, L. (1633-1660)

Drolet, A.: Louis Chartier. DCB 1:201, 1966 ⟨I-00932⟩

Chaudillon, A. (1643-1707)

Biron, H.: Antoine Chaudillon. DCB 2:140-141, 1969 ⟨I-01017⟩

Cheadle, W.B. (1836-1910)

Stanley, G.D.: Dr. W.B. Cheadle. CACHB 3(1):307, 1938 ⟨I-00916⟩

Thorington, J.M.: Four Physicians-Explorers of the Fur Trade Days. Annals of Medical History, ser. 3, 4:294-301, 1942 ⟨I-04906⟩

Chipman, W.W. (1866-1950)

Philpott, N.W.: Dr. Walter William Chipman. CMAJ 62:519-20, 1950 ⟨I-04485⟩

Chisholm, G.B.

Howard-Jones, N.: What was WHO -- Thirty Years Ago?. Dialogue 59:28-34, 1979 ⟨I-00894⟩

Senex (N. Howard-Jones): Fifteen Words that Saved Humanity. WHO Dialogue 73:7-8, 1979 ⟨I-00895⟩

Chisholm, M. (1848-1929)

Hattie, W.H.: Dr. Murdoch Chisholm. CMAJ 22:295-96, 1930 ⟨I-03010⟩

Chisholm, T. (1842-1931)

Clarkson, F.A.: Dr. Thomas Chisholm, M.P. 1842-1931. CMAJ 29:82-86, 1933 ⟨I-03009⟩

Chown, H.H. (1859-1944)

Mitchell, R.: H.H. Chown, Third Dean of Manitoba Medical College 1859-1944. Manitoba Medical Review 39:189-191, 1959 ⟨I-01702⟩

Mitchell, R.: Manitoba Surgical Pioneers James Kerr (1849-1911) and H.H. Chown (1859-1944). Canadian Journal of Surgery 3:281-285, 1960 ⟨I-03556⟩

Christie, A.J. (1787-1843)

Bond, C.C.J.: Alexander James Christie, Bytown Pioneer -- His Life and Times, 1787-1843. Ontario History 56(1):16-36, 1964 〈I-01704〉

Hill, H.P.: The Bytown Gazette: A Pioneer Newspaper. Ontario Historical Society Papers and Records 27:407-423, 1931 〈I-01302〉

Cipriani, A.J. (1908-1956)

Keys, D.A.: Andre Joseph Cipriani, 1908-1956. Proceedings and Transactions of the Royal Society of Canada Series 3, 50:65-9, 1956 〈I-04775〉

Keys, D.A.: Dr. Andre Joseph Cipriani. CMAJ 74:590, 1956 〈I-04743〉

Clark, D. (1835-1912)

Clarkson, F.A.: Dr. Daniel Clark: A Physician of old Ontario. CACHB 22:157-170, 1957 〈I-01524〉

Clark, M.

Stanley, G.D.: Dr. Michael Clark. CMAJ 48:449-453, 1943 〈I-01525〉

Clarke, C.K. (1857-1924)

Falconer, R.A.: Charles Kirk Clarke, M.B., M.D., LL.D. CMAJ 14:349, 1924 〈I-02994〉

F[arrar], C.B.: I Remember C.K. Clarke, 1857-1957. American Journal of Psychiatry 114:368-370, 1957 〈I-02007〉

Greenland, C.: C.K. Clarke: A Founder of Canadian Psychiatry. CMAJ 95:155-160, 1966 〈I-00901〉

Greenland, C.: Charles Kirk Clarke, A Pioneer of Canadian Psychiatry. Toronto, Clarke Institute of Psychiatry, 1966. 31 p. 〈I-00900〉

Greenland, C.: Three Pioneers of Canadian psychiatry. JAMA 200:833-842, 1967 〈I-00903〉

Mott, F.W.: Charles Kirk Clarke, M.D., LL.D. British Medical Journal 1:219, 1924 〈I-02006〉

Primrose, A.: C.K. Clarke, M.D., LL.D.: A Man of Many Parts. University of Toronto Monthly 24:223-224, 1924 〈I-01515〉

Clegg, F.R. (1890-1966)

Tew, W.P.: Dr. Frank R. Clegg. CMAJ 95:1045, 1966 〈I-02044〉

Cleland, F.A. (1874-1933)

Hutchison, H.S.: Dr. Frederick Adam Cleland. CMAJ 30:107-108, 1934 〈I-03542〉

Clinch, J. (1748/49-1819)

Davies, J.W.: A Historical Note on the Reverend John Clinch, First Canadian Vaccinator. CMAJ 102(9):957-61, 1970 〈I-05292〉

Jones, F.: John Clinch. DCB 5:189-190, 1983 〈I-05314〉

Cluff, W.A. (1873-1940)

Baltzen, D.M.: Dr. William Alexander Cluff. CMAJ 44:431-432, 1941 〈I-03350〉

Cogswell, C. (1813-1892)

Campbell, D.A.: Charles Cogswell (1813-1892). In Kelly HW, Burrage WL: Dictionary of American Medical Biography. New York and London, D. Appleton and Co., 1928. p. 243. 〈I-00923〉

Colbeck, J.C. (-1964)

E., G.B.: Dr. J. Christopher Colbeck. CMAJ 91:403, 1964 〈I-02040〉

Colby, M.F. (1795-1863)

Phelps, M.L.: Moses French Colby. DCB 9:144-145, 1976 〈I-00927〉

Coleman, W.F. (1838-1917)

Shastid, T.H.: W. Franklin Coleman (1838-1917). In Kelly HW, Burrage WL: Dictionary of American Medical Biography. New York and London, D. Appleton and Co., 1928. p. 247. 〈I-00922〉

Collip, J.B. (1892-1965)

Barr, M.L., Rossiter,R.J.: James Bertram Collip 1892-1965. Biographical Memoirs of Fellows of the Royal Society 19:235-267, 1973 〈I-02008〉

Barr, M.L.: James Bertram Collip (1892-1965); A Canadian Pioneer in Endocrinology. In International Congress for the History of Medicine, 25th, Quebec, 1976. Proceedings, volume II, 1976. p. 469-476 〈I-00896〉

Hall, G.E.: James Bertram Collip:1892-1965. CMAJ 93:673, 1965 〈I-02010〉

Keys, D.A.: James Bertram Collip, C.B.E., M.D., Ph.D., D.Sc., F.R.S. CMAJ 93:774-775, 1965 〈I-02004〉

Noble, R.L.: Memories of James Bertram Collip. CMAJ 93:1356-1364, 1965 〈I-02009〉

Noble, R.L.: James Bertram Collip. Dictionary of Scientific Biography 3:351-354, 1971 〈I-02762〉

Thomson, D.L.: Dr. James Bertram Collip. Canadian Journal of Biochemistry and Physiology 35:1-5, 1957 〈I-02011〉

Warwick, O.H.: James Bertram Collip -- 1892-1965. CMAJ 93:425-426, 1965 〈I-02005〉

Collison, J. (1873-1930)

Learmonth, G.E.: Dr. John Collison. CMAJ 23:116, 1930 〈I-03022〉

Comfort, W.M. (1822-1899)

Peer, E.T.: A Nineteenth Century Physician of Upper Canada and His Library. Bulletin of the Cleveland Medical Library 19:78-85, 1972 〈I-04908〉

Compain, P-J. (1740-1806)

Janson, G.: Pierre-Joseph Compain. DCB 5:201-202, 1983 〈I-05313〉

Cone, W.V. (1897-1959)

Entin, M.A.: Dr. William Vernon Cone: an appreciation. McGill Medical Journal 29:63-69, 1960 〈I-02012〉

Connell, J.C. (1863-1947)

Lynn, R.B.: James Cameron Connell:1863-1947. Canadian Journal of Surgery 2:336-339, 1968 〈I-02013〉

Cordeau, J-P. (1922-1971)

Leduc, J.: La vie et l'ouevre de Jean-Pierre Cordeau, 1922-1971. L'UMC 101:2641-5, 1972 〈I-05294〉

Cote, C.-H.-O. (1809-1850)

LeBlond, S.: Docteur Cyrille Hector Octave Cote (1809-1850). L'UMC 102:1572-1574, 1973 〈I-00928〉

Cotton, R.B. (-1903)
    Hamilton, Z.M.: Dr. R.B. Cotton (In Regina from 1882-1902). CACHB 8:7-10, 1943 ⟨I-02036⟩

Coulter, J.E. (1869-1929)
    Mitchell, R.: Dr. John Ernest Coulter. CMAJ 21:747-748, 1929 ⟨I-02034⟩

Covernton, C.F. (1879-1958)
    MacD, J.H.: Dr. Charles F. Covernton. CMAJ 79:1026-1027, 1958 ⟨I-02033⟩

Cowie, A.J. (1836-1929)
    Walker, S.L.: Andrew James Cowie, M.D. CMAJ 20:449-450, 1929 ⟨I-02031⟩

Craigie, W. (1799-1863)
    Greenfield, K.: William Craigie. DCB 9:165-166, 1976 ⟨I-00930⟩

Craik, R. (1829-1906)
    H., W.H.: Dr. Craik. Montreal Medical Journal 35:539-543, 1906 ⟨I-02015⟩
    Macphail, A.: Robert Craik (1829-1907). In Kelly HW, Burrage WL: Dictionary of American Medical Biography. New York and London, D. Appleton and Co., 1928. p. 265. ⟨I-00914⟩

Crane, J.W. (1877-1959)
    Bates, D.G.: Dr. J.W. Crane -- A Biography. University of Western Ontario Medical Journal 28:125-130, 1958 ⟨I-02016⟩

Crawford, T.H. (1871-1925)
    Learmonth, G.E.: Dr. Thomas Henry Crawford. CMAJ 15:1281-1282, 1925 ⟨I-01593⟩

Cream, T.N. (1850-1892)
    Bensley, E.H.: McGill University's Most Infamous Medical Graduate. CMAJ 109:1024, 1973 ⟨I-05377⟩
    Cashman, J.: The Gentleman from Chicago. New York/Evanston/San Francisco/London, Harper and Row, Publishers, 1973. 310 p. ⟨I-00907⟩
    Jenkins, E.: Neill Cream, Poisoner. In: Reader's Digest, 1978. pp 67-156 ⟨I-00917⟩
    Scatliff, H.K.: A Doctor Specializes -- in Crime. Chicago Medicine 69(16):691-698, 1966 ⟨I-00908⟩

Creelman, P.A. (-1957)
    F., E.M., S., W.R.: Dr. P.A. Creelman, an appreciation, CMAJ 76:998, 1957 ⟨I-04733⟩

Crevier, J-A. (1824-1889)
    Desjardins, E.: Un precurseur de la recherche medicale au XIX siecle: le docteur Joseph-Alexandre Crevier. L'UMC 101:708-11, 1972 ⟨I-05376⟩
    Lortie, L.: Joseph-Alexandre Crevier. DCB 11:217-18, 1982 ⟨I-04863⟩

Cryderman, W.J. (1893-1966)
    Harris, C.W.: Dr. Wilbur James Cryderman. CMAJ 95:1271, 1966 ⟨I-02028⟩

Cumming, A. (1877-1926)
    Hardisty, R.H.M.: Dr. Alison Cumming. CMAJ 16:859, 1926 ⟨I-01619⟩
    M., A.S.: Dr. Alison Cumming. CMAJ 16:990-991, 1926 ⟨I-01618⟩

Cunningham, G.S. (1895-1972)
    Hellstedt, L. McG (edit): Gladys Story Cunningham. In: Women Physicians of the World: Autobiographies of Medical Pioneers New York, McGray-Hill Book Co., 1978. pp 123-7 ⟨I-03918⟩

Cunningham, H.M. (1865-1930)
    Bastin, C.H.: Dr. Henry Mortimer Cunningham. CMAJ 23:726, 1930 ⟨I-03024⟩

Curry, W.A. (1888-1966)
    Ross, E.F.: Wilfred Alan Curry, BA, MD, FRCS(Eng.), FRCS(C), FACS. CMAJ 96:62-63, 1967 ⟨I-02026⟩

Cushing, H.B. (1873-1947)
    Goldbloom, A: Pediatrics and Medical Practice. CMAJ 60:620-623, 1949 ⟨I-03933⟩
    M[acDermot], H.E.: Dr. Harold Beveridge Cushing. CMAJ 57:606-7, 1947 ⟨I-04400⟩

D

Dafoe, A.R. (1884-1943)
    Cameron, M.H.V.: Allan Roy Dafoe, OBE, MB. CMAJ 49:149, 1943 ⟨I-01514⟩

Dagneau, P.C. (1877-1940)
    LeBlond, S.: Le Docteur P.C. Dagneau. CMAJ 43:193-194, 1940 ⟨I-03340⟩

Darby, G.E. (1889-1962)
    Gunn, S.W.A.: George Elias Darby: 1889-1962. Canadian Journal of Surgery 10:275-280, 1967 ⟨I-04227⟩
    McKervill, H.W.: Darby of Bella Bella. Toronto, Ryerson Press, 1964 ⟨I-02986⟩

Darrah, R.J. (1842-)
    Watson, I.A.: Robert J. Darragh. In: Physicians and Surgeons of America. Concord, Republican Press Association, 1896. p. 66 ⟨I-02514⟩

David, A.H. (1812-1882)
    Ballon, H.C.: Aaron Hart David, M.D. (1812-1882). CMAJ 86:115-122, 1962 ⟨I-01574⟩
    David, A.H.: Reminiscences Connected with the Medical Profession in Montreal During the Last Fifty Years. Canada Medical Record 11:1-8, 1882 ⟨I-01206⟩

David, F.R. (-1948)
    Fraser, H.A., Schwartz, H.W., Bethune, C.M., Atlee, H.B.: In Memoriam: Frank Roy David, MD, CM(Dal), FACS. Nova Scotia Medical Bulletin 27:237-240, 1948 ⟨I-01464⟩

Davies, J.A. (1889-1964)
    B., J.W.: Dr. John Angus Davies. CMAJ 90:1479, 1964 ⟨I-05229⟩

Davison, J.L. (1853-1917)
    Anderson, H.B.: John L. Davison, M.D. CMAJ 7:549-551, 1917 ⟨I-01511⟩

Deadman, W.J. (1886-1965)
    Bensley, E.H.: Dr. William James Deadman. CMAJ 92:1138-1139, 1965 ⟨I-01465⟩
    Farmer, G.R.D.: Dr. William James Deadman. CMAJ 92:1322, 1965 ⟨I-01466⟩
    K(elly), A.D.: Dr. William James Deadman. CMAJ 92:1138, 1965 ⟨I-01507⟩

Deane, R.B. (1870-1941)
Scarlett, E.P.: Reginald Burton Deane 1870-1941. CACHB 6(3):9-16, 1941 ⟨I-02489⟩

Dearin, J.J. (1818-1890)
Hiller, J.K.: John Joseph Dearin. DCB 11:239-40, 1982 ⟨I-04865⟩

De Gaspe, P.A.
De Gaspe, P.A.: Memoires. Montreal, Bibliotheque Canadienne-Francaise, 1971. 435 p. ⟨I-00891⟩

Delahaye, G.
Dumas, P.: Un Medecin-Psychiatre Qui Avait Ete Poete, Gullaume LaHaise et Son Double, Guy Delahaye. L'UMC 100:321-326, 1971 ⟨I-02231⟩

Delany, M.R. (1812-1885)
Cameron, S., Falk, L.A.: Some Black Medical History: Dr. Martin R. Delany's Canadian Years as Medical Practitioner and Abolitionist (1856-1864). In International Congress for the History of Medicine, 25th, Quebec, 1976. Proceedings, volume II, 1976. p. 537-545 ⟨I-00883⟩

Delarue, N.C. (1915-)
Gray, C.: Norman Charles Delarue. CMAJ 128:185, 1983 ⟨I-05046⟩

Demosny, J. (1643-1687)
Boissonnault, C.M.: Jean Demosny. DCB 1:255-256, 1966 ⟨I-01006⟩

Denechaud, J. (1728-1810)
Desjardins, E.: Jacques Denechaud. DCB 5:248-249, 1983 ⟨I-05312⟩

Dennison, J.H. (-1966)
Hogarth, W.P.: Dr. John Hoyle Dennison. CMAJ 96:120-121, 1967 ⟨I-01506⟩

Derome, W. (1877-1931)
Fontaine, R.: Professor Wilfrid Derome. CMAJ 26:122, 1932 ⟨I-01035⟩

Descouts, M. (1682-1745)
Belanger, H.: Martin Descouts. DCB 3:182, 1974 ⟨I-01014⟩

Desjardins, L.E. (1837-1919)
Desjardins, E.: L.E. Desjardins (1837-1919): Un Des Pionniers De L'Opthalmologie Au Canada Francais. Canadian Journal of Surgery 12:165-171, 1969 ⟨I-04660⟩

Desmarets, C.D.
Massicotte, E.Z.: L'Engagement d'un Chirurgien Pour L'Ouest au Dix-Huitieme Siecle. L'UMC 49:204-205, 1920 ⟨I-01774⟩

DeVeber, L.G. (1849-1925)
Campbell, P.M.: Leverett George DeVeber. CMAJ 15:971, 1925 ⟨I-01504⟩
Learmonth, G.E.: Dr. Leverett George De Veber. CMAJ 15:868, 1925 ⟨I-01503⟩
Stanley, G.D.: Hon. L.G. DeVeber. CACHB 2(1):11-12, 1937 ⟨I-01208⟩

Dickson, J.R. (1819-1882)
Angus, M.S.: John Robinson Dickson. DCB 11:263-264, 1982 ⟨I-04864⟩
Gibson, T.: A Sketch of the Career of Doctor John Robinson Dickson. CMAJ 38:493-494, 1938 ⟨I-03370⟩

Dickson, W.H. (1878-1932)
Richards, G.E.: William Howard Dickson, MD. CMAJ 29:690-91, 1933 ⟨I-03049⟩

Diereville (fl.1699-1711)
Rousseau, J.: Diereville. DCB 2:188-189, 1969 ⟨I-01018⟩

Dill, W.
LeBlond, S.: Le Dr. Dill. CMAJ 79:55-57, 1958 ⟨I-01502⟩

Dobbs, H. (1808-1887)
Angus, M.S.: Harriet (Cartwright) Dobbs. DCB 11:265-66, 1982 ⟨I-04860⟩

Dorion, J. (1797-1877)
Galarneay, C.: Jacques Dorion. DCB 10:236, 1972 ⟨I-01204⟩

Douglas, A.J. (1874-1940)
Mitchell, R.: Dr. Alex. J. Douglas 1874-1940. Manitoba Medical Review 38:47-48, 1948 ⟨I-01467⟩

Douglas, G.M. (1804-1864)
LeBlond, S.: George Mellis Douglas. DCB 9:217-218, 1976 ⟨I-00880⟩

Douglas, J. (1800-1886)
Atwater, E.C.: The protracted labor and brief life of a country medical school: the Auburn Medical Institution, 1825. JHMAS 34:334-352,1979 ⟨I-01202⟩
Bayne, J.R.D.: A Defence of Dr. James Douglas. CMAJ 51:277-278, 1944 ⟨I-04441⟩
Douglas, J.: Journals and reminiscences. New York, 1910 Privately printed ⟨I-03243⟩
LeBlond, S.: James Douglas, M.D. (1800-1886). CMAJ 66:283-287, 1952 ⟨I-01201⟩
LeBlond, S.: Le Dr. James Douglas, de Quebec, remonte le Nil en 1860-61. Les Cahiers Des Dix 42:101-123, 1979 ⟨I-01665⟩
LeBlond, S.: James Douglas. DCB 11:271-272. 1982 ⟨I-04866⟩
Russel, C.K.: Dr. James Douglas, 1800-1886, Adventurer. Transactions of the American Neurological Association, pp 2-6, 1935 ⟨I-04834⟩
Stone, A.C.: The Life of James Douglas, M.D. McGill Medical Undergraduate Journal 8:6-20, 1938 ⟨I-01469⟩

Douglas, M.S. (-1961)
L., E.K.: Dr. Murray Scott Douglas. CMAJ 85:761-762, 1961 ⟨I-01496⟩

Douglas, G.M. (1804-1864)
LeBlond, S.: Le Docteur George Douglas (1804-1864). Cahier des Dix 34:144-164, 1969 ⟨I-00881⟩
LeBlond, S.: Ne a La Grosse-Ile. Cahier des Dix 40:113-139, 1975 ⟨I-00882⟩

Swinton, W.E.: George Mellis Douglas: typhus and tragedy. CMAJ 125:1284-6, 1981 ⟨I-04561⟩

Doupe, J. (1910-1966)
Hildes, J.A.: Recollections of Joseph Doupe. CMAJ 96:63, 1967 ⟨I-01500⟩
Klass, A.: Dr. Joseph Doupe, an appreciation. CMAJ 95:1329-1331, 1966 ⟨I-01472⟩
Naimark, A.: About Joe (Joseph Doupe). University of Manitoba Medical Journal 28:1, 1966 ⟨I-01474⟩

Doust, J.W.L. (1914-1980)
C., R.A., H., R.C.A.: Memory and Appreciation: John William Lovett Doust 1914-1980. Canadian Journal of Psychiatry 25:683, 1980 ⟨I-02880⟩

Drew, C. (1904-1950)
Montagnes, J.: McGill Grad Honored by U.S. [C.R. Drew]. Canadian Doctor 48(7):33, 1982 ⟨I-04952⟩

Drummond, W.H. (1859-1907)
C[ampbell], W.W.: William Henry Drummond. PTRSC 3d. Series, vol. 1, viii-ix, 1907 ⟨I-01197⟩
Craig, R.H.: Reminiscences of W.H. Drummond. The Dalhousie Review 5:161-169, 1925-6 ⟨I-01694⟩
Fish, A.H.: Dr. William Henry Drummond 1854-1907. CACHB 12:1-8, 1947 ⟨I-01196⟩
McDonald, J.F.: William Henry Drummond. Toronto, The Ryerson Press, n.d., 132 p. ⟨I-02145⟩
McNally, L.B.: Dr. William Drummond; Poet - Physician to the " Habitant". CAMSI Journal 22:9-16, 1963 (Feb.) ⟨I-01198⟩
Swinton, W.E.: William Henry Drummond -- A Master of the Peasant Thought. CMAJ 114:265-6, 1976 ⟨I-01477⟩

Duchesne, A. (?-post 1656)
Cadotte, M.: Le Docteur Adrien Duchesne, Le Premier Expert Medico-Legal de La Nouvelle-France (1639). L'UMC 104:276-278, 1975 ⟨I-01008⟩
Drolet, A.: Adrien Du Chesne. DCB 1:287, 1966 ⟨I-01007⟩

Dufault, P. (1895-1969)
Nadeau, G.: Le Docteur Paul Dufault (1895-1969). L'UMC 99:1672-1673, 1970 ⟨I-01052⟩

Duff, G.L. (1904-1956)
Hamilton, J.: George Lyman Duff, 1904-1956. PTRSC Series 3, 51:89-93, 1957 ⟨I-04776⟩
M[artin], C.P.: Dr. George Lyman Duff. CMAJ 75:964, 1956 ⟨I-04738⟩

Duff, G.L. (1904-1958)
Boyd, W.: George Lyman Duff: In Memoriam. CMAJ 78:962-963, 1958 ⟨I-01581⟩

Dugay, J. (1647-1727)
Douville, R.: Jacques Dugay. DCB 2:202-203, 1969 ⟨I-01019⟩

Duncombe, C. (1792-1867)
Cross, M.S.: Charles Duncombe. DCB 9:228-232, 1976 ⟨I-00884⟩
Landon, F.: The Duncombe Uprising of 1837 and Some of its Consequences. PTRSC series 3, vol. 25:83-98, 1931 ⟨I-03367⟩

Read, C.: The Duncombe rising, its aftermath, anti-Americanism, and sectarianism. Histoire Sociale/Social History 9(17):47-69, 1976 ⟨I-03003⟩
Read, C.F.: The Rising in Western Upper Canada, 1837-38. Thesis (Ph.D.), University of Toronto, 1976. Microfiche #2795 ⟨I-00885⟩

Dunlop, D.R. (1870-1927)
Learmonth, G.E.: Dr. Daniel Rolston Dunlop. CMAJ 18:356, 1928 ⟨I-01627⟩

Dunlop, W. (1792-1848)
Dunlop, A.: Dunlop of that Ilk. Glasgow, Kerr and Richardson, Ltd., 1898, 150 p. ⟨I-04436⟩
Dunlop, W.: Recollections of the American War 1812-1814. Toronto, Historical Publishing Co., 1905. 112 p. ⟨I-01176⟩
Ford, F.S.L.: William Dunlop. Toronto, Murray Printing Co., 1931. 57 p. ⟨I-01960⟩
Ford, F.S.L.: William Dunlop, 1792-1848. CMAJ 25:210-19, 1931 ⟨I-03153⟩
Ford, F.S.L.: William Dunlop. Toronto, Albert Britnel Book Shop, 1934. 60 p. ⟨I-00888⟩
Graham, W.H.: The Tiger of Canada West. Toronto/Vancouver, Clarke, Irwin and Co. Ltd., 1962. 308 p. ⟨I-00889⟩
Kelly, H.A.: William Dunlop (1791-1848). In Kelly HW, Burrage WL: Dictionary of American Medical Biography. New York and London, D. Appleton and Co., 1928. pp 358-359 ⟨I-00887⟩
Klinck, C.F.: William "Tiger" Dunlop. "Blackwoodian Backwoodsman". Toronto, Ryerson Press, 1958. 185 p. ⟨I-00890⟩
Ladell, M.: 'The Tiger': A Giant of a Man. The Medical Post, October 1983. p. 2 ⟨I-05217⟩
Russell, G.: Phrenological Sketch of the Character of Dr. Wm. Dunlop, Late Member of Parliament for the County of Huron. British American Journal of Medical and Physical Science 4:153-154, 1848-9 ⟨I-01497⟩
Stewart, I.A.: The 1841 Election of Dr. William Dunlop as Member of Parliament for Huron County. Ontario Historical Society Papers and Records 39:51-62, 1947 ⟨I-02018⟩
Swinton, W.E.: Physician contributions to nonmedical science: William "Tiger" Dunlop, soldier, editor, lecturer and warden of the forests. CMAJ 115:690-4, 1976 ⟨I-01480⟩

E

Earle, S.Z. (1822-1888)
McGahan, E.W.: Sylvester Zobieski Earle. DCB 11:295-96, 1982 ⟨I-04867⟩

Eberts, E.M. (1873-1945)
Roman, C.L.: Dr. E.M. Eberts. CMAJ 53:412, 1945 ⟨I-04343⟩

Eccles, F.R. (1843-1924)
Bateson, U.E.: Dr. F.R. Eccles. CMAJ 14:764, 1924 ⟨I-02777⟩

Edward, M.L. (1885-)
Edward, M.L.: Reflections of Dr. Mary Lee Edward. N,p., 1977. ⟨I-05379⟩

Effner, B. (-)
Rehwinkel, B.L.: Dr. Bessie. The Life Story and Romance of a Pioneer Lady Doctor on our Western and the Canadian Frontier. St. Louis, Mo., Concordia Pub. House, 1963 ⟨I-05059⟩

Egbert, W.E. (1871-1936)
L., G.: Honourable William E. Egbert. CMAJ 36:210, 1937 ⟨I-03437⟩

Elliott, J.H. (1873-1942)
Clarkson, F.A.: Jabez Henry Elliott. CMAJ 50:264-267, 1944 ⟨I-02778⟩
Clarkson, F.A.: Jabez Henry Elliott: 1873-1942. Bulletin of the Academy of Medicine [Toronto] 17:95-100, 1944 ⟨I-04420⟩
Parfitt, C.D.: Dr. Jabez Henry Elliott. CMAJ 48:181-2, 1943 ⟨I-04250⟩

Emery, A.F. (1856-1933)
Kirkland, A.S.: Dr. Alban Frederick Emery. CMAJ 30:108-109, 1934 ⟨I-03544⟩

Emery-Coderre, J. (1813-1888)
Desjardins, E.: Joseph Emery-Coderre. DCB 11:302-303, 1982 ⟨I-04869⟩

Erad, J.B. (1695-1757)
Romkey, R.: Johann Burghard Erad. DCB 3:212, 1974 ⟨I-01015⟩

Evans, D.J. (1868-1928)
Dube, J.E.: Dr. David James Evans, an appreciation. CMAJ 19:501-502, 1928 ⟨I-03496⟩
Hamilton, H.D.: Dr. David James Evans. CMAJ 19:501, 1928 ⟨I-03495⟩

F

Fafard, T. (1855-1890)
Painchaud, R.: Theogene Fafard. DCB 11:306-307, 1982 ⟨I-04836⟩

Fahrni, G.S. (1887-)
Carpenter, P.: Gordon Samuel Fahrni. CMAJ 123:1060, 1980 ⟨I-02773⟩
Fahrni, G.: Dr. Gordon Fahrni: reminiscing on 70 years of medicine. CMAJ 125:94-97, 1981 ⟨I-04555⟩
Fahrni, G.S.: Prairie Surgeon. Winnipeg, Queenston House Publishing Inc., 1976. 138 p. ⟨I-01404⟩

Farish, H.G. (1770?-1856)
Campbell, D.A.: Henry Greggs Farish (1770?-1856). In Kelly HW, Burrage WL: Dictionary of American Medical Biography. New York and London, D. Appleton and Co., 1928. p. 395. ⟨I-01209⟩
Farish, G.W.T.: A medical biography of the Bond-Farish family. CMAJ 23:696-698, 1930 ⟨I-03169⟩

Farley, F.J. (-1930)
Young, G.: Dr. Frank Jones Farley. CMAJ 22:742, 1930 ⟨I-03014⟩

Farquharson, R.F. (1897-1965)
Dauphinee, J.A.: Ray Fletcher Farquharson, 1897-1965. PTRSC series 4, 4:83-9, 1966 ⟨I-04774⟩

Hamilton, J.D.: Tributes presented at the memorial service for Professor R.F. Farquharson. CMAJ 93:234-235, 1965 ⟨I-02813⟩
Wightman, K.J.R.: Tributes presented at the memorial service for Professor R.F. Farquharson. CMAJ 93:233-234, 1965 ⟨I-02781⟩

Farrar, C.B. (1874-1970)
S., A.B.: Clarence B. Farrar. CMAJ 103:307, 1970 ⟨I-02783⟩

Farrell, E. (1843-1901)
Campbell, D.A.: Edward Farrell (1843-1901). In Kelly HW, Burrage WL: Dictionary of American Medical Biography. New York and London, D. Appleton and Co., 1928. p. 399. ⟨I-01211⟩

Farris, H.A. (1881-1953)
Kirkland, A.S.: Dr. Hugh A. Farris. CMAJ 68:625-6, 1953 ⟨I-04528⟩

Fenwick, G.E. (1825-1894)
Kelly, H.A.: George Edgeworth Fenwick (1825-1894). In Kelly HW, Burrage WL: Dictionary of American Medical Biography. New York and London, D. Appleton and Co., 1928. p. 403. ⟨I-01214⟩
MacDermot, H.E.: George Edgeworth Fenwick (1825-1894). Canadian Journal of Surgery 11:1-4, 1968 ⟨I-04229⟩

Ferguson, A.H (1853-1911)
Mitchell, R., Ferguson, C.C.: Alexander Hugh Ferguson 1853-1911. Canadian Journal of Surgery 6:1-4, 1963 ⟨I-02785⟩

Ferguson, J. (1850-1939)
Routley, T.C.: Dr. John Ferguson. CMAJ 42:94, 1940 ⟨I-01219⟩

Ferguson, J.Y. (1875-1965)
Plewes, B.: Dr. James Young Ferguson: an appreciation. CMAJ 92:896, 1965 ⟨I-02819⟩

Ferguson, R.G. (1884-1964)
Wherrett, G.J.: Dr. Robert G. Ferguson. CMAJ 90:995-996, 1964 ⟨I-05224⟩

Ferris, W.D. (1870-1927)
Whitelaw, W.H.: Lieutenant-Colonel W.D. Ferris, MB. CMAJ 17:1233, 1927 ⟨I-02815⟩

Fiddes, J.
Fiddes, J., Jaques, L.B.: Reminiscences. Saskatoon, University of Saskatchewan (Dept. of Physiology and Pharmacology), 1970. 101 p. ⟨I-03242⟩

Fife, J.K.M. (1898-1947)
Huckell, R.G.: John Keith Munroe Fife. CMAJ 56:585, 1947 ⟨I-02816⟩

Finley, F.G. (-1940)
Gordon, A.H.: Dr. Frederick Gault Finley. CMAJ 43:193, 1940 ⟨I-01048⟩
MacLaren, M.: Col. F.G. Finley. CMAJ 43:193, 1940 ⟨I-03339⟩
Fischer, W.J. (-1920) G., K.L.: Dr. W.J. Fischer, MA. CMAJ 10:1144, 1920 ⟨I-02818⟩

FitzGerald, J.G. (1882-1940)

Defries, R.D.: Dr. John Gerald FitzGerald. CMAJ 43:190-192, 1940 ⟨I-03362⟩

F[arrar], C.B.: I. Remember J.G. Fitzgerald. American Journal of Psychiatry 120:49-52, 1963 ⟨I-02791⟩

Fraser, D.T.: John Gerald Fitzgerald (1882-1940). PTRSC 35:113-115, 1941 ⟨I-03572⟩

Mullin, J.H.: Dr. John Gerald FitzGerald. CMAJ 43:192, 1940 ⟨I-01218⟩

Fleet, G.A. (-1943)

M[acDermot], H.E.: Dr. George A. Fleet. CMAJ 49:149, 1943 ⟨I-02175⟩

Fleming, A.G. (1887-1943)

Hincks, C.M.: Dr. A. Grant Fleming. CMAJ 48:548, 550, 1943 ⟨I-02787⟩

Pedley, F.D.: Grant Fleming. CMAJ 48:464, 1943 ⟨I-02788⟩

Fletcher, A.A. (1889-1964)

Campbell, W.R.: Andrew Almon Fletcher. CMAJ 92:145-146, 1965 ⟨I-02790⟩

Harris, R.I.: Almon Fletcher. CMAJ 92:198, 1965 ⟨I-02789⟩

Foigny, G. de (-1770)

Nadeau, G.: Un Medecin de Roi a Quebec Qui Ne Vint Pas au Canada: Gandoger de Foigny. L'UMC 100:1990-1992, 1971 ⟨I-02233⟩

Forbes, A.E.G. (1881-1927)

W., S.L.: Arthur Edward Grant Forbes, MD, CM. Nova Scotia Medical Bulletin 6:29-31, 1927 ⟨I-02807⟩

Forbes, A.M. (1874-1929)

Cushing, H.B.: Dr. A. MacKenzie Forbes. CMAJ 21:109, 1929 ⟨I-02793⟩

MacDermot, H.E.: Dr. Mackenzie Forbes and his hospital. McGill News 37:35, 62, 1956 ⟨I-02792⟩

Ford, F.S.L. (1868-1944)

Deadman, W.J.: Frederick Samuel Lampson Ford, CMG, MD. CMAJ 52:109, 1945 ⟨I-02125⟩

Forestier, A. (1646-1717)

Boissonnault, C.M.: Antoine Forestier. DCB 2:226, 1969 ⟨I-01020⟩

Forestier, A.-B. (1687-1742)

Moogk, P.N.: Antoine-Bertrand Forestier. DCB 3:220-221, 1974 ⟨I-01016⟩

Forster, F.J.R. (1876-1967)

Ingham, G.H.: Dr. Frederick Joseph Richardson Forster. CMAJ 98:63-64, 1968 ⟨I-02172⟩

Fortier, L-E. (1865-1947)

Fortier, A.: Bio-Bibliographie du Professeur L.-E. Fortier. Ecole de Bibliothecaires, de l'Universite de Montreal, 1952. 39 p. n.p. ⟨I-02261⟩

Fortin, P-E. (1823-1888)

Bilas, I.: Pierre-Etienne Fortin. DCB 11:320-21, 1982 ⟨I-04837⟩

Foster, S. (1792-1868)

MacKinnon, C.: Sewell Foster. DCB 9:276-277, 1976 ⟨I-01213⟩

Fotheringham, J.T. (1861-1940)

C., C.J.: Major-General John Taylor Fotheringham, CMG, MD. CMAJ 43:87-88, 1940 ⟨I-01216⟩

Foucher, A.A. (1856-)

Watson, I.A.: Auguste Achille Foucher. In: Physicians and Surgeons of America. Concord, Republican Press Association, 1896. pp 207-208 ⟨I-02515⟩

Found E.M. (1905-)

Gray, C.: Eric MacLean Found. CMAJ 127:322, 1982 ⟨I-04902⟩

Fox, J. (1793-1866)

MacKenzie, K.A.: Doctor John Fox: 1793-1866. Nova Scotia Medical Bulletin 33:302-303, 1954 ⟨I-02820⟩

Francis, W.W. (1878-1959)

Fulton, J.F.: William Willoughby Francis, 1878-1959. JHMAS 15:1-6, 1960 ⟨I-02798⟩

M., H.E.: William W. Francis. CMAJ 81:516, 1959 ⟨I-02821⟩

MacDermot, H.E.: Dr. William W. Francis 1878-1959. McGill News 61:16-17, 1959 ⟨I-02796⟩

Simpson, E.E.: William Willoughby Francis. Placerville, California, Blackwood Press, 1981, 7 p. ⟨I-04362⟩

Stevenson, L.G.: Dr. William W. Francis 1878-1959. CMAJ 81:515-516, 1959 ⟨I-02797⟩

Stevenson, L.G.: W.W. Francis 1878-1959. BHM 34:373-378, 1960 ⟨I-02795⟩

Frappier, A.

Robillard, D.: Armand Frappier. CMAJ 123:807, 1980 ⟨I-02020⟩

Fraser, A.H. (1827-)

Stanley, G.D.: Surgeon-General A.H. Fraser. CACHB 12:83-84, 1948 ⟨I-01210⟩

Fraser, D.B. (1848-1933)

Fisher, A.W.: Dr. Donald Blair Fraser, An Ontario Physician. CACHB 13(2):35-38, 1948 ⟨I-01215⟩

Fraser, D.T. (1888-1954)

Cameron, G.D.W.: The First Donald Fraser Memorial Lecture. Canadian Journal of Public Health 51:341-348, 1960 ⟨I-02800⟩

Fraser, R. (-1957)

T., M.W.: Roy Fraser, BSA, MA, FRMS, LLD, an appreciation. CMAJ 77:357-58, 1957 ⟨I-04753⟩

Fraser, R.L. (-1925)

Leeder, F.: Dr. R.L. Fraser. CMAJ 16:99, 1926 ⟨I-01606⟩

Thomas, M.W.: Dr. R.L. Fraser. CMAJ 16:99, 1926 ⟨I-01608⟩

Fraser, T. (-1954) Defries, R.D.: Dr. Thomas Fraser. CMAJ, 71:401, 1954 ⟨I-04567⟩

Freeman, C. (1827-1895)

Corrigan, S.H.: Doctor Clarkson Freeman 1827-1895: a sketch. CMAJ 23:438-440, 1938 ⟨I-03030⟩

Freeze, D.D. (1885-1962)

G., H.B.: Doctor David Dawson Freeze. Canadian Anaesthetist's Society Journal 9:560, 1962 ⟨I-02826⟩

Fremont, C.-J. (1806-1862)
Boissonnault, C.M.: Charles-Jacques Fremont. DCB 9:286-287, 1976 ⟨I-02232⟩

Fulton, J. (1837-1887)
Kelly, H.A.: John Fulton (1837-1887). In Kelly HW, Burrage WL: Dictionary of American Medical Biography, New York and London, D. Appleton and Co., 1928. pp. 442-443. ⟨I-01212⟩
Roland, C.G.: John Fulton. DCB 11:328-29, 1982 ⟨I-04838⟩

G

Gaboury, C-P. (1902-)
LeSage, A.: Docteur Charles-Paul Gaboury, Colonel R.C.A.M.C. L'UMC 71:447-449, 1942 ⟨I-01767⟩

Gairdner, M. (1809-1837)
Harvey, A.G.: Meredith Gairdner: Doctor of Medicine. British Columbia Historical Quarterly 9:89-111, 1945 ⟨I-02802⟩

Galbraith, W.S. (1866-1939)
Stanley, G.D.: Dr. Walter S. Galbraith of Lethbridge. CACHB 13:79-82, 1949 ⟨I-01380⟩

Gallie, W.E. (1882-1959)
Harris, R.I.: As I remember him: William Edward Gallie, Surgeon, Seeker, Teacher, Friend. Canadian Journal of Surgery 10:135-150, 1967 ⟨I-02803⟩
Harris, R.I.: William Edward Gallie, 1882-1959: an appreciation. CMAJ 81:766-770, 1959 ⟨I-02143⟩
Mercer, W.: William Edward Gallie. CMAJ 81:691-692, 1959 ⟨I-02171⟩
Plewes, B.: William Edward Gallie: A Tribute by a Gallie Slave. CMAJ 81:692, 1959 ⟨I-02123⟩
Ziegler, H.R.: Dr. W.E. Gallie. CMAJ 81:854-855, 1959 ⟨I-02827⟩

Gamache, J. (1879-1933)
Learmonth, G.E.: Dr. Joseph Gamache. CMAJ 30:226, 1934 ⟨I-03551⟩

Gamelain Fontaine, M (1640-1676)
Boissonnault, C.M.: Michel Gamelain de la Fontaine. DCB 1:320-321, 1966 ⟨I-01398⟩

Gardner, W. (1845-1926)
Chipman, W.W.: William Gardner, M.D. CMAJ 16:1284, 1926 ⟨I-01612⟩
Shepherd, F.J.: William Gardner, M.D. CMAJ 16:1284-1285, 1926 ⟨I-01611⟩

Garneau, P. (1897-1941)
LeBlond, S.: Dr. Paul Garneau. CMAJ 45:89, 1941 ⟨I-03534⟩

Garnier, J.H. (1823-1898)
Johnston, W.V.: John Hutchison Garnier a Canadian naturalist and physician. CMAJ 29:314-316, 1933 ⟨I-03008⟩
Johnston, W.V.: John Hutchison Garnier of Lucknow, Ont.: A Canadian Naturalist and Physician. Bulletin of the Academy of Medicine, Toronto 7:11-20, 1933 ⟨I-04964⟩

Mackenzie, A.J.: A Canadian Naturalist; John Hutchison Garnier of Lucknow. CMAJ 17:355-356, 1927 ⟨I-02805⟩

Garrett, R.W. (1853-1925)
Howard, C.A.: Dr. Richard William Garrett. CMAJ 15:329, 1925 ⟨I-02829⟩

Garrow, A.E. (1862-1923)
Stewart, W.G.: Dr. Alexander Esselmont Garrow. CMAJ 13:931, 1923 ⟨I-02998⟩

Gaschet, R. (1665-1744)
Paquin, M.: Rene Gaschet. DCB 3:236-237, 1974 ⟨I-02258⟩

Gaspe, P.A. de (1786-1871)
Cadotte, M.: Les Memoires de Philippe Aubert de Gaspe et Les Medecins. L'UMC 105:1250-1268, 1976 ⟨I-02259⟩
Gaspe, P.A. de: Memoires. Montreal, Bibliotheque Canadienne-Francaise, 1971. 435 p. ⟨I-01026⟩

Gaultier, J-F. (1708-1756)
Ahern, M.J.: Ahern, G.: Jean Francois Gaultier (1708-1756). In Kelly HW, Burrage WL: Dictionary of American Medical Biography. New York and London, D. Appleton and Co., 1928. pp. 457-458. ⟨I-01396⟩
Boivin, B.: Jean-Francois Gaultier. DCB 3:241, 675-681, 1974 ⟨I-01397⟩
Lessard, R.: Un De Nos Illustres Devanciers: Jean-Francois Gaultier. L'UMC 95:676-678, 1966 ⟨I-02237⟩

Gauthier, C.A. (1901-1983)
LeBlond, S.: Dr. Charles Auguste Gauthier. CMAJ 129:771-772, 1983 ⟨I-05163⟩

Gendron, F. (1618-1688)
Nadeau, G.: Francois Gendron. DCB 1:328, 1966 ⟨I-01402⟩
Prieur, G.O.: Francois Gendron: the First Physician of Old Huronia. CACHB 21:1-7, 1956 ⟨I-01403⟩

Genest, J. (1919-)
Gray, C.: Jacques Genest. CMAJ 126:1216, 1982 ⟨I-04831⟩

George, H. (1864-1932)
Stanley, G.D.: Dr. Henry George. CACHB 2(2):8-10, 1937 ⟨I-01381⟩

Gerin-Lajoie, L. (1895-1959)
Dufresne, R.R.: Leon Gerin-Lajoie. CMAJ 80:398, 1959 ⟨I-02248⟩
Routley, T.C.: Dr. Leon Gerin-Lajoie. CMAJ 80:397-398, 1959 ⟨I-02247⟩

Gervais, T. (-1940)
Gervais-Roy, C.: Un Medecin de Campagne d'autrefois. Revue d'Ethnologie du Quebec 7:85-102, 1981 ⟨I-04939⟩

Gesner, A. (1797-1864)
Campbell, D.A.: Abraham Gesner (1797-1864). In Kelly HW, Burrage WL: Dictionary of American Medical Biography. New York and London, D. Appleton and Co., 1928. pp. 462-463 ⟨I-01392⟩

Gray, F.W.: Pioneer Geologists of Nova Scotia. Dalhousie Review 26:10-25, 1946-47 ⟨I-02023⟩

Johnson, G.R., Oborne, H.V.: Abraham Gesner - 1797-1864: A Forgotten Physician-Inventor. CACHB 13:30-34, 1948 ⟨I-01393⟩

MacKenzie, K.A.: Abraham Gesner, M.D., Surgeon Geologist, 1797-1864. CMAJ 59:384-387, 1948 ⟨I-04480⟩

Russell, L.S.: Abraham Gesner. DCB 9:308-312, 1976 ⟨I-01394⟩

Scarlett, E.P.: A Forgotten Figure. Group Practice, pp 24, 26, 1970 ⟨I-03412⟩

Swinton, W.E.: Abraham Gesner, inventor of kerosene. CMAJ 115:1126-9, 1976 ⟨I-04429⟩

Giard, L. (1809-1887)

Audet, L.-P.: Louis Giard. DCB 11:345-46. 1982 ⟨I-04845⟩

Gibson, A. (1883-1956)

Boyd, W.: Cause and Effect: The Fifth Alexander Gibson Memorial Lecture. CMAJ 92:868-874, 1965 ⟨I-03186⟩

M., R.: Dr. Alexander Gibson. CMAJ 74:852, 1956 ⟨I-02776⟩

Mercer, W.: Edinburgh and Canadian Medicine: The First Alexander Gibson Memorial Lecture, part 1. CMAJ 84:1241-1257, 1313-1317, 1961 ⟨I-01573⟩

Gibson, T. (1865-1941)

Chevrier, G.R.: Dr. Thomas Gibson. CMAJ 45:193, 1941 ⟨I-03518⟩

Miller, J.: Dr. Thomas Gibson. CMAJ 45:192-193, 1941 ⟨I-03519⟩

Giffard, R. (1587-1668)

Besnard, J.: Les diverses professions de Robert Giffard. Nova Francia 4:322-329, 1929 ⟨I-04937⟩

Giffard R. (1587-1668)

Provost, H.: Robert Giffard de Moncel. DCB 1:330-331, 1966 ⟨I-01399⟩

Gilchrist, J. (1792-1849)

Elliott, J.H.: John Gilchrist: A pioneer New England Physician in Canada. BHM 7:737-750, 1939 ⟨I-02775⟩

Gilchrist, S. (1901-1970)

Archibald, F.E.: Salute to Sid: The Story of Dr. Sidney Gilchrist. Windsor, Lancelot Press, 1970. 127 pp. ⟨I-03936⟩

Gillam, G.J. (1886-1941)

F.A.C.: Dr. George Joshua Gillam. CMAJ 46:200, 1942 ⟨I-04274⟩

Gillespie, A. (1854-1937)

Wright, J.S.: Dr. Alexander Gillespie. CMAJ 36:99, 1937 ⟨I-02875⟩

Gillespie, J. (1927-1981)

Howell, J.M.: Gillespie, J. CMAJ 126:205, 1982 ⟨I-04718⟩

Gillespie, W.

Gillespie, R.: The unforgettable Doctor (William Gillespie, Kitchener). Kitchener-Waterloo Academy of Medicine, K-W Hospital, Kitchener, Ontario, 11 p. Unpublished ⟨I-01372⟩

Gillespie, W.F. (1891-1949)

McGugan, A.C.: Dr. W. Fulton Gillespie. CMAJ 62:208-9, 1950 ⟨I-04484⟩

Gilmour, C. (-1952)

Bell, L.G.: Dr. Clifford Gilmour. CMAJ, 67:483, 1952 ⟨I-04554⟩

Gilmour, C.H. (1879-1933)

Wales, H.C.: Dr. Charles Hawkins Gilmour 1879-1933. CMAJ 27:689, 1933 ⟨I-02809⟩

Gilpin, J.B. (1810-1892)

Campbell, D.A.: John Bernard Gilpin (1810-1892). In Kelly, H.W., Burrage, W.L.: Dictionary of American Med Bio. New York and London, D. Appleton and Co., 1928. p. 470. ⟨I-01388⟩

Ginsburg, B.J. (1894-1962)

M[itchell], R.: Dr. B.J. Ginsburg. CMAJ 86:796, 1962 ⟨I-02808⟩

Goldbloom, A. (1890-1968)

Goldbloom, A.: Small Patients. The Autobiography of a children's doctor. Toronto, Longmans, Green and Co., 1959. 316 p. ⟨I-01369⟩

Gomery, M. (1875-1967)

Bensley, E.H.: Dr. Minnie Gomery. CMAJ 96:1294,1967 ⟨I-02493⟩

Good, J.W. (1852-1926)

Blanchard, R.J.: James Wilford Good, M.B, L.R.C.P. (Edin), F.A.C.S. CMAJ 16:1283, 1926 ⟨I-01614⟩

Gemmell, J.P.: "Good -- Doctor" Dr. J. Wilford Good, Dean of Manitoba Medical College, 1887-1898. University of Manitoba Medical Journal 51:98-103, 1981 ⟨I-04832⟩

Mitchell, R.: James Wilford Good, M.B., L.R.C.P.(Edin), F.A.C.S. CMAJ 16:1283, 1926 ⟨I-02137⟩

Montgomery, E.W.: J.W. Good - The Most Unforgettable Character I Have Known. University of Manitoba Medical Journal 21:27-34, 1949 ⟨I-01582⟩

Goodall, J.R. (1878-1947)

Campbell, A.D.: The Late Dr. J.R. Goodall. CMAJ 58:304, 1948 ⟨I-02152⟩

Gordon, A.H. (1876-1953)

M[acDermot], H.E.: Dr. Alvah Hovey Gordon. CMAJ 68:300, 1953 ⟨I-04531⟩

Goupil, R. (1608-1642)

Pouliot, L.: Rene Goupil. DCB 1:343-344, 1966 ⟨I-02260⟩

Prieur, G.O.: Rene Goupil, Surgeon: The First of the Jesuit Martyrs. CACHB 12:25-31, 1947 ⟨I-02112⟩

Gove, S.T. (1813-1897)

Oborne, H.G.: Samuel Tilley Gove 1813-1897: The Chronicle of a Canadian Doctor of a Century Ago. CACHB 12:31-38, 1947 ⟨I-02113⟩

Grafton, H.F.P. (1903-1962)

R., I.: Dr. Hartley Frederic Patterson Grafton: an appreciation. CMAJ 86:995-996, 1962 ⟨I-02150⟩

Graham, C.W. (1881-1946)
Wilson, C.: Colin W. Graham: a tribute. CMAJ 55:315, 1946 ⟨I-02149⟩

Graham, D.C.
[Godden, J.]: A Nosegay for Donald C. Graham. CMAJ 94:298, 1966 ⟨I-02115⟩

Graham, G.W. (1876-1926)
L., J.: Dr. George Wilbur Graham. CMAJ 17:128, 1927 ⟨I-02148⟩

Graham, J.E. (1847-1899)
Morrow, P.A.: James Elliott Graham (1847-1899). In Kelly HW, Burrage WL: Dictionary of American Medical Biography. New York and London, D. Appleton and Co., 1928. pp. 486-487. ⟨I-01386⟩

Graham, J.W. (1906-1962)
Cecil, R.L.: Dr. J. Wallace Graham: an appreciation. CMAJ 88:107, 1963 ⟨I-02163⟩
Copeman, W.S.C.: Dr. Wallace Graham: an appreciation. CMAJ 88:168, 1963 ⟨I-02161⟩
Fletcher, A.: Dr. Wallace Graham: an appreciation. CMAJ 88:222-223, 1963 ⟨I-02140⟩
Hollander, J.L.: Dr. Wallace Graham: an appreciation. CMAJ 88:168-169, 1963 ⟨I-02138⟩
Kellgren, J.J.: Dr. Wallace Graham: an appreciation. CMAJ 88:168, 1963 ⟨I-02160⟩
Lenoch, F.: Dr. Wallace Graham: an appreciation. CMAJ 88:167-168, 1963 ⟨I-02139⟩
McEwan, C.: Dr. Wallace Graham: an appreciation. CMAJ 88:107, 1963 ⟨I-02162⟩
Svartz, N.: Dr. Wallace Graham: an appreciation. CMAJ 88:222, 1963 ⟨I-02141⟩
Walters, A.: James Wallace Graham, M.D., F.R.C.P.(Lond), F.R.C.P.(C). CMAJ 88:104-106, 1963 ⟨I-02116⟩
Woodside, M.St.A.: Dr. Wallace Graham: an appreciation. CMAJ 88:223, 1963 ⟨I-02159⟩

Grant, H.G. (1889-1954)
A[tlee], H.B.: Harry Goudge Grant. Nova Scotia Medical Bulletin 33:168-170, 1954 ⟨I-02157⟩
Routley, T.C.: Harry Goudge Grant. Nova Scotia Medical Bulletin 33:165, 1954 ⟨I-02158⟩
Scammell, H.L.: Harry Goudge Grant. Nova Scotia Medical Bulletin 33:167-168, 1954 ⟨I-02156⟩
Stewart, C.B.: Harry Goudge Grant. Nova Scotia Medical Bulletin 33:166-167, 1954 ⟨I-02154⟩
Tompkins, M.G.: Harry Goudge Grant. Nova Scotia Medical Bulletin 33:165-166, 1954 ⟨I-02155⟩

Grant, J. (1887-1947)
Bensley, E.H.: James Grant: ship's surgeon on the ill-fated Empress of Ireland. CMAJ 126:318-9, 1982 ⟨I-04757⟩

Grant, J.A. (1830-1920)
Watson, I.A.: Sir James A. Grant. In: Physicians and Surgeons of America. Concord, Republican Press Association, 1896. pp 402-403 ⟨I-02516⟩

Grant, J.C.B.
Sauerland, E.K.: Dr. J.C. Boileau Grant, Anatomist Extraordinaire. JAMA 232:1347-1348, 1975 ⟨I-01373⟩

Grasett, F.L. (1851-1930)
Fotheringham, J.T.: Frederick LeMaitre Grasett. CMAJ 22:596, 1930 ⟨I-03012⟩
Ryerson, E.S.: Frederick LeMaitre Grasett. CMAJ 22:594-95, 1930 ⟨I-03028⟩

Gray, J.C. (1910-1978)
Henderson, R.D.: Dr. Jessie Gray (1910-1978). Canadian Journal of Surgery 23:220, 1980 ⟨I-02878⟩

Grenfell, W.T. (1865-1940)
Duncan, N.: Dr. Grenfell's Parish: the deep sea fisherman. New York/Chicago/Toronto, Fleming H. Revell Co., 1905. 155 p. ⟨I-01389⟩
Grenfell, W.T.: A Labrador Doctor (The Autobiography of Wilfred Thomason Grenfell). Boston/New York, Houghton Mifflin Co., 1919. 441p. ⟨I-01390⟩
Grenfell, W.T.: Forty Years for Labrador. London, Hodder and Stoughton Ltd., 1934, 365 p. ⟨I-04421⟩
Kerr, J.L.: Wilfred Grenfell: His Life and Work. New York, Dodd, Mead and Company, 1959, 270 p. ⟨I-04479⟩
Moore, T.: Wilfred Grenfell. Toronto, Fitzhenry and Whiteside Limited, 1950, p.64. ⟨I-04519⟩
Stuart, H.A.: Sir Wilfred Thomason Grenfell, 1865-1940. CACHB 5(3):1-3, 1940 ⟨I-02182⟩
Thomas, G.W.: Wilfred T. Grenfell, 1865-1941 [sic]. Founder of the International Grenfell Association. Canadian Journal of Surgery 9:125-130, 1966 ⟨I-02119⟩

Grenier, G. (1847-1876)
Laramee, A.: Georges Grenier, M.D. L'UMC 5:286-88, 1876 ⟨I-04829⟩

Grisdale, L.C. (1919-)
Gray, C.: Lloyd Carl Grisdale. CMAJ 125:1360, 1981 ⟨I-04716⟩

Gross, L. (1895-1937)
Libman, E.: Louis Gross, May 5, 1895 - October 17, 1937. Journal of the Mount Sinai Hospital 4, 1938 ⟨I-02120⟩
Oertel, H.: Louis Gross. McGill Medical Undergraduate Journal 7:8-10, 1937 ⟨I-02121⟩
Segall, H.N.: Dr. Louis Gross. CMAJ 37:609, 1937 ⟨I-02142⟩
White, P.D.: A Tribute to Louis Gross. CMAJ 37:609, 1937 ⟨I-02153⟩

Groves, A. (1847-1935)
Harris, C.W.: Abraham Groves of Fergus: The First Elective Appendectomy?. Canadian Journal of Surgery 4:405-410, 1961 ⟨I-01377⟩
Mestern, P.M.: Clara: an Historical Novel of an Ontario Town 1879-1930 [Fiction]. Guelph, Ontario, Back Door Press, 1979. 187 p. ⟨I-01375⟩
Stanley, G.D.: Dr. Abraham Groves 1847-1935: A Great Crusader of Canadian Medicine. CACHB 13:4-10, 1948 ⟨I-01376⟩

Gunn, J. N. (-1937)
L., G.E.: Lieutenant-Colonel John Nisbet Gunn, DSO, MB. CMAJ 37:510-511, 1937 ⟨I-02882⟩

Gunn, W. R. L. (1900-1965)
MacDermot, J.H.: Dr. Robert Lynn Gunn: an appreciation. CMAJ 92:897, 1965 ⟨I-02178⟩

Gurd, F. B. (1884-1948)
McKim, L.H.: Fraser Baillie Gurd: an appreciation. CMAJ 58:394-395, 1948 ⟨I-02177⟩

Gwyn, N. B. (1875-1952)
Farrar, C.B.: Dr. Norman B. Gwyn. CMAJ 66:401-2, 1952 ⟨I-04542⟩
M[acDermot], H.E.: Dr. Norman Gwyn. CMAJ 66:402-3, 1952 ⟨I-04541⟩

Gwynne, W. C. (1806-1875)
Dyster, B.: William Charles Gwynne. DCB 10:325-326, 1972 ⟨I-01387⟩

H

Hale, R. (1702-1767)
Wagner, R.L.: Robert Hale. DCB 3:274-275, 1974 ⟨I-01365⟩

Hall, A. (1812-1868)
Bensley, E.H.: Archibald Hall. DCB 9:357-358, 1976 ⟨I-01345⟩

Hall, W. (1856-1933)
Ferguson, R.G.: Dr. William Hall. CMAJ 30:578, 1934 ⟨I-03539⟩

Halpenny, G. (1908-)
Gray, C.: Gerald Halpenny. CMAJ 127:157, 1982 ⟨I-04909⟩

Halpenny, J. (1869-1930)
Brandson, B.J.: Dr. Jasper Halpenny: an appreciation. CMAJ 24:324, 1931 ⟨I-03068⟩
Mitchell, R.: Dr. Jasper Halpenny. CMAJ 24:323-24, 1931 ⟨I-03045⟩

Hamilton, J. (1797-1877)
[Osler, W.]: James Hamilton, L.R.C.S. Canada Medical and Surgical Journal 5:478-80, 1876-77 ⟨I-04959⟩

Hamilton, J. S. (1805-1897)
Kennedy, J.E.: Jane Soley Hamilton, Midwife. Nova Scotia Historical Review 2:6-30, 1982 ⟨I-05070⟩

Hamilton, T. G. (1874-1935)
Chown, B.: Dr. T. Glendenning Hamilton, (an appreciation). CMAJ 32:710-711, 1935 ⟨I-01343⟩
Mitchell, R.: Dr. T. Glen Hamilton: The Founder of the Manitoba Medical Review. Manitoba Medical Review 40:219-221, 1960 ⟨I-02131⟩
Rankin, L: A Many Sided Man. The Alumni Journal [University of Manitoba] 41:4-7, 1981 ⟨I-03934⟩

Hamman, A. (1866-1958)
Stanley, G.d.: Dr. Alfred Hamman of Taber, Alberta. CACHB 13:39-40, 1948 ⟨I-01339⟩

Hannah, J. A. (1899-1977)
Paterson, G.R.: Jason A. Hannah: Pathologist, Economist, Historian. CMAJ 117:193, 1977 ⟨I-02133⟩

Harding, W. S.
Cushing, J.E., Casey, T., Robertson, M.: A Chronicle of Irish Emigration to Saint John, New Brunswick, 1847. New Brunswick, The New Brunswick Museum, 1979. 77 p. ⟨I-01361⟩

Hardisty, R. H. M. (1879-1947)
Wright, H.P.: Dr. Richard Henry Moore Hardisty, D.S.O., M.C. CMAJ 56:114. 1947 ⟨I-04403⟩

Harris, J. (1739-1802)
Hattie, W.H.: Dr. John Harris, 1739-1802. CMAJ 18:214-215, 1928 ⟨I-01628⟩

Harwood, L. de L. (1866-1934)
Gerin-Lajoie, L.: Dr. Louis de Lotbiniere Harwood. CMAJ 31:106, 1934 ⟨I-01730⟩
LeSage, A.: Le Decanat a la Faculte de Medecine de L'Universite de Montreal: Trois Doyens (1880-1934) -- Rottot, Lachapelle, Harwood. L'UMC 68:166-178, 1939 ⟨I-02265⟩
Nicholls, A.G.: The Late Louis de Lotbiniere Harwood. CMAJ 31:539-541, 1934 ⟨I-02136⟩

Hastings, C. J. O. (1858-1931)
Fleming, G.: Dr. Charles John Collwell Oliver Hastings. CMAJ 24:473, 1931 ⟨I-03044⟩

Hattie, W. H. (1870-1931)
Royer, B.F.: Dr. William Harop Hattie, (an appreciation). CMAJ 26:121-122, 1932 ⟨I-01341⟩

Hebert, C-E. (-1968)
Desjardins, E.: Dr. Charles-Edouard Hebert. CMAJ 98:796-797, 1968 ⟨I-02492⟩

Hebert, L. (1575-1627)
Bennett, E.M.G.: Louis Hebert. DCB 1:367-368, 1966 ⟨I-01366⟩
Charlton, M.: Louis Hebert. Johns Hopkins Hospital Bulletin 25:158-160, 1914 ⟨I-04652⟩
Charlton, M.: Louis Hebert (-1627). In Kelly HW, Burrage WL: Dictionary of American Medical Biography. New York and London, D. Appleton and Co., 1928. pp. 549-551. ⟨I-01367⟩
Hattie, W.H.: Canada's First Apothecary. Dalhousie Reiew 10:376-381, 1930-31 ⟨I-02017⟩
Hattie, W.H.: On Apothecaries, Including Louis Hebert. CMAJ 24:120-123, 1931 ⟨I-01009⟩

Hebert, P. Z. (1850-1942)
White, W.: Paul Z. Hebert, M.D.: "The Last Leaf" of Oslers's McGill Class of 1872. The Bulletin of the Los Angeles County Medical Association 71:520-527, 1941 ⟨I-04654⟩
White, W.: Medical Education at McGill in the Seventies: Excerpts From the "Autobiographie" of the late Paul Zotique Hebert, M.D. BHM 13:614-626, 1943 ⟨I-02483⟩

Hector, J. (1834-1907)
Ballon, H.C.: Sir James Hector, M.D. 1834-1907. CMAJ 87:66-74, 1962 ⟨I-02484⟩
Mitchell, R.: Sir James Hector. CMAJ 66:497-499, 1952 ⟨I-02485⟩
Patterson, H.S.: Sir James Hector, M.D. 1834-1906. CACHB 6(3):2-10, 1941 ⟨I-01353⟩

Thorington, J.M.: Four Physicians-Explorers of the Fur Trade Days. Annals of Medical History, ser. 3, 4:294-301, 1942 ⟨I-04907⟩

Helmcken, J.S. (1825-1920)

Kidd, H.M.: The William Osler Medal Essay: Pioneer Doctor John Sebastian Helmcken. BHM 21:419-461, 1947 ⟨I-02487⟩

MacDermot, J.H.: J.S. Helmcken, MRCP(Lond.), LSA. CMAJ 55:166-171, 1946 ⟨I-02486⟩

Smith, D.B. (Edit.): The Reminiscences of Doctor John Sebastian Helmcken. British Columbia, University of British Columbia Press, 1975. 373 p. ⟨I-01359⟩

Henderson, A.

Stanley, G.D.: Andrew Henderson. CACHB 5(3):5-7, 1940 ⟨I-01344⟩

Henderson, D.A. (-1966)

H., G.: Dr. David A. Henderson, an appreciation. CMAJ 96:171-172, 1967 ⟨I-02490⟩

Henderson, V.E. (1877-1945)

Wasteneys, H.: Velyien Ewart Henderson, 1877-1945. PTRSC 40:91-93, 1946 ⟨I-04386⟩

Hendry, W.B. (1874-1939)

Brodie, F.: Col. William Belfry Hendry, DSO, VD, MB, FRCS(C), FCOG. CMAJ 40:524+526, 1939 ⟨I-01735⟩

Henry, W. (1791-1860)

Hayward, P.: Surgeon Henry's Trifles: Events of a Military Life. London, Chatto and Windus, 1970. 281 p. ⟨I-01364⟩

Henry, W.: Trifles from my port-folio. Quebec, William Neilson (Printers), 1839. Vol 1, 251 p. Vol 2. 252 p. ⟨I-01363⟩

Howell, W.B.: Walter Henry, Army Surgeon. CMAJ 36:302-310, 1937 ⟨I-02764⟩

Mitchell, C.A.: Walter Henry et l'Autopsie de l'Empereur Napoleon I. L'UMC 94:1651-1653, 1965 ⟨I-01521⟩

Mitchell, CA: Walter Henry and the Autopsy of Emperor Napoleon I. University of Ottawa Medical Journal 9:3-8. 1965 ⟨I-03927⟩

Roland, C.G.: Doctors Afield: Walter Henry -- a Very Lilyputian Hero. New England Journal of Medicine 280:31-33, 1969 ⟨I-04870⟩

Hepburn, J. (1888-1956)

Farquharson, R.F.: Dr. John Hepburn, an appreciation. CMAJ 74:943, 1956 ⟨I-04727⟩

Hill, H.W. (1873-1947)

Murphy, H.H.: Dr. H. W. Hill. CMAJ 57:607, 1947 ⟨I-04417⟩

Hilliard, A.M. (1902-1958)

D., J.F.: Dr. Anna Marion Hilliard. CMAJ 79:295, 1958 ⟨I-04896⟩

Robinson, M.O.: Give my Heart; The Dr. Marion Hilliard Story. New York, Doubleday and Co., Inc., 1964. 348 p. ⟨I-01199⟩

Wilson, M.C.: Marion Hilliard. Toronto, Fitzhenry and Whiteside Limited, 1977, p. 64 ⟨I-04520⟩

Hillsman, J.B. (1901-)

Hillsman, J.B.: Eleven Men and a Scalpel. Winnipeg, Columbia Press Ltd., 1948. 144 p. ⟨I-04935⟩

Hiltz, J.E. (1909-1969)

G., A.R., J., C.W.L.: Dr. J. Earle Hiltz. CMAJ 100:1065, 1969 ⟨I-05037⟩

Hincks, C.M. (1885-1964)

Roland, C.G.: Dr. Clarence Meredith Hincks. CMAJ 92:305, 1965 ⟨I-01663⟩

Roland, C.G.: Clarence Hincks in Manitoba, 1918. Manitoba Medical Review 46:107-113, 1966 ⟨I-03415⟩

Hingston, D.A. (1868-1950)

Desjardins, E.: Donald A. Hingston, 1868-1950. L'UMC 80:3-5, 1951 ⟨I-02527⟩

Hingston, W.H. (1829-1907)

Desjardins, E.: Sir William Hales Hingston (1829-1907). Canadian Journal of Surgery 2:225-232, 1958-9 ⟨I-04236⟩

Desjardins, E.: Deux Medecins Montrealais du XIX Siecle Adeptes de la Pensee Ecologique. L'UMC 99:487-492, 1970 ⟨I-01348⟩

Macphail, A.: William Hales Hingston (1829-1907). In Kelly, HW, Burrage WL: Dictionary of American Medical Biography. New York and London, D. Appleton and Co., 1928. pp. 569-570. ⟨I-01349⟩

[Osler, W.]: Sir William Hales Hingston, M.D., LL.D., D.C.L., F.R.C.S., Eng. Lancet 1:770, 1907 ⟨I-05179⟩

Power, D'Arcy: The Hon. Sir William Hales Hingston. In : Plarr's Lives of the Fellows of the Royal College of Surgeons of England. Bristol and London, The Royal College of Surgeons, 1930. Vol. 1:545-6 ⟨I-02758⟩

Hodder, E.M. (1810-1878)

[Osler, W.]: Edward Mulberry Hodder, M.D. Canada Medical and Surgical Journal 6:428-31, 1877-88 ⟨I-04960⟩

Pilon, H.: Edward Mulberry Hodder. DCB 10:350-351, 1972 ⟨I-01354⟩

Hogan, E.V. (1875-1933)

Gosse, N.H.: Edward Vincent Hogan, CBE, MD, CM, FACS, FRCS(C). CMAJ 28:342, 1933 ⟨I-03054⟩

Hoig, D.S. (1853-)

Hoig, D.S.: Reminiscences and Recollections. Oshawa, Mundy-Goodfellow Printing Co. Ltd., 1933, 227 p. ⟨I-04816⟩

Holbrook, J.H. (1876-1958)

Campbell, M.F.: Holbrook of the San. Toronto, The Ryerson Press, 1953. 212 p. ⟨I-03419⟩

Hollis, K.E. (-1964)

Taylor, W.I.: Dr. Karl Edward Hollis. CMAJ 92:198-199, 1965 ⟨I-02282⟩

Holmes, A.F. (1797-1860)

Abbott, M.E.: Andrew Fernando Holmes (1797-1860). In Kelly HW, Burrage WL: Dictionary of American Medical Biography. New York and London, D. Appleton and Co., 1928. pp. 581-582. ⟨I-01360⟩

Houssaye, J.C-F. (1719-)
Massicotte, E.Z.: Le Sieur de la Houssaye. L'UMC 50:302-303, 1921 ⟨I-01771⟩

Howard, H. (1815-1887)
Shastid, T.H.: Henry Howard (1815-1889). In Kelly HW, Burrage WL: Dictionary of American Medical Biography. New York and London, D. Appleton and Co., 1928. pp. 604-605. ⟨I-01350⟩

Howard, R.P. (1823-1889)
Bensley, E.H.: Robert Palmer Howard. DCB 11:428-29, 1982 ⟨I-04846⟩
Macphail, A.: Robert Palmer Howard (1823-1889). In Kelly HW, Burrage WL: Dictionary of American Medical Biography. New York and London, D. Appleton and Co., 1928. p. 606. ⟨I-01351⟩
McEwen, D.: Robert Palmer Howard. McGill Medical Journal 34:141-145, 1965 ⟨I-02557⟩
[Osler, W.]: Robert Palmer Howard, M.D. Medical News 54:419, 1889 ⟨I-05182⟩

Howell, W.B. (1874-1947)
M[acDermot], H.E.: Dr. William Boyman Howell. CMAJ 57:177-8, 1947 ⟨I-04411⟩

Howland, F.L. (1842-)
Watson, I.A.: Francis L. Howland. In: Physicians and Surgeons of America. Concord, Republican Press Association, 1896. p 156 ⟨I-02517⟩

Howley, T. (1842-1889)
Baker, M.: Thomas Howley. DCB 11:429-30, 1982 ⟨I-04847⟩

Huestis, F.
Roberts, W.: Six New Women: A Guide to the Mental Map of Women Reformers in Toronto. Atlantis 3:145-164, 1977-8 ⟨I-01978⟩

Hunter, A.J. (1868-1940)
Mitchell, R.: Alexander Jardine Hunter, MD, DD, MBE. CMAJ 43:396, 1940 ⟨I-03344⟩

Husband, H.A. (1843-)
Watson, I.A.: Henry Aubrey Husband. In: Physicians and Surgeons of America. Concord, Republican Press Association, 1896. p 329 ⟨I-02518⟩

Hutchison, H.S. (1880-1934)
Armour, R.G.: Dr. Henry Seaton Hutchison. CMAJ 30:337, 1934 ⟨I-03537⟩

Hutchison, J.A. (1864-1929)
Finley, F.G.: Col. James Alexander Hutchison, MD: an appreciation. CMAJ 21:237, 1929 ⟨I-01740⟩

Hyland, H.H. (1900-1977)
R., J.C.: Herbert Hylton Hyland. Canadian Journal of Neurological Science 5:51, 1978 ⟨I-01337⟩

I

Iffland, A von (1798-1876)
Hertzman, L.: Anthony von Iffland. DCB 10:375-376, 1972 ⟨I-01336⟩

Inglis, M.S. (-1938)
Tait, R.: The First Western Canadian X-Ray Specialist. University of Manitoba Medical Journal 45:57-59, 1975 ⟨I-01335⟩

Ingvaldsen, T. (1886-1930)
Cameron, A.T.: Dr. Thorsten Ingvaldsen. CMAJ 23:116-117, 1930 ⟨I-03021⟩

Irving, J.F. (1877-1941)
Houston, C.J.: James Franklin Irving. CMAJ 44:640-641, 1941 ⟨I-03355⟩

J

Jackes, A.G. (-1888)
Ferguson, A.H.: Apneumatosis. Manitoba, Northwest and B.C. Lancet 1:163-165, 1888 ⟨I-01332⟩

Jackson, F.W. (1889-1958)
Wilton, M.H.: Dr. Frederick Wilbur Jackson, an appreciation. CMAJ 78:296-297, 1958 ⟨I-02555⟩

Jackson, M.P.
Jackson, M.P.: On the Last Frontier: Pioneering in the Peace River Block. Letters of Mary Percy Jackson. London, The Sheldon Press, 1933. 118 p. ⟨I-01326⟩
Jackson, M.P.: My Life at Keg River. Journal of the Medical Women's Federation 38:40-55, 1956 ⟨I-01327⟩
Keywan, Z.: Mary Percy Jackson: pioneer doctor. The Beaver pp. 41-48, Winter 1977 ⟨I-01328⟩

Janes, E.C. (1898-1966)
Kelly, A.D.: Dr. Ernest Clifford Janes, an appreciation. CMAJ 95:1163-1164, 1966 ⟨I-02552⟩
Orr, W.J.: Dr. Ernest Janes: an appreciation. CMAJ 96:64, 1967 ⟨I-01742⟩
Romanov, A.: Dr. Ernest Clifford Janes: an appreciation. CMAJ 96:64, 1967 ⟨I-01741⟩

Janes, R.M. (1894-1966)
Delaney, R.J.: Dr. Robert Meredith Janes: an appreciation. CMAJ 95:1400, 1966 ⟨I-01745⟩
Delaney, R.J.: Dr. Robert Meredith Janes (1894-1966): Professor of Surgery, University of Toronto (1947-1957). Canadian Journal of Surgery 12:1-11, 1969 ⟨I-02551⟩
Kergin, F.G.: Robert Meredith Janes: an appreciation. CMAJ 95:1399-1400, 1966 ⟨I-02550⟩
Kergin, F.G.: Robert Meredith Janes 1894-1966. Canadian Journal of Surgery 10:1-2, 1967 ⟨I-02549⟩
Low, D.M.: Robert Meredith Janes: The Man (an appreciation). CMAJ 95:1400, 1966 ⟨I-02278⟩
Wales, W.F.: Dr. Robert Meredith Janes: an appreciation. CMAJ 95:1401, 1966 ⟨I-01744⟩

Jaques, L.B. (1911-)
Fiddes, J.: Jaques, L.B.: Reminiscences. Saskatoon, University of Saskatchewan (Dept. of Physiology and Pharmacology), 1970. 101 p. ⟨I-01324⟩
Jaques, L.B.: Reminiscences on completing twenty-five years of research in the blood coagulation field. University of Saskatchewan Medical Journal 3:4-6, 1960 ⟨I-01325⟩

Jenkins, S.R. (1858-1929)
Dewar, G.F.: Dr. Stephen Rice Jenkins: an appreciation. CMAJ 21:620-621, 1929 ⟨I-02275⟩
McKenzie, J.W.: Dr. Stephen Rice Jenkins, FACS. CMAJ 21:620, 1929 ⟨I-02276⟩

Jeremie, C. (1644-1744)
Fortin-Morisset, C.: Catherine Jeremie. DCB 3:314-315, 1974 ⟨I-01011⟩

Johns, E.M. (1879-1968)
Street, M.M.: Watch-Fires on the Mountains: The Life and Writings of Ethel Johns. Toronto, University of Toronto Press, 1973. 336 p. ⟨I-03939⟩

Johnson, G.R. (1877-1956)
M., W.B.: Dr. George Ray Johnson. CMAJ 74:590-591, 1956 ⟨I-02274⟩

Johnson, H.D. (1863-1944)
MacMillan, W.J.P.: Dr. Harry Dawson Johnson. CMAJ 51:186-7, 1944 ⟨I-04256⟩

Johnson, J. (-1926)
Gwyn, N.B.: The letters of a devoted Father to an Unresponsive Son. BHM 7:335-351, 1939 ⟨I-03877⟩

Johnston, G.M. (1817-1877)
Blakeley, P.R.: George Moir Johnston. DCB 10:382-383, 1972 ⟨I-01330⟩

Johnston, S. (1868-1946)
Shields, H.J.: Pioneers of Canadian Anaesthesia: Dr. Samuel Johnston: A Biography. Canadian Anaesthetist's Society Journal 19:589-593, 1972 ⟨I-02574⟩

Johnston, W.G. (1859-1902)
Macphail, A.: Wyatt Galt Johnston (1859-1902). In Kelly HW, Burrage WL: Dictionary of American Medical Biography. New York and London, D. Appleton and Co., 1928. p. 670. ⟨I-01329⟩
Sexton, A.M.: Wyatt Galt Johnston and the Founding of the Laboratory Section. American Journal of Public Health 40:160-164, 1950 ⟨I-02572⟩

Jones, R.O. (1914-)
Gray, C.: Robert Orville Jones. CMAJ 127:528, 1982 ⟨I-04958⟩

Jones, S. (-1822)
Pierce, L.: Some Unpublished Letters of John Strachan, First Bishop of Toronto. Proceedings and Transactions of the Royal Society of Canada, series 3, vol. 23:25-35, 1929 ⟨I-03338⟩

Jukes, A.L. (1821-1905)
Deane, R.B.: Augustus L. Jukes: A Pioneer Surgeon. CACHB 2(4):1-4, 1938 ⟨I-01334⟩

K

Keenan, C.B. (1867-1953)
Lewis, D.S.: Campbell B. Keenan, D.S.O., M.D., C.M., F.R.C.S. [C], 1867 to 1953. Canadian Journal of Surgery 15:287-294, 1972 ⟨I-04225⟩

Keith, H.W. (1873-1933)
Kidston, J.: Harry Wishart Keith, M.D. 1873-1933. Okanagan Historical Society Annual Report 30L145-147, 1966 ⟨I-05069⟩

Kennedy, E. (1850-1930)
Walker, S.L.: Evan Kennedy, MD. CMAJ 22:743, 1930 ⟨I-03015⟩

Kennedy, G.A. (1858-1913)
Ritchie, J.B.: Early Surgeons of the North West Mounted Police. III Doctor George Alexander Kennedy, Part 2. CACHB 22:201-218, 1957 ⟨I-01322⟩
Ritchie, J.B.: Early Surgeons of the North West Mounted Police. III Doctor George Alexander Kennedy. CACHB 22:171-181, 1957 ⟨I-01323⟩
Ritchie, J.B.: George Alexander Kennedy, M.D. 1858-1913. CMAJ 1:279-286, 1958 ⟨I-01575⟩

Kenney, W.W. (-1931)
Scammell, H.L.: Remember "Pa" Kenney?. Nova Scotia Medical Bulletin 32:260-265, 1953 ⟨I-02570⟩

Kerr, J. (1849-1911)
Mitchell, R.: Manitoba Surgical Pioneers James Kerr (1849-1911) and H.H. Chown (1859-1944). Canadian Journal of Surgery 3:281-285, 1960 ⟨I-03555⟩
Mitchell, R., Thorlakson, T.K.: James Kerr, 1849-1911 and Harry Hyland Kerr, 1881-1963: Pioneer Canadian-American Surgeons. Canadian Journal of Surgery 9:213-220, 1966 ⟨I-02569⟩

Kerr, R. (1755-1824)
Colgate, W.: Dr. Robert Kerr: An Early Practitioner of Upper Canada. CMAJ 64:542-546, 1951 ⟨I-02568⟩

Kerr, R.B. (1908-)
Gray, C.: Robert Bews Kerr. CMAJ 130:194, 1984 ⟨I-05380⟩

Kidd, J.F. (1863-1933)
Small, H.B.: John Franklin Kidd, CMG, MD, LLD. CMAJ 29:452-53, 1933 ⟨I-03073⟩

Kilborn, L.G. (1895-1967)
Walmsley, L.C.: Dr. Leslie Gifford Kilborn: an appreciation. CMAJ 97:490-491, 1967 ⟨I-02566⟩

King, R. (1810-1876)
Cooke, A.: Richard King. DCB 10:406-408, 1972 ⟨I-01321⟩
Swinton, W.E.: Physicians as Explorers: Richard King: Argumentative Cassandra in the Search for Franklin. CMAJ 117:1330-7, 1977 ⟨I-02575⟩

Kirkland, A.S. (1890-1963)
Ross, A.: Dr. A. Stanley Kirkland: an appreciation. CMAJ 89:733-734, 1963 ⟨I-01746⟩

Kittson, J.G. (1846-1884)
Ritchie, J.B.: Early Surgeons of the North West Mounted Police, II: Doctor John George Kittson: First Surgeon. CACHB 22:130-143, 1957 ⟨I-02589⟩

Klotz, O. (1878-1936)
Holman, W.L.: Oskar Klotz, 1878-1936. Archives of Pathology 22:840-845, 1936 ⟨I-02588⟩
Holman, W.L.: Prof. Oskar Klotz. CMAJ 36:97-98, 1937 ⟨I-01734⟩
Oertel, H.: Prof. Oskar Klotz. CMAJ 36:98-99, 1937 ⟨I-02863⟩

Knox, W.J. (1878-1967)

Green, D.: Dr. William John Knox, 1878-1967: Beloved Doctor of the Okanagan. Okanagan Historical Society Annual Report 33:8-18, 1969 ⟨I-05068⟩

L

Labillois, C.-M. (1793-1868)

Goyer, G.: Charles-Marie Labillois. DCB 9:438-439, 1976 ⟨I-01309⟩

Labrie, J. (1784-1831)

Desjardins, E.: Le Destin Tragique de Manuscript Historique de Labrie. L'UMC 98:1119-1125, 1969 ⟨I-01772⟩

Gosselin, A.: Un Historien Canadien Oublie: le Dr. Jacques Labrie (1784-1831). PTRSC Volume 11, section I, 33-64, 1893 ⟨I-02255⟩

Lachapelle, E.P. (1845-1918)

Watson, I.A.: Emmanuel P. Lachapelle. In: Physicians and Surgeons of America. Concord, Republican Press Association, 1896. p 19 ⟨I-02519⟩

Lachapelle, E.-P. (1880-1934)

LeSage, A.: Le Decanat a la Faculte de Medecine de L'Universite de Montreal: Trois Doyens (1880-1934) -- Rottot, Lachapelle, Harwood. L'UMC 68:166-178, 1939 ⟨I-02264⟩

La Croix, H.-J. de (1703-1760)

Fortin-Morisset, C.: Hubert-Joseph de la Croix. DCB 3:334, 1974 ⟨I-01316⟩

Lafferty, J.D. (1850-1920)

Elliott, J.H., Revell, D.G.: Medical Pioneering in Alberta (James Delamere Lafferty). CACHB 6(1):11-12, 1941 ⟨I-01306⟩

Stanley, G.D.: James Delamere Lafferty. CACHB 5(4):12-16, 1941 ⟨I-01307⟩

Lafleur, H.A. (1863-1939)

Gordon, A.H.: Dr. Henri A. Lafleur. CMAJ 41:96, 1939 ⟨I-03393⟩

Peters, C.A.: Henri Amedee LaFleur. CMAJ 62:607-8, 1950 ⟨I-04936⟩

LaHaise, F.G.

Dumas, P.: Un Medecin-Psychiatre Qui Avait Ete Poete, Gullaume LaHaise et Son Double, Guy Delahaye. L'UMC 100:321-326, 1971 ⟨I-02230⟩

Laidlaw, W.C. (1874-1926)

Orr, H.: Dr. William Charles Laidlaw. CMAJ 16:1285, 1926 ⟨I-01610⟩

Lajus, J. (1673-1742)

Moogk, P.N.: Jordain Lajus. DCB 3:344-345, 1974 ⟨I-01010⟩

Lamberd, G. (-1982)

White, J.: Gordon Lamberd. University of Manitoba Medical Journal 52:66, 1982 ⟨I-04966⟩

Landry, J-E (1815-1884)

Sylvain, P.: Jean-Etienne Landry. DCB 11:483-86, 1982 ⟨I-04848⟩

Lang, H. (1845-1918)

Stanley, G.D.: Dr. Hugh Lang of Granton: A Family Physician on the Old Ontario Strand. CACHB 16:82-87, 1951 ⟨I-01314⟩

Langis, H.E. (1857-1937)

Andrews, M.W.: Medical Attendance in Vancouver, 1886-1920. B.C. Studies 40:32-56, 1978-1979 ⟨I-03552⟩

Langstaff, L. (1883-1978)

Langstaff, J.R.: Dr. Lillian: A Memoir. Ontario, The Langstaff Medical Heritage Committee, 1979, 44 p. ⟨I-04432⟩

La Rue, F-A-H (1833-1881)

Lortie, L.: Francois-Alexandre-Hubert La Rue. DCB 11:495-97, 1982 ⟨I-04849⟩

Wahl, P., Greenland, C.: Du Suicide: F.A.H. LaRue, M.D. (1833-1881). Canadian Psychiatric Association Journal 15:95-97, 1970 ⟨I-04717⟩

Laterriere, M-P.deS. (1792-1872)

Desjardins, E.: La Profession de foi Politique du Docteur Marc-Pascal Laterriere. L'UMC 99:1294-3000, 1970 ⟨I-02243⟩

Gagnon, J.P.: Marc-Pascal de Sales Laterriere. DCB 10:431-432, 1972 ⟨I-02253⟩

La Terriere, P. de S. (1743-1815)

Belanger, L.F.: Un Ancetre de la Medecine Trifluvienne: Pierre de Sales La Terriere (1743-1815). L'UMC 69:860-863, 1940 ⟨I-02240⟩

Belanger, L.F.: A Canadian physician in the 18th century. University of Ottawa Medical Journal 14(4):13-15, 1972 ⟨I-02700⟩

Desjardins, E: Le Docteur Pierre La Terriere et ses Traverses. L'UMC 98:797-801, 1969 ⟨I-02239⟩

Dufour, P., Hamelin, J.: Pierre de Sales Laterriere. DCB 5:735-738, 1983 ⟨I-05298⟩

Fitz, R.: The Surprising Career of Peter la Terriere, Bachelor in Medicine. Annals of Medical History 3rd series, 3:265-282, 395-417, 1941 ⟨I-01974⟩

Guerra, F.: Les Medecins Patriotes. In International Congress for the History of Medicine, 25th, Quebec, 1976. Proceedings, Volume II, 1976. p. 746-754 ⟨I-01023⟩

Laterriere, P. de S.: Memoires de Pierre de Sales Laterriere et de ses Traverses. Quebec, L'Imprimerie de L'Evenement, 1873. pp 271 ⟨I-02257⟩

Shipton, C.K.: Peter de Sales Laterriere. Sibley's Harvard Graduates 16(1764-67):492-9, 1972 ⟨I-05378⟩

Latreille, E. (1879-1928)

Rheaume, P.Z.: Dr. Eugene Latreille. CMAJ 19:738, 1928 ⟨I-03492⟩

Rheaume, P.Z.: Latreille, 1879-1928. L'UMC 57:699-702, 1928 ⟨I-01769⟩

Simard, L.C.: Le Docteur Eugene Latreille. L'UMC 58:55-56, 1929 ⟨I-01768⟩

Lawford, C.H. (-1952)

Shortliffe, E.C.: Dr. Charles H. Lawford. Alberta Medical Bulletin 18:50-51, 1953 ⟨I-03225⟩

Leathes, J.B. (1864-1956)
  Graham, D.: John Beresford Leathes, 1864-1956. PTRSC Series 3, 52:89-90, 1958 ⟨I-04777⟩

Le Beau, F. (1720-1777)
  Nadeau, G.: Francois le Beau, Medecin du Roi. L'UMC 82:312-316, 1953 ⟨I-02242⟩

Leech, B.C. (1898-1960)
  G., H.B.: Beverly Charles Leech. Canadian Anaesthetist's Society Journal 7:351-352, 1960 ⟨I-03238⟩

Leeder, F.B. (1865-1945)
  Murphy, H.H.: Dr. Forrest B. Leeder. CMAJ 52:644, 1945 ⟨I-04371⟩

Leger de la Grange,J (1663-1736?)
  Lee, D.: Jean Legere de la Grange. DCB 2:387-388, 1969 ⟨I-01021⟩

Lehmann, J.E. (1868-1934)
  Hunter, C.: Dr. Julius Edward Lehmann. CMAJ 31:227, 1934 ⟨I-03528⟩
  Mathers, A.T.: Dr. Julius Edward Lehmann. CMAJ 31:227, 1934 ⟨I-03527⟩

LeMesurier, A.B. (1889-1982)
  Keith, W.S.: Dr. Arthur B. LeMesurier. CMAJ 126:1353, 1982 ⟨I-04835⟩

Lemieux, R. (1900-)
  Robillard, D.: Profil: Renaud Lemieux. CMAJ 125:383, 1981 ⟨I-04556⟩

Lesslie, R.B. (-1893)
  Elliott, J.H.: Rolph Bidwell Lesslie, MA, MD. CMAJ 49:527-529, 1943 ⟨I-03037⟩

Lewis, D.S. (1886-1976)
  R., H.R.: David Sclater Lewis: student and maker of history. CMAJ 116:314, 1977 ⟨I-03883⟩

Lindsay, J.G.K. (1902-1946)
  Anderson, J.F.C.: Dr. James George Keber Lindsay. CMAJ 55:416, 1946 ⟨I-03084⟩

Lindsay, L.M. (1886-1966)
  Ross, S.G.: Dr. Lionel Mitcheson Lindsay: an appreciation. CMAJ 95:738-739, 1966 ⟨I-03085⟩

Lindsay, N.J. (1845-1925)
  Learmonth, G.E.: Dr. Neville James Lindsay. CMAJ 16:204, 1926 ⟨I-01601⟩
  Stanley, G.D.: Dr. Neville James Lindsay. CACHB 4(2):6-9, 1939 ⟨I-01308⟩

Litchfield, J.P. (1808-1868)
  Gibson, T.: The Astonishing Career of John Palmer Litchfield. CMAJ 70:326-330, 1954 ⟨I-03229⟩
  Rasporich, A.W., Clarke, I.H.: John Palmer Litchfield. DCB 9:470-471, 1976 ⟨I-01313⟩

Livingston, N.
  MacDermot, H.E.: Nora Livingston and Maude Abbott. CACHB 22:228-235, 1958 ⟨I-01305⟩

Livingstone, L.D. (1889-1964)
  Copland, D.: Livingstone of the Arctic. Ottawa, D. Copland, 1967. 183 p ⟨I-03940⟩

Locke, M.W. (1880-1943)
  Beach, R.: The Hands of Dr. Locke. New York, Farrar and Rinehart, 1932. 56 p. ⟨I-01304⟩
  Carter, J.S.: Doctor M.W. Locke and the Williamsburg Scene. Toronto, Life Portrayal Series, 1933. 138 p. ⟨I-01303⟩
  Kiely, E.B.: Dr. M.W. Locke Heals with his Hands. 1937. n.p., no pagination (first published as a series of articles in the Montreal Daily Herald). ⟨I-01519⟩
  MacDonald, J.: Dr. Locke, Healer of Men. Toronto, Maclean Publishing Co., 1933. 83 p. ⟨I-01520⟩

Lockhart, F.A.L. (1864-1925)
  Little, H.M.: Dr. Frederick Albert Lawton Lockhart. CMAJ 15:220, 1925 ⟨I-03083⟩

Lockman, L. (1697-1769)
  Blakeley, P.R.: Leonard Lockman. DCB 3:405, 1974 ⟨I-01317⟩

Loedel, H.N.C.
  Richard, L.: La Famille Loedel. Le Bulletin des Recherches Historiques 56:78-79, 1950 ⟨I-01315⟩

Logie, W.L. (1811-1879)
  Tunis, B., Bensley, E.H.: A La Recherche de William Leslie Logie, Premier Diplome de L'Universite McGill. L'UMC 100:536-538, 1971 ⟨I-02227⟩
  Tunis, B.R.: Bensley, E.H.: William Leslie Logie: McGill University's first graduate and Canada's first medical graduate. CMAJ 105:1259-1263, 1971 ⟨I-01312⟩
  Tunis, B.R.: Tribute to William Leslie Logie. CMAJ 122:273, 1980 ⟨I-01311⟩

Longmore, G. (1758-1811)
  Tunis, B.R.: George Longmore. DCB 5:501-503, 1983 ⟨I-05311⟩

Longmore, H.B. (1872-1952)
  Anderson, J.R.: Dr. H.B. Longmore. CMAJ 67:71, 1952 ⟨I-04539⟩

Longtin, L. (1907-1979)
  Denis, R.: Leon Longtin, M.D., F.R.C.P.(C), 1907-1979. Canadian Anaesthetists Society Journal 27:181-182, 1980 ⟨I-01053⟩

Low, D. (-1941)
  Moore, S.E.: David Low, MD. CMAJ 44:534, 1941 ⟨I-03351⟩

Lowrie, H.A. (1888-)
  Repka, W.: Howard Lowrie M.D.: Physician Humanitarian. Toronto, Progress Books, 1977 104p. ⟨I-04240⟩

Lowry, W.H. (1880-1942)
  MacDonald, A.E.: William Herbert Lowry, M.D., C.M., M.R.C.S., F.R.C.S. (C),. CMAJ 47:384, 1942 ⟨I-04277⟩

Lyon, E.K.
  Carpenter, P.: E. Kirk Lyon. CMAJ 123:1265, 1980 ⟨I-02884⟩

Lyons, J.N. (-1930)
  Walker, S.L.: James Norbert Lyons, MD, CM. CMAJ 22:743, 1930 ⟨I-03016⟩

M

Mabane, A. (1734-1792)

Neatby, H.: The political career of Adam Mabane. CHR 16:137-150, 1935 ⟨I-01454⟩

Warren, F.C., Fabre-Surveyer, E.: From Surgeon's Mate to Chief Justice - Adam Mabane (1734-1792). PTRSC 3rd series, 24(II): 189-210, 1930 ⟨I-03038⟩

Macallum, A.B. (1858-1934)

Richardson, R.A.: Archibald Byron Macallum. In: Dictionary of Scientific Biography 8:583-4, 1973 ⟨I-05293⟩

Macallum, A.B. (1885-1976)

Barr, M.L.: Archibald Bruce Macallum, 1885-1976. PTRSC series IV, 15:99-100, 1977 ⟨I-03036⟩

MacAlpine, J. (1850-1925)

Hall, G.E.: Dr. John MacAlpine -- Physician and Surgeon. Canada Lancet and Practitioner 77:47-52, 1931 ⟨I-02839⟩

MacArthur, J.A. (1848-1934)

Mitchell, R.: Dr. John Alexander MacArthur. CMAJ 31:453, 1934 ⟨I-02846⟩

MacCallum, D.C. (1825-1904)

Watson, I.A.: Duncan Campbell MacCallum. In: Physicians and Surgeons of America. Concord, Republican Press Association, 1896. p 34 ⟨I-02521⟩

MacCallum, G.A. (1843-1936)

Malloch, A.: Dr. George Alexander MacCallum: an appreciation. CMAJ 37:200-202, 1937 ⟨I-03050⟩

MacCallum, J.B. (1876-1906)

Bardeen, C.R.: John Bruce MacCallum (1876-1906). In Kelly HW, Burrage WL: Dictionary of American Medical Biography. New York and London, D. Appleton and Co., 1928. pp. 769-770 ⟨I-01434⟩

Malloch, A.: Short Years: The Life and Letters of John Bruce MacCallum, M.D., 1876-1906. Chicago, Normandie House, 1938. 343 p. ⟨I-01435⟩

[Osler, W.]: John Bruce MacCallum, B.A., M.D. British Medical Journal 1:955-956, 1906 ⟨I-05180⟩

Roland, C.G.: Maude Abbott and J.B. MacCallum: Canadian Cardiac Pioneers. Chest 57:371-77, 1970 ⟨I-03564⟩

MacCallum, J.M. (1860-1943)

Matthews, R.M.: James Metcalfe MacCallum, BA, MD, CM (1860-1943). CMAJ 114:621-624, 1976 ⟨I-01426⟩

MacDermot, H.E. (1888-1983)

Bensley, E.H.: Dr. Hugh Ernest MacDermot. CMAJ 128:860-861, 1983 ⟨I-05071⟩

MacDermot, J.H. (1883-1969)

K[elly], A.D.: John H. MacDermot, M.D. CMAJ 100:922, 1969 ⟨I-05039⟩

Macdonald, A. (1784-1859)

Campbell, D.A.: Alexander Macdonald (1784-1859). In Kelly HW, Burrage WL: Dictionary of American Medical Biography. New York and London, D. Appleton and Co., 1928. pp. 780-781. ⟨I-01452⟩

MacDonald, R.H. (1884-1949)

Mullally, E.J.: Dr. Ronald Hugh MacDonald. CMAJ 61:641-2, 1949 ⟨I-04492⟩

MacDonnell, R.L. (1818-1878)

Chalifoux, J.P.: Robert Lea MacDonnell. DCB 10:470-471, 1972 ⟨I-01437⟩

MacDonnell, R.L. (1855-1890)

[Osler, W.]: Richard Lea MacDonnell. New York Medical Journal 54:162, 1891 ⟨I-05181⟩

MacDougall, J.G. (1869-1950)

Morton, C.S.: John George MacDougall, MD, CM(McGill), FACS, FRCS(Can), 1897-1947. Nova Scotia Medical Bulletin 26:105-110, 1947 ⟨I-03233⟩

Morton, C.S.: John George MacDougall, MD, CM (McGill), FACS, FRCS(C). Nova Scotia Medical Bulletin 29:185-194, 1950 ⟨I-03221⟩

Scammell, H.L.: John George MacDougall, M.D.C.M., F.A.C.S., F.R.C.S. [C.]. CMAJ 63:314-5, 1950 ⟨I-04512⟩

MacFarlane, J.A. (-1966)

Hamilton, J.: Dr. Joseph Arthur MacFarlane; an appreciation. CMAJ 94:1069-1070, 1966 ⟨I-01732⟩

Kelly, A.D.: Dr. Joseph Arthur MacFarlane: an appreciation. CMAJ 94:1070, 1966 ⟨I-01757⟩

MacDonald, R.I.: Dr. Joseph Arthur MacFarlane, an appreciation. CMAJ 94:1067-1069, 1966 ⟨I-01054⟩

Porter, D.: Dr. Joseph Arthur MacFarlane, an appreciation. CMAJ 94:1070, 1966 ⟨I-01406⟩

Macgregor, J.A. (1857-1939)

Watson, E.M.: John Alexander Macgregor, MD. CMAJ 41:518, 1939 ⟨I-03397⟩

Mack, T. (1820-1881)

Godfrey, C.M.: Theophilus Mack. DCB 11:558-559, 1982 ⟨I-04850⟩

Runnalls, J.L.: A Century with the St.Catharines General Hospital. St. Catharines, St. Catharines General Hospital, 1974. 150 p. ⟨I-01526⟩

Mackay, F.H. (1884-1947)

Gordon, A.H.: Doctor F.H. Mackay: an appreciation. CMAJ 58:393-394, 1948 ⟨I-03220⟩

M[acDermot], H.E.: Dr. Fred Holland Mackay. CMAJ 57:408-9, 1947 ⟨I-04402⟩

MacKay, M.A. (1880-1934)

Chase, L.A.: Dr. Murdoch Angus MacKay. CMAJ 31:107-108, 1934 ⟨I-03526⟩

MacKay, W.M. (1836-1917)

Jamieson, H.C.: The Pioneer Doctor of Alberta: William Morrison MacKay. CMAJ 37:388-393, 1937 ⟨I-02843⟩

Stanley, G.D.: Doctor William Morrison MacKay. CACHB 4(3):13-15, 1939 ⟨I-01447⟩

MacKeen, R.A.H. (-1957)

T., J.: Dr. R.A.H. MacKeen, an appreciation. CMAJ 77:522, 1957 ⟨I-04754⟩

MacKellar, M. (1861-1941)

Oliver, B.C.: Dr. Margaret MacKellar: The Story of Her Early Years. Canada, Women's Missionary Society of the Presbyterian Church in Canada, 1920. 42 p. ⟨I-01425⟩

Mackenzie, A.J. (1873-1939)
Elliott, J.H.: Colonel Alexander John Mackenzie, BA, LLB, MB, FACP, VD. CMAJ 40:409, 1939 ⟨I-02842⟩

Mackenzie, I. (1910-1966)
Stewart, C.B.: Ian MacKenzie, MBE, MB, ChB, FRCS(Edin), FRCS(C), FACS. CMAJ 95:1218-1219, 1966 ⟨I-03409⟩

Mackenzie, J.J. (1865-1922)
Mackenzie, K.C.: #4 Canadian Hospital: The Letters of Professor J.J. Mackenzie from the Salonika Front. Toronto, Macmillan Co. of Canada Ltd., 1933. pp 247 ⟨I-02000⟩

MacKenzie, K.A.
MacKenzie, K.A.: In Retrospect. Dalhousie Medical Journal II:18-20, 1958 ⟨I-01410⟩

MacKenzie, W.C. (1909-1978)
Baker, J.: Tributes from the United States [W.C. MacKenzie]. Canadian Journal of Surgery 22,307-308, 1979 ⟨I-04287⟩
Graham, J.H.: A proud Scottish Canadian. CMAJ 120:988, 1979 ⟨I-01415⟩
Grisdale, L.: Walter MacKenzie: a gift for friendship. CMAJ 120:985, 988, 1979 ⟨I-01414⟩
Kay, D.: A Tribute from Scotland [W.C. MacKenzie]. Canadian Journal of Surgery 22:309, 1979 ⟨I-04286⟩
Lougheed, P.: Inspiration and a source of pride. CMAJ 120:988, 1979 ⟨I-01413⟩
Louw, J.: A Tribute from South Africa [W.C. MacKenzie]. Canadian Journal of Surgery 22:310, 1979 ⟨I-04285⟩
Macbeth, R.A.: Walter C. MacKenzie, OC, BSc, MD, CM. MS, FACS, FRCS C, Hon FRCS, Hon FRCS (Edin), Hon FRCS (Ire), Hon FRCS (Glas), LLD (McGill), LLD (Dalhousie), LLD (Manitoba), 1909-1978. Canadian Journal of Surgery 22:303-307, 1979 ⟨I-04290⟩
Ong, E.G.: A Tribute from Hong Kong [W.C. MacKenzie]. Canadian Journal of Surgery 22:311-312, 1979 ⟨I-04284⟩
Porritt, A.: A Tribute from England [W.C. MacKenzie]. Canadian Journal of Surgery 22:312-313, 1979 ⟨I-04283⟩
Rudowski, W.: A tribute from Poland [W.C. MacKenzie]. Canadian Journal of Surgery 22:313-314, 1979 ⟨I-04282⟩

Mackid, H.G. (1858-1916)
Gunn, J.N.: Harry Goodsir Mackid, M.D., LRCP and S.(Edin), FACS. CMAJ 22:700-701, 1930 ⟨I-02180⟩

MacKieson, J. (1795-1885)
Lea, R.G.: Dr. John MacKieson (1795-1885): Strangulated Hernia in the Early 19th Century. Canadian Journal of Surgery 8:1-9, 1965 ⟨I-04232⟩
Roger, I.L.: John Mackieson. DCB 11:565-66, 1982 ⟨I-04851⟩

MacKinnon, A. (1846-1929) McCrae, T.: Dr. Angus MacKinnon. CMAJ 21:110, 1929 ⟨I-02848⟩

MacKinnon, W.F. (-1952)
Murphy, G.H.: Dr. William F. MacKinnon. CMAJ 67:379, 1952 ⟨I-04535⟩

Macklin, C.C. (1883-1959)
Thompson, I.M.: Charles Clifford Macklin. PTRSC 54:133-135, 1960, 3d series ⟨I-01407⟩

MacLaren, M. (1861-1942)
Baxter, J.B.M.: Colonel Murray MacLaren. CMAJ 48:180-181, 1943 ⟨I-01751⟩

MacLean, H. (1887-1958)
MacLean, H.: A Pioneer Prairie Doctor. Saskatchewan History 15:58-66, 1962 ⟨I-01297⟩

Maclean, N.J. (1870-1946)
Chase, L.A.: Dr. Neil John MacLean. CMAJ 56:115, 1947 ⟨I-03406⟩
Montgomery, E.W.: Dr. Neil John Maclean. CMAJ 56:115, 1947 ⟨I-03408⟩

MacLeod, E.J. (1909-)
Hellstedt, L.McG. (edit): Enid MacLeod. In: Women Physicians of the World: Autobiographies of Medical Pioneers New York, McGraw-Hill Book Co., 1978. pp 383-85 ⟨I-03923⟩

MacLeod, J.W.
B., B.: John Wendell MacLeod. CMAJ 123:557, 1980 ⟨I-01584⟩

MacMillan, C.L.
MacMillan, C.L.: Memoirs of a Cape Breton Doctor. Toronto, Montreal, New York, McGraw-Hill Ryerson Limited, 1975. 177 p. ⟨I-01411⟩

MacMillan, H.A. (1920-1964)
K., J.D.: Dr. Hugh Alexander MacMillan. CMAJ 92:641-642, 1965 ⟨I-02838⟩

MacMillan, W.J.P. (1881-1958)
M., J.A.: Dr. W.J.P. MacMillan. CMAJ 78:71, 1958 ⟨I-02836⟩

MacMurchy, H. (1862-1953)
Buckley, S.: Efforts to Reduce Infant Maternity Mortality in Canada Between the Two World Wars. Atlantis 2(2):76-84, 1977 ⟨I-01661⟩
McConnachie, K.: Methodology in the Study of Women in History: A Case Study of Helen MacMurchy, M.D. Ontario History 75:61-70, 1983 ⟨I-05055⟩
Roberts, W.: Six New Women: A Guide to the Mental Map of Women Reformers in Toronto. Atlantis 3:45-164, 1977-8 ⟨I-01977⟩

Macnab, D.S. (1879-1951)
Scarlett, E.P.: "The Macnab". CACHB 16:21-24, 1951 ⟨I-01417⟩
Stanley, G.D.: Daniel Stewart Macnab, October 28, 1879 - February 2, 1951. CACHB 16;10-20, 1951 ⟨I-01416⟩

Macnaughton, B.F. (-1941)
Roman, C.R.: Dr. Benjamin Franklin Macnaughton. CMAJ 45:468-469, 1941 ⟨I-03523⟩

MacNeill, A. (1853-1926)

MacMillan, W.J.: Alexander MacNeill , MD, CM, FACS. CMAJ 16:707, 1926 ⟨I-01598⟩

Macphail, A. (1864-1938)

Edgar, P.: Sir Andrew Macphail 1864-1938. PTRSC 33:147-149, 1939 ⟨I-03573⟩

Edgar, P.: Sir Andrew Macphail. Queen's Quarterly 54:8-22, 1947 ⟨I-02128⟩

Leacock, S.: Andrew Macphail. Queen's Quarterly 45:445-463, 1938 ⟨I-02129⟩

Macphail, A.: The Master's Wife. Toronto, McClelland and Stewart Limited, 1977. 173 p. ⟨I-01424⟩

Martin, C.F.: Sir Andrew Macphail. CMAJ 39:508-509, 1938 ⟨I-03373⟩

Shortt, S.E.D.: Andrew Macphail: The Ideal in Nature. In: The Search for an Ideal: Six Canadian Intellectuals and Their Convictions in An Age of Transition 1890-1930. Toronto/Buffalo, Univ. of Toronto Press, 1976. pp. 13-38 ⟨I-01419⟩

Shortt, S.E.D.: Sir Andrew Macphail: Physician, Philosopher, Founding Editor of CMAJ. CMAJ 118.323-325, 1978 ⟨I-01516⟩

Stuart, H.A.: Sir Andrew Macphail (1864-1938). CACHB 9:61-67, 1945 ⟨I-01421⟩

Thompson, I.M.: Sir Andrew MacPhail, 1864-1938. Winnipeg Clinic Quarterly 20(1and2):20-32, 1967 ⟨I-01420⟩

Thompson, I.M.: Sir Andrew Macphail, 1864-1938. CMAJ 98:40-44, 1968 ⟨I-02833⟩

Macpherson, C. (1879-1966)

Marrie, T.: In Retrospect (Cluny Macpherson). Dalhousie Medical Journal 20:89 + 91, 1967 ⟨I-02301⟩

McGrath, J.: Dr. Cluny Macpherson. CMAJ 96:172-174, 1967 ⟨I-03421⟩

MacTaggart, D.D. (1863-1929)

Oertel, H.: Dr. D. D. MacTaggart. CMAJ 20:214-215, 1929 ⟨I-01754⟩

Madry, J. (ca.1625-1669)

Nadeau, G.: Jean Madry. DCB 1:478-479, 1966 ⟨I-01455⟩

Mahaffy, A.F. (1891-1962)

McK, N.: Alexander Francis Mahaffy, CMG, BA, MB, DPH; an appreciation. CMAJ 88:906-907, 1963 ⟨I-03424⟩

Maheut, L. (1650-1683)

Drolet, A.: Louis Maheut. DCB 1:479-480, 1966 ⟨I-01456⟩

Mainprize, W.G. (1911-1974)

Chatenay, H.P.: Echoes of Silence. The Chronicles of William Graham Mainprize, M.D., 1911-1974. Edmonton, H.P. Chatenay, 1978. ⟨I-05061⟩

Malcolmson, G. (1868-1936)

Stanley, G.D.: Dr. George Malcolmson. CACHB 14:78-85, 1950 ⟨I-01430⟩

Malcolmson, H. (1912-1964)

Johnson, G.: Dr. Hugh Malcolmson. CMAJ 91:92, 1964 ⟨I-03425⟩

Malhiot, C-C. (1808-1874)

Crete-Begin, L.: Charles-Christophe Malhiot. DCB 10:490-491, 1972 ⟨I-01438⟩

Malloch, T.A. (1887-1953)

F(ulton), J.F.: T. Archibald Malloch. JHMAS 8:449, 1953 ⟨I-01296⟩

M[acDermot], H.E.: Dr. Archibald Malloch. CMAJ 69:543-4, 1953 ⟨I-04523⟩

Malloch, W.J.O. (1872-1919)

Power, D'Arcy: William John Ogilvie Malloch. In: Plarr's Lives of the Fellows of the Royal College of Surgeons of England. Bristol and London, The Royal College of Surgeons, 1930. Vol. 2:18-19 ⟨I-02757⟩

Mance, J. (1606-1673)

Atherton, W.H.: The Saintly Life of Jeanne Mance: first Lay Nurse in North America. Hospital Progress 26:182-190, 192-201, 234-243, 1945 ⟨I-03427⟩

D'Allaire, M.: Jeanne-Mance a Montreal en 1642: une femme d'action qui force les evenements. Forces 23:38-46, 1973 ⟨I-04658⟩

Daveluy, M.C.: Jeanne Mance. DCB 1:483-487, 1966 ⟨I-01457⟩

Foran, J.K.: Jeanne Mance or "The Angel of the Colony" Foundress of the Hotel Dieu Hospital, Montreal, Pioneer Nurse of North America 1642-1673. Montreal, The Herald Press, Ltd., 1931, 192 p. ⟨I-04427⟩

MacDermot, H.E.: Jeanne Mance. CMAJ 57:67-73, 1947 ⟨I-03426⟩

Manchester, G.H. (1872-)

Donaldson, B.: Dr. Manchester of New Westminster. CACHB 20:81-88, 1956 ⟨I-03428⟩

Manion, R.J. (1881-)

Manion, R.J.: A Surgeon in Arms. New York, D. Appleton and Co., 1918. 310 p. ⟨I-03417⟩

Manion, R.J.: Life is an Adventure. Toronto, The Ryerson Press, 1936, 360 p. ⟨I-04780⟩

Mann, J.B. (1885-1925)

Cameron, J.S.: Dr. John Burritt Mann. CMAJ 16:333, 1926 ⟨I-01599⟩

Marien, A. (1886-1936)

Desjardins, E.: L'Ecole D'Amedee Marien Et Ses Eleves Rheaume Et Pare. Canadian Journal of Surgery 9:325-331, 1966 ⟨I-04659⟩

Marion, D. (1897-1971)

Amyot, R.: Donation Marion, 1897-1971. L'UMC 100:1197-1198, 1971 ⟨I-01298⟩

Marlow, F.W. (1877-1936)

Anderson, H.B.: Frederick William Marlow, MD, CM. CMAJ 35:463, 1936 ⟨I-02869⟩

Cosbie, W.G.: Frederick Marlow (1877-1936) and the Development of the Modern Treatment of Carcinoma of the Cervix. Canadian Journal of Surgery 5:357-365, 1962 ⟨I-03429⟩

Marot, B. (fl.1610-1650)

MacBeath, G.: Bernard Marot. DCB 1:490, 1966 ⟨I-01458⟩

Marsden, W. (1807-1885)

Kelly, A.D.: Our Forgotten Man. CMAJ 96:1485-86, 1967 ⟨I-03916⟩

LeBlond, S.: William Marsden (1807-1885): Essai Biographique. Laval Medical 41:639-658, 1970 ⟨I-02263⟩

Martin, C.F. (1868-1953)

Meakins, J.C.: Charles Ferdinand Martin. CMAJ, 70:95-6, 1954 ⟨I-04562⟩

Routley, T.C.: Dr. Charles Martin. CMAJ, 70:96-7, 1954 ⟨I-04563⟩

Martinet Fonblanche (1645-1701)

Boissonnault, C.M.: Jean Martinet de Fonblanche. DCB 2:465-566, 1969 ⟨I-01022⟩

Masson, L-H. (1811-1880)

Desilets, A.: Luc-Hyacinthe Masson. DCB 10:499-500, 1972 ⟨I-01439⟩

Masson, P. (1880-1959)

Simard, L.C.: Le Professeur Pierre Masson a L'Academie de Medecine de Paris. L'UMC 64:1401-1404, 1935 ⟨I-02228⟩

Simard, L.C.: Le Professeur Pierre Masson, Medecin Honoraire a L'Hospital Notre-Dame (de Montreal). L'UMC 83:194-195, 1954 ⟨I-02229⟩

Masson, R. (1875-1928)

Lapierre, G.: Dr. Raoul Masson. CMAJ 19:739, 1928 ⟨I-03493⟩

Letondal, P.: Raoul Masson (1875-1928): Pionnier de la pediatrie au Canada francais. L'UMC 108:1-4, 1979 ⟨I-01422⟩

Mathers, A.T. (1888-1960)

Adamson, J.D.: Dr. A.T. Mathers -- The Retiring Dean. University of Manitoba Medical Journal 21:4-7, 1950 ⟨I-01583⟩

Bell, L.G.: Dr. Alvin Mathers: an appreciation. CMAJ 82:336, 339, 1960 ⟨I-03430⟩

Mathers, R.E. (1875-1957)

MacKenzie, L., Johnston, S.R.: Dr. Robert Evatt Mathers. CMAJ 76:592, 1957 ⟨I-04732⟩

Matheson, E. (1866-1958)

Buck, R.M.: The Doctor Rode Side-Saddle. McClelland and Steward Ltd., 1974, 175 p. ⟨I-04426⟩

Matheson, E.B. (1866-1958)

Mitchell, R.: Pioneer! Dr. Elizabeth Beckett Matheson, 1866-1958. Manitoba Medical Review 40:617 + 619, 1960 ⟨I-05058⟩

McCallum, H.A. (1860-1921)

Spence, E.: Hugh A. McCallum, M.D., FRCP, LL.D. CMAJ 15:1173, 1925 ⟨I-02298⟩

McClure, R. (1900-)

Scott, M.: McClure: The China Years of Dr. Bob McClure. Toronto, Canec Publishing and Supply House, 1977. 409 p. ⟨I-01278⟩

Scott, M.: McClure: Years of Challenge. Toronto, Canec Publishing and Supply House, 1979, 295 pp. ⟨I-04439⟩

McClure, W. (1856-1956)

H., L.W.: Salute to a Centenarian (William McClure). CMAJ 74:654-655, 1956 ⟨I-03175⟩

McConnell, J.B. (1851-1930)

Reddy, H.L.: J. Bradford McConnell, MD, DCL. CMAJ 22:893, 1930 ⟨I-03017⟩

McConney, F. (1894-)

Hellstedt, L.McG (edit): Florence McConney. New York, McGraw-Hill Book Co., 1978. pp 120-22 ⟨I-03944⟩

McCormick, N.A. (1901-1967)

Brien, W.P.: Dr. Norman Arnold McCormick. CMAJ 98:64, 1968 ⟨I-01762⟩

Lyon, E.K.: Dr. Norman Arnold McCormick. CMAJ 98:64-65, 1968 ⟨I-01761⟩

Maus, J.H.: Dr. Norman Arnold McCormick. CMAJ 98: 65-66, 1968 ⟨I-01760⟩

McCormick, R. (1800-1890)

Swinton, W.E.: Physicians as Explorers: Robert McCormick: Travels by Open Boat in Arctic Canada. CMAJ 117:1205-8, 1977 ⟨I-03171⟩

McCoy, E.C. (1911-)

Gray, C.: Edwin Clarence McCoy. CMAJ 129:1139, 1983 ⟨I-05319⟩

McCrae, J. (1872-1918)

Dubin, I.N.: A Letter From John McCrae to Maude Abbott: January 9, 1918. Perspectives in Biology and Medicine 24:667-669, 1981 ⟨I-04193⟩

Johnson, A.L.: John McCrae of Poppy Day: an overdue revelation. London, The British Legion, 1968 ⟨I-01289⟩

Kelly, H.A.: John McCrae (1872-1918). In Kelly HW, Burrage WL: Dictionary of American Medical Biography. New York and London, D. Appleton and Co., 1928. pp. 777-778 ⟨I-01291⟩

Leacock, S.: The Death of John McCrae. University Monthly [Toronto], April 1918, pp 245-248 ⟨I-03165⟩

McCrae, J.: In Flanders Fields. New York/London, G.P. Putnam's Sons, 1919. 141 p. ⟨I-01293⟩

Prescott, J.F.: The Extensive Medical Writings of Soldier-Poet John McCrae. CMAJ 122:110, 113-114, 1980 ⟨I-01290⟩

Rodin, A.E.: John McCrae, Poet-Pathologist. CMAJ 88:204-205, 1963 ⟨I-01292⟩

Swinton, W.E.: John McCrae, physician, soldier, poet. CMAJ 113:900-2, 1975 ⟨I-04442⟩

McCreary, J.F.

G., D.C., E., G.R.F.: John Ferguson McCreary: A Man for all Seasons. CMAJ 122:123-124, 1980 ⟨I-01279⟩

McDiarmid, A. (1854-)

Watson, I.A.: Andrew McDiarmid. In: Physicians and Surgeons of America. Concord, Republican Press Association, 1896. pp 585-6 ⟨I-02520⟩

McDonald, S.H. (1878-1936)

Kirkland, A.S.: Dr. Stephen Henry McDonald, an appreciation. CMAJ 34:358-359, 1936 ⟨I-03447⟩

McEachern, D. S. (1905-1951)

Bell, L.G.: Doctor Donald McEachern. University of Manitoba Medical Journal 23:64-65, 1951 ⟨I-03211⟩

Mitchell, R.: Dr. Donald S. McEachern. CMAJ 66:82-3, 1952 ⟨I-04522⟩

McEachern, J. S. (-1948)

Routley, T.C.: John Sinclair McEachern. CMAJ 58:290, 1948 ⟨I-03178⟩

McGeachy, J. A. (1905-1966)

Bailey, A.A.: Dr. Jessie A. McGeachy. CMAJ 94:923, 1966 ⟨I-03210⟩

Forgues, L.C.: Dr. Jessie A. McGeachy. CMAJ 94:923-924, 1966 ⟨I-03209⟩

McGregor, H. (1889-1943)

Howe, J.: Dr. and Mrs. H. McGregor. Okanagan Historical Society Annual Report 41:114-125, 1977 ⟨I-05065⟩

McGuinness, F. G. (1891-1968)

B[lack], E.F.E.: Dr. Frederick Gallagher McGuinness: an appreciation. CMAJ 99:145, 1968 ⟨I-03206⟩

McIlwraith, D. G. (1879-1948)

Deadman, W.J.: Douglas Gordon McIlwraith, M.B. CMAJ 58:414, 1948 ⟨I-04510⟩

McIntyre, L. C. (1891-1967)

Dollar, H.: Dr. Lillias Cringan McIntyre. CMAJ 97:760, 1967 ⟨I-02849⟩

McIvor, N. K. (1875-1931)

Mitchell, R.: Dr. Norman Kitson McIvor. CMAJ 26:259, 1932 ⟨I-03060⟩

McKechnie, R. E. (1861-1944)

M, J.H.: Robert E. McKechnie, C.B.E., M.D., C.M. (McGill), LL.D. (McGill and U.B.C.), F.A.C.S., F.R.C.S. (C). CMAJ 51:81-90, 1944 ⟨I-04246⟩

McKee, C. S. (-1961)

M., J.H.: Dr. Charles S. McKee: an appreciation. CMAJ 86:141, 1962 ⟨I-03204⟩

McKenzie, K. G. (1893-1964)

Alexander, E.: Kenneth George McKenzie, Canada's First Neurosurgeon. Journal of Neurosurgery 41:1-9, 1974 ⟨I-05371⟩

Botterell, E.H.: Dr. Kenneth George McKenzie. CMAJ 91:880-881, 1964 ⟨I-03200⟩

Turnbull, F.A.: Kenneth George McKenzie as the Young Chief: Retrospect. CMAJ 92:146, 1965 ⟨I-03179⟩

McKenzie, R. T. (1867-1938)

Boucot, K.R.: R. Tait McKenzie: A Biographical Sketch. Archives of Environmental Health 14:652-656, 1967 ⟨I-03219⟩

Brown, J.: R. Tait McKenzie, on the Centennial of His Birth. Archives Environmental Health 14:651, 1967 ⟨I-03217⟩

Buffam, F.: Robert Tait McKenzie. McGill Medical Journal 37:225-232, 1968 ⟨I-03199⟩

De Santana, H.: Danby: Images of Sport. Toronto, Amerley House Limited, 1978. 64 p. ⟨I-01280⟩

Gerber, E.W.: Robert Tait McKenzie 1867-1938. In: Innovators and Institutions in Physical Education Philadelphia, Lea and Febiger, 1971, 339-347 ⟨I-04518⟩

Gunter, J.U.: Burial of a Heart (R.T. McKenzie). Hospital Tribune, September 25, 1967, page 11 ⟨I-03216⟩

Harshman, J.P.: Robert Tait McKenzie: Another Canadian Centennial. Ontario Medical Review 34:443-448 + 452, 1967 ⟨I-03174⟩

Hussey, C.: Tait McKenzie, A Sculptor of Youth. Philadelphia, J.B. Lippincott Co., 1930. 107 p. ⟨I-01287⟩

Kozar, A.J.: R. Tait McKenzie, The Sculptor of Athletes. Knoxville, University of Tennessee Press, 1975. 118 p. ⟨I-01286⟩

Krumbhaar, E.B.: Memoir of R. Tait McKenzie, M.D. Transactions and Studies of the College of Physicians of Philadelphia 6:260-270, 1938 ⟨I-03218⟩

McGill, J.: The Joy of Effort: A Biography of R. Tait McKenzie. Sewdley, Ontario, Clay Publishing Company Limited, 1980. 241 p. ⟨I-03002⟩

McKenzie, R.T.: Compensations at 70. Transactions and Studies of the College of Physicians of Philadelphia 6:271-181, 1938 ⟨I-03488⟩

Thompson, I.M.: Robert Tait McKenzie. CMAJ 93:551-555, 1965 ⟨I-01281⟩

McKeown, P. W. (1866-1925)

Magner, W.: Dr. P.W. McKeown, CBE, BA, MD, CM, MRCS. CMAJ 15:1281, 1925 ⟨I-01594⟩

McKibben, P. S. (1886-1941)

Macklin, C.C.: Paul Stilwell McKibben 1886-1941. PTRSC 37:79-85, 1943 ⟨I-03571⟩

McKinnon, F. L. (1879-1929)

Mitchell, R.: Dr. Frank L. McKinnon. CMAJ 21:350, 1929 ⟨I-02847⟩

McLarren, P. D. (1896-1928)

Walker, S.L.: Philip Doane McLarren, MD, CM. CMAJ 19:124-125, 1928 ⟨I-03501⟩

McLay, J. F. (1885-1932)

Deadman, W.J.: James Franklin McLay. CMAJ 26:379, 1932 ⟨I-03062⟩

McLeod, S. H.

McLeod, S.H.: Nova Scotia Farm Boy to Alberta M.D. np., 1970. 110 p. ⟨I-03411⟩

McLoughlin, J. (1784-1857)

Greve, A.: Dr. McLoughlin's house. The Beaver 272(2):32-35, 1941 ⟨I-03240⟩

Marquis, A.S.: Dr. John McLoughlin (The Great White Eagle). Toronto, The Ryerson Press, 1929, 31 p. ⟨I-03172⟩

Morrison, D.N.: The Eagle and The Fort: The Story of John McLoughlin. New York, Atheneum, 1979. 119 p. ⟨I-01586⟩

Thorington, J.M.: Four Physicians-Explorers of the Fur Trade Days. Annals of Medical History, ser. 3, 4:294-301, 1942 ⟨I-04904⟩

McLoughlin, J. (1784-1857)

Rich, E.E. (edit): The Letters of John McLoughlin from Fort Vancouver to the Governor and Committee, first series, 1825-38; second series 1839-44; third series 1844-46. Toronto, The Champlain Society 1941; 1943; 1944 ⟨I-05173⟩

McMillan, D.S. (-1932)

Paterson, A.O.: Dr. Daniel S. McMillan. CMAJ 27:109, 1933 ⟨I-02542⟩

McMurrich, J.P. (1859-1939)

Macklin, C.C.: James Playfair McMurrich. CMAJ 40:409-410, 1939 ⟨I-02841⟩

McNabb, A.M. (1899-1962)

B., A.A.: Dr. Atholl Munro McNabb: an appreciation. CMAJ 86:1042-1043, 1962 ⟨I-02543⟩

McNaughton, G.A. (1908-1966)

Chute, A.L.: Dr. George A. McNaughton. CMAJ 96:381, 1967 ⟨I-02544⟩

Cox, M.A.: Dr. George Alfred McNaughton. CMAJ 96:380, 1967 ⟨I-02304⟩

McNichol, V.E. (1910-)

McNichol, V.E.: Smiling through Tears. Bloomingdale, Ont., One M Printing Co., 1970, 1:256p. Bridgeport, Ont., Union Print, 1971, 2:408 p., 3:489 p., 4:494 p. 5:379 p. ⟨I-04891⟩

McNulty, P.H. (-1967)

MacCharles, M.R.: Dr. Patrick H. McNulty. CMAJ 98:328-329, 1968 ⟨I-02303⟩

Mitchell, R.: Dr. Patrick H. McNulty. CMAJ 97:1429-1430, 1967 ⟨I-01764⟩

McPhedran, A. (1847-1935)

Foerster, D.K.: Alexander McPhedran. University of Toronto Medical Journal 28:244-248, 1951 ⟨I-02302⟩

Goldie, W.: Dr. Alexander McPhedran. CMAJ 32:222, 1935 ⟨I-01283⟩

McCrae, T.: Dr. Alexander McPhedran. CMAJ 32:222-223, 1935 ⟨I-01284⟩

McQueen, J.D. (1887-1948)

Best, B.D.: Dr. John D. McQueen. CMAJ 60:102, 1949 ⟨I-04504⟩

Mead, H.R. (-1898)

Stanley, G.D.: Herbert Rimington Mead (? - 1898). CACHB 6(3):10-14, 1941 ⟨I-01448⟩

Meakins, J.C. (1882-1959)

C., R.: Dr. Jonathan C. Meakins. CMAJ 81:857, 1959 ⟨I-01755⟩

D., D.M.: Dr. Jonathan C. Meakins. CMAJ 81:857, 1959 ⟨I-01756⟩

Horsfall, F.L.: Dr. Jonathan Campbell Meakins: an appreciation. CMAJ 81:956, 1959 ⟨I-03457⟩

Long, C.N.H.: Dr. Jonathan Campbell Meakins: an appreciation. CMAJ 81:955-956, 1959 ⟨I-03456⟩

Neufeld, A.H.: Seventy-fifth birthday of Dr. Jonathan C. Meakins. CMAJ 77:58, 1957 ⟨I-03456⟩

Medd, A.E. (-1946)

Haig, K.M.: Dr. A.E. Medd. CMAJ 56:115-6, 1947 ⟨I-04405⟩

Medovy, H. (1904-)

Gray, C.: Harry Medovy. CMAJ 129:375, 1983 ⟨I-05215⟩

Medovy, H.: Blue Babies and Well Water. Alumni Journal [University of Manitoba] 38:4-7, 18-19, 1978 ⟨I-04962⟩

Meilleur, J-B (1796-1878)

Audet, L.-P.: Index Analytique du Memorial de l'Education dans le Bas-Canada du Dr. Jean-Baptiste Meilleur. PTRSC. Series 4, 2:49-62, 1964 ⟨I-04949⟩

Audet, L.-P.: Jean-Baptiste Meilleur etait-il un candidat valable au poste de Surintendant de l'Education pour les Bas -Canada en 1842?. Cahier Des Dix 31:163-201, 1966 ⟨I-04656⟩

Dumas, P.: Jean-Baptiste Meilleur, medecin, chimiste, publiciste et educateur. L'UMC 102:406-13, 1973 ⟨I-05375⟩

Lortie, L.: Jean-Baptiste Meilleur. DCB 10:504-509, 1972 ⟨I-01440⟩

Melancon, M-V. (1754-1817)

Rousseau, F.: Marie-Venerande Melancon. DCB 5:587-588, 1983 ⟨I-05310⟩

Melanson, J.A. (-1969)

Maddison, G.E.: Dr. J. Arthur Melanson. CMAJ 100:543-544, 1969 ⟨I-05044⟩

Meltzer, S. (1900-1942)

Boyd, W.: Dr. Sara Meltzer. CMAJ 47:600, 1942 ⟨I-04279⟩

Metcalf, W.G. (1847-1885)

Greenland, C.: William George Metcalf. DCB 11:590-91, 1982 ⟨I-04852⟩

Mewburn, F.H. (1858-1929)

Campbell, P.M.: Frank Hamilton Mewburn. CACHB 15:61-69, 1951 ⟨I-01431⟩

Coulson, F.S.: Frank Hamilton Mewburn (1858-1929). CACHB 10:120-125, 1945 ⟨I-01733⟩

Deane, R.B.: Frank Hamilton Mewburn. CMAJ 20:306-308, 1929 ⟨I-03453⟩

Galbraith, W.S.: Frank Hamilton Mewburn. CMAJ 20:329, 1929 ⟨I-03454⟩

Jamieson, H.C.: Frank Hamilton Mewburn. CMAJ 20:328, 1929 ⟨I-03433⟩

Rankin, A.C.: Dr. Frank Hamilton Mewburn. CMAJ 20:328-329, 1929 ⟨I-03506⟩

Rawlinson, H.E.: Frank Hamilton Mewburn, OBE, MD, CM, LLD, LT.-COL., CAMC, Professor of Surgery, University of Alberta, Pioneer Surgeon. Canadian Journal of Surgery 2:1-5, 1958 ⟨I-03432⟩

Mewburn, F.H.H. (1889-1954)

Hepburn, H.H.: Dr. F. Hastings Mewburn. CMAJ, 71:633, 1954 ⟨I-04570⟩

Meyers, D.C. (1863-1927)

Barker, L.F.: Dr. Campbell Meyers. CMAJ 17:968, 1927 ⟨I-01428⟩

Pos, R., Walters, J.A., Sommers, F.G.: D. Campbell Meyers, M.D., L.R.C.P., M.R.C.S. (Eng.): 1863-1927 Pioneer of Canadian General Hospital Psychiatry. Canadian Psychiatric Association Journal 20:393-403, 1975 ⟨I-05290⟩

Miller, A.F. (-1965)
Hiltz, J.E.: Dr. Arthur Frederick Miller, an appreciation. CMAJ 93:1374, 1965 ⟨I-03180⟩

Miller, G.G. (1893-1964)
Luke, J.C.: Dr. George Gavin Miller, an appreciation. CMAJ 92:247, 1965 ⟨I-03198⟩

Miller, G.W. (1905-1980)
Hart, G.D.: George Wesley Miller. CMAJ 123:940, 1980 ⟨I-02507⟩

Mills, J.R.F. (1909-1981)
Delarue, N.C.: Dr. J.R. Frank Mills. CMAJ 125:112, 1981 ⟨I-04557⟩

Mills, T.W. (-1915)
[Osler, W.]: Thomas Wesley Mills. Lancet 1:466, 1915 ⟨I-05178⟩

Milne, G.L. (1850-)
Watson, I.A.: George Lawson Milne. In: Physicians and Surgeons of America. Concord, Republican Press Association, 1896. p 649 ⟨I-02522⟩

Mitchell, R.B. (1880-1972)
Mitchell, J.R.: Alexandra Park -- Johnston Park: "One Man's Fight to Save a Park" [Dr. Ross Mitchell]. University of Manitoba Medical Journal 51:61-69, 1981 ⟨I-04713⟩
Thorlakson, P.H.T.: A Tribute to Dr. Ross B. Mitchell. Winnipeg Clinic Quarterly 23:65-68, 1970 ⟨I-03181⟩

Moffat, A.K. (1905-)
Hellstedt, L. McG.(edit): Agnes K. Moffat. In: Women Physicians of the World: Autobiographies of Medical Pioneers New York, Mcgraw-Hill Book Co, 1978. pp 220-223 ⟨I-03920⟩

Moffatt, G.M. (1921-1980)
Snidal, D.P.: Garfield M. Moffatt. CMAJ 124:516, 1981 ⟨I-03163⟩

Moir, D.M. (1798-1851)
Scarlett, E.P.: Delta: A Problem in Authorship. CMAJ 55:299-304, 1946 ⟨I-04363⟩

Mondelet, D. (1734-1802)
Janson, G.: Dominique Mondelet. DCB 5:599-600, 1983 ⟨I-05309⟩

Montgomery, E.W. (1863-1948)
Gunn, J.A.: Dr. Edward William Montgomery. CMAJ 59:494-5, 1948 ⟨I-04481⟩

Montizambert, F. (1843-1929)
McCullough, J.W.S.: Dr. Frederick Montizambert, CMG, ISO, FRCSE, DCL (an appreciation). CMAJ 21:747, 1929 ⟨I-01759⟩
Watson, I.A.: Frederick Montizambert. In: Physicians and Surgeons of America. Concord, Republican Press Association 1896. pp 27-28 ⟨I-02508⟩

Moody, J.P. (1920-)
Moody, J.P., de Grott van Embden, W.: Arctic Doctor. New York, Dodd, Mead and Company, 1955, 274 p. ⟨I-04433⟩

Moore, D.F. (1911-1974)
W., J.D.: Dr. Donald F. Moore. CMAJ 111:171, 1974 ⟨I-05169⟩

Moreau de Bresoles,J (1620-1687)
Lefebvre, E.: Judith Moreau de Bresoles. DCB 1:512, 1966 ⟨I-01459⟩

Morgentaler, H. (1923-)
Pelrine, E.W.: Morgentaler: The Doctor who couldn't turn away. Canada, Gage Publishing Ltd., 1975. 210 p. ⟨I-01299⟩

Morisette, L. (1911-1970)
LeClair, M.: Leopold Morisette (1911-1970). L'UMC 100:770-2, 1971 ⟨I-02262⟩

Morrin, J. (1794-1861)
Boissonnault, C.M.: Joseph Morrin. DCB 9:572-573, 1976 ⟨I-01451⟩

Morris, F.W. (1802-1867)
Blakeley, P.R.: Frederick William Morris. DCB 9:573-574, 1976 ⟨I-01453⟩

Morrison, M.D. (-1946)
Scammell, H.L.: Dr. Murdock Daniel Morrison. CMAJ 55:88, 1946 ⟨I-03193⟩

Morrow, W.S. (1869-1920)
Segall, H.N.: William Stairs Morrow, Canada's First Physiologist-cardiologist. CMAJ 114:543-545, 1976 ⟨I-03182⟩

Morse, H.D. (1893-1966)
Mitchell, R.: Dr. Harry D. Morse. Winnipeg Clinic Quarterly 19:105-109 ⟨I-02531⟩
S., C.B.: Dr. Harry Dodge Morse, an appreciation. CMAJ 95:885, 1966 ⟨I-03194⟩

Morse, L.R. (1833-1903)
Morse, F.W.: A Country Doctor's Life, 1855-1898. Nova Scotia Medical Bulletin 46:169-175, 1967 ⟨I-03183⟩

Mowbray, F.B. (1883-1931)
D., W.J.: Dr. Frederick Bruce Mowbray. CMAJ 25:749, 1931 ⟨I-03152⟩

Muir, W.S. (1853-1902)
Campbell, D.A.: William Scott Muir (1853-1902). In Kelly HW, Burrage WL: Dictionary of American Medical Biography. New York and London, D. Appleton and Co., 1928. pp. 883-884. ⟨I-01446⟩

Mullin, R.H. (1879-1924)
G., N.B.: Dr. Robert Hyndman Mullin. CMAJ 14:889, 1924 ⟨I-02993⟩

Mundie, G.S. (1885-1926)
Martin, C.F.: Dr. Gordon Stewart Mundie. CMAJ 16:608, 1926 ⟨I-01423⟩

Munro, H. (1770-1854)
Warren, M.R.: Dr. Henry Munro -- An elusive Figure. CMAJ 92:377-378, 1965 ⟨I-03191⟩

Munroe, A.R. (1879-1965)
Macbeth, R.A.: Alexander Russell Munroe: 1879-1965. Canadian Journal of Surgery 10:3-10, 1967 ⟨I-03184⟩

Munson, L. (1820-1882)
Richardson, G.: Mrs. Letitia (Lecitia) Munson. DCB 11:629-30, 1982 〈I-04853〉

Murray, E.G.D. (1890-1964)
Collip, J.B.: Professor E.G.D. Murray, an appreciation. CMAJ 92:95-97, 1965 〈I-03215〉

Murray, F. J. (1894-)
Murray, F.J.: At the Foot of Dragon Hill. New York, E.P. Dutton and Co., 1975. 240 p. 〈I-03935〉

Murray, G.
Murray, G.: Medicine in the making. Toronto, Ryerson Press, 1960. 235 p. 〈I-01409〉
Murray, G.: Quest in Medicine. Toronto, Ryerson Press, 1963. 185 p. 〈I-01408〉

Murray, G. (1825-1888)
Beck, J.M.: George Murray. DCB 11:633, 1982 〈I-04854〉

Murray, L.M. (1875-1931)
Caulfield, A.H.W.: Dr. Leonard Milton Murray. CMAJ 25:503, 1931 〈I-03159〉

Musgrove, W.W.L. (1882-1947)
Mitchell, R.: Dr. William Wesley Lorne Musgrove. CMAJ 56:349, 1947 〈I-04408〉

Mustard, R.A. (1913-)
Gray, C.: Robert Alexander Mustard. CMAJ 127:1216, 1982 〈I-04961〉

N

Neilson, W.J. (1854-1903)
Halpenny, J.: William Johnston Neilson (1854-1903). In Kelly HW, Burrage WL: Dictionary of American Medical Biography. New York and London, D. Appleton and Co., 1928. pp. 899-900 〈I-01272〉

Neish, J. (1834-1908)
Roland, C.G.: James Neish and the Canadian Medical Times. McGill Medical Journal 36:107-125, 1967 〈I-01271〉

Nelles, T.R.B. (1883-1967)
MacDermot, J.H.: Dr. Thomas R.B. Nelles, an appreciation. CMAJ 98:180, 1968 〈I-01766〉

Nelson, R. (1793-1844)
Burrage, W.L.: Robert Nelson (1793-1844). In Kelly HW, Burrage WL: Dictionary of American Medical Biography. New York and London, D. Appleton and Co., 1928. p. 900 〈I-01275〉
Chabot, R., Monet, J., Roby, Y.: Robert Nelson. DCB 10:544-547, 1972 〈I-01270〉

Nelson, R. (1794-1873)
Lusignan, C.A.: Dr. Robert Nelson. Canada Medical Record 1:213-14, 1872-3 〈I-04826〉

Nelson, W. (1792-1863)
Guerra, F.: Les Medecins Patriotes. In International Congress for the History of Medicine, 25th, Quebec, 1976. Proceedings, Volume II, 1976. p. 746-754 〈I-01277〉

Thompson, J.B.: Wolfred Nelson. DCB 9:593-597, 1976 〈I-01274〉

Nevitt, R.B. (1850-1928)
Cameron, I.H.: Richard Barrington Nevitt, an appreciation. CMAJ 19:382-383, 1928 〈I-03503〉
Ritchie, J.B.: Early Surgeons of the North West Mounted Police: V. Doctor Richard Barrington Nevitt. CACHB 22:249-265, 1958 〈I-02540〉
Ritchie, J.B.: Early Surgeons of the North-West Mounted Police (R.B. Nevitt). RCMP Quarterly 24:61-65, 1958 〈I-02541〉

Newcombe, C.F. (1851-1924)
Low, J.: Dr. Charles Frederick Newcombe. The Beaver, Spring 1982, pp 32-39 〈I-04833〉

Nichols, R.B. (-1966)
S, H.L.: Dr. Roberta Bond Nichols. CMAJ 96:234, 1967 〈I-02537〉
W., A.S., P., I.E.: Dr. Roberta Bond Nichols, an appreciation. Canadian Anaesthetists Society Journal 14:152, 1967 〈I-02538〉

Nooth, J.M. (1737-1828)
Nadeau, G.: Un Savant Anglais a Quebec a La Fin du XVIIIe Siecele le Docteur John-Mervin Nooth. L'UMC 74:49-74, 1945 〈I-02249〉

Normand, L.P. (1863-1928)
St. Jacques, E.: Hon. Dr. L.P. Normand. CMAJ 19:260-261, 1928 〈I-03502〉

O

O'Brien, L.J. (1797-1870)
Armstrong, F.H.: Lucius James O'Brien. DCB 9:606-607, 1976 〈I-01263〉
Stanley, G.D.: Dr. Louis J. O'Brien. CACHB 15:72-80, 1951 〈I-01244〉

O'Brien, M. (1867-1955)
Tyre, R.: Saddlebag Surgeon. The story of Murrough O'Brien M.D. Toronto, J.M. Dent and Sons (Canada) Limited, 1954, 261 p. 〈I-04515〉

O'Callaghan, E.B. (1797-1880)
Durley, M.S.: Dr. Edmund Bailey O'Callaghan, His Early Years in Medicine, Montreal 1823-1828. Canadian Catholic Historical Association 47:23-40, 1980 〈I-04558〉
Monet, J.: Edmund Bailey O'Callaghan. DCB 10:554-556,1972 〈I-01262〉

O'Donnell, J.H. (1838-1912)
Mitchell, R.: John Harrison O'Donnell, M.D. (1838-1912). Canadian Journal of Surgery 10:399-402, 1967 〈I-02535〉

O'Donnell, J.M. (-1912)
Watson, I.A.: John Morrison O'Donnell. In: Physicians and Surgeons of America. Concord, Republican Press Association, 1896. pp 772-3 〈I-03246〉

Oertel, H. (1872-1956)
M[acDermot], H.E.: Professor Horst Oertel. CMAJ 74:485, 1956 〈I-04742〉

Oille, J.A. (1876-1962)

G[raham], D.: Dr. John A. Oillie, an appreciation. CMAJ 87:881-882, 1962 ⟨I-02293⟩

Oillie, J.A.: My experiences in medicine. CMAJ 91:855-860, 1964 ⟨I-02307⟩

Oille, L.S.

Dittrick, H.: Our family doctor, the Mayor. CACHB 10:160-163, 1946 ⟨I-01266⟩

Olmsted, I. (1864-1936)

Malloch, A.: Dr. Ingersoll Olmsted, an appreciation. CMAJ 37:93-94, 1937 ⟨I-03445⟩

Olmsted, A.I.: Ingersoll Olmsted (1864-1937). Canadian Journal of Surgery 3:1-4, 1959-60 ⟨I-04235⟩

Olszewski, J. (1913-1964)

R., A.C.: Professor J. Olszewski, M.D., Ph.D. CMAJ 90:1379, 1964 ⟨I-05227⟩

O'Neill, H.P. (1877-1966)

E., H.S.: Dr. Hugh Pius O'Neill. CMAJ 95:1331, 1966 ⟨I-02291⟩

O'Reilly, G. (1806-1861)

Roland, C.G.: Gerald O'Reilly. DCB 9:611-612, 1976 ⟨I-01267⟩

Orr, H. (1889-1952)

Marshall, M.R.: Dr. Harold Orr. CMAJ 68:185, 1953 ⟨I-04550⟩

Orton, G.T. (1837-1901)

Halpenny, J.: George Turner Orton (1837-1901). In Kelly HW, Burrage WL; Dictionary of American Medical Biography. New York and London, D. Appleton and Co., 1928. p. 921. ⟨I-01268⟩

Osler, W. (1849-1919)

Abbott, M.E.: Sir William Osler Memorial Volume. Montreal, International Association of Medical Museums, Bull No. IX, 1926. 634 p. ⟨I-01250⟩

Abbott, M.E.: More about Osler. Bulletin of the Institute of the History of Medicine 5:765-796, 1937 ⟨I-02534⟩

Abbott, M.E. (Edit.): Classified And Annotated Bibliography of Sir William Osler's Publications. Montreal, Medical Museum, McGill University, 1939. 163 p. ⟨I-01256⟩

Cushing, H.: The Life of Sir William Osler. Oxford, Claredon Press, 1925; 2 Vols., 685 p., 728 p. ⟨I-01257⟩

Dumas, P.: William Osler et la Bibliotheca Osleriana. L'UMC 100:539-545, 1971 ⟨I-01251⟩

Elliott, J.H.: Osler's Class at the Toronto School of Medicine. CMAJ 47:161-165, 1942 ⟨I-01252⟩

Gwyn, N.B.: Osler, student of the Toronto School of Medicine: a detail of the personal side of teaching. Annals of Medical History 5:305-308, 1923 ⟨I-02532⟩

Gwynn, N.B.: Some Details of Osler's Early Life as Collected by a Near Relation. North Carolina Medical Journal 10:491-496, 1949 ⟨I-01124⟩

Howard, R.P.: William Osler: " A Potent Ferment" at McGill. Archives of Internal Medicine 84:12-15, 1949 ⟨I-02533⟩

Kelly, H.A.: Sir William Osler (1849-1919). In Kelly HW, Burrage WL: Dictionary of American Medical Biography. New York and London, D. Appleton and Co., 1928. pp. 921-923. ⟨I-01254⟩

Linell, E.A.: A Cairn to the memory of Osler. CMAJ 85:1347-1350, 1961 ⟨I-02290⟩

Nation, E.F., Roland, C.G., McGovern, J.P.: An Annotated Checklist of Osleriana. Kent State University Press, 1970. 289 p. ⟨I-01255⟩

Reid, E.G.: The Great Physician. (A Short Life of Sir William Osler). London/New York/Toronto, Oxford University Press, 1931. 299 p. ⟨I-01253⟩

Rodin, A.E.: Canada's Foremost Pathologist of the Nineteenth Century -- William Osler. CMAJ 107:890-896, 1972 ⟨I-01259⟩

Rodin, A.E.: Osler's Autopsies: Their Nature and Utilization. Medical History 17:37-48, 1973 ⟨I-01247⟩

Saunders, L.Z.: Some Pioneers in Comparative Medicine. Canadian Veterinary Journal 14:27-35, 1973 ⟨I-01260⟩

Scott, J.W.: Osler and the Science of Medicine. In International Congress for the History of Medicine, 25th, Quebec, 1976. Proceedings, Volume III, 1976. p. 1244-1252 ⟨I-01269⟩

Stewart, W.G.: Personal reminiscences of Sir William Osler. Bulletin IX, International Association of Medical Museums, 1927, pp. 4381-j. ⟨I-02289⟩

Owen, T. (-1964)

Farrar, C.B.: Trevor Owen, M.B., FRCP (Lond), FRCP (C), an appreciation. CMAJ 93:1375-1376, 1965 ⟨I-02287⟩

Owens, M. (1892-)

Hellstedt, L. McG (edit): Margaret Owens. In: Women Physicians of the World: Autobiographies of Medical Pioneers New York, McGraw-Hill Book Co., 1978. pp 79-84 ⟨I-03943⟩

Ower, J.J. (1886-1962)

MacG., J.W.: Dr. John James Ower, an appreciation. CMAJ 86:796-797, 1962 ⟨I-02530⟩

Ower, J.J.: Pictures on Memory's Walls. CACHB 19:1-22, 1954 ⟨I-01245⟩

Ower, J.J.: Pictures on Memory's Walls, Part II (Army Days). CACHB 19:35-62, 1954 ⟨I-01246⟩

P

Painchaud, J. (1787-1871)

Boissonnault, C.M.: Joseph Painchaud. DCB 10:563-564, 1972 ⟨I-01237⟩

LeBlond, S.: Joseph Painchaud. L'UMC 82:182-187, 1953 ⟨I-02002⟩

LeBlond, S.: Une Conference Inedite du Docteur Joseph Painchaud. Laval Medical 39:355-360, 1968 ⟨I-04711⟩

LeBlond, S.: Le docteur Joseph Painchaud (1787-1871) conferencier populaire. Cahier des Dix 36:120-138, 1971 ⟨I-01238⟩

Paine, W.

Chaisson, A.F.: Dr. William Paine -- Loyalist. CMAJ 69:446-447, 1953 ⟨I-02286⟩

Palmer, D. D. (1845-)

Gielow, V.: Daniel David Palmer: Rediscovering the Frontier Years, 1845-1887. Chiropractic History 1:11-14, 1981 ⟨I-04840⟩

Parfitt, C. D. (1872-1951)

Farrar, C.B.: Dr. Charles D. Parfitt M.D. CMAJ 66:294, 1952 ⟨I-04548⟩

Wetherell, A.: Charles Daniel Parfitt. Ontario History 44:45-56, 1952 ⟨I-02564⟩

Pariseau, L. E. (1882-1944)

Desjardins, E.: Et Avant L'Acfas, Il Y Eut La Spaslac. L'UMC 100:1402-1406, 1971 ⟨I-01234⟩

Jutras, A.: Dr. Leo Erol Pariseau, an appreciation. CMAJ 50:187-188, 1944 ⟨I-01697⟩

Park, A. W.

Fish, A.H.: Doctor Park of Cochrane. CACHB 13:55-61, 1948 ⟨I-01230⟩

Parker, D. McN. (1822-1907)

Campbell, D.A.: Daniel McNeil Parker (1822-1907). In Kelly HW, Burrage WL: Dictionary of American Medical Biography. New York and London, D. Appleton and Co., 1928. pp. 937-938. ⟨I-01242⟩

Parker, W.F.: Daniel McNeill Parker, M.D.: His ancestry and a memoir of his life. Toronto, William Briggs, 1910. pp. 604 ⟨I-01032⟩

Parsons, R. (1875-1944)

Anderson, W.G.: Dr. Richard Parsons. CMAJ 52:111, 1945 ⟨I-04359⟩

Stanley, G.D.: Dr. Richard Parsons of Red Deer. CACHB 15:41-51, 1950 ⟨I-02562⟩

Patch, F. S. (1878-1953)

M[acDermot], H.E.: Dr. Frank S. Patch. CMAJ 69:79-80, 1953 ⟨I-04526⟩

Paterson, D. H. (1890-1968)

K[elly], A.D.: Donald Hugh Paterson, M.D. CMAJ 100:466, 1969 ⟨I-05042⟩

Patrick, T. A. (1864-1943)

Houston, C.J., Houston, C.S.: Pioneer of vision: The Medical and political memoirs of T.A. Patrick, M.D. CMAJ 119:964-967, 1978 ⟨I-01232⟩

Houston, C.J., Houston, C.S.: Pioneer of Vision: The Reminiscences of T.A. Patrick, M.D. Saskatoon, Western Producer Prairie Books, 1980. 149 p. ⟨I-01231⟩

Seaborn, E.: Doctor Thomas Patrick: A Pioneer Saskatchewan Doctor. CACHB 10:83-88, 1945 ⟨I-02561⟩

Payen de Noyan, M-C. (1730-1818)

Plamondon, L.: Marie-Catherine Payen de Noyan. DCB 5:661-662, 1983 ⟨I-05308⟩

Pearson, J. M. (1869-1935)

Keith, W.D.: John Mawer Pearson Lecture. Bulletin of the Vancouver Medical Association 25:60-64, 1949 ⟨I-02560⟩

Peikoff, S. S.

Peikoff, S.S.: Yesterday's Doctor: An Autobiography. Winnipeg, The Prairie Publishing Company, 1980. 145 p. ⟨I-01058⟩

Pelletier, A (1876-1917)

Gouin, J.: Antonio Pelletier, La vie et l'oeuvre d'un medecin et poete meconnu (1876-1917). Montreal, Editions du Jour, 1975. 202 p. ⟨I-05211⟩

Peltier, H. (1822-1878)

Audet, L.-P.: Hector Peltier. DCB 10:588-589, 1972 ⟨I-01239⟩

Penfield, W. G. (1891-1976)

Feindel, W.: Wilder Penfield (1891-1976): The Man and His Work. Neurosurgery 1:93-100, 1977 ⟨I-01228⟩

Feindel, W.: The Contributions of Wilder Penfield and the Montreal Neurological Institute to Canadian Neurosciences. In: Roland, C.G. (ed): Health, Disease and Medicine: Essays in Canadian History. Toronto, Hannah Institute for the History of Medicine, 1984, 347-358. ⟨I-05369⟩

Lewis, J.: Something Hidden: A Biography of Wilder Penfield. Toronto, Doubleday Canada Ltd., 1981, 311 p. ⟨I-04765⟩

Penfield, W.: No Man Alone. Boston/Toronto, Little, Brown and Co., 1977. 398 p. ⟨I-01229⟩

Penfield, W.: Penfield Remembered. The Review [Imperial Oil Ltd.] 66(2):26-29, 1982 ⟨I-04771⟩

Perrault, J-F. (1753-1844)

Bender, L.P.: Old and New, Canada 1753-1844: Historic Scenes and Social pictures, or The Life of Joseph-Francois Perrault. Montreal, Dawson Brothers, Publishers, 1882, 291 p. ⟨I-04438⟩

Perrigo, J. (1845-1928)

England, F.R.: Dr. James Perrigo. CMAJ 18:757, 1928 ⟨I-02586⟩

McConnell, J.B.: Dr. James Perrigo. CMAJ 18:757-758, 1928 ⟨I-01620⟩

Peters, G. A. (1859-1907)

Gallie, W.E.: George Armstrong Peters: (As I remember him). Canadian Journal of Surgery 2:119-122, 1959 ⟨I-02585⟩

Philipps, J. (1736-1801)

Kernaghan, L.K.: John Philipps. DCB 5:670, 1983 ⟨I-05307⟩

Phlem, Y. (? -1749)

Blais, M.C.: Yves Phlem. DCB 3:518-520, 1974 ⟨I-01012⟩

Pigarouich, E. (fl. 1639)

Monet, J.: Etienne Pigarouich. DCB 1:548-549, 1966 ⟨I-01000⟩

Pilcher, S. (1906-1954)

S[carlett], E.P.: Frederick Pilcher 1906-1954. CACHB 19:63-4, 1954 ⟨I-04387⟩

Pinard, L. (1663-1695)

Nadeau, G.: Louis Pinard. DCB 1:550, 1966 ⟨I-01005⟩

Piuze, L. (1754-1813)
Morin, J.: Liveright Piuze. DCB 5:676, 1983 ⟨I-05306⟩

Playter, E. (1834-1909)
Defries, R.D.: Dr. Edward Playter - A Vision Fulfilled. Canadian Journal Public Health 50:368-377, 1959 ⟨I-02582⟩
Watson, I.A.: Edward Playter. In: Physicians and Surgeons of America. Concord, Republican Press Association, 1896. p 199 ⟨I-02523⟩

Popham, E.S. (1856-1930)
Mitchell, R.: Dr. Edwin S. Popham. CMAJ 22:443, 1930 ⟨I-02581⟩

Porter, A.E. (1855-1940)
Stanley, G.D.: Andrew Everett Porter (1855-1940). CACHB 6(2):5-11, 1941 ⟨I-01236⟩

Potts, J. (? -1764)
Williams, G.: John Potts. DCB 3:533-534, 1974 ⟨I-01243⟩

Powell, G. (1779-1873)
Powell, R.W.: Dr. Grant Powell. CMAJ 18:213-214, 1928 ⟨I-02299⟩

Powell, I.W. (1836-1915)
McKelvie, B.A.: Lieutenant-Colonel Israel Wood Powell, M.D., C.M. British Columbia Historical Quarterly 11:33-54, 1947 ⟨I-05064⟩

Powell, N.A. (1851-1935)
McCulloch, E.A.: That Reminds Me of N.A.P. Toronto, The Ryerson Press, 1942, 78 p. ⟨I-04517⟩

Powell, R.H.W. (1856-1935)
Argue, J.F.: Dr. Robert Henry Wynyard Powell. CMAJ 32:590, 1935 ⟨I-01034⟩

Prevost, Albert (-1926)
Montpetit, E.: Albert Prevost. L'Union Medicale du Canada 55:675-680, 1926 ⟨I-05062⟩

Price, L.H. (1868-)
McGuire, C.R.: The Canadian Connection with St. Helena. Stampex Canada Catalogue 1981, pp [6] - [13], [16] ⟨I-03873⟩

Primrose, A. (1861-1944)
Harris, R.I.: Alexander Primrose, 1861-1944. Canadian Journal of Surgery 1:183-8, 1957-8 ⟨I-04241⟩
Young, G.S.: Dr. Alexander Primrose, C.B., LL.D.,. CMAJ 50:389-390, 1944 ⟨I-04247⟩

Prowse, S.W. (1869-1931)
MacLean, J.A.: Dr. Samuel Willis Prowse. CMAJ 25:366, 1931 ⟨I-03158⟩
Mitchell, R.: Samuel Willis Prowse, MD 1869-1931: Fourth Dean of Medicine. Manitoba Medical Review 38:551-553, 1958 ⟨I-02694⟩
Mitchell, R.: Samuel Willis Prowse. Manitoba Medical Review 41:455-459, 1961 ⟨I-02695⟩
Smith, W.H.: Dr. Samuel Willis Prowse. CMAJ 25:366-67, 1931 ⟨I-03157⟩

Puddicombe, J.F. (1901-1966)
Whyte, J.C.: Dr. John Francis Puddicombe. CMAJ 96:507, 1967 ⟨I-02771⟩

R

Rabinovitch, R. (1909-1965)
Gibson, W.C.: Dr. Reuben Rabinovitch, an appreciation. CMAJ 93:988, 1965 ⟨I-02696⟩

Radford, J.H. (1856-1937)
Woolner, W.: Dr. Joseph Henry Radford. CMAJ 36:99, 1937 ⟨I-02876⟩

Rae, J. (1813-1893)
Fortuine, R.: Doctors Afield: John Rae, Surgeon to the Hudson's Bay Company. New England Journal of Medicine 268:37-39, 1963 ⟨I-01577⟩
Hamilton, Z.W.: Admiralty documents concerning Dr. John Rae. CACHB 9:32-35, 1944 ⟨I-02769⟩
Mitchell, R.: Physician, fur trader and explorer. The Beaver 267(2):16-20 ⟨I-03227⟩
Mitchell, R.: Dr. John Rae, Arctic explorer, and his search for Franklin. CMAJ 28:85-90, 1933 ⟨I-03004⟩
Richards, R.L.: Rae of the Arctic. Medical History 19:176-193, 1975 ⟨I-01127⟩
Swinton, W.E.: Physicians as explorers: the contribution of John Rae to Canada's development. CMAJ 117:531-6 and 541, 1977 ⟨I-04385⟩

Raynor, M. (1879-1925)
Leeder, F.: Dr. Melbourne Raynor. CMAJ 16:100, 1926 ⟨I-01605⟩
Thomas, T.A.: Dr. Melbourne Raynor. CMAJ 16:100, 1926 ⟨I-01604⟩

Rees, W. (Ca.1800-1874)
Canniff, W.: William Rees. In Kelly HW, Burrage WL: Dictionary of American Medical Biography. New York and London, D. Appleton and Co., 1928. pp. 1020-1021 ⟨I-01225⟩
Ormsby, W.: William Rees. DCB 10:610-611, 1972 ⟨I-01128⟩

Revell, D.G. (1869-)
Stanley, G.D.: Dr. Daniel Graisberry Revell: Medical teacher, scholar and gentleman. CACHB 14:48-54, 1949 ⟨I-01119⟩

Rhea, L.J. (1877-1944)
M, H.E.: Dr. Lawrence J. Rhea. CMAJ 51:184-5, 1944 ⟨I-04258⟩

Richards, G.E. (1885-1949)
Cosbie, W.G.: The Gordon Richards Memorial Lecture: Gordon Richards and the Ontario Cancer Foundation. Journal of the Canadian Association of Radiologists 9:1-7, 1958 ⟨I-02498⟩
Jones, W.A.: Gordon Earle Richards -- a little about his life and times. Journal of the Canadian Association of Radiologists 6:1-7, 1955 ⟨I-02497⟩

Richardson, J. (1787-1865)
Johnson, G.R.: Sir John Richardson (1787-1865). CACHB 7(1):1-10, 1942 ⟨I-01227⟩
Johnson, R.E.: Sir John Richardson. DCB 9:658-661, 1976 ⟨I-01222⟩

Richardson, J.H. (1823-1910)

Hunter, J.: Dr. J.H. Richardson, (an appreciation). Canadian Practitioner and Review 35:121-122, 1910 ⟨I-01131⟩

Montgomery, W.D.: Dr. J.H. Richardson. Canada Lancet and Practitioner 66:18-21, 1926 ⟨I-02765⟩

Y[oung], W.A.:: The Death of Dr. James H. Richardson. Canadian Journal of Medicine and Surgery 27:111-113, 1910 ⟨I-02499⟩

Richmond, G. (1904-)

Richmond, G.: Prison Doctor. Surrey, Nunaga Publishing, 1975. 186 p. ⟨I-04197⟩

Riddell, W.R. (1852-1945)

Neary, H.B.: William Renwick Riddell: Judge, Ontario Publicist and Man of Letters. Law Society of Upper Canada Gazette 11:144-174, 1977 ⟨I-01122⟩

Surveyer, E.F.: The Honourable William Renwick Riddell 1852-1945. PTRSC 39:111-114, 1945 ⟨I-03576⟩

Ridewood, H.E. (1878-1952)

Murphy, H.H.: Dr. Harold Edward Ridewood. CMAJ 68:186, 1953 ⟨I-04534⟩

Ridge, J. (1913-1967)

N., J.E., W., J.C., W., P.: Dr. John Ridge: an appreciation. CMAJ 97:1496, 1967 ⟨I-02504⟩

Rieutord, J-B. (1733-1818)

Cadotte, M., Lessard, R.: Jean-Baptiste Rieutord. DCB 5:712-713, 1983 ⟨I-05305⟩

Roach, R.D. (-1952)

Gass, C.L.: Dr. R.D. Roach. CMAJ 67:484, 1952 ⟨I-04533⟩

Roberts, H.D. (1908-)

Gray, C.: Harry Duncan Roberts. CMAJ 126:710, 1982 ⟨I-04778⟩

Roberts, J. (1877-1940)

Gagan, R.R.: Disease, Mortality and Public Health, Hamilton, Ontario, 1900-1914. Thesis, McMaster University, School of Graduate Studies, Master of Arts, April, 1981. 225 pages ⟨I-04894⟩

Roberts, J.B. (1907-1980)

Buffam, G.B.B.: James Boyd Roberts. CMAJ 123:695, 1980 ⟨I-01579⟩

Roberts, W.F. (1869-1938)

Kirkland, A.S.: Hon. Dr. W.F. Roberts. CMAJ 38:303, 1938 ⟨I-03371⟩

Robertson, A.A. (1871-1925)

Gordon, A.H.: Dr. Andrew Armour Robertson. CMAJ 15:556, 1925 ⟨I-01588⟩

Robertson, D.E. (1884-1944)

Brown, A.: Dr. David Edwin Robertson, an appreciation. CMAJ 50:391, 1944 ⟨I-02500⟩

Robertson, H.R. (1912-)

Gray, C.: Harold Rocke Robertson. CMAJ 125:916, 1981 ⟨I-04418⟩

Robertson, J.S. (1878-)

Hellstedt, L.McG. (edit): Jeannie Smillie Robertson. In: Women Physicians of the World: Autobiographies of Medical Pioneers New York, McGraw-Hill Book Co., 1978. pp 1-4 ⟨I-03941⟩

Robertson, W. (1784-1844)

Ruttan, R.F.: William Robertson (1784-1844). In Kelly HW, Burrage WL: Dictionary of American Medical Biography. New York and London, D. Appleton and Co., 1928. p. 1044 ⟨I-01224⟩

Roche, W.J. (1859-1937)

Roche, W.J.: Reminiscences. University of Western Ontario Medical Journal 1:8-10, 1930 ⟨I-04761⟩

Rochfort, J. (? -1865)

Davis, D.J.: John Rochfort. DCB 9:681-682, 1976 ⟨I-01226⟩

Roddick, T.G. (1846-1923)

MacDermot, H.E.: Sir Thomas Roddick. His Work in Medicine and Public Life. Toronto, Macmillan Co. of Canada Ltd., 1938. 160 p. ⟨I-01120⟩

MacDermot, H.E.: Thomas George Roddick (1846-1923). Canadian Journal of Surgery 4:1-3, 1960-61 ⟨I-04238⟩

Power, D'Arcy: Sir Thomas George Roddick. In: Plarr's Lives of the Fellows of the Royal College of Surgeons of England. Bristol and London, The Royal College of Surgeons, 1930. Vol 2:236-37 ⟨I-02763⟩

Shepherd, F.J.: Sir Thomas George Roddick, M.D., LL.D., F.R.C.S.(Eng.). CMAJ 13:283-284, 1923 ⟨I-03001⟩

Rolph, J. (1793-1870)

Canniff, W.: John Rolph (1793-1870). In Kelly HW, Burrage WL: Dictionary of American Medical Biography. New York and London, D. Appleton and Co., 1928. pp. 1055-1056. ⟨I-01135⟩

Craig, G.M.: Two Contrasting Upper Canadian Figures: John Rolph and John Strachan. PTRSC IV, 12:237-248, 1974 ⟨I-01405⟩

Craig, G.M.: John Rolph. DCB 9:683-690, 1976 ⟨I-01132⟩

Gryfe, A.: Dr. John Rolph -- physician, lawyer and rebel. CMAJ 113:971-974, 1975 ⟨I-01133⟩

Gwyn, N.B.: The Chapter from the Life of John Rolph. Bulletin of the Academy of Medicine, Toronto 9:137-144, 1936 ⟨I-04965⟩

Riddell, [W.R.]: The Court of King's Bench in Upper Canada, 1824-1827. N.P./n.d. pp. 1-28 ⟨I-01136⟩

Roland, C.G.: When Did John Rolph First Practice Medicine in Upper Canada?. Canadian Society for the History of Medicine Newsletter, Autumn, 1982. pp 24-25 ⟨I-04975⟩

Sissons, C.B.: Dr. John Rolph's own account of the Flag of Truce incident in the Rebellion of 1837. CHR 19:56-59, 1938 ⟨I-01134⟩

Stanley, G.D.: Dr. John Rolph: Medicine and Rebellion in Upper Canada. CACHB 9:1-13, 1944 ⟨I-01137⟩

Romieux, P. (Ca. 1636-1675)

Hutcheson, M.M.: Pierre Romieux. DCB 1:578-579, 1966 ⟨I-01004⟩

Rorke, R.F. (1864-1948)

Day, O.J.: Dr. Robert Francis Rorke. CMAJ 60:203-4, 1949 ⟨I-04493⟩

Rose, W.O. (-1936)

A., F.M.: Dr. William Oliver Rose. CMAJ 34:595-596, 1936 ⟨I-03449⟩

Rosebrugh, A.M. (1835-1914)

Houston, P.J.F.: Early Ophthalmology in Toronto. CMAJ 24:708-710, 1931 ⟨I-01138⟩

Ross, A.M. (1832-1892)

Ross, A.M.: Recollections and Experiences of an Abolitionist; from 1885 to 1865. Toronto, Rowsell and Hutchison, 1875. 224 p. ⟨I-01641⟩

Ross, A.M.: Memoirs of a Reformer (1832-1892). Toronto, Hunter Rose and Co., 1893. 271 p. ⟨I-01643⟩

Ross, C. (1843-1916)

Currie, M.G.: A Pioneer Woman in Canadian Medicine. Nova Scotia Medical Bulletin 33:266-267, 1954 ⟨I-03930⟩

Douglass, M.E.: A pioneer woman doctor of Western Canada (C. Ross). Manitoba Medical Review 27:255-256, 1947 ⟨I-02577⟩

Ross, C.W. (1843-1916)

Angel, B., Angel, M.: Charlotte Whitehead Ross. Winnipeg, Pegius Publishers Limited, 1982. ⟨I-05053⟩

McFarlane, C.J.: Manitoba's First Woman Doctor. University of Manitoba Medical Journal 53:11-14, 1983 ⟨I-05130⟩

Ross, G. (1834-1892)

Macphail, A.: George Ross (1834-1892). In Kelly HW, Burrage WL: Dictionary of American Medical Biography. New York and London, D. Appleton and Co., 1928. p. 1058 ⟨I-01140⟩

Ross, H. (1845-1928)

Thaler, A.F.: Dr. Hugh Ross. CMAJ 19:738, 1928 ⟨I-03491⟩

Ross, J.B. (1902-1942)

H.E.M.: Dr. James Brodie Ross. CMAJ 46:399-400, 1942 ⟨I-04273⟩

Ross, J.W.

Ross, J.W.: A Half-Century in Medicine. Bulletin of the Academy of Medicine, Toronto 25:28-32, 1951 ⟨I-01050⟩

Ross, J.F.W. (1857-1911)

Davison, J.L.: Dr. Ross as a Man. Canada Lancet 45:331-334, 1912 ⟨I-01146⟩

Marlow, F.W.: A Few Notes Referring to the Contributions to Medical Literature and the Writings of the late Dr. James F.W. Ross, Toronto. Canada Lancet 45:334-337, 1912 ⟨I-01144⟩

Powell, N.A.: In Memoriam of Dr. J.F.W. Ross. Canada Lancet 45:327-329, 1912 ⟨I-01143⟩

Powell, N.A.: James Frederick William Ross (1857-1911). In Kelly HW, Burrage WL: Dictionary of American Medical Biography. New York and London, D. Appleton and Co., 1928. pp. 1058-1059. ⟨I-01141⟩

Stanley, G.D.: Dr. J.F. ("Windy") Ross. Medical Recollections of Toronto Varsity. CACHB 18:88-95, 1954 ⟨I-01142⟩

Temple, J.A.: Dr. Ross as a Surgeon. Canada Lancet 45:329-330, 1912 ⟨I-01147⟩

Rottot, J.P. (1827-1910)

LeSage, A.: Les Debuts de L'Union Medicale Durant L'Annee 1872. Le Dr. Rottot. L'UMC 61:78-95, 1932 ⟨I-02226⟩

LeSage, A.: Le Decantat a la Faculte de Medecine de L'Universite de Montreal: Trois Doyens (1880-1934) -- Rottot, Lachapelle, Harwood. L'UMC 68:166-178, 1939 ⟨I-02266⟩

Rouleau, E.H. (1843-1912)

Stanley, G.D.: Edward Hector Rouleau. CACHB 5(1):4-10, 1940 ⟨I-01221⟩

Roussel, T. (1639-1700)

Nadeau, G.: Timothee Roussel. DCB 1:583, 1966 ⟨I-01003⟩

Routley, T.C. (1889-1963)

Clegg, H.: Dr. T. Clarence Routley, an appreciation. CMAJ 88:1046, 1963 ⟨I-01673⟩

Editorial: T.C. Routley. CMAJ 88:816, 1963 ⟨I-02600⟩

Gear, H.: Dr. Thomas Clarence Routley, an appreciation. CMAJ 88:953, 1963 ⟨I-02599⟩

Gilder, S.S.B.: Dr. T. Clarence Routley, an appreciation. CMAJ 88:1131, 1963 ⟨I-02598⟩

K[elly], A.D.: Thomas Clarence Routley: an appreciation. CMAJ 88:860, 1963 ⟨I-01695⟩

MacDermot, H.E.: Dr. T. Clarence Routley, an appreciation. CMAJ 88:1046, 1963 ⟨I-01672⟩

S[awyer], G.: Thomas Clarence Routley, MD, FRCP(C), LLD, DSc, CBE. Ontario Medical Review 30:202-203, 1963. ⟨I-02601⟩

Stewart, B.: CMA's Dr. T. Clarence Routley: 34 Years of Devoted Service. CMAJ 129:642-643, 645, 1983 ⟨I-05171⟩

Walker, E.R.C.: Dr. T. Clarence Routley, an appreciation. CMAJ 88:1223, 1963 ⟨I-02597⟩

Rowand, A. (1816?-1889)

Mitchell, R.: Doctor Alexander Rowand 1816(?)-1889. CACHB 7(4):1-5, 1943 ⟨I-01126⟩

Thorington, J.M.: Four Physicians-Explorers of the Fur Trade. Annals of Medical History, ser. 3, 4:294-301, 1942 ⟨I-04905⟩

Roy, F. (1898-1974)

S., E.: Le docteur Francois Roy. CMAJ 111:569, 1974 ⟨I-05170⟩

Russel, C.K. (1877-1956)

Francis, W.W.: Colin Russel, the Man. CMAJ 77:716-718, 1957 ⟨I-04714⟩

McNaughton, F.L.: Colin Russel, a pioneer of Canadian neurology. CMAJ 77:719-723, 1957 ⟨I-02576⟩

Penfield, W., Francis, W.W., Russell, C.: Tributes to Colin Kerr Russel 1877-1956. CMAJ 77:715-723, 1957 ⟨I-02590⟩

Ruttan, R.F. (1856-1930)

Macallum, A.B.: Robert Fulford Ruttan. CMAJ 22:596-97, 1930 ⟨I-03029⟩

Tory, H.M.: Robert Fulford Ruttan. CMAJ 22:597, 1930 ⟨I-03013⟩

Ryerson, G.S. (1855-1925)

Anderson, H.B.: George Sterling Ryerson. CMAJ 15:971, 1925 ⟨I-01183⟩

Ryerson, G.S.: Looking backward. Toronto, The Ryerson Press, 1924. 264 p. ⟨I-01148⟩

Watson, I.A.: George Sterling Ryerson. In: Physicians and Surgeons of America. Concord, Republican Press Association, 1896. pp 545 ⟨I-02524⟩

S

Salter, R.B.

McCaffery, M.: Missionary Doctor -- In Deepest Toronto [Dr. Robert B. Salter]. Canadian Family Physician 25:487-490, 1979 ⟨I-01078⟩

Sampson, J. (1789-1861)

Angus, M.S.: James Sampson. DCB 9:699-701, 1976 ⟨I-01113⟩

Samson, J.E. (1894-1963)

Favreau, J.C.: Dr. J. Edouard Samson, an appreciation. CMAJ 89:832, 1963 ⟨I-01991⟩

Sarrazin, M. (1659-1734)

Abbott, M.E.: An early Canadian biologist -- Michel Sarrazin (1659-1735) his life and times. CMAJ 19:600-607, 1928 ⟨I-01982⟩

Coulson, F.: Michel Sarrazin (1659-1734). CACHB 7(2):1-6, 1942 ⟨I-01118⟩

Kelly, H.A.: Michel S. Sarrazin (1659-1734). In Kelly HW, Burrage WL: Dictionary of American Medical Biography. New York and London, D. Appleton and Co., 1928. pp. 1077-1078 ⟨I-01117⟩

Laflamme, M.L.: I -- Michel Sarrazin: Materiaux pour servir a l'histoire de la science en Canada. PTRSC 5:1-23, 1887 ⟨I-01969⟩

LeBlond, S.: Michel Sarrazin: un document inedit. Laval Medical 31(3):1-8, 1961 ⟨I-01981⟩

LeBlond, S.: Le testament de Michel Sarrazin. La Vie medicale au Canada francais 3:510-513, 1974 ⟨I-04655⟩

Massicotte, E.Z.: Un Document du Docteur Sarrazin. L'UMC 49:418-420, 1920 ⟨I-01770⟩

Tondreau, R.L.: Michel Sarrazin (1659-1734): the father of French Canadian science. Trans. and Studies of the College of Physicians of Philadelphia 31:124-127, 1963 ⟨I-01983⟩

Vallee, A.: Un Biologiste Canadien, Michel Sarrazin (1659-1739). Quebec, Archives de Quebec, 1927. 291 pp ⟨I-01968⟩

Vallee, A.: Michel Sarrazin (1659-1734). The Crest 5(5):9-10, 1962 ⟨I-01990⟩

Saucier, J. (1899-1968)

Desjardins, E.: Le Docteur Jean Saucier. CMAJ 100:446-447, 1969 ⟨I-05043⟩

Savage, M.S. (1901-1970)

McFadden, I.: The Indomitable Savage. Toronto, United Church of Canada, Board of Information and Stewardship, 1963. ⟨I-05060⟩

Sawyer, G.I.

Gray, C.: Glenn Ivan Sawyer. CMAJ 124:514, 1981 ⟨I-03164⟩

Scarlett, E.P. (1896-1982)

Roland, C.G.: Dr. Earle Scarlett: melding tradition and beauty in historical writing. CMAJ 122:822-826, 1980 ⟨I-01074⟩

Schoenfeld, R.W. (1906-)

Hellstedt, L.McG. (edit): Rebe Willits Schoenfeld. In: Women Physicians of the World: Autobiographies of Medical Pioneers New York, McGraw-Hill Book Co., 1978. pp 326-32 ⟨I-03922⟩

Schultz, J.C. (1840-1896)

Campbell, M.: Dr. J.C. Schultz. Historical and Scientific Society of Manitoba Papers, series 3, No. 20:7-12, 1965 ⟨I-02579⟩

Halpenny, J.: Sir John Christian Schultz (1840-1896). In Kelly HW, Burrage WL: Dictionary of American Medical Biography, New York and London, D. Appleton and Co., 1928. pp. 1083-1084. ⟨I-01104⟩

Scarlett, E.P.: Sir John Christian Schultz (1840-1896). CACHB 8(2):1-7, 1943 ⟨I-01979⟩

Scott, E. (1866-1958)

Buck, R.M.: The Mathesons of Saskatchewan Diocese. Saskatchewan History 13:41-62, 1960 ⟨I-03560⟩

Scott, J. (1816-?1865)

Rasporich, A.W., Clarke, I.H.: John Scott. DCB 9:706-707, 1976 ⟨I-01114⟩

Scrimger, F.A.C. (1878-1937)

Archibald, E.: Dr. Francis Alexander Carron Scrimger. CMAJ 36:323, 1937 ⟨I-03435⟩

Howell, W.B.: Colonel F.A.C. Scrimger, V.C. CMAJ 38:279-281, 1938 ⟨I-03372⟩

Secord, W.H. (1883-1936)

M., R.: Dr. Wesley Herbert Secord. CMAJ 35:105, 1936 ⟨I-02870⟩

Selby, G. (1759-1835)

Lefebvre, J.J., Desjardins, E.: Le Docteur George Selby, Medecin de L'Hotel-Dieu de 1807 a 1829, et sa Famille. L'UMC 100:1592-1594, 1971 ⟨I-02244⟩

Selye, H. (1907-1982)

B., B.: Hans Selye. CMAJ 123:316, 1980 ⟨I-02853⟩

Goupil, G: Hans Selye: La Sagesse du Stress. Nouvelle Optique, 1981, 169 p. ⟨I-04196⟩

Selye, H.: The story of the adaptation syndrome. Montreal, ACTA, Inc., Medical Publishers, 1952. 225 p. ⟨I-01076⟩

Selye, H.: From dream to discovery: on being a scientist. New York/Toronto, McGraw-Hill Book Co., 1964. 419 p. ⟨I-01075⟩

Selye, H: The Stress of My Life: A Scientist's Memories. Toronto, McClelland and Stewart, 1977/ 272 p. ⟨I-03938⟩

Serres, A. (1732-1812)
Lessard, R.: Alexandre Serres. DCB 5:752, 1983 ⟨I-05304⟩

Shadd, A.S. (1870-1915)
Thomson, C.A.: Doc Shadd. Saskatchean History 30:41-55, 1977 ⟨I-01029⟩
Thomson, C.A.: Saskatchewan's black pioneer doctor [Alfred Schmitz Shadd]. Canadian Family Physician 23:1343-1351, 1977 ⟨I-01980⟩

Shaner, R.F. (1893-1976)
Collier, H.B.: Ralph Faust Shaner 1893-1976. PTRSC series 4, 16:113-114, 1978 ⟨I-04957⟩

Sharpe, E.M. (1862-1947)
Stanley, G.D.: Dr. Edward M. Sharpe. CACHB 11:57-63, 1946 ⟨I-02169⟩

Shaw, J.H. (1907-1957)
K[elly], A.D.: Dr. J. Harold Shaw. CMAJ 77:276, 1957 ⟨I-04752⟩

Shenstone, N.S. (1881-1970)
C, W.G.: Dr. Norman Strahan Shenstone. CMAJ 102:1112-1113, 1970 ⟨I-01675⟩

Shepherd, F.J. (1851-1929)
Bazin, A.T.: Francis J. Shepherd. McGill News 36:25, 55, 57-59, 1955 ⟨I-01693⟩
Blackader, A.D.: Dr. Francis J. Shepherd. CMAJ 20:210-211, 1929 ⟨I-01677⟩
Howell, W.B.: F.J. Shepherd: His Life and Times. Toronto and Vancouver, J.M. Dent and Sons Ltd., 1934. 251 p. ⟨I-01639⟩
MacDermot, H.E.: Francis J. Shepherd, M.D. LL.D. (Harvard, McGill, Queen's), Hon. F.R.C.S. Engl, Hon. F.A.C.S. Canadian Journal of Surgery 1:5-7, 1957-8 ⟨I-04242⟩
Macphail, A.: Howell's "Shepherd". CMAJ 669-672, 1934 ⟨I-01676⟩
Mills, J.A.: Dr. Francis John Shepherd. McGill Medical Journal 22:67-72, 1953 ⟨I-01678⟩
Primrose, A.: Dr. Francis J. Shepherd, an appreciation. CMAJ 20:211-212, 1929 ⟨I-01691⟩
Shepherd, F.J.: Reminiscences of Student Days and Dissecting Room. Montreal, 1919. Printed for private circulation only. 28 p. ⟨I-01640⟩
Stewart, J.: Dr. Francis J. Shepherd, an appreciation. CMAJ 20:212, 1929 ⟨I-01692⟩
Thompson, I.M.: F.J. Shepherd as anatomist. CMAJ 39:287-290, 1938 ⟨I-01679⟩

Shulman, M. (1925-)
Shulman, M.: Coroner. Toronto/Montreal/Winnipeg/Vancouver, Fitzhenry and Whiteside, 1975. 154 p. ⟨I-01081⟩
Shulman, M.: Member of the legislature. Toronto/Montreal/Winnipeg/Vancouver, Fitzhenry and Whiteside, 1979. 226 p. ⟨I-01079⟩

Silver, L.M. (1864-1951)
Scammell, H.L.: Dr. Louis Morton Silver. Nova Scotia Medical Bulletin 30:165-167, 1951 ⟨I-01689⟩

Silverthorn, G. (1889-1926)
Cameron, M.H.V.: Dr. Gideon Silverthorn. CMAJ 17:129, 1927 ⟨I-01688⟩

Simard, L.-C. (1900-1970)
Lauze, S: Louis-Charles Simard, 1900-1970. L'UMC 1314-1315, 1970 ⟨I-01077⟩

Simpson, J.C. (1876-1944)
Martin, C.F.: Dean J.C. Simpson. McGill Medical Journal 13:257-260, 1944 ⟨I-01680⟩

Simpson, T. (1833-1918)
Claxton, B.: Dr. Thomas Simpson (1833-1918; McGill, Med. 1854). Canadian Services Medical Journal 13:420-438, 1957 ⟨I-01681⟩
MacDermot, H.E.: The papers of Dr. Thomas Simpson (1833-1918). CMAJ 77:266-267, 1957 ⟨I-01687⟩

Skinner, H.A.L. (1899-1967)
Barry, J.L., Carr, D.H., Buck, R.C.: Dr. Henry Alan Lawson Skinner. CMAJ 96:1182, 1967 ⟨I-01686⟩

Slayter, W.B. (1841-1898)
Campbell, D.A.: William B. Slayter (1841-1898). In Kelly HW, Burrage WL: Dictionary of American Medical Biography. New York and London, D. Appleton and Co., 1928. p. 1120 ⟨I-01098⟩

Smallwood, C. (1812-1873)
Marshall, J.S.: Charles Smallwood. DCB 10:658-659, 1972 ⟨I-01096⟩

Smith, E. (1859-1949)
Strong-Boag, V.(edit.): A Woman with a Purpose: The Diaries of Elizabeth Smith 1872-1884. Toronto/Buffalo/London, University of Toronto Press, 1980. 298 p. ⟨I-02592⟩

Smith, F. (1903-1949)
Murray, E.G.D.: Frederick Smith. McGill Medical Journal 18:155-157, 1949 ⟨I-01631⟩

Smith, H.
Morton, C.S.: Doctor Herbert Smith. Nova Scotia Medical Bulletin 28:122-124, 1949 ⟨I-01997⟩

Smith, H. (1790-1872)
Spack, V.M.: The story of a pioneer doctor -- Harmaunus Smith. Wentworth Bygones 5:40-43, 1964 ⟨I-01630⟩

Smith, H.R. (1873-1928)
Whitelaw, T.H.: Dr. Henry Richard Smith. CMAJ 19:737-738, 1928 ⟨I-03490⟩

Smith, H.W. (1914-1967)
Ferguson, J.K.W.: Dr. H. Ward Smith, an appreciation. CMAJ 97:552-553, 1967 ⟨I-01674⟩
Lucas, D.M.: H. Ward Smith. CMAJ 97:363-364, 1967 ⟨I-01684⟩
Smith, J.F. (1858-) Smith, J.F.: Life's Waking Part. Toronto, Thomas Nelson and Sons, Ltd., 1937. 345 p. ⟨I-02306⟩

Smith, W. (fl. 1784-1803)
Morgan, R.J.: William Smith. DCB 5:766-67, 1983 ⟨I-05303⟩

Smith, W.E.
Smith, W.E.: A Canadian Doctor in West China: Forty Years under Three Flags. Toronto, Ryerson Press, 1939. 278 p. ⟨I-01092⟩

Smith, W.H. (1868-1940)
Martin, C.F.: William Harvey Smith, an appreciation. CMAJ 43:87, 1940 ⟨I-03357⟩
Mitchell, R.: William Harvey Smith. CMAJ 43:86-87, 1940 ⟨I-03364⟩

Smith, W.H. (fl. 1843-1973)
Morley, W.F.E.: William Henry Smith. DCB 10:660-661, 1972 ⟨I-01101⟩

Smyth, C.E. (1870-)
Stanley, G.D.: Dr. Charles Ernest Smyth: pioneer doctor of Medicine Hat. CMAJ 58:200-204, 1948 ⟨I-01660⟩

Smyth, H. (1941-)
O'Malley, M.: A Doctor's Dilemma. Saturday Night, May 1983, pp 19-29, 1983 ⟨I-05073⟩

Smyth, W.H. (1873-1941)
MacDermot, H.E.: Dr. Walter H. Smyth. CMAJ 45:287-288, 1941 ⟨I-03521⟩

Somers, J. (1840-1898)
Campbell, D.A.: John Somers (1840-1898). In Kelly HW, Burrage WL: Dictionary of American Medical Biography. New York and London, D. Appleton and Co., 1928. p. 1142 ⟨I-01099⟩

Souart, G. (ca. 1611-1691)
Maurault, O.: Gabriel Souart. DCB 1:612-613, 1966 ⟨I-01001⟩

Soupiran, S. (1704-1764)
Moogk, P.N.: Simon Soupiran. DCB 3:595-596, 1974 ⟨I-01106⟩

Spagniolini, J.-F. (1704-1764)
Moogk, P.N.: Jean-Fernand Spagniolini. DCB 3:597-598, 1974 ⟨I-01107⟩

Sparks, W.E.L. (-1963)
C., G.C.: Dr. Willmot E.L. Sparks, an appreciation. CMAJ 89-99, 1963 ⟨I-01658⟩

Speakman, T.J. (1924-1969)
Macbeth, R.A.: Dr. Thomas John Speakman: an appreciation. CMAJ 100:782-783, 1969 ⟨I-05045⟩

Speechly, H.M. (1866-1951)
Mitchell, R.: Dr. H.M. Speechly. CMAJ 64:460, 1951 ⟨I-04546⟩

Spence, P.M. (1913-1958)
H., W.P.: Dr. Peter McKellar Spence. CMAJ 78:811, 1958 ⟨I-04749⟩

Spencer, B. (1853-1902)
Clarkson, F.A.: Dr. Bertram Spencer, MB, MRCS. CACHB 7(3):1-5, 1942 ⟨I-01102⟩

Spilsbury, E.A. (1855-)
Watson, I.A.: Edward Attrill Spilsbury. In:Physicians and Surgeons of America. Concord, Republican Press Association, 1896. p 45 ⟨I-02525⟩

Stalker, M.R. (1901-1965)
Quintin, T.J.: Dr. Murray Stalker, an appreciation. CMAJ 92:437, 1965 ⟨I-01632⟩

Stanbury, W.S. (1905-1962)
M., G.W.: Dr. W. Stuart Stanbury. CMAJ 87:1208, 1962 ⟨I-01633⟩

Stanley, G.D. (1876-1954)
Clarkson, F.A.: Douglass Stanley: An Appreciation. CACHB 19(1):27-30, 1954 ⟨I-01086⟩
Scarlett, E.P.: Salutation to an elder. CACHB 17:59-60, 1952 ⟨I-01083⟩
Scarlett, E.P.: And...at the last. No Marble, No Conventional Phrase. CACHB 19:32-34, 1954 ⟨I-01087⟩
Stanley, G.D.: A Medical Pilgrim's Progress. CACHB 3(2):5-9, 1938 ⟨I-01084⟩
Stanley, G.D.: A pioneer funeral. CACHB 11:13-15, 1946 ⟨I-01088⟩
Stanley, G.D.: One physician's honeymoon. CACHB 11:47-48, 1946 ⟨I-01090⟩
Strachan, M.: "Dr. Stanley" 1876-1954. CACHB 19:23-26, 1954 ⟨I-01085⟩

Stanton, A.T. 1875-1938
Keith, W.D.: Some Early Canadian Ships' Surgeons. B.C. Medical Journal 1:103-116, 1959 ⟨I-04199⟩

Starr, C.L. (1868-1928)
Janes, R.M.: Dr. Clarence Leslie Starr. Canadian Journal of Surgery 3:109-111, 1959-60 ⟨I-04237⟩
Primrose, A.: Dr. Clarence L. Starr. CMAJ 20:212, 1929 ⟨I-01634⟩

Starr, F.N.G. (1867-1934)
Berube, B.: Dr. F.N.G. Starr: in memory of the medical statesman. CMAJ 127:417, 419-421, 1982 ⟨I-04890⟩
Graham, R.R.: Frederic Newton Gisborne Starr, CBE, MB, MD, CM, FRGS. CMAJ 30:694-695, 1923 ⟨I-01636⟩

Steiman, I. (1898-1981)
Gibson, W.C.: Pioneer Physician and Scientific Translator: Dr. Iser Steiman. Canadian Family Physician 28:549-50, 1982 ⟨I-04773⟩

Stephenson, J. (1797-1842)
Francis, W.W.: Repair of Cleft Palate by Philibert Roux in 1819. A Translation of John Stephenson's De Velosynthesi. JHMAS 18:209-219, 1963 ⟨I-01111⟩
Macphail, A.: John Stephenson (1797-1842). In Kelly HW, Burrage WL: Dictionary of American Medical Biography. New York and London, D. Appleton and Co., 1928. p. 1157 ⟨I-01108⟩
Stephenson, J.: Repair of Cleft Palate by Philibert Roux in 1819. Plastic and Reconstructive Surgery 47:277-283, 1971 ⟨I-01109⟩
Wallace, A.B.: Canadian-Franco-Scottish co-operation: A Cleft-Palate Story. British Journal of Plastic Surgery 19(1):1-14, 1966 ⟨I-01110⟩
Whiteford, W.: Reminiscences of Dr. John Stephenson, one of the founders of McGill Medical Faculty. Canadian Medical and Surgical Journal 11:728-731, 1883 ⟨I-01112⟩

Stevenson, G.H. (1894-1976)

Barrt, M.L.: George Herbert Stevenson 1894-1976. PTRSC series 4, 15:114-116, 1977 ⟨I-01646⟩

Stevenson, R.A. (1848-1919)

S, F.J.: Robert A. Stevenson, M.D. CMAJ 10:207-208, 1920 ⟨I-01651⟩

Stewart, C.B. (1902-)

Swartz, D.: An appreciation of C.B. Stewart. Manitoba Medical Review 46:486-487, 1966 ⟨I-01647⟩

Stewart, C.C. (1888-1958)

F., R.: Dr. Charles C. Stewart. CMAJ 78:551-552, 1958 ⟨I-01655⟩

Stewart, D.A. (1874-1937)

Ferguson, R.G.: Dr. D.A. Stewart. CMAJ 36:435, 1937 ⟨I-03441⟩

Gordon, A.H.: Dr. D.A. Stewart. CMAJ 36:435-436, 1937 ⟨I-03440⟩

Mitchell, R.: Dr. D.A. Stewart. CMAJ 36:435, 1937 ⟨I-03879⟩

Morgan, H.V.: David Alexander Stewart (1874-1937). CACHB 6(2):1-5, 1941 ⟨I-01094⟩

Stewart, J. (1846-1906)

Macphail, A.: James Stewart (1846-1906). In Kelly HW, Burrage WL: Dictionary of American Medical Biography New York and London, D. Appleton and Co., 1928. p 1166-1167 ⟨I-01097⟩

Stewart, J. (1848-1933)

Falconer, J.W.: Dr. John Stewart. CMAJ 30:224, 1934 ⟨I-01717⟩

Fraser-Harris, D.F.: Dr. John Stewart. CMAJ 30:223-224, 1934 ⟨I-01716⟩

Gass, C.L.: John Stewart Memorial Lecture. Nova Scotia Medical Bulletin 41:188-196, 1962 ⟨I-01637⟩

Murphy, G.H.: John Stewart. CMAJ 30:222-223, 1934 ⟨I-03549⟩

Scammell, H.L.: John Stewart. Canadian Journal of Surgery 4:263-237, 1960-61 ⟨I-04239⟩

Thomson, St. C.: Dr. John Stewart. CMAJ 30:222, 1934 ⟨I-01718⟩

Stewart, O.W. (-1950)

Elliott, H.: Dr. O.W. Stewart. CMAJ, 63:618, 1950 ⟨I-04513⟩

Moorman, L.J.: Bill Stewart as Student, Patient and Friend. CMAJ 63: 618-9, 1950 ⟨I-04514⟩

Stewart, W.G. (1860-1928)

Hamilton, W.F.: Dr. William Grant Stewart. CMAJ 18:630, 1928 ⟨I-01623⟩

Martin, C.F.: Dr. William Grant Stewart, an appreciation. CMAJ 18:630-631, 1928 ⟨I-01652⟩

Stimson, E. (1792-1869)

Godfrey, C.M.: Elam Stimson. DCB 9:748-749, 1976 ⟨I-01103⟩

St. Martin, A. (1794-1880)

Bensley, E.H.: Alexis St. Martin. CMAJ 80:907-909, 1959 ⟨I-01971⟩

LeBlond, S.: AlexisSt-Martin: Sa Vie et Son Temps. Laval Medical 33:578-585, 1962 ⟨I-01970⟩

Stokes, A.B. (1906-1978)

Sarwer-Foner, G.J.: In Memoriam: Professor Aldwyn Brockway Stokes, CBE, MA, BM, BCH (Oxon), DCH, DPM, FRCP (Lond), FRCP (C), February 23, 1906 - May 3, 1978. Psychiatric Journal of the University of Ottawa 3:235-236, 1978 ⟨I-01080⟩

Stowe, E.H. (1831-1903)

Montagnes, J.: Emily Howard Stowe, physician and social reformer. Canadian Doctor 47(2):27, 1981 ⟨I-04195⟩

Roberts, W.: Six New Women: A Guide to the Mental Map of Women Reformers in Toronto. Atlantis 3:145-164, 1977-8 ⟨I-01975⟩

Thompson, J.E.: The influence of Dr. Emily Howard Stowe on the woman suffrage movement in Canada. Ontario History 54:253-266, 1962 ⟨I-01638⟩

Waxman, S.B.: Dr. Emily Stowe: Canada's First Female Practitioner. Canada West 10(1) 17:23, 1980 ⟨I-04764⟩

Stowe-Gullen, A.S. (1857-1943)

Roberts, W.: Six New Women: A Guide to the Mental Map of Women Reformers in Toronto. Atlantis 3:145-164, 1977-8 ⟨I-01976⟩

Smith, K.: Dr. Augusta Stowe-Gullen: A Pioneer of Social Conscience. CMAJ 126:1465-1467, 1982 ⟨I-04900⟩

Strathy, G.S. (1843-1925)

Hutchison, H.S.: Dr. George Stewart Strathy. CMAJ 15:1172-1173, 1925 ⟨I-02300⟩

Strong, G.F. (-1957)

K[elly], A.D.: Dr. George Frederick Strong. CMAJ 76:517, 1957 ⟨I-04731⟩

Struthers, E.B. (1886-)

Struthers, E.B.: A Doctor Remembers: Days in China and Korea. 1976, 146 p. ⟨I-04435⟩

Sullivan, M.T. (1874-1928)

Walker, S.L.: Michael Thomas Sullivan, MD. CMAJ 19:739-740, 1928 ⟨I-03494⟩

Suzor, F-M. (1756-1810)

Lessard, R.: Francois-Michel Suzor. DCB 5:788-89, 1983 ⟨I-05302⟩

Sylvain, T.

Desjardins, E.: L'Odyssee du Sieur Timothee Sylvain, Medecin de Montreal. L'UMC 98:91-94, 1969 ⟨I-02245⟩

T

Tache, E.-P. (1795-1865)

Desilets, A.: Sir Etienne-Paschal Tache. DCB 9:774-779, 1976 ⟨I-02251⟩

Tailhandler, M. (1665-1738)

Neatby, L.H.: Marien Tailhandler. DCB 2:617-618, 1969 ⟨I-01193⟩

Tait, J. (1878-1944)

Scratch, G.W.: John Tait 1878-1944. PTRSC 39:119-122, 1945 ⟨I-03570⟩

Taylor, G.H. (1790-1890)

Taylor, H.L.: Henry Taylor (1790-1890). In Kelly H.W., Burrage W.L.: Dictionary of American Medical Biography. New York and London, D. Appleton and Co., 1928. p. 1188 ⟨I-01158⟩

Taylor, H.I. (1862-1943)

Kirkland, A.S.: Dr. H.I. Taylor. CMAJ 48:464-465, 1943 ⟨I-02698⟩

Taylor, W.O. (1859-1943)

Taylor, R.B.: Dr. William Oliver Taylor. CMAJ 49:150, 152, 1943 ⟨I-02756⟩

Tehorenhaegnon (fl. 1628-37)

Jury, E.M.: Tehorenhaegnon. DCB 1:634-635, 1966 ⟨I-01002⟩

Tempest, W. (1819-1871)

Elliott, J.H.: William Tempest, MB, LMB, UC 1819-1871. Ontario Medical Association Bulletin 5:37-47, 1938 ⟨I-04762⟩

Temple, J.A. (1843-1931)

Anderson, H.B.: Dr. James Algernon Temple. CMAJ 26:258, 1932 ⟨I-03042⟩

Templeman, W. (1907-1966)

Miller, L.A.: Dr. Walter Templeman, an appreciation. CMAJ 95:1219, 1966 ⟨I-02753⟩

Templeton, C.P. (1874-1929)

Edmison, J.H., Baragar, C.A.: Charles Perry Templeton, CBE, DSO, VD, MD, CM. CMAJ 21:238, 1929 ⟨I-02699⟩

Thackeray, J.B. (1890-1955)

D., J.K.M.: Dr. Joseph Bulmer Thackeray. CMAJ, 72:713-4, 1955 ⟨I-04576⟩

Thomas, M.W. (1882-1944)

M., J.H.: Morris W. Thomas, M.D., C.M. CMAJ 52:112, 1945 ⟨I-04361⟩

Thompson, E. (fl.1725-1749)

Williams, G.: Edward Thompson. DCB 3:624-625, 1974 ⟨I-01195⟩

Thompson, I.M. (-1981)

Moore, K.L.: Dr. Ian MacLaren Thompson. University of Manitoba Medical Journal 52:9, 1982 ⟨I-04971⟩

Sigurdson, L.A.: Dr. Ian MacLaren Thompson. University of Manitoba Medical Journal 52:8-9, 1982 ⟨I-04970⟩

Sirluck, E.: Dr. Ian MacLaren Thompson. University of Manitoba Medical Journal 52:7-8, 1982 ⟨I-04969⟩

Thompson, W.E. (1859-1953)

Thompson, I.M.: A doctor of the old school. CMAJ 69:74-75, 1953 ⟨I-02749⟩

Thomson, J. (1808-1884)

McGahan, E.W.: John Thomson. DCM 11:878-888, 1982 ⟨I-04855⟩

Thorlakson, P.H.T. (1895-)

Gray, C.: Paul H.T. Thorlakson. CMAJ 128:1211, 1983 ⟨I-05056⟩

Tiffany, O. (1763-1835)

Farmer, M.H.: The ledger of an early doctor of Barton and Ancaster, 1798-1801. Wentworth Bygones 8:34-38, 1969 ⟨I-02987⟩

Tiffin, E.R. (1903-1964)

S., L.J.: Dr. E.R. Tiffin. CMAJ 90:1139, 1964 ⟨I-05226⟩

Tilley, A.R. (-1983)

Gray, C.: A. Ross Tilley. CMAJ 129:154, 1983 ⟨I-05216⟩

Tisdall, F.F. (1893-1949)

Brown, A.: Frederick F. Tisdall, MD, MB(Tor), MRCS (Eng), LRCP (Lond) FRCP(C). CMAJ 64:263-265, 1951 ⟨I-02701⟩

Brown, A., Drake, T.G.H., Ebbs, J.H.: Dr. Fred F. Tisdall. CMAJ 61:86, 1949 ⟨I-04502⟩

Todd, J.L. (1876-1949)

Fallis, A.M.: John L. Todd: Canada's First Professor of Parasitology. CMAJ 129:486, 488-89, 1983 ⟨I-05213⟩

Todd, J.O. (1864-1929)

Mitchell, R.: Dr. John Orchard Todd. CMAJ 21:748, 1929 ⟨I-02746⟩

Tofield, J.H. (1840-1918)

Newerla, G.J.: Canadian Medical History: James Henry Tofield. M.D. September 1967, page 31 ⟨I-02745⟩

Tolmie, W.F. (1812-1886)

Hopwood, V.: William Fraser Tolmie: Natural Scientist and Patriot. British Columbia Studies, 5:45-51, 1970. ⟨I-03167⟩

Johansen, D.O.: William Fraser Tolmie of the Hudson's Bay Company 1833-1870. The Beaver 268(2):29-32, 1937 ⟨I-03230⟩

Jones, O.M.: William Fraser Tolmie (1812-1886). In Kelly HW, Burrage WL: Dictionary of American Medical Biography. New York and London, D. Appleton and Co., 1928. p. 1216. ⟨I-01153⟩

Lamb, W.K.: William Fraser Tolmie. DCB 11:885-888, 1982 ⟨I-04856⟩

Scarlett, E.P.: A Doctor of the Frontier. Group Practice 16:659-664, 1967 ⟨I-03554⟩

Tolmie, S.F.: My Father: William Fraser Tolmie, 1812-1886. British Columbia Historical Quarterly 1:227-240, 1937 ⟨I-05066⟩

Trainor, W.C. (1895-1957)

M[itchell], R.M.: Dr. Owen C. Trainor,. CMAJ 76:165, 1957 ⟨I-04756⟩

Treleaven, G.W. (-1931)

Webster, W.: Major George Willard Treleaven. CMAJ 24:475, 1931 ⟨I-03066⟩

Trout, J. (1841-1921)

Hacker, C.: Jennie Trout: An Indomitable Lady Doctor Whose History Was lost for a Half-Century. CMAJ 110:841-3, 1974 ⟨I-05370⟩

Truax, W.

Truax, W.: Reminiscences of a Country Doctor. CMAJ 60:411-415, 1949 ⟨I-01051⟩

Tufts, W.B. (1906-1982)

Cooper, R.C.: Dr. William Burton Tufts. CMAJ 127:309, 1982 ⟨I-04901⟩

Tupper, C. (1821-1915)

Longley, J.W.: Sir Charles Tupper. Toronto, Makers of Canada (Morang) Ltd., 1916. 304 p. ⟨I-05051⟩

McInnis, R.: Sir Charles Tupper -- Nova Scotia's Father of Confederation. Dalhousie Medical Journal 20:99-106, 1967 ⟨I-03562⟩

McIntosh, A.W.: The Career of Sir Charles Tupper in Canada, 1864-1900. Thesis, University of Toronto, Ph.D., 1970, 598 pages ⟨I-04893⟩

O., W.: Sir Charles Tupper, Bart. Lancet 2:1049-50, 1915 ⟨I-05177⟩

O[sler], W.: The Right Hon. Sir Charles Tupper, Bart. M.D., Edin. The Lancet, 2:1049-50, 1915 ⟨I-05218⟩

Sanders, E.M. (Edit.): The Life and Letters of the Rt. Hon. Sir Charles Tupper, Bart., K.C.M.G., Vol. 1 and Vol. 2. New York, Frederick A. Stokes Co., 1916. 319 p. -- Vol. II 298 p. ⟨I-01155⟩

Simpson, J.H.L.: The life of Sir Charles Tupper. CMAJ 40:606-610, 1939 ⟨I-03375⟩

Stanley, G.D.: Sir Charles Tupper 1812-1915. CACHB 6(4):1-9, 1942 ⟨I-01157⟩

Tait, D.H.: Dr. Charles Tupper: A Father of Confederation. Collections of the Nova Scotia Historical Society 36:279-300, 1968 ⟨I-01156⟩

Tupper, C.: Recollections of Sixty Years. Cassell and Company, Ltd, London, New York, Toronto, and Melbourne, 1914, 414p. ⟨I-04553⟩

Turcot, J. (-1977)

Dionne, L.: Hommage Au Docteur Jacques Turcot. Canadian Journal of Surgery 20:567, 1977 ⟨I-04289⟩

V

Vail, E.A. (1817-1885)

Whalen, J.M.: Edwin Arnold Vail. DCB 11:896-97, 1982 ⟨I-04857⟩

Vaisrub, S. (1906-1980)

Blum, A.: Vaisrub: Good Language with a Light Touch. CMAJ 127:307-308, 1982 ⟨I-04903⟩

Blum, A.: Remembering Sam Vaisrub. University of Manitoba Medical Journal 53:17-19, 1983 ⟨I-05132⟩

[Blum, A.]: Samuel Vaisrub, M.D., Clinician, Editor, 'Amateur'. University of Manitoba Medical Journal 53:16-17, 1983 ⟨I-05131⟩

Blum, A.: Vaisrub: Good Language with a Light Touch. University of Manitoba Medical Journal 53:14-15, 1983 ⟨I-05133⟩

Vallee, A. (1882-1939)

Delage, C.F.: Arthur Vallee (1882-1939). PTRSC 33:155-157, 1939 ⟨I-03577⟩

LeBlond, S.: Arthur Vallee, M.D. Newsletter, Canadian Society for the History of Medicine, 6:15-16, 1981 ⟨I-04767⟩

Valois, M.-F. (1801-1869)

Chabot, R.: Michel-Francois Valois. DCB 9:802-803, 1976 ⟨I-01192⟩

Seguin, R-L.: Le docteur Valois, un patriote ignore. Le Bulletin des Rechereches Historiques 60:85-91, 1954 ⟨I-01024⟩

Van Cortlandt, E. (1805-1875)

Bond, C.C.J.: Edward van Cortlandt. DCB 10:691-692, 1972 ⟨I-01189⟩

Vango, H.M. (1895-1931)

Ower, J.J.: Dr. Harold Main Vango. CMAJ 26:377, 1932 ⟨I-03061⟩

VanWart, G.C. (1868-1938)

Kirkland, A.S.: Dr. George Clowes VanWart. CMAJ 39:510, 1938 ⟨I-03329⟩

Verey, G. (1830-1881)

Rasporich, A.W., Getty, I.A.L.: George Verey. DCB 11:900-901, 1982 ⟨I-04858⟩

Verge, W.

Verge, W.: Mon Cinquantenaire de Pratique Medico-Chirurgicale. L'UMC 87:958-962, 1958 ⟨I-01057⟩

Veronneau, A. (1707-1764)

Duclos, L.: Agathe Veronneau. DCB 3:643, 1974 ⟨I-01194⟩

Vincent, T.S. (1868-1933)

Cameron, A.T.: The late Professor Swale Vincent. CMAJ 30:335, 1934 ⟨I-03535⟩

Vineberg, H.N. (1857-1945)

Ballon, H.C., Ballon, S.C.: Hiram Nahum Vineberg 1857-1945. Canadian Jewish Historical Society Journal 3:1-9, 1979 ⟨I-02865⟩

Vogl, J.F. (1888-1963)

Sabia, M.J.: Dr. Joseph F. Vogl, an appreciation. CMAJ 89:834, 1963 ⟨I-02739⟩

W

Waddell, J. (1810-1878)

Spray, W.A.: John Waddell. DCB 10:695-696, 1972 ⟨I-01190⟩

Wade, M.S. (1858-1929)

Murphy, H.H.: Dr. M.S. Wade. CMAJ 20:682, 1929 ⟨I-02738⟩

Waldron, J. (1744-1818)

Handcock, W.G.: John Waldron. DCB 5:837-839, 1983 ⟨I-05301⟩

Wallace, J.B. (1919-1974)

W., J.D.: Dr. J. Beatty Wallace. CMAJ 111:171, 1974 ⟨I-05168⟩

Walton, C.H.A. (1906-)

Walton, C.H.A.: A Medical Odyssey. Winnipeg, The Winnipeg Clinic, 1980 ⟨I-05052⟩

Walton, G. (1894-1963)

K[elly], A.D.: Dr. George Walton. CMAJ 90:704, 1964 ⟨I-05222⟩

Warner, W.P. (1896-1955)

M., R.I.: Wilfred Parsons Warner, DSC, CBE, MB, FRCP(c), LL.D.(Tor). CMAJ 74:167-168, 1956 ⟨I-04741⟩

Warwick, W. (1881-1943)

Kirkland, A.S.: Dr. William Warwick. CMAJ 49:68, 1943 ⟨I-04267⟩

Watson, A.D. (1859-1926)

Chant, C.A.: Albert Durrant Watson. Journal of the Royal Astronomical Society of Canada 20:153-157, 1926 ⟨I-02706⟩

Elliott, J.H.: Albert Durrant Watson, M.D. CMAJ 16:991-992, 1926 ⟨I-01954⟩

Pierce, L.: Albert Durrant Watson (1859-1926). Toronto, 1924. 30 p. n.p. ⟨I-03420⟩

Weaver, M. McD. (1901-1963)

Mather, J.M.: Myron McDonald Weaver, AB, MS, PhD, MD, DSc, FACP, FRCP(C). CMAJ 90:750, 1964 ⟨I-02704⟩

Webster, I. (1766-1851)

MacKenzie, K.A.: Dr. Isaac Webster, 1766-1851. Nova Scotia Medical Bulletin 33:215-219, 1954 ⟨I-02734⟩

Webster, J. (1863-)

Gordon, K.: Miss Webster of the Montreal General Hospital. CMAJ 28:552-556, 1933 ⟨I-02705⟩

Webster, J.C. (1863-1950)

Heaney, N.S.: John Clarence Webster 1863-1950. Proceedings of the Institute of Medicine of Chicago 18:174-176, 1950- 51. ⟨I-01175⟩

Kirkland, A.S.: Dr. John Clarence Webster, M.D.C.M., C.M.G., D. Sc., LL.D., F.R.C.P., F.A.C.S., F.R.S.,. CMAJ 62:521-2, 1950 ⟨I-04486⟩

Mitchell, R.: Dr. John Clarence Webster (1863-1950) Man of Two Careers. Canadian Journal of Surgery 6:407-413, 1963 ⟨I-04234⟩

Priest, F.O.: Dr. John Clarence Webster. CMAJ 64:351-353, 1951 ⟨I-01070⟩

Stanley, G.F.G.: John Clarence Webster the Laird of Shediac. Acadiensis 3:51-71, 1973-4 ⟨I-01174⟩

Webster, J.C.: Those Crowded Years 1863-1944: An Octogenarian's Record of Work. Shediac, New Brunswick. Privately printed for His Family 1944. 51 p. ⟨I-01172⟩

Webster, W. (1865-1934)

Aikenhead, D.C.: William Webster, MD, Anesthetist: an appreciation. Anesthesia and Analgesia 16:312-317, 1937 ⟨I-02733⟩

Galloway, H.P.H.: Dr. William Webster, an appreciation. CMAJ 31:691, 1934 ⟨I-01719⟩

Minuck, M.: [Dr. W. Webster]. Manitoba Medical Review 47:315-316, 1967 ⟨I-03561⟩

Minuck, M.: Pioneers of Canadian Anaesthesia -- Dr. William Webster. Canadian Anaesthetists Society Journal 19:322-6, 1972 ⟨I-05373⟩

Mitchell, R.: Dr. William Webster. CMAJ 31:691, 1934 ⟨I-01668⟩

Montgomery, E.W.: Dr. William Webster, an appreciation. CMAJ 31:691, 1934 ⟨I-01669⟩

Webster, W.B. (1798-1861)

Tracy, M.: William Bennett Webster. DCB 9:824-825, 1976 ⟨I-01191⟩

Wesbrook, F.F. (1868-1918)

Gibson, W.C.: Frank Fairchild Wesbrook (1868-1918). A Pioneer Medical Educator in Minnesota and British Columbia. JHMAS 22:357-379, 1967 ⟨I-01161⟩

Gibson, WC: President Wesbrook -- His University, His Profession and the Community. British Columbia Medical Journal 9:10-20, 1967 ⟨I-03932⟩

Gibson, W.C.: Wesbrook and His University. Vancouver, Library of the University of British Columbia, 1973. 204 p. ⟨I-01162⟩

Wetmore, F.H. (1861-1938)

Kirkland, A.S.: Dr. Frederick Henry Wetmore. CMAJ 39:510, 1938 ⟨I-03330⟩

Wheeler, B.W. (1910-1963)

Cameron, M.: Captain B.W. Wheeler, MBE, M.D., FRCP(C), Late Indian Medical Service. Alberta Medical Bulletin 29:57-58, 1964 ⟨I-05187⟩

Collins, R.: A Man Sent From God. Reader's Digest, August 1983. pp 144-175. ⟨I-05172⟩

Wheeler, D. (1892-1955)

M [itchell] R.: Dr. Digby Wheeler. CMAJ, 73:920, 1955 ⟨I-04582⟩

Whetham, G.J. (1882-1930)

Chase, L.A.: Dr. George Jamieson Whetham. CMAJ 24:476, 1931 ⟨I-03067⟩

White, C.C. (-1963)

L., E.K.: Dr. C. Carman White, an appreciation. CMAJ 89:99-100, 1963 ⟨I-02707⟩

White, E.H. (1877-1933)

Birkett, H.S.: Dr. Ernest Hamilton White. CMAJ 29:218, 1933 ⟨I-01722⟩

Currie, A.: Dr. Ernest Hamilton White. CMAJ 29:218, 1933 ⟨I-01720⟩

Whiteside, W.C. (1901-1967)

Whiteside, C.: The Nomadic Life of a Surgeon. Edmonton, Alberta, Douglas Printing Co., 1950. 89 p. ⟨I-01173⟩

Whittaker, M. (-1952)

Smith, F.E.: Dr. Mary Whittaker. CMAJ 67:378-9, 1952 ⟨I-04536⟩

Widmer, C. (1780-1858)

Charlton, M.: Christopher Widmer. Annals of Medical History 4:346-350, 1922 ⟨I-04899⟩

Harris, R.I.: Christopher Widmer, 1780-1858 and the Toronto General Hospital. York Pioneer 61:3-11, 1965 ⟨I-03414⟩

McFall, W.A.: The Life and Times of Dr. Christopher Widmer. Annals of Medical History, ser. 3, 4:324-334, 1942 ⟨I-04898⟩

Powell, N.A.: Christopher Widmer (1780-1858). In Kelly HW, Burrage WL: Dictionary of American Medical Biography. New York and London, D. Appleton and Co., 1928. pp. 1299-1300. ⟨I-01160⟩

Wiebe, C.W. (1893-)

Reimber, M.: Cornelius W. Wiebe: A Beloved Physician. Winnipeg, Hyperion Press Limited, 1983 ⟨I-05054⟩

Wilkinson, F.A.H. (1906-1959)

H., W.H.P.: Dr. F. Arthur H. Wilkinson. CMAJ 80:921-922, 1959 ⟨I-02728⟩

Noble, A.B.: Frederick Arthur Harvey Wilkinson. Canadian Anaesthetists Society Journal 6:292-293, 1959 ⟨I-02727⟩

Williamson, A.R.B. (1876-1928)

Connell, J.C.: Dr. A.R.B. Williamson. CMAJ 20:213-214, 1929 ⟨I-02729⟩

Willinsky, A.I. (1885-1976)

Willinsky, A.I.: A Doctor's Memoirs. Toronto, Macmillian Co. of Canada Ltd., 1960. 183 p. ⟨I-01177⟩

Wilson, D.B. (1895-1963)

McK., N.: David Bruce Wilson, BA, MB, DPH: an appreciation. CMAJ 88:639, 1963 ⟨I-02710⟩

Wilson, W. (1888-1966)

Elliot, G.R.F.: (Wallace Wilson). British Columbia Medical Journal 8:233, 1966 ⟨I-03401⟩

Fahrni, G.S.: (Wallace Wilson). British Columbia Medical Journal 8:231, 1966 ⟨I-03403⟩

Gibson, W.C.: (Wallace Wilson). British Columbia Medical Journal 8:234, 1966 ⟨I-03400⟩

Gunn, S.W.A.: (Wallace Wilson). British Columbia Medical Journal 8:236, 1966 ⟨I-03398⟩

Kelly, A.D.: (Wallace Wilson). British Columbia Medical Journal 8:229, 1966 ⟨I-03405⟩

K(elly), A.D.: Dr. Wallace Wilson: an appreciation. CMAJ 94:1021, 1966 ⟨I-02726⟩

Kerr, R.B.: (Wallace Wilson). British Columbia Medical Journal 8:232, 1966 ⟨I-03402⟩

Mackenzie, N.: (Wallace Wilson). British Columbia Medical Journal 8:228, 1966 ⟨I-03320⟩

McCoy, E.C.: (Wallace Wilson). British Columbia Medical Journal 8:235, 1966 ⟨I-03399⟩

McCreary, J.F.: (Wallace Wilson). British Columbia Medical Journal 8:230, 1966 ⟨I-03404⟩

Turnbull, F.: (Wallace Wilson). British Columbia Medical Journal 8:226-227, 1966 ⟨I-03321⟩

Woodley, J.W. (1875-1929)

Thomson, A.R.: James Walter Woodley. CMAJ 20:682, 1929 ⟨I-02722⟩

Woolverton, J. (1811-1883)

Roland, C.G.: Diary of a Canadian Country Physician: Jonathan Woolverton (1811-1883). Medical History 14:168-180, 1971 ⟨I-04872⟩

Workman, J. (1805-1894)

Boyle, D.: Notes on the Life of Dr. Joseph Workman. Toronto, Arbuthnot Bros. and Co., 1894. pp 8 ⟨I-02720⟩

Editorial: Doctor Joseph Workman. Canadian Practitioner 14:14, 1889 ⟨I-04422⟩

Greenland, C.: Three pioneers of Canadian psychiatry. JAMA 200:833-842, 1967 ⟨I-01167⟩

Worthington, E.D. (1820-1895)

Worthington, E.D.: Reminiscences of student life and practice. Sherbrooke, Quebec, 1897. ⟨I-01644⟩

Wright, A.H. (1846-1930)

Cameron, I.H.: Dr. Adam Henry Wright. CMAJ 23:725-726, 1930 ⟨I-01149⟩

Wright, H.P. (1851-1898)

P., R.W.: Henry P. Wright, M.D. Montreal Medical Journal 27:879-880, 1898 ⟨I-02718⟩

Wright, H.P. (1888-1952)

M[acDermot], H.E.: Dr. H.P. Wright. CMAJ 66:295, 1952 ⟨I-04543⟩

Wright, R.R. (1852-1933)

McM., J.P.: Prof. R. Ramsay Wright. Nature 132:631, 1933 ⟨I-02719⟩

Wright, W. (1825-1908)

S, F.J.: Rev. Prof. Wm. Wright, M.D. Died, April 15th, 1908, Aet. 81. Montreal Medical Journal 37:366-368, 1908 ⟨I-01169⟩

Wright, W.W. (1882-1967)

Elliot, A.J.: Dr. Walter Walker Wright. CMAJ 98:1157-1158, 1968 ⟨I-01723⟩

Macrae, H.M.: Dr. Walter Walker Wright. CMAJ 98:1158, 1968 ⟨I-01724⟩

Y

Yates, H. (1821-1882)

Angus, M.S.: Horatio Yates. DCB 11:940-41, 1982 ⟨I-04859⟩

Yonge, J. (1647-1721)

Poynter, F.N.L.: James Yonge. DCB 2:670-672, 1969 ⟨I-01013⟩

Poynter, F.N.L. (Edit.): The Journal of James Yonge (1647-1721). Hamden, Conneticut, Archon Books, 1963 ⟨I-02712⟩

Young, A.M. (1878-1939)

Valens, J.A.: Dr. Alexander MacGillvray Young. CMAJ 41:213, 1939 ⟨I-03395⟩

Young, H.G. (1890-1967)

Heal, F.C.: Dr. Harvey Gordon Young. CMAJ 96:1544, 1967 ⟨I-02715⟩

Young, M.A.R. (1894-1981)

Weatherilt, J.L.: Morley Alphonse Ryerson Young. CMAJ 125:218, 1981 ⟨I-04194⟩

Z

Zimmerman, R. (-1878)

Osler, W.: Obituary of Richard Zimmerman of the Toronto School of Medicine. Canada Medical and Surgical Journal 16:510-511, 1887-88 ⟨I-05183⟩

Zumstein, G.T. (-1961)

S., M.J.: Dr. George T. Zumstein, an appreciation. CMAJ 85:1215, 1961 ⟨I-02714⟩

SUBJECT LISTING

Aerospace Medicine

1919-1945
Canada
Stewart, C.B.: Canadian Research in Aviation Medicine. Nova Scotia Medical Bulletin 26:86-95, 1947 ⟨II-03838⟩

1946-1979
British Columbia
Foulkes, R.G.: Medics in the North. Medical Services Journal, Canada 18:523-550, 1962 ⟨II-04045⟩

Anatomy

1816-1867
Quebec
Bensley, E.H.: Sculduggery in the Dead House. CACHB 22:245-248, 1958 ⟨II-00033⟩

Lawrence, D.G.: "Resurrection" and legislation or body-snatching in relation to the anatomy act in the Province of Quebec. BHM 32:408-424, 1958 ⟨II-00035⟩

LeBlond, S.: Au Quebec, on volait aussi des cadavres. La Vie medicale au Canada francais 3:1210-1213, 1974 ⟨II-04669⟩

LeBlond, S.: Le vol des cadavres dans la legende au Quebec. La Vie medicale au Canada francais 3:67-68, 1974 ⟨II-02413⟩

1868-1918
Manitoba
Mitchell, R.: Manitoba Anatomists. Canadian Journal of Surgery 11:123-134, 1968 ⟨II-04304⟩

Persaud, T.V.N.: A Brief History of Anatomy at the University of Manitoba. Anatomischer Anzeiger 153:3-31, 1983 ⟨II-05121⟩

Quebec
Thompson, I.M.: F.J. Shepherd as anatomist. CMAJ 39:287-290, 1938 ⟨II-01945⟩

United States
Bardeen, C.R.: John Bruce MacCallum (1876-1906). In Kelly HW, Burrage WL: Dictionary of Amer Med Biog. New York/London, D. Appleton and Co., 1928. pp 769-770 ⟨II-00036⟩

Malloch, A.: Short Years: The Life and Letters of John Bruce MacCallum, M.D. 1876-1906. Chicago, Normandie House, 1938. 343 p. ⟨II-01850⟩

Anesthesiology

1816-1867
Canada
Connor, J.T.H.: To be Rendered Unconscious of Torture: Anesthesia and Canada, 1847-1920. Thesis (M. Phil.), Waterloo, University of Waterloo, 1983 ⟨II-05079⟩

Gordon, R.A.: A Capsule History of Anesthesia in Canada. Canadian Anesthetists' Society Journal 25:75-83, 1978 ⟨II-04125⟩

Griffith, H.R.: Some Canadian Pioneers in Anesthesia. Canadian Anesthetists' Society Journal 11:557-566, 1964 ⟨II-04172⟩

Griffith, H.R.: Anesthesia in Canada, 1847-1967: II. the Development of Anesthesia in Canada. Canadian Anesthetists' Society Journal 14:510-518, 1967 ⟨II-04174⟩

Jacques, A: Anaesthesia in Canada, 1847-1967: The Beginnings of Anaesthesia in Canada. Canadian Anaesthetists' Society Journal 14:500-509, 1967 ⟨II-03984⟩

Johnston, S: The Growth of the Specialty of Anesthesia in Canada. CMAJ 17:163-165, 1927 ⟨II-03979⟩

Matsuki, A., Zsigmond, E.K.: A bibliography of the history of surgical anaesthesia in Canada (supplement to Dr. Roland's Checklist). Canadian Anesthetists' Society Journal 21:427-430. 1974 ⟨II-00040⟩

Matsuki, A.: A Chronology of the Very Early History of Inhalation Anaesthesia in Canada. Canadian Anaesthetists Society Journal 21:92-5, 1974 ⟨II-05439⟩

Matsuki, A., Zsigmond, E.K.: The Early Anesthesia Chart in Canada. Anaesthesist 23:268-9, 1974 ⟨II-05452⟩

Roland, C.G.: Bibliography of the History of Anesthesia in Canada: Preliminary Checklist. Canadian Anesthetists' Society Journal 15:202-214, 1968 ⟨II-04884⟩

Shields, H.J.: The History of Anaesthesia in Canada. Canadian Anesthetists' Society Journal 2:301-307, 1955 ⟨II-03700⟩

Nova Scotia
H., W.H.: Early Adventures with Chloroform in Nova Scotia. CMAJ 14:254-255, 1924 ⟨II-03098⟩

Ontario
Colbeck, W.K.: The First Record of an Anesthetic in Ontario. CMAJ 32:84-85, 1935 ⟨II-04091⟩

Matsuki, A., Zsigmond, E.K.: The first fatal case of chloroform anaesthesia in Canada. Canadian Anesthetists' Society Journal 20:395-397, 1973 ⟨II-00041⟩

Roland, C.G.: The First Death From Chloroform at the Toronto General Hospital. Canadian Anesthetists' Society Journal 11:437-439, 1964 ⟨II-03799⟩

Steward, D.J.: The Early History of Anaesthesia in Canada: The Introduction of Ether to Upper Canada, 1847. Canadian Anaesthesist Society Journal 24(2):153-61, 1977 ⟨II-05326⟩

Quebec
Jacques, A.: The Hotel-Dieu de Quebec, 1639-1964, 325th Anniversary: Anesthesia, Past and Present. Anesthesia and Analgesia -- Current Researches 45:15-20, 1966 ⟨II-04695⟩

1868-1918
Canada
Griffith, H.R.: Fifty Years of Progress in Surgery and Anesthesia. Canadian Nurse 54:540-542, 1958 ⟨II-04173⟩

Griffith, H.R.: An Anesthetist's Valediction. Canadian Anesthetists' Society Journal 4:373-381, 1967 ⟨II-04178⟩

Manitoba

Minuck, M.: Recent advances in anaesthesia in Manitoba. Manitoba Medical Review 47:146-148, 1967 ⟨II-03647⟩

Webster, W.: Notes on the development of anaesthesia in Western Canada. CMAJ 17:727-728, 1927 ⟨II-03583⟩

Ontario

Shields, H.J.: Pioneeers of Canadian Anaesthesia: Dr. Samuel Johnston: A Biography. Canadian Anaesthetist Society Journal 19:589-593, 1972 ⟨II-02670⟩

Stringer, R.M., Catton, D.V.: The history of anaesthesia in Hamilton, Ontario, Canada. October 1977. 45p. n.p. ⟨II-00042⟩

1919-1945

Canada

Gordon, R.A.: A Report on Canadian Anesthesia and the Canadian Anesthetists Society. Canadian Anesthetists' Society Journal 3:182-86, 1956 ⟨II-04122⟩

Griffith, H.R.: The Early Clinical Use of Cyclopropane. Anesthesia and Analgesia....Current Researches 40;28-31, 1961 ⟨II-04176⟩

Ontario

Griffith, H.R.: Cyclopropane: A Revolutionary Anesthetic Agent. CMAJ 36:496-500, 1937 ⟨II-04175⟩

Henderson, V.E.: The Search for an Ideal Anaesthetic. PTRSC, Ser.3, 32:1-19, 1938 ⟨II-00043⟩

Lucas, G.H.W.: The Discovery and Pharmacology of Cyclopropane. Canadian Anesthetists' Society Journal 7:237-256, 1960 ⟨II-03746⟩

Lucas, G.H.W.: The discovery of cyclopropane. Anesthesia and Analgesia...Current Researches, 40:15-27, 1961 ⟨II-03851⟩

Quebec

Griffith, H.R.: The Evolution of the Use of Curare in Anesthesiology. Annals of the New York Academy of Science 54:493-497, 1951 ⟨II-04177⟩

1946-1979

British Columbia

Graves, H.B.: The B.C. Division of the Canadian Anesthetists Society, 1945-1964. B.C. Medical Journal 6:478-481, 1964 ⟨II-04182⟩

Animals

1816-1867

Nova Scotia

Campbell, D.A.: John Bernard Gilpin (1810-1892). In Kelly, H.W., Burrage, W.L.: Dictionary of American Med Biog. New York/London, D. Appleton and Co., 1928, p. 470. ⟨II-00044⟩

Art and Medicine

1760-1815

British Columbia

Cole, D.: Sigismund Bacstrom's northwest coast drawings and an account of his curious career. British

Columbia Studies, No. 46, pp 61-86, 1980 ⟨II-03249⟩

1868-1918

Canada

Harshman, J.P.: Robert Tait McKenzie: Another Canadian Centennial. Ontario Medical Review 34:443-448, 452, 1967 ⟨II-01781⟩

McGill, J.: Medals and Medallions of R. Tait McKenzie. Canadian Collector, July/August 1976. pages 21-23 ⟨II-04808⟩

Alberta

Oko, A.J.: The Frontier art of R.B. Nevitt: Surgeon, North-West Mounted Police, 1874-78. Calgary, Glenbow-Alberta Institute, n.d.,n.p. ⟨II-00045⟩

British Columbia

Low, J.: Dr. Charles Frederick Newcombe. The Beaver, Spring 1982, pp 32-39 ⟨II-04874⟩

1919-1945

Ontario

Jackson, A.Y.: Banting: As an Artist. Toronto, Ryerson Press, 1943. 37 p. ⟨II-00046⟩

All embracing

Canada

Gunn, S.W.A.: Medicine in primitive Indian and Eskimo Art. CMAJ 14:513-514, 1970 ⟨II-04168⟩

British Columbia

Gunn, S.W.A.: A Complete Guide to the Totem Poles in Stanley Park, Vancouver, B.C. Vancouver, W.E.G. MacDonald, Publisher, 1965. 24p. ⟨II-04179⟩

Balneology, Hydrotherapy and Health Resorts
1700-1759

Quebec

Nadeau, G.: Histoire de la Medecine Dans la Nouvelle-France: L'Alkermes et le Kermes Mineral. L'UMC 79:924-928, 1950 ⟨II-02354⟩

1760-1815

Ontario

Connor, J.T.H.: Preservatives of Health: Mineral Water Spas of Nineteenth Century Ontario. Ontario History 75:135-152, 1983 ⟨II-05207⟩

1946-1979

British Columbia

Sismey, E.D.: Quil'-Sten Okanagan Steam Bath. The Beaver 297(1):41-43, 1966 ⟨II-03317⟩

Biology

1700-1759

Quebec

Abbott, M.E.: An Early Canadian Biologist -- Michel Sarrazin (1659-1735) His Life and Times. CMAJ 19:600-607, 1928 ⟨II-02064⟩

Laflamme, M.L.: I -- Michel Sarrazin: Materiaux pour servir a l'histoire de la science en Canada. PTRSC 5:1-23, 1887 ⟨II-02062⟩

Tondreau, R.L.: Michel Sarrazin (1659-1734): the Father of French Canadian Science. Trans. and Studies of the College of Physicians of Philadelphia 31:124-127, 1963 ⟨II-02074⟩

Vallee, A.: Un Biologiste Canadien, Michel Sarrazin (1659-1739). Archives de Quebec. 1927. 1927. 291 pp. ⟨II-02062⟩

Birth Control

1868-1918
Canada

McLaren, A.: Birth Control and Abortion in Canada, 1870-1920. CHR 59:319-340, 1978. ⟨II-00047⟩

McLaren, A.: What Has This to Do with Working Class Women?: Birth Control and the Canadian Left, 1900-1939. Histoire Sociale/Social History 14:435-454, 1981 ⟨II-04792⟩

1919-1945
Canada

Bain, I.: The Development of Family Planning in Canada. Canadian Journal of Public Health 55:334-340, 1964 ⟨II-04796⟩

Kaufman, A.R.: History of Birth Control Activities in Canada. International Planned Parenthood Federation 4th Report of the Proceedings, August 1953, pp 17-22 ⟨II-05031⟩

Ontario

Bailey, T.M.: For the Public Good. Hamilton, The Planned Parenthood Society of Hamilton, 1974 37 p. ⟨II-05000⟩

Dodd, D.: The Hamilton Birth Control Clinic of the 1930's. Ontario History 75:71-86, 1983 ⟨II-05093⟩

Quaggin, A.: 'For the Public Good': Early Birth control Clinics in Canada. Canadian Family Physician 28:1868-1869, 1982 ⟨II-05024⟩

Stortz, G.: Of Tactics and Prophylactics. Canadian Lawyer 6(2):4-6, 1982 ⟨II-05002⟩

Blood Transfusion

1868-1918
Ontario

Gunson, H.H.: Blood Transfusions in 1875. CMAJ 80:130-131, 1959 ⟨II-02333⟩

Other

Guiou, N.M.: Haemorrhage at the Outposts. CMAJ 23:679-681, 1930 and 30:449, 1934 ⟨II-00363⟩

1919-1945
Other

Weil, P.: Norman Bethune and the Development of Blood Transfusion Services. In: Shephard, D.A.E.; Levesque. A.(edit): Norman Bethune: His Times and His Legacy. Ottawa, Canadian Public Health Association, 1982. pp 177-181 ⟨II-04923⟩

Botany

1700-1759
Quebec

Ahern, M.J., Ahern, G.: Jean Francois Gaultier (1708-1756). In Kelly HW, Burrage WL: Dictionary of Amer Med Biog. New York/ London, D. Appleton and Co., 1928. pp 457-458 ⟨II-00048⟩

LeBlond, S.: Michel Sarrazin: un document inedit. Laval Medical 31(3):1-8, 1961 ⟨II-02072⟩

1816-1867
Ontario

Collard, E.: Flowers to heal and comfort: Mrs. Traill's Books for Collectors. Canadian Collector, May/June 1978. pages 32-36 ⟨II-04805⟩

All embracing
Canada

Erichsen-Brown, C.: Use of Plants for the past 500 years. Aurora, Breezy Creeks Press, 1979. 510 p. ⟨II-00051⟩

Cardiology and Circulatory System

1760-1815
Quebec

Lessard, R.: Les Debuts de la Cardiologie a Quebec. CSHM Newsletter, Spring 1982, pp 17-18 ⟨II-04943⟩

1816-1867
Canada

Segall, H.N.: L'Introduction du Stethoscope et de L'Auscultation Clinique au Canada. L'UMC 97:1115-1117, 1968 ⟨II-02346⟩

1868-1918
Canada

Roland, C.G.: Maude Abbott and J.B. MacCallum: Canadian Cardiac Pioneers. Chest 57:371-377, 1970 ⟨II-03854⟩

Quebec

MacDermot, H.E.: Maude Abbott: A Memoir. Toronto, Macmillan Co. of Canada Ltd., 1941. 264 p. ⟨II-00055⟩

Segall, H.N.: William Stairs Morrow, Canada's First Physiologist-cardiolgist. CMAJ 114:543-545, 1976 ⟨II-03277⟩

1919-1945
Canada

Segall, H.N.: Histoire de la Societe Canadienne de Cardiologie. L'UMC 89:82-85, 1960 ⟨II-04681⟩

Segall, H.N.: History of the Canadian Heart Association. Mantioba Medical Review 40:94-96, 1960 ⟨II-03265⟩

Quebec

Boyd, W.: George Lyman Duff: In Memoriam. First Annual George Lyman Duff Memorial Lecture. CMAJ 798:962-963, 1958 ⟨II-02225⟩

MacDermot, H.E.: Nora Livingston and Maude Abbott. CACHB 22:228-235, 1958 ⟨II-00056⟩

Chemistry and Biochemistry

1816-1867
Quebec

Nicholls, R.V.V.: McGill University and the Teaching of Chemistry in Canada. Chemistry and Industry, August 1958, pp 1106-1107 〈II-03788〉

1919-1945
Canada

Quastel, J.H.: Fifty Years of Biochemistry. A Personal Account. Canadian Journal of Biochemistry 52:71-82, 1974 〈II-05450〉

Child Health

1760-1815
Canada

Siegel, L.S.: Child Health and Development in English Canada, 1790-1850. In: Roland, C.G.(ed.): Health, Disease and Medicine: Essays in Canadian History. Toronto, Hannah Institute for the History of Medicine, 1984, 360-380 〈II-05407〉

1816-1867
North West Territories

Helm, J.: Female infanticide, European diseases, and population levels among the Mackenzie Dene. American Ethnologist 7:259-285, 1980 〈II-04203〉

1868-1918
Canada

Sutherland, N.: To create a Strong and Healthy Race.: School Children in the Public Health Movement, 1880-1914. History of Education Quarterly, ser.3, 12:304-333, 1972. 〈II-00059〉

Sutherland, N.: To create a strong and health race: school children in the Public Health Movement, 1880-1914. In Katz, Michael B., Mattingly, Paul H. (ed.) Education and social change: themes from Ontario's past. New York, New York University Press, 1975. pp. 133-166 〈II-00058〉

Ontario

Jones, A., Rutman, L.: In the Children's Aid: J.J. Kelso and Child Welfare in Ontario. Toronto, University of Toronto Press, 1981. 210 p. 〈II-04989〉

Saskatchewan

Telford, G.S.: The First Child Welfare Conferences in Saskatchewan. Saskatchewan History 4:57-61, 1951 〈II-00060〉

1919-1945
Canada

Buckley, S.: Efforts to Reduce Infant and Maternal Mortality in Canada between the World Wars. Atlantis 2:76-84, 1977 〈II-00061〉

Ontario

Blatz, W.E., Chant, N., et al: Collected Studies on the Dionne Quintuplets. Toronto, The University of Toronto Press, 1937. Discontinuous pagination. 〈II-01545〉

Blatz, W.E.: The Five Sisters: A Study of Child Psychology. Toronto, McClelland and Stewart Ltd., 1938. 209 p. 〈II-01544〉

All embracing
Canada

Chapman, M.: Infanticide and Fertitlity Among Eskimos: A Computer Simulation. American Journal of Physical Anthropology 53:317-327, 1980 〈II-04202〉

Climate

1700-1759
Quebec

Boivin, B.: Jean-Francois Gaultier. DCB 3:241, 675-681, 1974 〈II-00348〉

1816-1867
Quebec

Desjardins, E.: Deux Medecins Montrealais du XIX Siecle Adeptes da la Pensee Ecologique. L'UMC 99:487-492, 1970 〈II-02411〉

1868-1918
Canada

Hingston, W.H.: The climate of Canada and its relations to life and health. Montreal, Dawson Brothers, Publishers, 1884. 266 p. 〈II-00065〉

Communicable Disease Control

1816-1867
New Brunswick

Cushing, J.E., Casey, T., Robertson, M.: A Chronicle of Irish Emigration to Saint John, New Brunswick, 1847. New Brunswick, The New Brunswick Museum, 1979. 77 p. 〈II-00066〉

Quebec

Mitchell, C.A.: Events Leading up to and the Establishment of the Grosse Ile Quarantine Station. Medical Services Journal, Canada 23:1436-1444, 1967 〈II-03644〉

Montizambert, F.: The Story of Fifty-Four Years' Quarantine Service from 1866-1920. CMAJ 16:314-319, 1926 〈II-01804〉

1868-1918
Saskatchewan

Middleton, F.C.: Evolution of Tuberculosis Control in Saskatchewan. Canadian Public Health Journal 24:505-513, 1933 〈II-00067〉

1919-1945
Ontario

Cameron, G.D.W.: The First Donald Fraser Memorial Lecture. Canadian Journal of Public Health 51:341-348, 1960 〈II-02936〉

Congresses

1816-1867
Other

Kelly, A.D.: Hands Across the Sea. CMAJ 97:1494, 1967 〈II-03968〉

Death

1760-1815

Ontario

Osborne, B.S.: The Cemeteries of the Midland District of Upper Canada: A Note on Mortality in a Frontier Society. Pioneer America 6:46-55, 1974 ⟨II-05267⟩

1816-1867

Ontario

Bowden, B., Hall, R.: The Impact of Death: An Historical and Archival Reconnaissance into Victorian Ontario. Archivaria 14:93-105, 1982 ⟨II-05264⟩

Dentistry

1816-1867

Canada

G., M.H.: The History of Dental Journalism in Canada. Journal of the Canadian Dental Association 18:335-38, 1952 ⟨II-05201⟩

Quebec

Fortier, A.: Histoire de la profession dentaire dans la metropole. Journal of the Canadian Dental Association 18:384-387, 1952 ⟨II-05198⟩

1868-1918

Canada

Bagnall, J.S.: Dental Education in Canada. Journal of the Canadian Dental Association 18:310-314, 1952 ⟨II-05204⟩

Dale, J.: 100 Years of Dental Education in Canada: 1875-1975. Ontario Dentist 53(6):33-39, 1976 ⟨II-05457⟩

Gullett, D.W.: Notes on the Development of the Canadian Dental Association. Journal of the Canadian Dental Association 18:303-309, 1952 ⟨II-05205⟩

Johnson, J.H.: The History of Dental Research in Canada. Journal of the Canadian Dental Association 18:315-320, 1952 ⟨II-05203⟩

Wansbrough, E.M.: Royal Canadian Dental Corps. Journal of the Canadian Dental Association 18:322-27, 1952 ⟨II-05202⟩

Ontario

McKenna, C.A.: Toronto in 1896. Journal of the Canadian Dentistry Association 19:133-136, 1953 ⟨II-03776⟩

Quebec

Hamel, P.: Evolution de la dentisterie dans Quebec et la region, de 1902 a nos jours. Journal of the Canadian Dental Association 18:372-378, 1952 ⟨II-05200⟩

1919-1945

Quebec

Geoffrion, P.: Evolution de l'enseignement a la Faculte de Chirurgie Dentaire de l'Universite de Montreal. Journal of the Canadian Dental Association 18:379-381, 1952 ⟨II-05199⟩

Toket, M.H.: Highlights of a Half Century. Journal Dentaire du Quebec Dental Journal 8:7, 13, 1971 ⟨II-03756⟩

All embracing

Canada

Gullett, D.W.: A History of Dentistry in Canada. Toronto, University of Toronto Press, 1971. 308 p. ⟨II-00068⟩

Dermatology

1919-1945

Canada

Birt, A.R.: The Canadian Dermatological Association: First 50 Years. International Journal of Dermatology 16:289-295, 1977 ⟨II-00071⟩

Forsey, R.R.: History of the Canadian Dermatological Association. Archives of Dermatology 91:486-492, 1965 ⟨II-04048⟩

1946-1979

Canada

Cleveland, D.E.H.: The Canadian Dermatological Association -- First 25 Years. CMAJ 75:863-865, 1956 ⟨II-04095⟩

Diseases and Injuries

Adrenal Gland

1919-1945

Quebec

Selye, H.: The story of the adaptation syndrome. Montreal, ACTA, Inc., Medical Publishers, 1952. 225 p. ⟨II-00073⟩

Selye, H.: From dream to discovery: on being a scientist. New York/Toronto, McGraw-Hill Book Co., 1964. 419 p. ⟨II-00072⟩

Alcoholism

1700-1759

Manitoba

Pannekoek, F.: "Corruption" at Moose. Beaver, Spring 1979, pp. 4-11 ⟨II-00074⟩

1816-1867

Canada

Henry, W.: Statistics of Delirium Tremens amongst the Troops in Canada for the last thirty years, with some observations on the Disease. Medical Chronicle 1:321-327, 1854 ⟨II-00076⟩

New Brunswick

Chapman, J.K.: The mid-nineteenth-century temperance movement in New Brunswick and Maine. CHR 35:43-60, 1954 ⟨II-00075⟩

Ontario

Garland, M.A., Talman, J.J.: Pioneer Drinking Habits and the Rise of the Temperance Agitation in Upper Canada Prior to 1840. Ontario Historical Society 27:341-364, 1931 ⟨II-04065⟩

1868-1918

Canada

Gray, J.H.: Bacchanalia Revisited. Western Canada's Boozy Skid to Social Disaster. Saskatoon, Western Producer Prairie Books, 1982. 206 p. ⟨II-05015⟩

Manitoba

Thompson, J.H.: The Voice of Moderation: The Defeat of Prohibition in Manitoba. Mercury Series, History Div. Paper No. 1, The Twenties in Western Canada, 1972. pp 170-190. ⟨II-00077⟩

1919-1945

Ontario

Hallowell, G.A.: Prohibition in Ontario. Ontario Historical Society, 1972. 180 p. ⟨II-00078⟩

Anemia

1919-1945

New Brunswick

Everett, H.S.: The First Case of Pernicious Anaemia Successfully Treated in Canada. CMAJ 75:449-450, 1956 ⟨II-01793⟩

Appendicitis

1868-1918

Quebec

Murphy, D.A.: James Bell's Appendicitis. Canadian Journal of Surgery 15:335-338, 1972 ⟨II-04291⟩

Beriberi

1868-1918

Newfoundland

MacPherson, C.: The First Recognition of Beri-beri in Canada?. CMAJ 95:278-279, 1966 ⟨II-03687⟩

Other

Keith, W.D.: Some Early Canadian Ships' Surgeons. B.C. Medical Journal 1:103-116, 1959 ⟨II-04220⟩

Cholera

1816-1867

Canada

Bilson, G.: Cholera!. Canadian Historical Magazine 1(2):41-55, 1973 ⟨II-03107⟩

Bilson, G.: Canadian Doctors and the Cholera. Historical Papers, CHA, 1977. pp 104-119. ⟨II-00079⟩

Marsden, W.: An Essay on the Contagion, Infection, Portability, and Communicability of the Asiatic Cholera in its Relations to Quarantine; with a brief History of its Origin and Course in Canada, from 1832. Canada Medical Journal and Monthly Record of Medical and Surgical Science. 4:529-543, 1868; 5:1-7, 49-53,101-108, 145-151, 195-203, 243-250, 1868-1869. ⟨II-00090⟩

Tache, J.C.: Memorandum On Cholera, Adopted at a Medical Conference held in the Bureau of Agriculture, in March, 1866. Bureau of Agriculture and Statistics, 1866. (Ottawa) ⟨II-00092⟩

Workman, J.: Cholera in Canada in 1832 and 1834. Canada Medical Journal and Monthly Record of Medical and Surgical Science 2:485-489, 1865-1866 ⟨II-00093⟩

New Brunswick

Bilson, G.: The Cholera Epidemic in Saint John, N.B., 1854. Acadiensis 4:85-99, 1974-5 ⟨II-00080⟩

Death, J.: My Cholera Experiences. St. John, N.B., Sun, 1892 ⟨II-00084⟩

Kennedy, E.: Immigrants, Cholera and the Saint John Sisters of Charity. Canadian Catholic Historical Association, Study Sessions 44, 1977. pp 25-44 ⟨II-00088⟩

Nova Scotia

Bilson, G.: Two Cholera Ships in Halifax. Dalhousie Review 53:449-459, 1973 ⟨II-00082⟩

Ontario

Bilson, G.: Cholera in Upper Canada, 1832. Ontario History 67:15-30, 1975 ⟨II-00081⟩

Dade, C.: Notes on the Cholera Seasons of 1832 and 1834. Canadian Journal of Industry, Science, and Art, No. 37:17-28, 1862 ⟨II-04801⟩

Godfrey, C.M.: The cholera epidemics in Upper Canada 1832-1866. Toronto and Montreal, Seccombe House, 1968. pp.72 ⟨II-00086⟩

Hodder, E.M.: Transfusion of Milk in Cholera. Practitioner 10:14-16, 1873 ⟨II-04148⟩

Loeb, L.J.: The Cholera Epidemics in Upper Canada 1832-1834. Western Ontario Historical Notes 11:44-54, 1953 ⟨II-04988⟩

Patterson, M.A.: The Cholera Epidemic of 1832 in York, Upper Canada. Bulletin of the Medical Library Association 46:165-184, 1958 ⟨II-00091⟩

Seaborn, E.: The Asiatic Cholera in 1832 in the London District. PTRSC 31:153-169, 1931 ⟨II-03871⟩

Quebec

Bilson, G.: The first epidemic of Asiatic Cholera in Lower Canada, 1832. Medical History 21:411-433, 1977 ⟨II-00083⟩

Dechene, L., Robert, J.-C.: Le cholera de 1832 dans le Bas-Canada: Mesure des inegalites devant la mort. In: The Great Mortalities: Methodological Studies of Demographic Cries in the Past, edited by H. Charbonneau and A. Larose, pp. 229-56. Liege: Ondina, 1979. ⟨II-05139⟩

Desjardins, E.: L'Epidemie de Cholera de 1832. L'UMC 100:2395-2401, 1971 ⟨II-02410⟩

Giroux, S.: Le cholera a Quebec. National Gallery of Canada Bulletin 20:3-12, 1972 ⟨II-02409⟩

LeBlond, S.: Cholera in Quebec in 1849. CMAJ, 71:288-292, 1954 ⟨II-04647⟩

LeBlond, S.: Le Cholera A Quebec En 1849. CMAJ, 71:292-296 1954 ⟨II-04710⟩

LeBlond, S.: Quebec en 1832. Laval Medical 38:183-191, 1967 ⟨II-02408⟩

Cleft Palate

1816-1867
Other

Francis, W.W.: Repair of Cleft Palate by Philibert Roux in 1819. A Translation of John Stephenson's De Velosynthesi. JHMAS 18:209-219, 1963 ⟨II-00094⟩

[Roland, C.G.]: The First Operation for Cleft Palate. CMAJ 89:825-826, 1963 ⟨II-00095⟩

Stephenson, J.: Repair of Cleft Palate by Philibert Roux in 1819. Plastic and Reconstructive Surgery 47:277-283, 1971 ⟨II-00096⟩

Wallace, A.B.: Canadian-Franco-Scottish Co-operation: A Cleft-Palate Story. British Journal of Plastic Surgery 19:1-14, 1966 ⟨II-00097⟩

Congenital Malformations

1868-1918
Ontario

Greenland, C., Griffin, J.D.: The Honorable Mary MacDonald: a lesson in attitude. CMAJ 25:305-308, 1981 ⟨II-04221⟩

Diabetes

1868-1918
Canada

Allan, F.N.: Diabetes Before and After Insulin. Medical History 16:266-73, 1972 ⟨II-05437⟩

Ontario

Campbell, W.R.: Anabasis. CMAJ 87:1055-1061, 1962 ⟨II-04105⟩

Saskatchewan

Chase, L.A.: The Trend of Diabetes in Saskatchewan 1905 to 1934. CMAJ 36:366-369, 1937 ⟨II-04099⟩

1919-1945
Canada

Best, C.H.: The First Clinical Use Of Insulin. Diabetes 5:65-67, 1956 ⟨II-00103⟩

Pratt, J.H.: A reappraisal of researches leading to the discovery of Insulin. JHMAS 9:281-289, 1954 ⟨II-00105⟩

Ontario

Banting, F.G.: Diabetes and Insulin. Stockholm, P.A. Norstedt and Fils, 1925. pp 1-20 ⟨II-00099⟩

Banting, F.G.: The History of Insulin. Edinburgh Medical Journal 36:1-18, 1929 ⟨II-00098⟩

Best, C.H.: A Canadian Trail of Medical Research. Journal of Endocrinology 19:1-17, 1959 ⟨II-00101⟩

Best, C.H.: Diabetes since Nineteen Hundred and Twenty. CMAJ 82(21):1061-1066, 1960. ⟨II-00102⟩

Best, C.H.: Forty Years of Interest in Insulin. British Medical Bulletin 16(3):179-182, 1960 ⟨II-00100⟩

Bliss, M.: The Discovery of Insulin. Toronto, McClelland and Stewart Limited, 1982. 304 p. ⟨II-05020⟩

Collip, J.B.: Reminiscences on the Discovery of Insulin. CMAJ 87:1045, 1962 ⟨II-04092⟩

Feasby, W.R.: The Discovery of Insulin. JHMAS 13:68-84, 1958 ⟨II-00104⟩

Fletcher, A.A.: Early Clinical Experiences with Insulin. CMAJ 87:1052-1055, 1962 ⟨II-04049⟩

Laugier, H.: Banting et la Decouverte de L'Insuline. L'UMC 70:347-351, 1941 ⟨II-02407⟩

Rafter, G.W.: Banting and Best and the Sources of Useful Knowledge. Perspectives in Biology and Medicine 26:281-286, 1983 ⟨II-05049⟩

Shortt, S.E.D.: Banting, Insulin and the Question of Simultaneous Discovery. Queen's Quarterly 89:260-273, 1982 ⟨II-04981⟩

Williams, J.R.: The Most Important Dog in History. The Bulletin, volume 3, number 9, 1946 ⟨II-00106⟩

United States

Joslin, E.P.: A Personal Impression. Diabetes 5:67-68, 1956 ⟨II-02907⟩

Diphtheria

1868-1918
Canada

Dolman, C.E.: The Donald T. Fraser Memorial Lecture, 1973. Landmarks and Pioneers in the Control of Diptheria. Canadian Journal of Public Health 64:317-36, 1973 ⟨II-05443⟩

Ontario

Phair, J.T., McKinnon, N.E.: Mortality Reductions in Ontario 1900-1942 V. Diptheria. Canadian Journal of Public Health 37:69-73, 1946 ⟨II-04455⟩

Quebec

Foley, A.R.: Half a Century of Diptheria Prevalence in Quebec. Canadian Public Health Journal 33:198-204, 1942 ⟨II-04047⟩

Drug Addiction

1868-1918
Alberta

Chapman, T.L.: Drug Use in Western Canada. Alberta History 24(4):18-27, 1976 ⟨II-00107⟩

Encephalitis

1868-1918
Manitoba

Medovy, H.: The History of Western Encephalomyelitis in Manitoba. Canadian Journal of Public Health 67 Suppl. 1:13-4, 1976 ⟨II-05235⟩

Fractures

All embracing
Canada

Couch, J.H.: History of Fractures in Canada. CMAJ 45:174-177, 1941 ⟨II-03669⟩

Goiter

1500-1699
Canada

Greenwald, I.: The History and Character of Goitre in Canada. CMAJ 84:379-388, 1961 ⟨II-00108⟩

Gonorrhea

1700-1759

Quebec

LeBlond, S.: Le genou malade de Madame d'Youville. Cahier des Dix 41:43-49, 1976 ⟨II-00109⟩

Hernia

1816-1867

Prince Edward Island

Lea, R.G.: Dr. John Mackieson (1795-1885): Strangulated Hernia in the Early 19th Century. Canadian Journal of Surgery 8:1-9, 1965 ⟨II-04299⟩

Iatrogenic

1700-1759

Nova Scotia

Bedwell, S.F.: D'Anville's Doom. A Neurological Vignette from Historic Halifax. The Canadian Journal of Neurological Sciences 7:1-8, 1980 ⟨II-00345⟩

Influenza

1868-1918

Canada

McGinnis, J.P.D.: The Impact of Epidemic Influenza: Canada, 1918-1919. Historical Papers, CHA, 1977. pp 120-140 ⟨II-00820⟩

Pettigrew, E.: The Silent Enemy: Canada and the Deadly Flu of 1918. Saskatoon, Western Producer Prairie Books, 1983. pp 156 ⟨II-05368⟩

Alberta

McGinnis, J.P.D.: A City Faces an Epidemic. Alberta History 24(4):1-11, 1976 ⟨II-00819⟩

British Columbia

Andrews, M.W.: Epidemic and Public Health: Influenza in Vancouver, 1918-1919. B.C. Studies 34:1-24, 1977 ⟨II-04031⟩

Ontario

Oliver, E.B.: The Influenza Epidemic of 1918-19. Thunder Bay Historical Society Annual 10:9-10, 1919 ⟨II-03827⟩

Quebec

LeSage, A.: L'epidemie de grippe a Montreal en 1918. L'UMC 48:1-10, 1919 ⟨II-02388⟩

Leprosy

1760-1815

New Brunswick

Whitehead, F.L.: Leprosy in New Brunswick: the end of an era. CMAJ 97:1299-1300, 1967 ⟨II-03589⟩

1816-1867

Canada

Brown, C.P.: Leprosy in Canada. Canadian Journal of Public Health 43:252-58, 1952 ⟨II-04015⟩

McGinnis, J.D.: "Unclean, Unclean": Canadian Reaction to Lepers and Leprosy. In: Roland, C.G.(ed.): Health, Disease and Medicine: Essays in Canadian History. Toronto, Hannah Institute for the History of Medicine, 1984, 250-275 ⟨II-05402⟩

Ruttan, H.R.: The Leprosy Problem in Canada with Report of a Case. CMAJ 78:19-21, 1958 ⟨II-03713⟩

New Brunswick

Kalisch, P.A.: Tracadie and Penikese Leprosaria: a Comparative Analysis of Societal Response to Leprosy in New Brunswick, 1844-1880, and Massachusetts, 1904-1921. BHM 47:480-512, 1973 ⟨II-04887⟩

Kato, L, Marchand, J: Leprosy: "Loathsome Disease in Tracadie, New Brunswick" -- a glimpse into the past century. CMAJ 114:440-442, 1976 ⟨II-03993⟩

Kelly, A.D.: Unclean no More. CMAJ 97:1298, 1967 ⟨II-03967⟩

Kelly, C.M.: An Account of Canadian Leprosy. Montreal Medical Journal 38:387-392, 1909 ⟨II-03969⟩

Malaria

1760-1815

Ontario

Riddell, W.R.: The Mosquito in Upper Canada. Ontario Historical Society Papers and Records 17:85-89, 1919 ⟨II-00111⟩

Roland, C.G.: "Sunk under the Taxation of Nature": Malaria in Upper Canada. In: Roland, C.G. (ed.): Health, Disease and Medicine: Essays in Canadian History. Toronto, Hannah Institute for the History of Medicine, 1984, 154-170 ⟨II-05397⟩

1816-1867

Canada

Fisk, G.H.: Malaria and the Anopheles Mosquito in Canada. CMAJ :679-683, 1931 ⟨II-01839⟩

Ontario

McMaster, J.: Despite Tempest and Ague: an 1844 letter to the folks at home. York Pioneer 74:1-4, 1979 ⟨II-03285⟩

Wylie, W.N.T.: Poverty, Distress, and Disease: Labour and the Construction of the Rideau Canal, 1826-32. Journal of Canadian Labour Studies, Spring 1983. pp 7-30 ⟨II-05275⟩

1868-1918

Ontario

Stewart, D.A.: Malaria in Canada. CMAJ 26:239:241, 1932 ⟨II-00364⟩

Measles

1868-1918

Ontario

McKinnon, N.E.: Mortality Reductions in Ontario, 1900-45 VII. Measles and Whooping Cough. Canadian Journal of Public Health 39:95-8, 1948 ⟨II-04476⟩

Mental Disorders
1500-1699
Canada

Griffin, J.D., Greenland, C.: Manifestations of Madness in New France. In International Congress for the History of Medicine, 25th, Quebec, 1976. Proceedings, Volume II, 1976. p. 727-745 ⟨II-00112⟩

Neoplasms
1700-1759
Quebec

Blais, M.C.: Yves Phlem. DCB 3:518-520, 1974 ⟨II-00113⟩

1919-1945
Manitoba

Israels, L.G.: 1930-1980: From the Minutes of Early Years [Cancer Relief and Research Institute]. University of Manitoba Medical Journal 52:37-39, 1982 ⟨II-05004⟩

Ontario

DeLarue, N.C.: Lung Cancer in Historical Perspective: Lessons from the Past, Implications of Present Experience, Challenges for the Future. Canadian Journal of Surgery 23:549-557, 1980 ⟨II-04331⟩

Saskatchewan

Shephard, D.A.E.: First in Fear and Dread -- Cancer Control in Saskatchewan: A History of the Saskatchewan Cancer Commission, 1929-1979. [Saskatchewan Cancer Commission, 1982] pp 354 + [75] ⟨II-05009⟩

1946-1979
Canada

Hildes, J.A., Schaefer, O.: The Changing Picture of Neoplastic Disease in the Western and Central Canadian Arctic (1950-1980). CMAJ 130:25-32, 1984 ⟨II-05321⟩

Parasitic
1868-1918
Alberta

Eaton, R.D.: Taeniasis in Southern Alberta, 1894-1900. CMAJ 115(10):976, 979, 981; 1976 ⟨II-05252⟩

Plague
1700-1759
Canada

Heagerty, J.J.: Plague in Canada. CMAJ 16:452-454, 1926 ⟨II-01803⟩

Poliomyelitis
1919-1945
British Columbia

Mackie, H.G.: The Polio Epidemic of 1927. Okanagan Historical Society Annual Report 29:43-48, 1965 ⟨II-05116⟩

1946-1979
Manitoba

Sherman, L.R.: Manitoba's Response to a Major Epidemic of Poliomyelitis and the Consequences for Rehabilitation Services. University of Manitoba Medical Journal 50:80-83, 1980 ⟨II-03734⟩

Rabies
1816-1867
Canada

Tabel, H., Corner, A.H., Webster, W.A., Casey, C.A.: History and Epizootiology of Rabies in Canada. Canadian Veterinary Journal 15:271-81, 1974 ⟨II-05441⟩

Ontario

Hayes, J.: The Death of the Duke of Richmond from Hydrophobia in 1820. CMAJ 16:319, 1926 ⟨II-04163⟩

Quebec

Anderson, W.J.: The Life of F.M., H.R.H. Edward, Duke of Kent. Ottawa/Toronto, Hunter, Rose and Co., 1870. 241 p. ⟨II-00114⟩

Mitchell, C.A.: Rabies in Quebec City: Case Report 1839. Medical Services Journal of Canada, 23:809-812, 1967 ⟨II-03643⟩

Respiratory Tract
1868-1918
Ontario

McKinnon, N.E.: Mortality Reductions in Ontario, 1900-1945 VIII. Respiratory Disease. Canadian Journal of Public Health 39:417-21, 1948 ⟨II-04457⟩

Scarlet Fever
1868-1918
Ontario

McKinnon, N.E.: Mortality Reductions in Ontario, 1900-42 VI. Scarlet Fever. Canadian Journal of Public Health 37:407-10, 1946 ⟨II-04454⟩

Scurvy
Pre-1500
Canada

Beeuwkes, A.M.: The Prevalence of Scurvy Among Voyageurs to America -- 1493-1600. Journal of American Dietetic Association 24:300-303, 1948 ⟨II-04027⟩

1500-1699
Nova Scotia

Murphy, A.L.: The Anti-Scurvy Club, 1606 AD. CMAJ 82:541-43, 1960 ⟨II-03753⟩

Quebec

Desjardins, E.: Les Observations Medicales de Jacques Cartier et de Samuel de Champlain. L'UMC 99:677-681, 1970 ⟨II-02351⟩

Riddell, W.R.: Sidelights on disease in French Canada before the conquest. Canadian Journal of Medicine and Surgery 69:5-12, 1931 ⟨II-03793⟩

Wells, D.B.: Scurvy: The First Disease Found in North America. CAMSI Journal 20:30-31, 1961 (Feb) ⟨II-00116⟩

1868-1918
North West Territories

Martin, K.R.: Life and Death at Marble Island, 1864-73. The Beaver, Spring 1979, pp 48-56 ⟨II-00117⟩

Smallpox

1500-1699
Canada

Stearn, E.W., Stearn, A.E.: The Effect of Smallpox on the Destiny of the Amerindian. Boston, Bruce Humphries, Inc., 1945. 153 p. ⟨II-03618⟩

1700-1759
Canada

Goodman, H: Inoculation in North America Prior to 1846. The Merck Report 58:15-21, 1949 ⟨II-04126⟩

Quebec

Gaumond, E: La Petite Verole. Laval Medical 18:3-13, 1953 ⟨II-04067⟩

1760-1815
Canada

Stewart, R.C.: Early Vaccinations in British North America. CMAJ 39:181-183, 1938 ⟨II-03840⟩

Newfoundland

Hewson, J.: What does Vaccination mean?. Newfoundland Quarterly 75(3):15-16, 1979 ⟨II-05122⟩

Roberts, K.B.: Smallpox: an Historic Disease. St. John's, Nfld.,Memorial University of Newfoundland, 1979. 49 p. ⟨II-00353⟩

Nova Scotia

Cash, P., Pine, C.: John Jeffries and the Sruggle Against Smallpox in Boston (1775-1776) and Nova Scotia (1776-1779). Bulletin of the History of Medicine 57:93-97, 1983 ⟨II-05113⟩

Hattie, W.H.: The Early Story of Vaccination on this Continent. CMAJ 14:255, 1924 ⟨II-03097⟩

Innis, M.Q.: The Record of an Epidemic. Dalhousie Review 16:371-375, 1936-7 ⟨II-02108⟩

Quebec

Tunis, B.: Inoculation for Smallpox in the Province of Quebec, a Re-appraisal. In: Roland, C.G.(ed.): Health, Disease and Medicine: Essays in Canadian History. Toronto, Hannah Institute for the History of Medicine, 1984, 171-193 ⟨II-05399⟩

1816-1867
Canada

Ray, A.J.: Smallpox: the epidemic of 1837-38. The Beaver, Autumn 1975, pp 8-13 ⟨II-00118⟩

Quebec

Tunis, B.R.: Public Vaccination in Lower Canada, 1815-1823: Controversy and a Dilemma. Historical Reflections 9:264-278, 1982 ⟨II-04995⟩

1868-1918
Canada

Bunn, J.: Smallpox Epidemic of 1869-70. Alberta Historical Review 11(2):13-19, 1963 ⟨II-02969⟩

British Columbia

Kidd, GA: Smallpox in Vancouver. Vancouver Medical Association Bulletin 23:86-88, 1946-47 ⟨II-03959⟩

Ontario

Craig, B.: Smallpox in Ontario: Public and Professional Perceptions of Disease, 1884-1885. In: Roland, C.G.(ed.): Health, Disease and Medicine: Essays in Canadian History. Toronto, Hannah Institute for the History of Medicine, 1984, 215-249 ⟨II-05401⟩

Graham, J.E.: A Brief History of the Recent Outbreak of Smallpox in Toronto. Dominion Medical Monthly 1:123-129, 1893 ⟨II-04185⟩

Spaulding, W.B.: Smallpox Control in the Ontario Wilderness, 1880-1910. In: Roland, C.G.(ed.): Health, Disease and Medicine: Essays in Canadian History. Toronto, Hannah Institute for the History of Medicine, 1984, 194-214 ⟨II-05400⟩

Quebec

Desjardins, E.: La Grande Epidemie de "Picote Noire". L'UMC 99:1470-1477, 1970 ⟨II-02406⟩

Duchesne, R.: Problemes d'histoire des sciences au Canada francais. Institut d'histoire et de sociopolitique des sciences/Universite de Montreal, 1978. 13 p. ⟨II-02404⟩

Firth, D.C.: A Tale of Two Cities: Montreal and the Smallpox Epidemic of 1885. Thesis (M.A.), Ottawa, University of Ottawa, 1983. ⟨II-05417⟩

Guyot, M.: A brief history of the smallpox epidemic in Montreal from 1871 to 1880 and the late outbreak of 1885. Montreal, s.n. 1886 ⟨II-01530⟩

Stewart, R.C.: Hospital Care of Smallpox in Montreal. CMAJ 43:381-383, 1940 ⟨II-03598⟩

Other

Taylor, J.G.: An Eskimo Abroad, 1880: His Diary and Death. Canadian Geographic 101(5):38-43, 1981 ⟨II-04980⟩

All embracing
Canada

Brown, J.R., McLean, D.M.: Smallpox -- A Retrospect. CMAJ 87:765-67, 1962 ⟨II-04014⟩

Syphilis

1760-1815
Quebec

Cochran, A.W.: Notes on the Measures Adopted by Government, between 1775 and 1786, to check the St. Paul's Disease. Transactions of the Literary and Historical Society of Quebec 4:139-152, 1841 ⟨II-00119⟩

Desjardins, E.: Le mal de la Baie Saint-Paul. L'UMC 102:2148-52, 1973 ⟨II-05445⟩

Gauvreau, J.: Le Mal de la Baie Saint-Paul. L'UMC 60:494-500, 1931 ⟨II-01870⟩

LeBlond, S.: Le Mal De La Baie Etait-Il La Syphilis?. In International Congress for the History of Medicine, 25th, Quebec, 1976. Proceedings, Volume II, 1976. p. 866-872 ⟨II-00120⟩

LeBlond, S.: La mal de la Baie: etait-ce la syphilis?. CMAJ 116:1284-88, 1977 ⟨II-00354⟩

Riddell, W.R.: La Maladie de la Baie de St. Paul. Public Health Journal 15:145-157, 1924 ⟨II-04473⟩

Sulte, B.: Le Mal De La Baie Saint-Paul. Le Bulletin des Recherches Historiques 22:36-39, 1916 ⟨II-00121⟩

1868-1918
Ontario

Casselman, J.I.: Venereal Disease in Ontario and Canada, 1900-1930. Thesis (M.A.), Kingston, Queen's University, 1981 ⟨II-04978⟩

1919-1945
Canada

Pierson, R.R.: The double bind of the double standard: V.D. control and the Canadian women's army corps in WWII. Presented at annual meeting of Can Hist Assoc, Saskatoon, 1979. Memorial Univ of Newfoundland, 1979. 41 p. n.p. ⟨II-00122⟩

Quebec

Desloges, A.H., Ranger, J.A.: Historique de la Lutte Antivenerienne dans la Province de Quebec. L'UMC 61:235-242, 1932 ⟨II-02442⟩

All embracing
Quebec

Gaumond, E.: La Syphilis au Canada Francais Hier et Aujourd'hui. Laval Medical 7:25-65, 1942 ⟨II-02405⟩

Tetanus
1816-1867
Ontario

Angus, M.S.: Lord Sydenham's one hundred and fifteen days in Kingston. Historic Kingston 15:36-49, 1967 ⟨II-03252⟩

Trichinosis
1500-1699
Manitoba

Young, D.: Was there an unsuspected killer aboard "The Unicorn". The Beaver 304(3):9-15, 1973 ⟨II-03315⟩

Tuberculosis
1500-1699
Canada

Baril, G., Boucher, R.: Resultats de Quelques Recherches Bibliographiques: Sur la Tuberculose des Indiens du Canada avant la Penetrasion Europeenne. L'UMC 55:519-521, 1926 ⟨II-02447⟩

1868-1918
Canada

McCuaig, K.: From Social Reform to Social Service. The Changing Role of Volunteers: the Anti-tuberculosis Campaign, 1900-30. CHR 71:480-501, 1980 ⟨II-02944⟩

McCuaig, K.: From "A Social Disease with a Medical Aspect" to "A Medical Disease with a Social Aspect": Fighting the White Plague in Canada, 1900-1940. In: Shephard, D.A.E.: Levesque, A.(edit): Norman Bethune: His Times and His Legacy, Ottawa, Canadian Public Health Assoc., 1982. pp 54-64 ⟨II-04925⟩

McCuaig, K.: Tuberculosis: The Changing Concepts of the Disease in Canada 1900-1950. In: Roland, C.G.(ed.): Health, Disease and Medicine: Essays in Canadian History. Toronto, Hannah Institute for the History of Medicine, 1984, 296-307 ⟨II-05404⟩

Moore, P.E.: No Longer Captain: A History of Tuberculosis and its Control Amongst Canadian Indians. CMAJ 84:1012-1015, 1961 ⟨II-03290⟩

Nadeau, G.: A T.B.'s Progress: The Story of Norman Bethune. BHM 8:1135-1171, 1940 ⟨II-00125⟩

Porter, G.D.: Pioneers in Tuberculosis Work in Canada. Canadian Public Health Journal 31:367-69, 1940 ⟨II-03790⟩

Ridge, J.M.: The Impact of a Great Discovery [TB Bacillus]. University of Manitoba Medical Journal 28:75, 77-78, 1957 ⟨II-05263⟩

Wherrett, G.J.: The Miracle of the Empty Beds: A History of Tuberculosis in Canada. Toronto/Buffalo, University of Toronto Press, 1977. 299 p. ⟨II-00383⟩

Alberta

McGinnis, J.P.D.: The White Plague in Calgary; Sanatorium Care in Southern Alberta. Alberta History 28(4):1-15, 1980 ⟨II-02945⟩

Manitoba

Morgan, H.V.: David Alexander Stewart (1874-1937). CACHB 6(2):1-5, 1941 ⟨II-00124⟩

Paine, A.L.: Manitoba Perspective on Tuberculosis. University of Manitoba Medical Journal 52:21-37, 1982 ⟨II-05005⟩

Ontario

Campbell, M.F.: Holbrook of the San. Toronto, The Ryerson Press, 1953. 212 p. ⟨II-03615⟩

Gale, G.L., DeLarue, N.D.: Surgical History of Pulmonary Tuberculosis: The Rise and Fall of Various Technical Procedures. Canadian Journal of Surgery 12:381-388, 1969 ⟨II-04303⟩

Gale, G.L.: Tuberculosis in Canada: a Century of Progress. CMAJ 126:526, 528-529, 1982 ⟨II-04822⟩

Holbrook, J.H.: Forty Years of Advance. Progress and evolution in the care of tuberculosis as exemplified in the story of the mountain Sanatorium at Hamilton. The Canadian Hospital 23:29-33, 92-93, 1946 ⟨II-00127⟩

McKinnon, N.E.: Mortality Reductions in Ontario 1900-1942 IV. Tuberculosis. Canadian Journal of Public Health 36:423-9, 1945 ⟨II-04451⟩

Stanley, G.D.: Early Days at the Muskoka San. CACHB 18(1):17-20, 1953 ⟨II-00126⟩

Quebec

Pierre-Deschenes, C.: La tuberculose au Quebec au debut au XXe Siecle: Probleme social et reponse reformiste. Thesis (M.A.) Quebec a Montreal, 1980 ⟨II-05146⟩

1919-1945

Alberta

McGinnis, J.P.D.: Records of Tuberculosis in Calgary. Archivaria 10:173-189, 1980 ⟨II-00369⟩

Ontario

Brink, G.C.: How Pasteurization of Milk Came to Ontario. CMAJ 91:972-973, 1964 ⟨II-04018⟩

Quebec

Nadeau, G.: Le Plus Illustre de Nos Poitrinaires: Sir Wilfred Laurier. L'UMC 73:404-433, 1944 ⟨II-01867⟩

Wherrett, G.J.: Norman Bethune and Tuberculosis. In: Shephard, D.A.E.; Levesque, A.(edit): Norman Bethune: His Times and His Legacy. Ottawa, Canadian Public Health Association, 1982. pp 65-70. ⟨II-04924⟩

Tularemia

1919-1945

British Columbia

Black, D.M.: Tularaemia in British Columbia. CMAJ 78:16-18, 1958 ⟨II-04021⟩

Typhoid

1868-1918

Canada

Meakins, J.C.: Typhoid Fever in the 1890's and the 1930's. CMAJ 42:81-82, 1940 ⟨II-03462⟩

British Columbia

Norris, J.: Typhoid in the Rockies: Epidemiology in a Constrained Habitat, 1883-1939. In: Roland, C.G.(ed.): Health, Disease and Medicine: Essays in Canadian History. Toronto, Hannah Institute for the History of Medicine, 1984, 276-295 ⟨II-05403⟩

Manitoba

Mitchell, R.: How Winnipeg Waged War on Typhoid. Manitoba Medical Review 49:166-67, 1969 ⟨II-05144⟩

Ontario

Lloyd, S.: The Ottawa Typhoid Epidemics of 1911 and 1912: A Case Study of Disease as a Catalyst for Urban Reform. Urban History Review 8:66-89, 1979 ⟨II-04209⟩

Ross, M.A.: Typhoid Fever Mortality in Ontario, 1880-1931. Canadian Public Health Journal 26:73-84, 1935 ⟨II-04878⟩

1919-1945

Quebec

Gordon, A.H.: Typhoid Fever from the Inside. CMAJ 48:358-362, 1943 ⟨II-04124⟩

Typhus

1700-1759

Quebec

Riddell, W.R.: A Case of 'Ship Fever' in French Canada. Canada Lancet and Practitioner 74:132-1934, 1930 ⟨II-00347⟩

1760-1815

Manitoba

Bumsted, J.M.: Lord Selkirk's Highland Regiment and the Kildonan Settlers. The Beaver, pp. 16-21, Autumn 1978 ⟨II-00339⟩

1816-1867

New Brunswick

Whalen, J.: "Almost as bad as Ireland": Saint John, 1847. Archivaria 10:85-97, 1980 ⟨II-00355⟩

Quebec

Desjardins, E.: Montreal aux Prises en 1847 Avec Les Victimes de la Faim. L'UMC 99:306-313, 1970 ⟨II-02438⟩

Nadeau, G.: Ledoyen and His Disinfectant: An Episode in the History of Typhus Fever in Quebec. CMAJ 50:471-476, 1944 ⟨II-04325⟩

Nadeau, G.: Un Episode de L'Histoire du Typhus a Quebec: Ledoyen et son Desinfectant. L'UMC 73:52-66, 1944 ⟨II-02450⟩

1919-1945

Other

Stiver, W.B.: Flight of the White Mice: A World War II Flashback. Ontario Medical Review 47:629-632, 1980 ⟨II-02977⟩

Whooping Cough

1868-1918

Ontario

McKinnon, N.E.: Mortality Reductions in Ontario, 1900-45 VII. Measles and Whooping Cough. Canadian Journal of Public Health 39:95-8, 1948 ⟨II-04477⟩

Wounds and Injuries

1919-1945

Alberta

McConnell, V.: An early venture in heteroplasty. CMAJ 83:609, 1960 ⟨II-03775⟩

Yellow Fever

1700-1759

Quebec

Heagerty, J.J.: Mal de Siam. CMAJ 15:1243-1245, 1925 ⟨II-04155⟩

Drugs and Chemicals

1500-1699

Quebec

Nadeau, G.: Les Vieux Remedes de la Nouvelle-France: l'huile de Petits Chiens. L'UMC 77:327-329, 1948 ⟨II-02349⟩

1700-1759

Canada

J[archo], S.: Drugs Used at Hudson Bay in 1730. Bulletin of the New York Academy of Medicine 47:838-42, 1971 ⟨II-02626⟩

1868-1918

Canada

Stieb, E.W., Quance, E.J.: Drug Adulteration: Detection and Control in Canada I: Beginnings: The Inland Revenue Act of 1875. Pharmacy in History 14:18-24, 1972 ⟨II-05433⟩

Stieb, E.W.: Drug Adulteration: Detection and Control in Canada. A Step Forward: The Adulteration Act of 1884. Pharmacy in History 18(1):17-24, 1976 ⟨II-05432⟩

1919-1945

Canada

Davidson, A.L.: Pharmacopoeial Drug Control in Canada. Canadian Pharmaceutical J 78:53, 73-74, 1945 ⟨II-00261⟩

Alberta

Parsons, W.B.: The day sulfanilamide came to town. Canadian Doctor 45:61-62,65, 1979 ⟨II-00262⟩

Economics, Medical

1500-1699

Quebec

Desjardins, E.: La Medecine a Forfait aux Debuts de Ville-Marie. L'UMC 98:239-242, 1969 ⟨II-02454⟩

Kelly, A.D.: Health Insurance in New France: A Footnote to the History of Medical Economics. BHM 28:535-541, 1954 ⟨II-00258⟩

Kelly, A.D.: Health Insurance in New France. CMAJ 82:1284-1286, 1960 ⟨II-00259⟩

1700-1759

Quebec

Desjardins, E.: Les Honoraries Medicaux D'Antan. L'UMC 99:897-902, 1970 ⟨II-02437⟩

Massicotte, E.Z.: Comptes de Chirurgiens Montrealais au 18eme Siecle. L'UMC 48:507-511, 1919 ⟨II-02360⟩

Massicotte, E.Z.: Documents pour L'Histoire de la Medecine au Canada. L'UMC 48:463-465, 1919 ⟨II-02387⟩

Massicotte, E.Z.: L'Engagement d'un Chirurgien Pour L'Ouest au Dix-Huitieme Siecle. L'UMC 49:204-205, 1920 ⟨II-01833⟩

1760-1815

Ontario

Farmer, M.H.: The ledger of an early doctor of Barton and Ancaster, 1798-1801. Wentworth Bygones 8:34-38, 1969 ⟨II-03100⟩

Riddell, W.R.: The First Medical Case in the Province. N.p. / n.d. ⟨II-00255⟩

Quebec

Fiset, P-A.: Une Correspondence Medicale Historique: Blake a Davidson. Laval Medical 23:419-448, 1957 ⟨II-02425⟩

1868-1918

Canada

Bothwell, R.S., English, J.R.: Pragmatic Physicians: Canadian Medicine and Health Care Insurance 1910-1945. Univ of Western Ontario Med J 46(3):14-17, 1976 ⟨II-00252⟩

MacDermot, H.E.: A Short History of Health Insurance in Canada. CMAJ 50:447-454, 1944 ⟨II-00253⟩

Naylor, C.D.: Canadian Doctors and State Health Insurance, 1911-1918. HSTC Bulletin 6:127-150, 1982 ⟨II-04991⟩

Shillington, C. H.: The Road to Medicare in Canada. Toronto, Del Graphics Pub. Dept., 1972, 208 p. ⟨II-04443⟩

Vandall, P.E.: History of the Canadian Medical Association's attitude toward health insurance. University of Western Ontario Medical Journal 20:42-53, 1950 ⟨II-00254⟩

British Columbia

Andrews, M.W.: Medical Attendance in Vancouver, 1886-1920. B.C. Studies 40:32-56, 1978-79 ⟨II-03698⟩

McDonnell, C.E.: Contract medicine before the railway. British Columbia Medical Journal 19:418-19, 1977 ⟨II-03119⟩

McDonnell, C.E.: CPR contract physicians and early hospital development in Vancouver. British Columbia Medical Journal 20:18-19, 1978 ⟨II-03118⟩

Nova Scotia

Crummey, J.M.: The daybooks of Robert MacLellan: a comparative study of a Nova Scotia family practice during World War 1. CMAJ 120:492-494, 497, 1979 ⟨II-00251⟩

Ontario

Matthews, R.M.: Philosophy of the Fee Schedule. Ontario Medical Review 31:21-23, 1964 ⟨II-03685⟩

1919-1945

Canada

Blishen, B.R.: Doctors and Doctrines. Toronto, University of Toronto Press, 1969. 202 p. ⟨II-00246⟩

Bothwell, R.S.: The Health of the Common People. In: English, J. and J.O. Stubbs, (eds.), Mackenzie King: Widening the Debate. The Macmillan Company of Canada Ltd., pp 191-220 ⟨II-04200⟩

Ettinger, G.H.: The Origins of Support for Medical Research in Canada. CMAJ 78:471-474, 1958 ⟨II-04060⟩

Harrison, H.M.: The End of an Era. CMAJ 82:1166-1167, 1960 ⟨II-00248⟩

Routley, T.C.: Canadian Experiments in Medical Economics. CMAJ 40:599-605, 1939 ⟨II-03778⟩

British Columbia

Andrews, M.W.: The Course of Medical Opinion on State Health Insurance in British Columbia, 1919-1939. Social History 16:129-41, 1983 ⟨II-05276⟩

Wilson, W.A.: Health Insurance -- A Flash-back. British Columbia Medical Journal 2:795-808, 1960 ⟨II-00250⟩

Manitoba

Moorhead, E.S.: A Page in Medical History Prepared by Request. Manitoba Medical Review 38:250 + 251, 1958 ⟨II-05088⟩

Thorlakson, P.H.T.: The History of Prepaid Hospital and Medical Care Plans in Manitoba. CMAJ 84:896-899, 1961 ⟨II-05082⟩

Ontario

Charles, C.A.: The Medical Profession and Health Insurance: an Ontario Case Study. Social Science and Medicine 10:33-38, 1976 ⟨II-05123⟩

Fisher, T.L.: Health Insurance and Associated Medical Services Incorporated. CMAJ 40:284-289, 1939 ⟨II-03592⟩

Hannah, J.A.: The Development of Associated Medical Services Inc. CMAJ 54:606-610, 1946 ⟨II-00247⟩

Robson, R.B.: Windsor Medical Services Incorporated. CMAJ 82:604-607, 1960 ⟨II-00249⟩

Routley, T.C.: Trial Plans in Health Insurance. Ontario Medical Review 34:315-319, 1967 ⟨II-03804⟩

Saskatchewan

Kelly, A.D.: The Swift Current Experiment. CMAJ 58:506-511, 1948 ⟨II-03962⟩

1946-1979
Canada

Gelber, S.M.: The First Decade: Ten Years of Hospital Insurance. Medical Services Journal of Canada 2:1134-1143, 1967 ⟨II-04138⟩

Ontario

Damude, E.F.: The First Ten Years. Toronto, The Physicians' Services Incorporated Foundation, 1980. 139 p. ⟨II-02909⟩

Dunham, H.S.: P.S.I. is born. Ontario Medical Review 35:151-52, 1968 ⟨II-03808⟩

Kelly, A.D.: The Great Medical Prepayment Debates. Ontario Medical Review 35:28-30, 1968 ⟨II-03805⟩

Saskatchewan

Blakeney, A.E.: Press Coverage of the Medicare Dispute in Saskatchewan: I. Queen's Quarterly 70:352-361, 1963-64 ⟨II-02322⟩

Peart, A.F.W.: The Medical Viewpoint. Journal of Public Health 53:724-728, 1963 ⟨II-03821⟩

Thomson, W.: Press Coverage of the Medicare Dispute in Saskatchewan: II. Queen's Quarterly 70:362-371, 1963-64 ⟨II-02323⟩

Education, Medical
1700-1759
Quebec

Seguin, R-L: "L'Apprentissage" de la Chirurgie en Nouvelle-France. Revue d'Histoire de l'Amerique Francaise 20:593-599, 1966-67 ⟨II-04940⟩

1760-1815
Canada

Comrie, J.D.: The part played by Scotland in early Canadian medical development. CMAJ 23:841-844, 1930 ⟨II-03147⟩

Fish, F.H.: Medical Education in Canada. CACHB 17:45-54, 1952 ⟨II-00245⟩

Geikie, W.B.: An Historical Sketch of Canadian Medical Education. Canada Lancet 34:225-287, 1901 ⟨II-04140⟩

MacDermot, H.E.: The Scottish Influence in Canadian Medicine. The Practitioner 183:84-91, 1959 ⟨II-03690⟩

Quebec

Tunis, B.R.: Medical Education and Medical Licensing in Lower Canada: Demographic Factors, Conflict and Social Change. Histoire Sociale/Social History 14:67-91, 1981 ⟨II-04793⟩

1816-1867
Canada

Cleveland, D.E.H.: The Edinburgh Tradition in Canadian Medical Education. Bulletin of the Vancouver Medical Association 28:216-220, 1952 ⟨II-04094⟩

Kett, J.F.: American and Canadian Medical Institutions, 1800-1870. JHMAS 22:343-356, 1967 ⟨II-00319⟩

MacDermot, H.E.: Early Medical Education in North America. CMAJ 67:370-375, 1952 ⟨II-03678⟩

MacDermot, H.E.: The Medical Faculties of Canadian Universities. CMAJ 73:101-103, 1955 ⟨II-03670⟩

McGhie, A.G.: The development of medical education in Canada. McGregor Clinic Bulletin 23(2):10-16, 1962 ⟨II-00328⟩

McGhie, A.G.: The growth of medical practice and medical education in Canada. Wentworth Bygones 9:48-55, 1971 ⟨II-03108⟩

Nova Scotia

Cameron, I.: One Hundred Years of Dalhousie. Dalhousie Medical Journal 21:5-9, 1967 ⟨II-04109⟩

Grant, H.D.: Greetings from the Medical Faculty of Dalhousie University. Nova Scotia Medical Bulletin 32:270-273, 1953 ⟨II-04184⟩

Hattie, W.H.: A note on the founding of Dalhousie University. CMAJ 20:192-193, 1929 ⟨II-03666⟩

MacKenzie, K.A.: The beginnings of Dalhousie Medical School. Dalhousie Med J 11(1):7-11, 1958 ⟨II-00324⟩

Ontario

Beatty, J.D.: History of Medical Education in Toronto. University of Toronto Medical Journal 47:152-57, 1970 ⟨II-05158⟩

Buehrle, R.: The Roots of our Medical School. University of Toronto Medical Journal 44:219-24, 1967 ⟨II-05350⟩

Cameron, M.H.V.: Medical Education in Toronto. CACHB 17:71-74, 1953 ⟨II-00297⟩

Clarkson, F.A.: The Medical Faculty of the University of Toronto. CACHB 13:21-30, 1948 ⟨II-00300⟩

Connell, W.T.: The Medical Faculty -- Queen's University. CACHB 13:45-50, 1948 ⟨II-00301⟩

Curtis, J.F.: The First Medical School in Upper Canada. Ontario Medical Review 34:449-452, 1967 ⟨II-01798⟩

Desjardins, E.: La vieille Ecole de Medecine Victoria. L'UMC 103:117-25, 1974 ⟨II-05453⟩

Desjardins, E.: Les conseillers en droit canonique de l'Ecole de Medecine Victoria. L'UMC 105:626-30, 1976 ⟨II-05233⟩

Dupuis, N.F.: A sketch of the history of the medical college at Kingston during the first 25 years of its existence. Kingston, s.n. 1879? ⟨II-00310⟩

Erb, T.: The Founding of the Medical School at Queen's. CAMSI Journal 24:39-40, 1965 (Apr) ⟨II-00311⟩

Ettinger, G.H.: Queen's University. CAMSI Journal 14:11-12, 1955 (Feb) ⟨II-00312⟩

Geikie, W.B.: Sketch of the Beginning of Medical Education in York, or as it is now called, Toronto. Canada Lancet 38:579-583, 1905 ⟨II-04139⟩

Gibson, T.: Notes on the Medical History of Kingston. CMAJ 18:331-334, 416-451, 1928 ⟨II-01808⟩

Godfrey, C.M.: Trinity Medical School. Applied Therapeutics 8:1024-1028, 1966 ⟨II-04127⟩

Godfrey, C.M.: King's College: Upper Canada's First Medical School. Ontario Medical Review 33:19-22, 26, 1967 ⟨II-04129⟩

Gundy, H.P.: Growing Pains: The Early History of Queen's Medical Faculty. Transactions of the Kingston Historical Society 4;14-25, 1954-55 ⟨II-04170⟩

Henderson, J.L.H.: The Founding of Trinity College, Toronto. Ontario History 44:7-14, 1952 ⟨II-01828⟩

Herald, J: History of Medical Education in Kingston,. Queen's Medical Quarterly 8:5-15, 1903 ⟨II-04152⟩

Hunstman, A.G.: The Jubilee Reunion of the Class of 1905: The Varsity Tree. Toronto, 1955, University of Toronto ⟨II-00316⟩

Jamieson, H.C.: Medical Teaching in Canada in 1824 and 1834. CMAJ 17:360-361, 1927 ⟨II-03983⟩

Kelly, A.D.: Ontario-1867: The Common Health. Ontario Medical Review 34:435-442, 1967 ⟨II-00318⟩

McConnell, F.: Highlights in the Early History of the Faculty of Medicine, the University of Toronto. CAMSI Journal 10:29, 1951 (Feb) ⟨II-00327⟩

Primrose, A.: The Faculty of Medicine. In: The University of Toronto and its Colleges, 1827-1906. Toronto, University Library, 1906. pp 168-179 ⟨II-02329⟩

Scott, J.W.: Medical Education Sites in Toronto Commemorated. Ontario Medical Review 47:452-454, 1980 ⟨II-01951⟩

Scott, J.W.: Rolph's Medical School. Ontario Medical Review 47:454-455, 1980 ⟨II-01952⟩

Spragge, G.W.: The Trinity Medical College. Ontario Historical Society Journal 58:63-98, 1966 ⟨II-00333⟩

Stanley, G.D.: Dr. John Rolph: Medicine and Rebellion in Upper Canada. CACHB 9(1):1-13, 1944 ⟨II-00334⟩

Sullivan, M.: Retrospect of Fifty Years of the Medical School of Kingston. Np, nd, pp. 35 ⟨II-03716⟩

[Travill, A.A.]: Queen's University at Kingston, Faculty of Medicine 1854-1979. One Hundred and Twenty-Five Years Dedicated to Education and Service. Kingston, Queen's University, 48 p. ⟨II-01852⟩

Wallace, W.S.: The Graduates of King's College, Toronto. Ontario History 42:163-4, 1950 ⟨II-03256⟩

Workman, J.: Discourse on Education. York Pioneer 67:32-38, 1971 ⟨II-03286⟩

Wright, A.H.: The Medical Schools of Toronto. CMAJ 18:616-620, 1928 ⟨II-01807⟩

Quebec

Abbott, M.E.: An Historical Sketch of the Medical Faculty of McGill University. Montreal Medical Journal 31:561-672, 1902 ⟨II-04213⟩

Abbott, M.E.: McGill's Heroic Past 1821-1921. Montreal, McGill University, 1921. 30 p. ⟨II-04120⟩

Abbott, M.E.: The Faculty of Medicine of McGill University. Surgery, Gynecology and Obstetrics 60:242-253, 1935 ⟨II-04038⟩

Audet, L.-P.: Index Analytique du Memorial de le'Education dans le Bas- Canada du Dr. Jean-Baptiste Meilleur. PTRSC. Series 4, 2:49-62, 1964 ⟨II-04950⟩

Bensley, E.H.: The Beginning of Teaching at McGill University. McGill Journal of Education 6:23-24, 1971 ⟨II-01542⟩

Boissonnault, C.M.: Histoire de la Faculte de Medecine de Laval. Quebec, Les Presses Universitaires Laval, 1953. 438 p. ⟨II-02427⟩

David, A.H.: Reminiscences Connected with the Medical Profession in Montreal During the Last Fifty Years. The Canada Medical Record 11:1-8, 1882 ⟨II-00307⟩

Desjardins, E.: L'Ecole de Medecine et de Chirurgie de Montreal: Ses Doyens. L'UMC 95:967-977, 1966 ⟨II-02389⟩

Desjardins, E.: L'Enseignement Medicale a Montreal au Milieu du XIX Siecle. L'UMC 100:305-309, 1971 ⟨II-02428⟩

Desjardins, E.: L'Universite Laval de Quebec. L'UMC 102:630-35, 1973 ⟨II-05345⟩

Douglas, J.: Journals and Reminiscences of James Douglas, M.D. New York, 1910. 254 p. ⟨II-04222⟩

Dufresne, R.: L'Ecole de Medecine et de Chirurgie de Montreal (1843-1891). L'UMC 75:1314-1325, 1946 ⟨II-02390⟩

Ewing, M.: Influence of the Edinburgh Medical School on the Early Development of McGill University. Canadian Journal of Surgery 18:287-296, 1975 ⟨II-04333⟩

Gauvreau, J.: L'Ecole de Medecine et de Chirurgie de Montreal Fondee en 1843: Le Docteur Thomas Arnoldi, son Premier President. L'UMC 60:818-827, 1931 ⟨II-02343⟩

Gauvreau, J.: Montreal Medical Institution Fondee en 1824 Par Les Medecins du Montreal General Hospital. L'UMC 60:732-736, 1931 ⟨II-01868⟩

Gibson, W.C.: Merchant Princes and Medicine. CMAJ 86:659-661, 1962 ⟨II-01789⟩

Hall, A.: On the Past, Present, and Future of the Faculty of Medicine of McGill University. Canadian Medical Journal and Monthly Record of Medical and Surgical Science 3:289-302, 1866-1867 ⟨II-00314⟩

Howard, R.P.: A Sketch of the Life of the Late G.W. Campbell A.M., LL.D., Late Dean of the Medical Faculty, and a Summary of the History of the Faculty; Being the Introductory Address of the Fiftieth Session of the Medical Faculty of McGill University. Montreal Gazette, 1882 ⟨II-00315⟩

Johnson, G.R.: McGill University -- Medical Faculty, Part 1. CACHB 14:41-47, 1949 ⟨II-00317⟩

LeBlond, S.: Pioneers of Medical Teaching in the Province of Quebec. JAMA 200:843-848, 1967 ⟨II-02429⟩

LeBlond, S.: William Marsden (1807-1885): Essai Biographique. Laval Medical 41:639-658, 1970 ⟨II-00321⟩

LeBlond, S.: Le docteur Joseph Painchaud (1787-1871) conferencier populaire. Cahier des Dix 36:120-138, 1971 ⟨II-00320⟩

LeBlond, S.: Le profession medicale sous l'Union (1840-1867). Cahier des Dix 38:165-203, 1973 ⟨II-02430⟩

Maheux, A.A.: Centenary of the Faculty of Medicine of Laval University. CMAJ 67:64-67, 1952 ⟨II-04629⟩

McGregor, M.: Le Troisieme Cinquantenaire de la Faculte de Medecine de McGill. L'UMC 100:435-437, 1971 ⟨II-02431⟩

Mignault, L.D.: Histoire de L'Ecole de Medecine et de Chirurgie de Montreal. L'Union Medicale du Canada 55:597-674, 1926 ⟨II-05110⟩

Mignault, L.D.: A Short History of the Medical Faculty of the University of Montreal. CMAJ 17:242-245, 1927 ⟨II-03645⟩

Quinn, R.W.: The Four Founders. McGill Medical Undergraduate Journal 5:5-11, 1936 ⟨II-00330⟩

Richard, L.: La Famille Loedel. Le Bulletin des Recherches Historiques 56:78-89, 1950 ⟨II-00331⟩

Shepherd, F.J.: The First Medical School in Canada. CMAJ 15:418-525, 1925 ⟨II-03702⟩

Tunis, B.R., Bensley, E.H.: A La Recherche de William Leslie Logie, Premier Diplome de L'Universite McGill. L'UMC 100:536-538, 1971 ⟨II-02456⟩

Tunis, B.R., Bensley, E.H.: William Lesley Logie: McGill University's first graduate and Canada's first medical graduate. CMAJ 105:1259-1263, 1971 ⟨II-00336⟩

Vallee, A.: The Medical Faculty of Laval University, Quebec. Surgery, Gynecology, and Obstetrics 60:1149-1150, 1935 ⟨II-05017⟩

Whiteford, W.: Reminiscences of Dr. John Stephenson, one of the Founders of McGill Medical Faculty. Canada Medical and Surgical Journal 11:728-731, 1883 ⟨II-00338⟩

United States

Cameron, M.H.V.: Jefferson Medical College in 1850 [for Canadian students]. CMAJ 66:73-75, + 82, 1952 ⟨II-04630⟩

1868-1918

Canada

MacDermot, H.E.: Sir Thomas Roddick. His Work in Medicine and Public LIfe. Toronto, Macmillan Co. of Canada Ltd., 1938. 160 p. ⟨II-00282⟩

McGovern, J.P., Roland, C.G.: William Osler: The Continuing Education. Springfield, Charles C. Thomas, Publisher, 1969 ⟨II-00279⟩

Alberta

Revell, D.G.: The Medical Faculty -- University of Alberta. CACHB 13:65-75, 1949 ⟨II-00284⟩

Scott, J.W.: Faculty of Medicine, University of Alberta. Alberta Medical Bulletin 20:58-61, 1955 ⟨II-03706⟩

Scott, J.W.: The History of the Faculty of Medicine of the University of Alberta 1913-1963. Alberta, The University of Alberta, 1963. 43 p. ⟨II-00286⟩

Stanley, G.D.: Dr. Daniel Graisberry Revell: Medical Teacher, Scholar and Gentleman. CACHB 14:48-54, 1949 ⟨II-00287⟩

British Columbia

Gibson, W.G.: Wesbrook and his University. Vancouver, Library of the University of British Columbia, 1973 ⟨II-00275⟩

Manitoba

Gemmell, J.P.: "Good -- Doctor" Dr. J. Wilford Good, Dean of Manitoba Medical College, 1887-1898. University of Manitoba Medical Journal 51:98-103, 1981 ⟨II-04873⟩

Mitchell, R.: Manitoba's medical school. CMAJ 706-708, 1930 Vol. 22 ⟨II-03111⟩

Mitchell, R.: Manitoba's Educational Institutions. CMAJ 22:705-708, 1930 ⟨II-03648⟩

Mitchell, R.: The Manitoba Medical College, 1883-1933. CMAJ 29:549-552, 1933 ⟨II-03087⟩

Mitchell, R.: Manitoba's Medical School. CACHB 12:66-69, 1948 ⟨II-03649⟩

Mitchell, R.: Samuel Willis Prowse, MD 1869-1931: Fourth Dean of Medicine. Manitoba Medical Review 38:551-553, 1958 ⟨II-02886⟩

Mitchell, R.: H.H. Chown, Third Dean of Manitoba Medical College 1859-1944. Manitoba Medical Review 39:189-191, 1959 ⟨II-01925⟩

Mitchell, R.: Samuel Willis Prowse. Manitoba Medical Review 41:455-459, 1961 ⟨II-02887⟩

Mitchell, R., Thorlakson, T.K.: James Kerr, 1848-1911 and Harry Hyland Kerr, 1881-1963: Pioneer Canadian-American Surgeons. Canadian Journal of Surgery 9:213-220, 1966 ⟨II-02665⟩

Montgomery, E.W.: J.W. Good -- The Most Unforgettable Character I Have Known. University of Manitoba Medical Journal 21:27-34, 1949 ⟨II-02190⟩

Peters, H.: A History of the Education of Selected Health Professions in Manitoba, Thesis (Master of Education). Department of Educational Foundation, University of Manitoba, January 1979 ⟨II-00281⟩

Wilt, J.C.: The History of Medical Education in Manitoba. University of Manitoba Medical Journal 39:125-132, 1968 ⟨II-03585⟩

Nova Scotia

Atlee, H.B.: Dalhousie Medical School 1907-1957. Dalhousie Medical Journal 11(1):21-33, 1958 ⟨II-00266⟩

Hattie, W.H.: Historical Sketch of the Dalhousie Medical School. CMAJ 15:539-541, 1925 〈II-01801〉

MacKenzie, K.A., Stewart, C.B.: Dalhousie University. CAMSI Journal 15:15-20, 1956 〈II-03676〉

McKenzie, K.A.: The Dalhousie Medical School. CACHB 11:78-81, 1947 〈II-00280〉

Scammell, H.L.: The Halifax Medical College. Dalhousie Medical Journal 11(1):12-17, 1958 〈II-00285〉

Ontario

Barr, M.L.: A Century of Medicine at Western. London, Ontario, University of Western Ontario, 1977. 672 p. 〈II-00267〉

Crane, J.W.: The University of Western Ontario, London, Ontario. CACHB 13:1-3, 1948 〈II-00270〉

Dittrick, H.: The Old Days in Toronto. CACHB 7(4):6-9, 1943 〈II-00271〉

Elliott, J.H.: Osler's Class at the Toronto School of Medicine. CMAJ 47:161-165, 1942 〈II-00272〉

Gray, W.A.: Early Years in our Medical School [U.W.O.]. University of Western Ontario Medical Journal 22:106-112, 1952 〈II-04183〉

Gullen, A.S.: A Brief History of the Ontario Medical College for Women, 1906. Canadian Journal of Medicine and Surgery 65:82-88, 1929 〈II-02339〉

Gwyn, N.B.: Osler, Student of the Toronto School of Medicine: a Detail of the Personal Side of Teaching. Annals of Medical History 5:305-308, 1923 〈II-02633〉

Gwyn, N.B.: The Medical Arena in the Toronto of Osler's Early Days in the Study of Medicine. Archives of Internal Medicine 84:2-6, 1949 〈II-00276〉

Lynn, R.B.: James Cameron Connell: 1863-1947. Canadian Journal of Surgery 11:336-339, 1968 〈II-02095〉

MacDonald, J.A.: The Daffydil Story. University of Toronto Medical Journal 31:64-67, 1953 〈II-03642〉

McCrae, T.: Some Medical Teachers of the Nineties. Canadian Journal of Medicine and Surgery 50:138-141, 1921 〈II-03773〉

Roche, W.J.: Reminiscences. University of Western Ontario Medical Journal 1:8-10, 1930 〈II-04797〉

Shortt, E.S.: Historical Sketch of Medical Education of Women in Kingston, Canada. N.p., Kingston, September, 1916, 24 p. 〈II-03701〉

Stevenson, L.G.: Canadian Medical Faculties through the years: University of Western Ontario. CAMSI Journal 13:17-21, 1954 〈II-03839〉

Stevenson, L.G.: University of Western Ontario. CAMSI Journal 13:17-18, 21, 1954 (Dec) 〈II-00289〉

Quebec

Gordon, A.H.: Medicine in Montreal in the Nineties. CMAJ 53:495-499, 1945 〈II-04123〉

Howard, R.P.: William Osler: "A Potent Ferment" at McGill. Archives of Internal Medicine 84:12-15, 1949 〈II-02634〉

Jobin, P.: La Faculte de Medecine de l'Universite Laval Depuis sa Fondation Jusqu'a 1875. L'UMC 75:1305-1313, 1946 〈II-02441〉

Johnson, G.R.: McGill University -- Medical Faculty, Part 11. CACHB 15:1-7, 1950 〈II-00277〉

LeSage, A.: Le Decanat a la Faculte de Medecine de L'Universite de Montreal: Trois Doyens (1880-1934) -- Rottot, Lachapelle, Harwood. L'UMC 68:166-178, 1939 〈II-02392〉

White, W.: Medical Education at McGill in the Seventies: Excerpts from the "Autobiographie" of the late Paul Zotique Hebert, MD. BHM 13:614-626, 1943 〈II-02606〉

Saskatchewan

Anderson, A.L.: The School of Medical Sciences and the Medical College of the University of Saskatchewan. CACHB 17:1-9, 1952 〈II-00265〉

1919-1945
British Columbia

Ranta, L.E.: The Medical School of British Columbia. CACHB 16:1-9, 1951 〈II-00243〉

Manitoba

Black, E.F.E.: Not So Long Ago. University of Manitoba Medical Journal 45:54-56, 1975 〈II-00242〉

Saunderson, H.H.: Class of '28 -- 50 Years Later. University of Manitoba Medical Journal 48:95-105, 1978 〈II-00244〉

Ontario

Eisen, D.: Diary of a Medical Student. Canadian Jewish Congress, 1974. 133 p. 〈II-05010〉

Tablyn, W.F.: Faculties of Medicine and Public Health, 1924-1938. In: These Sixty Years. London, Univ. of Western Ontario, 1938. pp 111-116 〈II-05360〉

Quebec

Bensley, E.H.: Bishop's Medical College. CMAJ 72:463-465, 1955 〈II-00268〉

LeBlond, S.: L'enseignement de la medecine a l'Universite Laval de 1923 a 1928. Canadian Society for the History of Medicine Newsletter, 1983. pp 1-5 〈II-05278〉

1946-1979
Ontario

Belanger, L.F.: On a Nickle and a Prayer. A Personal Outlook on the Early Days of the Medical School. Ottawa, University of Ottawa Press, 1978. 〈II-00240〉

Quebec

Maltais, R.: Le Centre Medical De L'Universite de Sherbrooke: Une esquisse de son histoire (1961-1979). Sherbrooke, de L'Universite de Sherbrooke, 1980. 〈II-04664〉

All embracing
Canada

MacFarlane, J.A.: Medical Education in Canada. Ottawa, Queen's Printer, 1965. 373 p. 〈II-00238〉

Emergency Care
1868-1918
Ontario

Hanna, J.A.: A Century of Red Blankets: A History of Ambulance Service in Ontario. Ontario, Boston Mills Press, 1982. 100 p. ⟨II-05260⟩

Endocrinology
1868-1918
Ontario

Best, C.H.: The Internal Secretion of the Pancreas. CMAJ 87:1046-1051, 1962 ⟨II-04022⟩

United States

Magner, L.N.: Ernest Lyman Scott's work with insulin: a reappraisal. Pharmacy in History 19:103-108, 1977 ⟨II-03620⟩

1919-1945
Canada

Barr, M.L.: James Bertram Collip (1892-1965); A Canadian Pioneer in Endocrinology. In International Congress for the History of Medicine, 25th, Quebec, 1976. Proceedings, volume 11, 1976. p. 469-476 ⟨II-00256⟩

Ontario

Allan, F.N.: The Discovery of Insulin. New England Journal of Medicine 297:283-4, 1977 ⟨II-05241⟩

Bastenie, P.A.: L'isolement de l'insuline. Bulletin Academie Royalle Medicine Belgique 11:321-8, 1971 ⟨II-05458⟩

Best, C.H.: Impact of Insulin on Metabolic Pathway. Recollections of 1921. Israel Journal of Medical Sciences 8:181-85, 1972 ⟨II-05352⟩

Best, C.H.: Nineteen Hundred Twenty-One in Toronto. Diabetes 21:385-95, 1972 ⟨II-05351⟩

Bliss, M.: The Aetiology of the Discovery of Insulin. In: Roland, C.G.(ed.): Health, Disease and Medicine: Essays in Canadian History. Toronto, Hannah Institute for the History of Medicine, 1984, 333-346 ⟨II-05405⟩

Cheymol, J.: A propos de la decouverte de l'insuline par Banting et Best, il y a cinquante ans. Bulletin de l'Academie Nationale de Medecine 155:836-52, 1971 ⟨II-05348⟩

Groen, J.J.: Discovery of Insulin Told as a Human Story. Israel Journal of Medical Sciences 8:476-83, 1972 ⟨II-05335⟩

Harris, S.: Banting's Miracle: The Story of the Discoverer of Insulin. Toronto/Vancouver, J.M. Dent and Sons (Canada) Ltd., 1946. 245 p. ⟨II-00234⟩

Harrison, R.C.: Canadian Contributions towards the Comprehension of Hyperinsulinism: the First Successful Excision of an Insulinoma. Canadian Journal of Surgery 23:401-403, 1980 ⟨II-02983⟩

Rowntree, L.G.: Banting's "Miracle". In: Amid Masters of Twentieth Century Medicine. Springfield, Charles C. Thomas Publisher, 1958. pp 339-354 ⟨II-02690⟩

Shaw, M.M.: He Conquered Death: The Story of Frederick Grant Banting. Toronto, Macmillan Co. of Canada Ltd., 1946. III p. ⟨II-00235⟩

Stevenson, L.G.: Sir Frederick Banting. Toronto, The Ryerson Press, 1946. 446 p. ⟨II-00236⟩

Wrenshall, G.A., Hetenyi, G., Feasby, W.R.: The Story of Insulin. Canada, Max Reinhardt, 1962. 232 p. ⟨II-00237⟩

Quebec

Goupil, G.: Hans Selye: La Sagesse du Stress. Nouvelle Optique, 1981 169 p. ⟨II-04218⟩

Other

Carr, F.H.: The early days of insulin manufacture. The Diabetic Journal 4:355-357, 1946 ⟨II-00233⟩

Epidemiology
1700-1759
Canada

Taylor, J.F.: Sociocultural Effects of Epidemics on the Northern Plains: 1734-1850. Western Canadian Journal of Anthropology 7(4):55-81, 1977 ⟨II-04205⟩

1760-1815
Canada

Drake, D.: A Systematic Treatise, historical, etiological and practical, on the Principal Diseases of the Interior Valley of North America, as they appear in the Caucasian, African, Indian, and Esquimaux Varieties of its Population. Cincinnati, Winthrop B. Smith and Co., Publishers, 1850, 878 p. ⟨II-00231⟩

1816-1867
Canada

Brown, C.P.: The Quarantine Service of Canada. Canadian Journal of Public Health 46:449-453, 1955 ⟨II-00228⟩

Ray, A.J.: Diffusion of Disease in the Western Interior of Canada, 1830-1850. Geographical Review 66:139-157, 1976 ⟨II-00230⟩

All embracing
Canada

Newman, M.T.: Aboriginal New World Epidemiology and Medical Care, and the Impact of Old World Disease Imports. American Journal of Physical Anthropology 45:667-672, 1976 ⟨II-04996⟩

Ethics, Medical
1816-1867
Ontario

Riddell, W.R.: A Medical Slander Case in 1831. Canada Lancet 48:501-3, 1915 ⟨II-04475⟩

Quebec

Bayne, J.R.D., Nadero, B.: A Defence of Dr. James Douglas. CMAJ 51:277-278, 1944 ⟨II-04472⟩

1868-1918

Canada

Sprague, J.D.: Medical Ethics and Cognate subjects. Toronto, Chas. P. Sparling and Co., Publishers, 1902. 248 p. 〈II-00227〉

1946-1979

Saskatchewan

Badgley, R.F., Wolfe, S: The Doctors' Right to Strike. In: Torrey, E.F. (edit): Ethical Issues in Medicine: The Role of Physician in Today's Society. Boston, Little, Brown and Company, 1968 pp 301-321 〈II-04028〉

1980-1989

Ontario

O'Malley, M.: A Doctor's Dilemma. Saturday Night, May 1983. pp 19-29, 1983 〈II-05129〉

Evolution

1919-1945

Other

Hood, D.: Davidson Black: A Biography. Toronto, University of Toronto Press, 1964. 145 p. 〈II-00226〉

Famous Persons

1816-1867

Other

Mitchell, C.A.: Walter Henry and the Autopsy of Emperor Napoleon I. University of Ottawa Medical Journal 9:3-8, 1965 〈II-04144〉

1868-1918

Canada

Anderson, F.W.: Louis Riel's insanity reconsidered. Saskatchewan History 3:104-110, 1950 〈II-02624〉

Clark, D.: A psycho-medical history of Louis Riel. American Journal of Insanity 44:33-51, 1887 〈II-026206U

Desjardins, E., Dumas, C.: Le complexe medical de Louis Riel. L'UMC 99:1656-61, 1970 〈II-05343〉

Flanagan, T.E.: Louis Riel: A Case Study in Involuntary Psychiatric Confinement. Canadian Psychiatric Association Journal 23:463-8, 1978 〈II-05256〉

Greenland, C.: The Life and Death of Louis Riel -- Part II -- Surrender, Trial, Appeal and Execution. Canadian Psychiatric Association Journal 10:253-259, 1965 〈II-04788〉

Knox, O.: The Question of Louis Riel's Insanity. Historical and Scientific Society of Manitoba. Papers, Series 3, No. 6:20-34, 1951 〈II-02102〉

Lehmann, P.O.: Louis Riel -- patriot or zealot?. B.C. Medical Journal 5:154-171, 1963 〈II-02619〉

Littmann, S.K.: A Pathography of Louis Riel. Canadian Psychiatric Association Journal 23:449-62, 1978 〈II-05257〉

Markson, E.R.: The Life and Death of Louis Riel: A Study in Forensic Psychiatry Part I. Canadian Psychiatric Association Journal 10:246-252, 1965 〈II-04789〉

Turner, R.E.: The Life and Death of Louis Riel -- Part III -- Medico-Legal Issues. Canadian Psychiatric Association Journal 10:259-264, 1965 〈II-04787〉

Alberta

Stanley, G.D.: 'Bob' Edwards again and his Eye-Opener!. CACHB 12:38-40, 1947 〈II-00224〉

Stanley, G.D.: The pioneer doctor and a famous newspaper editor. CACHB II:82-84, 1947 〈II-00225〉

Ontario

Livermore, J.D.: The Personal Agonies of Edward Blake. CHR 56:45-58, 1975 〈II-04876〉

Quebec

Bayne, J.R.D.: The Lot of Few Men [Murdo Morrison, the Megantic Outlaw]. CMAJ 66:178-180, 1952 〈II-04628〉

1980-1989

Canada

Lord, J.: The Song of Alopeix, and Other Poems [Terry Fox]. Hamilton, Epic Publishing Co., 1983. pp viii + 109 〈II-05283〉

Scrivener, L.: Terry Fox: His Story. Toronto, McClelland and Stewart, 1981, pp 176 〈II-05284〉

Folk and Popular Medicine

1500-1699

Quebec

Drolet, A.: Quelques remedes indigenes a travers la correspondance de Mere Sainte- Helene. Cahiers Histoire 22:30-7, 1970 〈II-05454〉

1760-1815

Nova Scotia

Blakeley, P.R.: And Having a Love for People. Nova Scotia Historical Quarterly 5:167-175, 1975 〈II-04013〉

1816-1867

Newfoundland

MacDonald, E.: Outport Medicine in Newfoundland. Canadian Pharmaceutical Journal 92(11):40-41, 1959 〈II-03689〉

Ontario

Aldren, B.: Life in Upper Canada in 1837. CMAJ 20:65-67, 1929 〈II-00356〉

Riddell, W.R.: Popular medicine in Upper Canada a century ago. Ontario Historical Society Papers and Records, 25:1-8, 1929 〈II-03791〉

Woolcock, H.R.: Attitudes to Health and Disease in London, Canada, 1826-1854. Thesis (M.A.), London, University of Western Ontario, 1977 〈II-05141〉

1868-1918

New Brunswick

Hoyt, J.: Great Grandmother's Medicine Ball. New Brunswick Historical Society Collections 17:41-43, 1961 〈II-04010〉

Thornton, L.A.: Grandmother's Pharmacy. New Brunswick Historical Society Collections 18:58-63, 1963 ⟨II-04011⟩

Ontario

Nyce, J.M.: The Gordon C. Eby Diaries, 1911-13: Chronicle of a Mennonite Farmer. Multicultural History Society of Ontario, 1982. 208 p. ⟨II-05268⟩

Quebec

Morisset, A.: Le Langage Populaire de la Medecine du Debut du Siecle au Canada Francais. La Vie Medicale 6:276-281, 1977 ⟨II-04945⟩

1946-1979
British Columbia

Layton, M.: Magico-Religious Elements in the Traditional Beliefs of Maillardville, B.C. British Columbia Studies 27:50-61, 1975 ⟨II-03255⟩

Quebec

Dulong, G.: Medecine Populaire au Canada Francais. In International Congress for the History of Medicine, 25th, Quebec, 1976. Proceedings, volume II, 1976. p. 625-633 ⟨II-00223⟩

All embracing
Canada

Cronin, F.: Elixir or not, Ginseng is a Lucrative Cash Crop. Canadian Geographic 102(6): 60-63, 1982 ⟨II-04994⟩

Langdon, E.: Medicines Out of the Earth. Canadian [Antique] Collector 13:28-31, 1978 ⟨II-00222⟩

Quebec

Desjardins, E.: La medecine populaire au Canada francais. L'UMC 101:1595-601, 1972;102:154-59, 1973 ⟨II-05344⟩

Lacourciere, L.: A Survey of Folk Medicine in French Canada from Early Times to the Present. In: Hand, W.D.: American Folk Medicine a Symposium. Berkeley, University of California Press, 1976. pp 203-214 ⟨II-02334⟩

Morin, V: Superstitions et Croyances Populaires. PTRSC 31 [1]:51:60, 1937 ⟨II-03985⟩

Foods and Food Supply
1760-1815
British Columbia

Archer, C.I.: Cannibalism in the Early History of the Northwest Coast: Enduring Myths and Neglected Realities. CHR 71:453-479, 1980 ⟨II-02943⟩

1816-1867
Ontario

Duncan, K.: Irish Famine, Immigration and the Social Structure of Canada West. Canadian Review of Sociology and Anthropology 2:19-40, 1964-5 ⟨II-00221⟩

Quebec

Desjardins, E.: Montreal aux Prises en 1847 Avec les Victimes de la Faim. L'UMC 99:305-313, 1970 ⟨II-02357⟩

1919-1945
Canada

Burgess, H.: Health by remote control. The Beaver 301(4):50-55, 1970 ⟨II-03308⟩

North West Territories

Whalley, G.(edit.): Death in the Barren Ground: Edgar Christian. Canada, Oberon Press, 1980 ⟨II-02618⟩

All embracing
Canada

Draper, H.H.: The Aboriginal Eskimo Diet in Modern Perspective. American Anthropologist 79:309-316, 1977 ⟨II-04998⟩

Rich, E.E.: The Fur Traders: Their Diet and Drugs. The Beaver, Summer 1976. pp 43-53 ⟨II-00220⟩

British Columbia

Edwards, G.T.: Indian Spaghetti. The Beaver, Autumn 1979. pp. 4-11. ⟨II-00219⟩

Forensic Medicine and Legal Medicine
1500-1699
Quebec

Cadotte, M.: Le Docteur Adrien Duchesne, Le Premier Expert Medico-Legal de La Nouvelle-France (1639). L'UMC 104:276-278, 1975 ⟨II-00344⟩

1816-1867
Ontario

Riddell, W.R.: A medical slander case in Upper Canada, 85 years ago. Canada Lancet 46:330-332, 1913 ⟨II-03834⟩

Quebec

LeBlond, S.: Le drame de Kamouraska: d'apres les documents de l'epoque. Cahier des Dix 37:239-273, 1972 ⟨II-02412⟩

1868-1918
Manitoba

Turner, R.E.: The life and death of Louis Riel: part III -- medico-legal issues. Canadian Psychiatric Association Journal 10:259-264, 1965 ⟨II-02623⟩

United States

Scammell, H.L.: Medicine Hat. Nova Scotia Medical Bulletin 28:146-148, 1949 ⟨II-03699⟩

Other

Jenkins, E.: Neill Cream, Poisoner. In: Reader's Digest, 1978. pp 67-156 ⟨II-00362⟩

1946-1979
Ontario

Scott, G.D.: Inmate: The Casebook Revelations of a Canadian Penitentiary Psychiatrist. Montreal, Optimum Publishing International Inc., 1982. 226 pages ⟨II-04818⟩

Gastroenterology and Digestive System
1816-1867
Canada

Bensley, E.H.: Alexis St. Martin. CMAJ 80:907-909, 1959 ⟨II-02068⟩

Bensley, E.H.: Alexis St. Martin and Dr. Bunting. BHM 44:101-8, 1970 ⟨II-05388⟩

Desjardins, E.: Le Cas D'Alexis Saint-Martin. L'UMC 100:964-968, 1971 ⟨II-00359⟩

LeBlond, S.: Alexis St. Martin: Sa Vie et Son Temps. Laval Medical 33:578-585, 1962 ⟨II-02067⟩

Martin, C.A.: Alexis le fistuleux. Vie Medicale au Canada Francais 2:378-83, 1973 ⟨II-05442⟩

Texter, J.H.: Misfortune to Fame. The Story of William Beaumont, M.D. and his Famous Patient Alexis St. Martin. Virginia Medical Monthly 102(10):821-6, 1975 ⟨II-05430⟩

General Practice and Family Medicine
1816-1867
Canada

Woods, D.: The family doctor in Canada evolves. CMAJ 112:92-95, 1975 ⟨II-00218⟩

1868-1918
Canada

Shortt, S.E.D.: "Before the Age of Miracles": The Rise, Fall, and Rebirth of General Practice in Canada, 1890-1940. In: Roland, C.G.(ed.): Health, Disease and Medicine: Essays in Canadian History. Toronto, Hannah Institute for the History of Medicine, 1984, 123-152 ⟨II-05398⟩

1946-1979
Canada

Woods, D.: Strength in Study. Toronto, College of Physicians of Canada, 1979. 248 p. ⟨II-00217⟩

Alberta

Dolgoy, M: The First Ten Years of the College of General Practice (Alberta Division). Canadian Family Physician 15:71-76, 1969 ⟨II-04081⟩

British Columbia

Wallace, A.W.: History of Family Practice in B.C. British Columbia Medical Journal 21:264-5, 1979 ⟨II-03248⟩

Ontario

McAuley, R.G., Moore, C.A.: Family Medicine in Hamilton 1965-1981: Change Over Time. Canadian Family Physician 28:556-558, 1982 ⟨II-04813⟩

Generation and Reproduction
1868-1918
Ontario

McConnachie, K.: A Note on Fertility Rates Among Married Women in Toronto, 1871. Ontario History 75:87-98, 1983 ⟨II-05087⟩

All embracing
Quebec

Bouvier, L.F.: The Spacing of Births Among French-Canadian families: An Historical Approach. Canadian Review of Social Anthropology 5(1):17-26, 1968 ⟨II-05455⟩

Genetics and Heredity
1919-1945
Alberta

Chapman, T.L.: Early Eugenics Movement in Western Canada. Alberta History 25(4):9-17, 1977 ⟨II-02980⟩

Gibson, D.: Involuntary Sterilization of the Mentally Retarded: A Western Canadian Phenomenon. Canadian Psychiatric Association Journal 19:59-63, 1974 ⟨II-05366⟩

Gynecology
1868-1918
Canada

Mitchinson, W.: Causes of Disease in Women: The Case of Late 19th Century English Canada. In: Roland, C.G.(ed.): Health, Disease and Medicine: Essays in Canadian History. Toronto, Hannah Institute for the History of Medicine, 1984, 381-395 ⟨II-05408⟩

Ontario

Cosbie, W.G.: Frederick Marlow (1877-1936) and the Development of the Modern Treatment of Carcinoma of the Cervix. Canadian Journal of Surgery 5:357-365, 1962 ⟨II-03629⟩

Yukon

Cruikshank, J.: Becoming a Woman in Athapaskan Society: Changing Traditions on the Upper Yukon River. Western Canadian Journal of Anthropology 5(2):1-14, 1975 ⟨II-04206⟩

1919-1945
Canada

Coshie, W.G.: The History of the Society of Obstetricians and Gynaecologists of Canada. 1944-1966. Toronto, N.P. 1968 p.65 ⟨II-04380⟩

Health Occupations and Professions
1816-1867
Canada

Nicholson, G.W.: The White Cross in Canada; A History of St. John Ambulance. Montreal, Harvest House, 1967. 206 p. ⟨II-05451⟩

1868-1918
Alberta

Browarny, L.: A Friend in Need. St. John Ambulance in Calgary. Calgary, Century Calgary Publications, 1975 ⟨II-05099⟩

Quebec

Gaucher, D.: La Formation des Hygienistes a L'Universite de Montreal, 1910-1975: De La Sante Publique a La Medecine Preventive. Recherches Sociographiques 20:59-85, 1979 ⟨II-04686⟩

Hematology

1868-1918
Manitoba

Mitchell, R.: The 55 "Hospitals" and nursing missions of greater Winnipeg. CMAJ 22:861-866, 1930 ⟨II-03145⟩

Mitchell, R.: Dr. F.W.E. Burnham 1872-1957. Manitoba Medical Review 46:549-550, 1966 ⟨II-03864⟩

1919-1945
Canada

Jaques, L.B.: Reminiscences on completing twenty-five years of research in the blood coagulation field. University of Saskatchewan Medical Journal 3:4-6, 1960 ⟨II-00216⟩

Manitoba

Chown, B: The Story of the Winnipeg Rh Laboratory. Journal-Lancet 87:38-40, 1967 ⟨II-04097⟩

Schmidt, A.: An Rh Retrospective. The Alumni Journal [U. Manitoba] 43:6-7, 1983 ⟨II-05209⟩

Histology

1946-1979
Ontario

Moore, K.L.: The Discovery of the Sex Chromatin. IN: the Sex Chromatin, Philadelphia, W.B. Saunders Co., 1966 ⟨II-03750⟩

Historiography and History of Medicine

1700-1759
Quebec

Bernier, J.: L'Histoire de la Medecine Quebecoise aux XVIIIe et XIXe siecles: Problems et Sources. Department d'Histoire, Universite Laval, 1978. 13 p. n.p. ⟨II-02424⟩

1760-1815
Canada

Ward, W.P.: Family Papers and the New Social History. Archivaria 14:63-73, 1982 ⟨II-05265⟩

Newfoundland

Lysaght, A.M.: Joseph Banks in Newfoundland and Labrador, 1766: His Diary, Manuscripts and Collections. Berkeley, University of California Press [1971], 512 p. ⟨II-05355⟩

1816-1867
Quebec

Desjardins, E.: Le Destin Tragique du Manuscript Historique de Labrie. L'UMC 98:1119-1125, 1969 ⟨II-01831⟩

Gosselin, A.: Un Historien Canadien Oublie:Le Dr.Jacques Labrie (1784-1831). PTRSC Volume 2, section I, 33-64, 1893 ⟨II-00215⟩

1868-1918
Canada

Abbott, M.E. (Edit.): Classified and Annotated Bibliography of Sir William Osler's Publications. Montreal, Medical Museum, McGill University, 1939. 163 p. ⟨II-00209⟩

Clarkson, F.A.: The Canadian Album -- Men of Canada. CACHB 14:17-25, 1949 ⟨II-00210⟩

Nation, E.F., Roland, C.G., McGovern, J.P.: An Annotated Checklist of Osleriana. Kent State University Press, 1970. 289 p. ⟨II-00212⟩

Ontario

Laver, A.B.: The Historiography of Psychology in Canada. Journal of the History of the Behavorial Sciences 13(3):243-41, 1977 ⟨II-05328⟩

Neary, H.B.: William Renwick Riddell: Judge, Ontario Publicist and Man of Letters. Law Society of Upper Canada Gazette II:144-174, 1977 ⟨II-00213⟩

Surveyer, E.F.: The Honourable William Renwick Riddell 1852-1945. PTRSC 39:111-114, 1945 ⟨II-03865⟩

1919-1945
Alberta

Roland, C.G.: Dr. Earle Scarlett: melding tradition and beauty in historical writing. Canadian Medical Association Journal 122:822-826, 1980 ⟨II-00206⟩

Manitoba

Thompson, I.M.: Dr. Adamson as a Medical Historian. Manitoba Medical Review 44(9):564-565, 1964 ⟨II-00208⟩

Thorlakson, P.H.T.: A Tribute to Dr. Ross B. Mitchell. Winnipeg Clinic Quarterly 23:65-68, 1970 ⟨II-03276⟩

New Brunswick

Stanley, G.F.G.: John Clarence Webster the Laird of Shediac. Acadiensis 3:51-71, 1973-4. ⟨II-00207⟩

Ontario

Bates, D.G.: Dr. J.W. Crane -- A Biography. University of Western Ontario Medical Journal 28:125-130, 1958 ⟨II-02098⟩

Gwyn, N.B.: A Short History of the Toronto Medical Historical Club. CMAJ 56:218-220, 1947 ⟨II-04167⟩

1946-1979
Canada

Gelfand, T.: Report on the Status of History of Medicine in Canadian Universities. In: Jarrell, R.A.; Ball, N.R.: Science, Technology, and Canadian History. Waterloo, Wilfrid Laurier Univ. Press, 1980. pp 199-200 ⟨II-00204⟩

LeBlond, S.: La Societe Canadienne D'Histoire de la Medecine. Cahier des Dix 39:1-32, 1974 ⟨II-02423⟩

British Columbia

Gibson, W.C.: History of the Health Sciences for Undergraduates. Journal of Medical Education 47:910-11, 1972 ⟨II-05336⟩

Ontario

Dunn, M.: The Medical Archives Inventory Project. In: Jarrell, R.A.; Ball, N.R.: Science, Technology, and Canadian History. Waterloo, Wilfrid Laurier Univ. Press, 1980. pp 202-205 ⟨II-00203⟩

P., G.R.: Jason A. Hannah: Pathologist, Economist, Historian. CMAJ 117:193, 1977 ⟨II-02212⟩

Paterson, G.R.: The Hannah Institute: Promoting Canadian History of Medicine. CMAJ 128:1325-1328, 1983 ⟨II-05078⟩

Other

Mazumdar, P.M.H.: History, science and the community. CMAJ 117:313-317, 1977 ⟨II-00205⟩

1980-1989
Canada

Shortt, S.E.D.: The New Social History of Medicine: Some Implications for Research. Archivaria 10:5-22, 1980 ⟨II-00201⟩

All embracing
Canada

Miller, G. (Edit.): Historiography of the History of Medicine of the United States and Canada, 1939-1960. Baltimore, John Hopkins Press, 1964. 428 p. ⟨II-00200⟩

Ray, A.J.: Opportunity and Challenge: The Hundson's Bay Company Archives and Canadian Science and Technology. In: Jarrell, R.A. Ball, N.R.: Science, Technology and Canadian History. Kingston, Wilfrid Laurier Univ. Press, 1980. pp 45-59 ⟨II-00374⟩

Roland, C.G.: Teaching Medical History in Canadian Universities. CMAJ 90:887, 1964 ⟨II-05282⟩

Shortt, S.E.D.: Antiquarians and Amateurs: Reflections on the Writing of Medical History in Canada. In: S.E.D. Shortt (edit.), Medicine in Canadian Society: Historical Perspectives. Montreal, McGill-Queen's University Press, 1981. pp 1-17 ⟨II-04880⟩

Alberta

Stanley, G.D.: Medical Archives and their Relation to the Profession. CACHB 15:28-35, 1950 ⟨II-00202⟩

Homeopathy
1816-1867
Quebec

LeBlond, S.: Homeopathie. Le Vie medicale au Canada Francais 7:1055-1061, 1978 ⟨II-04674⟩

Hospitals
1500-1699
Canada

Meiklejohn, M.L.: The early hospital history of Canada 1535-1875. Montreal Medical Journal 39:397-320, 1910 ⟨II-03794⟩

Nova Scotia

Hattie, W.H.: Early Acadian Hospitals. CMAJ 16: 707-708, 1926 ⟨II-01802⟩

Quebec

A., G.H.: Canada's First Hospital Celebrates its Tercentenary 300th Anniversary at Hotel Dieu, Quebec. Canadian Hospital 16:9-11, 1939 ⟨II-04041⟩

Allaire, M d': L'hopital-general de Quebec 1692-1764. Montreal, Fides [1971]. 251 p. ⟨II-05354⟩

Allard, S.: L'Hotel-Dieu de Montreal: Trois
Siecles de Devouement et de Progres. L'UMC 70:1271-1272, 1941 ⟨II-02363⟩

Beriner, J.: Trois siecles de charite a l'Hotel-Dieu de Montreal. Montreal, Therien, 1949 ⟨II-05149⟩

Casgrain, H.R.: L'Hotel-Dieu de Quebec. Mon
treal, C.O. Beauchemin and Fils, 1896, 592 p. ⟨II-04704⟩

Desjardins, E.: L'Hopital General des Freres Charon a Ville-Marie. L'UMC 98:2108-2112, 1969 ⟨II-02372⟩

Desjardins, E.: L'Hopital de Jeanne Mance: 1642-1673. L'UMC 102:1136-42, 1973 ⟨II-05346⟩

Desjardins, E.: Le role social du premier hopital de Montreal. L'UMC 102:1041-42, 1973 ⟨II-05341⟩

Donaldson, B.: L'Hotel Dieu de Quebec. CACHB 21:57-62, 1956 ⟨II-00198⟩

Donaldson, B.: Hotel Dieu de Montreal. CACHB 21:112-122, 1957 ⟨II-00197⟩

Dube, J.E.: Le Passe -- Leur Evolution -- Le Present. L'UMC 61:144-234, 1932 ⟨II-02373⟩

Dube, J.E.: 1636-1936: Celebration, A L'Hotel-Dieu de Montreal, du Tricentenaire de la Fondation de L'Institut des Religieuses Hospitalieres de Saint-Joseph, a la Fleche, France. L'UMC 65:547-556, 1936 ⟨II-02361⟩

Fauteux, A.E., Massicotte, E.Z., Bertrand, C. (editors): Annales De L'Hotel-Dieu de Montreal. Montreal, L'Imprimerie Des Editeurs Limitee, 1921, 252 p. ⟨II-04706⟩

Foran, J.K.: Jeanne Mance or "The Angel of the Colony" Foundress of the Hotel Dieu Hospital, Montreal Pioneer Nurse of North America 1642-1673. Montreal, The Herald Press, Ltd., 1931, 192 p. ⟨II-04468⟩

Fortier, L.E.: "Hotel-Dieu de Montreal". La Revue Medicale du Canada 6:350-354, 1902 ⟨II-02421⟩

Gerard, C: The History of Hotel-Dieu de Saint Joseph in Montreal, Quebec, Canada. Hospital Progress 23:68-71, 108-12, 165-69, 178-81, 1942 ⟨II-04137⟩

Howell, W.B.: L'Hotel Dieu de Quebec. Annals of Medical History 6:396-409, 1934 ⟨II-04143⟩

Lahaise, R.: L'Hotel-Dieu de Vieux-Montreal, 1642-1861. Montreal, Hurtubise HMH, 1973 ⟨II-05150⟩

LeBlond, S.: History of the Hotel-Dieu de Quebec. CMAJ 60:75-80, 1949 ⟨II-04678⟩

LeBlond, S.: L'Hotel-Dieu de Quebec. Laval Medical 16:5-17, 1951 ⟨II-04679⟩

LeSage, A.: Le Tricentenaire de la Fondation de L'Hotel-Dieu de Quebec 1639-1939. L'UMC 68:329-336, 1939 ⟨II-02368⟩

LeSage, A.: Le Tricentenaire de L'Hotel-Dieu et de Saint-Sulpice. L'UMC 70:1268-1270, 1941 ⟨II-02362⟩

MacDermot, H.E.: Jeanne Mance. CMAJ 57:67-73, 1947 〈II-03626〉

McCrae, J.: A Canadian Hospital of the 17th Century. Montreal Medical Journal 35:459-65, 1906 〈II-03774〉

Mercier, O.: Medecins et Chirurgeins de L'Hotel-Dieu. L'UMC 70:1273-1276, 1941 〈II-02364〉

Mercier, O.: Echo du Tricentenaire. L'UMC 71:608-609, 1942 〈II-02365〉

Nicholls, A.G.: L'Hotel-Dieu. CMAJ 47:372-374, 1942 〈II-04677〉

Raymond, R.: Hopital General de Montreal, Registre de lentree des pauvres (1691- 1741). Memories de la Societe Genealogique Canadienne-Francaise 20:238-42, 1969 〈II-05151〉

Rene, S.M.-C.: Soeurs Grises Nicoletaines; Mere Youville, Ses Auxiliaries, Son Oeuvre. Editions du Bien Public, Trois-Rivieres 1948. 355 p. 〈II-04671〉

Rousseau, F.: L'Hospitalisation en Nouvelle-France, l'Hotel-Dieu de Quebec, 1689- 1698. Thesis (M.A.), Laval University, 1975 〈II-05153〉

Rousseau, F.: Hopital et Societe en Nouvelle-France: L'Hotel-Dieu de Quebec a la Fin du XVIIe Siecle. Revue d'Histoire de l'Amerique Francaise 31:29-47, 1977-78 〈II-04692〉

Roy, P-G.: A Travers l'histoire de l'Hotel-Dieu de Quebec. Levis, 1939 〈II-05152〉

Schwitalla, A.M.: The Tercentenary of the Hotel-Dieu of Montreal 1642-1942. Hospital Progress 23:159-63, 235-44, 1942 〈II-04697〉

Wrenshall, E.: Hotel Dieu of Montreal Celebrates Three Hundred Years of Service. Canadian Hospital 19:13-15, 1942 〈II-03464〉

〈II-03464〉

Other

Marion-Landais, G.: The first European hospital in the Western hemisphere. Transactions and Studies of the College of Physicians of Philadelphia 4th Ser. 43(3):136-141, 1976 〈II-00199〉

1700-1759
Nova Scotia

Grant, M.H.L.: Historical Background of the Nova Scotia Hospital, Dartmouth and the Victoria General Hospital, Halifax. Nova Scotia Medical Bulletin 16:250-58, 314-319, 383-392, 1937 〈II-04181〉

Grant, M.H.L.: Historical Sketches of Hospitals and Alms Houses in Halifax, Nova Scotia, 1749-1859. Nova Scotia Medical Bulletin 27:229-38, 294-304, 491-512, 1938 〈II-05147〉

Hattie, W.H.: Early Acadian Hospitals. Nova Scotia Medical Bulletin 6:26-28, 1927 〈II-04160〉

Patton, W.W.: Hopital du Roy, Louisbourg. Nova Scotia Medical Bulletin 31:193-203, 1952 〈II-03786〉

Quebec

Casgrain, H.R.: Histoire de l'Hotel-Dieu de Quebec. Montreal, Beauchemin, 1894 〈II-02436〉

Rioux, C.: L'hopital militaire a Quebec: 1759-1871. Canadian Society for the History of Medicine Newsletter, 5:16-19, 1981 〈II-04673〉

1760-1815
Quebec

Desjardins, E.: L'hopital de la Misericorde de Montreal. L'UMC 102:400-05, 1973 〈II-05347〉

1816-1867
British Columbia

Young, E.M.: The Hospitals and Charities of Vancouver City. British Columbia Magazine 7:608-11, 1911 〈II-05154〉

New Brunswick

Bayard, W.: History of the General Public Hospital in the City of Saint John, N.B. Saint John, N.B., s.n. 1896 〈II-00183〉

Gibbon, A.D.: The Kent Marine Hospital. New Brunswick Historical Society Collection 14:1-19, 1955 〈II-04069〉

Nova Scotia

Fleming, M.W.: The Halifax Visiting Dispensary -- 100 Years Old. Nova Scotia Medical Bulletin 36:106-09, 1957 〈II-04050〉

Ontario

Angus, M.S.: Kingston General Hospital: A Social and Institutional History. Montreal/London, McGill-Queen's University Press, 1973. 205 p. 〈II-00182〉

Bigelow, W.G.: 150 Years 1829-1979: Toronto General Hospital. N.p. / n.d. 〈II-00185〉

Brown, J.N.E.: The Hospitals of Toronto. In: Middleton, J.E.: The Municipality of Toronto: A History. Toronto and New York, Dominion Publishing Co., vol II, 1923. pp 631-651. 〈II-00187〉

Clarke, C.K.: A History of the Toronto General Hospital. Toronto, William Briggs, 1913. 147 p. 〈II-00188〉

Cosbie, W.G.: The Toronto General Hospital 1819-1965: A Chronicle. Toronto, Macmillan of Canada Ltd., 1975. 373 p. 〈II-00189〉

Craig, H.: The Loyal and Patriotic Society of Upper Canada and its Still-Born Child: The "Upper Canada Preserved" Medal. Ontario History 52:31-52, 1960 〈II-00190〉

Gibson, T.: A Short Account of the Early History of the Kingston General Hospital. Kingston, Hanson and Edgar, 1935 〈II-05148〉

Harris, R.I.: Christopher Widmer, 1780-1858 and the Toronto General Hospital. York Pioneer 61:3-11, 1965 〈II-03610〉

[Hill, P.]: A Brief History of the Hamilton Civic Hospitals. Link II, January, February, March, April, 1982. 〈II-05006〉

Janes, [R.M.?]: The History of the Toronto General Hospital and Medical School. Middlesex Hospital Journal 57:74-76, 1957 〈II-03982〉

McConnell, D.: A Study of the British Military Buildings at Niagara-on-the-Lake, 1838-71. Manuscript Report No. 226, Parks Canada, 1977 〈II-00193〉

Reed, T.A.: "The Toronto General". CACHB 9(1):13-18, 1944 〈II-00196〉

Richardson, J.H.: The mystery of the medals. University of Toronto Monthly 2:130-135, 1902 〈II-02625〉

Quebec

Bensley, E.H.: The Caldwell - O'Sullivan Duel: A Prelude to the Founding of the Montreal General Hospital. CMAJ 100:1092-1095, 1969 〈II-00184〉

Bensley, E.H.: Pages of History. (Montreal, Montreal General Hospital), 1981. 40 p. 〈II-04216〉

Desjardins, E.: L'Hotel-Dieu, St. Patrick's Hospital et St. Lawrence School of Medicine. L'UMC 100:1794-1799, 1971 〈II-02418〉

Desjardins, E.: Un Duel Resulta D'Une Polemique Autour de L'Hotel-Dieu et du Montreal General Hospital. L'UMC 100:530-535, 1971 〈II-02359〉

Lapointe, M.: Hotel-Dieu Saint-Vallier de Chicoutimi. L'UMC 97:703-04, 1968 〈II-05422〉

LeBlond, S.: L'Hopital de la Marine de Quebec. L'UMC 80:616-626, 1951 〈II-02370〉

LeBlond, S.: The Marine Hospital of Quebec. CACHB 21:33-46, 1956 〈II-00191〉

MacDermot, H.E.: The Early Days of the Montreal General Hospital. Surgery, Gynecology, and Obstetrics 59:120-125, 1934 〈II-05018〉

MacDermot, H.E.: The early admission books of the Montreal General Hospital. CMAJ 36:524-529, 1937 〈II-03638〉

MacDermot, H.E.: A History of the Montreal General Hospital. Montreal, Montreal General Hospital, 1950. 135 p. 〈II-00192〉

Montague, J., Montague, S.: Impressions of Some Canadian Medical Institutions in 1837. Extracts from the Diary of Dr. James MacDonald. Canadian Psychiatric Association Journal 21:181-2, 1976 〈II-05323〉

Montizambert, L: An Account of the origin, rise and progress of the Montreal General Hospital. Canadian Magazine and Literary Repository 4:100-126, 1825 〈II-04002〉

Owen, M.: Annual Reports -- By-Laws and other Printed Documents of the Montreal General Hospital 1823-1971 Accession No. 1501/9 and 1501/75. Montreal, University Archives McGill University, January 1973, 62 p. 〈II-04608〉

Shepherd, F.J.: Origin and History of the Montreal General Hospital. N.p., n.d. 47 p. 〈II-04613〉

Stewart, R.C.: The Montreal General Hospital and the Care of Contagious Diseases 1822-1897. CMAJ 43:282-284, 1940 〈II-03597〉

Stone, A.C.: The Life of James Douglas, M.D. McGill Medical Undergraduate Journal 8:6-20, 1938 〈II-01879〉

Welch, C.E.: History of Canadian Surgery: The M.G.H. Twins. Canadian Journal of Surgery 8:325-331, 1965 〈II-03461〉

United States

Preston, R.A.: A Field Hospital in the American Civil War. CACHB 17:10-13, 1952 〈II-00195〉

1868-1918

Alberta

Dorward, C.: Below the Flight Path. A History of the Royal Alexandra Hospital and School of Nursing. Edmonton, Royal Alexandra Hospital, 1968. 〈II-05103〉

McGugan, A.C.: Hospitals and Hospital Administration Then and Now. Alberta Medical Bulletin 25:99-106, 1960 〈II-03695〉

McGugan, A.C.: The First Fifty Years. A History of the University of Alberta Hospital, 1914-1964. Edmonton, University of Alberta Hospital, 1964 〈II-05104〉

Price, H.W.: A Jubilee Survey of Alberta Hospitals. CACHB 20:62-67, 1955 〈II-00177〉

Ronaghan, A.: The Hospital on the Hill, 1912-1962. Islay, Municipal Hospital Board Historical Committee, 1962 〈II-05105〉

British Columbia

Carswell, S.: The Story of Lions Gate Hospital: The Realization of a Pioneer Settlement's Dream, 1908-1980. West Vancouver, Carswell, 1980. 〈II-05125〉

Fish, F.G.: The Vancouver General Hospital and its Forebears. Canadian Hospital 23:34-37, 1946 〈II-04051〉

John, (Sister): Vancouver Hospital Oldest in Northwest Area. Hospitals 18:36-38, 1945 〈II-03981〉

Large, R.G.: History of the Prince Rupert General Hospital. Vancouver, Mitchell Press Ltd., [1972?] 28 p. 〈II-04610〉

McDonnell, C.E.: The founding of St. Paul's hospital. British Columbia Medical Journal 20:112-4, 1978 〈II-03115〉

McDonnell, C.E.: The golden years and the founding of the Vancouver General Hospital. British Columbia Medical Journal 20:221-3, 1978 〈II-03112〉

Manitoba

Hiebert, M: Manitoba's Rural Hospitals. Canadian Nurse 53:294-296, 1957 〈II-04150〉

Medovy, H.: A Vision Fulfilled. The Story of the Children's Hospital of Winnipeg 1909-1973. Winnipeg, Peguis Publishers Limited, 1979. 156 p. 〈II-00176〉

Medovy, H.: Seven Decades of Service at the Children's Hospital of Winnipeg. CMAJ 123:1259-1261, 1980 〈II-02981〉

Newfoundland

Thomas, G.W.: The International Grenfell Association: Its Role in Northern Newfoundland and Labrador: part I: The Early Days. CMAJ 118:308-310, 326, 1978 〈II-02340〉

Nova Scotia

MacKenzie, K.A., Kirk, T.E., Lemoine, R.E.: Camp Hill Hospital: Its History and Development. Nova Scotia Medical Bulletin 36:369-74, 1957 〈II-03672〉

Murphy, G.H.: Golden Jubilee Saint Joseph's Hospital 1955. Nova Scotia Medical Bullletin 35:109-15, 1956 ⟨II-03754⟩

Ontario

Aldwinckle, J.: Oshawa General Hospital "Heart-beat of the Community". Oshawa, Oshawa General Hospital, 1975, 263 p. ⟨II-04606⟩

Braithwaite, M.: Sick Kids: The Story of the Hospital for Sick Children in Toronto. Toronto, McClelland and Stewart Ltd., 1974. 204 p. ⟨II-00173⟩

Cronin, G.: End of an Era; The story of Scarborough General Hospital. Toronto, Women's Auxiliary Scarborough General Hospital, [1974], 40 p. ⟨II-04607⟩

Cullen, T.S.: The House Surgeons of the Toronto General Hospital 1890, 1891. Canadian Journal of Medicine and Surgery 52:66-70, 1922 ⟨II-04086⟩

Denholm, K.A.: History of Parry Sound General Hospital. Margaret Higham, 1973, 44 p. ⟨II-04470⟩

Gale, G.L.: The Changing Years. The Story of Toronto Hospital and the Fight against Tuberculosis. Toronto, West Park Hospital, 1979. 134 p. ⟨II-00174⟩

Haffey, H.: Six Cots and a Prayer that became a Famous Children's Hospital. York Pioneer 71:15-25, 1975 ⟨II-03287⟩

Herrernan, M., McLaughlin, R.S.: A Short History of the Oshawa General Hospital. N.P., 1935, 61 p. ⟨II-04604⟩

Runnalls, J.L.: A Century with the St. Catharines General Hospital. St. Catharines, St. Catharines General Hospital, 1974. 150 p. ⟨II-01904⟩

Smith, A.S.: Thomas Dryburgh's Dream; A Story of the Sick Children's Hospital. Toronto, Briggs, 1889 ⟨II-00178⟩

Tompkins, G.: A History of the Kitchener-Waterloo Hospital. Waterloo Historical Society 52:44-60, 1964 ⟨II-04821⟩

Quebec

Archambault, P.-R.: L'Evolution d'un Hopital [l'hopital du Sacre-Couer, Montreal]. L'UMC 89:1076-1079, 1960 ⟨II-04662⟩

Beaumier-Paquet, M.: Une page memorable de la medecine a Quebec. Quebec, Editions Garneau, 1976. 121 p. ⟨II-04942⟩

Cauchon, R.: L'hopital St-Francois d'Assis: Souvenirs Personnels et Petite Histoire (1914-1954). [Np, nd, ca 1982] ⟨II-04941⟩

Lewis, D.S.: Royal Victoria Hospital 1887-1947. Montreal, McGill University Press, 1969, 327 p. ⟨II-00175⟩

Martin, C.F.: The Montreal General Hospital in Osler's Time. Montreal General Hospital Bulletin 2:11-15, 1955 ⟨II-03684⟩

Robillard, D.: L'Hopital Notre-Dame de Montreal celebre avec dynamisme 100 ans de progres. CMAJ 122:837-389, 1980 ⟨II-02417⟩

Salisbury, S.: The Montreal Children's Hospital. McGill Medical Journal 26:154-156, 1957 ⟨II-03727⟩

Scriver, J.B.: The Montreal Children's Hospital: Years of Growth. Montreal, McGill-Queen's University Press, 1979, 179 p. ⟨II-04614⟩

Saskatchewan

Thomas, L.H.: Early Territorial Hospitals. Saskatchewan History 2:16-20, 1949 ⟨II-00179⟩

1919-1945
Canada

Agnew, G.H.: Canadian Hospitals, 1920 to 1970, a Dramatic Half Century. Toronto, University of Toronto Press, 1974. 276 p. ⟨II-00169⟩

Woods, D.: Canadian Council on Hospital Accreditation. I: History and Philosophy of the Council. CMAJ 110:851-2, 1974 ⟨II-05440⟩

Alberta

Rothwell, A.: Love and Good Sense -- The First Half-Century of the Salvation Army Grace Hospital, Calgary 1926-1976. n.p., n.d. [ca. 1976] ⟨II-05016⟩

Newfoundland

Cant, D: The Cottage Hospital System in Newfoundland. Newfoundland Medical Association Newsletter 13:19-20, 23, 1971 ⟨II-04107⟩

Nova Scotia

Scammell, H.L.: The Old Lady Steps Back. Nova Scotia Medical Bulletin 26:266-269, 1947 ⟨II-03708⟩

Ontario

Jones, D.: Mount Sinai Hospital Began in an old Yorkville House. Ontario Medical Review 47:340, 1980 ⟨II-01840⟩

Quebec

Delva, P.: Norman Bethune: L'influence de l'hopital du Sacre-Coeur. In: Shephard, D.A.E.; Levesque, A.(edit.): Norman Bethune: His Times and His Legacy. Ottawa, Canadian Public Health Assoc., 1982. pp 85-91 ⟨II-04948⟩

Scriver, J.B.: The Royal Victoria Hospital, Montreal: Common Diseases in the 1920's and 1930's. In: Shephard, D.A.E.; Levesque, A.(edit): Norman Bethune: His Times and His Legacy. Ottawa, Canadian Public Health Assoc., 1982. pp 79-84 ⟨II-04927⟩

1946-1979
Ontario

Dunham, H.S.: Model Hospital By-Laws. Ontario Medical Review 35:417-18, 1968 ⟨II-04078⟩

Henry, S.: Mississauga Hospital: Largest Evacuation in Canada's History. CMAJ 122:582-585, 1980 ⟨II-00170⟩

Quebec

LeBlond, S.: Le Service de Sante des Anciens Combattants a Quebec en 1947. CSHM Newsletter, Spring 1982, pp 7-10 ⟨II-04944⟩

MacDermot, H.E.: The Years of Change (1945-70) [Montreal General Hospital]. Montreal General Hospital, [1970], 44 p. ⟨II-04615⟩

Hospitals, Psychiatric

1500-1699

Canada

Farrar, C.B.: The Early Days of Treatment of Mental Patients in Canada. CAMSI Journal 21:13-15, 1962 (Feb) ⟨II-00168⟩

Quebec

Griffin, J.D., Greenland, C.: Institutional Care of the Mentally Disordered in Canada - A 17th Century Record. Canadian Journal of Psychiatry 26:274-278, 1981 ⟨II-04215⟩

1700-1759

Nova Scotia

Scammell, H.L.: The Halifax Bridewell. CMAJ 64:163-15, 1951 ⟨II-01841⟩

Quebec

Porter, J.R.: L'Hopital-General de Quebec et le soin des alienes (1717-1845). La Societe Canadienne d'Histoire de l'Eglise Catholique, Study Session 44, pp 23-55, 1977 ⟨II-02416⟩

1760-1815

Ontario

Lavell, A.E.: The Beginning of Ontario Mental Hospitals. Queen's Quarterly 49:59-67, 1942 ⟨II-01842⟩

1816-1867

Canada

Allodi, F., Kedward, H.B.: The Evolution of the Mental Hospital in Canada. Canadian Journal of Public Health 68:219-24, 1977 ⟨II-05251⟩

Burgess, T.J.W.: Abstract of a Historical Sketch of Canadian Institutions for the Insane. American Journal of Insanity 55:667-711, 1899 ⟨II-00162⟩

New Brunswick

Francis, D.: The Development of the Lunatic Asylum in the Maritime Provinces. Acadiensis 6:23-38, 1976-77 ⟨II-01528⟩

Nova Scotia

Grant, D.M.: We Shall Conquer Yet. Nova Scotia Historical Quarterly 3:243-51, 1972 ⟨II-04012⟩

Ontario

Baird, G: 999 Queen: A Collective Failure of Imagination. City Magazine [Toronto] 2(3and4):34-59, 1976 ⟨II-03952⟩

Brown, T.E.: Architecture as Therapy. Archivaria 10:99-124, 1980 ⟨II-00161⟩

Carter-Edwards, D.: The Brick Barracks at Fort Malden. Research Bulletin 100:1-34, 1978. Ottawa, Parks Canada ⟨II-00163⟩

Clare. H.: Accomplishments of the Past, and Hopes for the Future. Ontario Journal of Neuro-Psychiatry 1:11-18, 1921 ⟨II-04464⟩

Gibson, T.: The Astonishing Career of John Palmer Litchfield. CMAJ 70:326-330, 1954 ⟨II-03301⟩

Lynch, D.O.: A century of psychiatric teaching at Rockwood Hospital, Kingston. CMAJ 70:283-87, 1954 ⟨II-03744⟩

Meyers, C: The historical development of the institutional care of the insane in Ontario. McMaster University, Hamilton, Ontario, 1978. 19 p. n.p. ⟨II-00165⟩

Price, G.A.: A History of the Ontario Hospital, Toronto. Thesis (M.S.W.), Toronto, University of Toronto, 1950 ⟨II-05161⟩

Price, G.C.: A History of the Ontario Hospital. Thesis (Ph.D.). University of Toronto, 1974. ⟨II-05032⟩

S., E.H.: Torono Insane Asylum. Canadian Journal of Medicine and Surgery 3:164-166, 1898 ⟨II-03704⟩

Sims, C.A.: An Institutional History of Rockwood Asylum at Kingston, 1856-1905. Thesis (M.A.), Kingston, Queen's University, 1981 ⟨II-04979⟩

1868-1918

Canada

Hurd, H.M., Drewry, W.F., Dewey, R., Pilgrim, C.W., Blumer, G.A., Burgess, T.J.W.: The Institutional Care of the Insane in the United States and Canada. Baltimore, Johns Hopkins Press, 1917, vol. 4. 352 pp. ⟨II-00155⟩

Mundie, G.S.: The Need of Psychopathic Hospitals in Canada. CMAJ 10:537-542, 1920 ⟨II-00157⟩

Tuke, D.H.: Chapter 5: The Insane in Canada. In The Insane in the United States and Canada. London, H.K. Lewis, 1885. pp. 189-259 ⟨II-00159⟩

Alberta

Clarke, I.H.: Public Provisions for the Mentally Ill in Alberta, 1907-1936. Thesis (M.A.) Calgary, University of Calgary, 1973. ⟨II-05023⟩

Manitoba

Griffin, J.D.: The Asylum at Lower Fort Garry. The Beaver, Spring 1980 pp 18-23 ⟨II-00153⟩

Musgrove, W.M.: The Progress of Mental Hygiene in Manitoba. CMAJ 14:377-378, 1924 ⟨II-00158⟩

Roland, C.G.: Clarence Hincks in Manitoba, 1918. Manitoba Medical Review 46:107-113, 1966 ⟨II-03611⟩

Ontario

B., H.E.: Hospital for the Insane, London, Ontario. Canadian Journal of Medicine and Surgery 4:44-48, 1898 ⟨II-04029⟩

Greenland, C.: The Compleat Psychiatrist: Dr. R.M. Bucke's Twenty-Five Years as Medical Superintendent, Asylum for the Insane, London, Ontario, 1877-1902. Canadian Psychiatric Association Journal 17:71-77, 1972 ⟨II-03855⟩

Griffin, J.D.: Psychiatry in Ontario in 1880: Some Personalities and Problems. Ontario Medical Review 47:271-274, 1980 ⟨II-00154⟩

Krasnick, C.L.: "In Charge of the Loons":A Portrait of the London, Ontario Asylum for the Insane in the Nineteenth Century. Ontario History 74:138-184, 1982 ⟨II-05011⟩

MacCallum, G.A.: History of the hospital for the insane (formerly the Military and Naval Depot), Penetanguishene, Ont. Ontario Historical Society Papers and Records 12:121-127, 1914 ⟨II-00156⟩

1919-1945

Manitoba

Hendrie, H.C., Varsamis, J.: The Winnipeg Psychopathic Hospital 1919-1969: an Experiment in Community Psychiatry. Canadian Psychiatric Association Journal 16:185-186, 1971 ⟨II-04784⟩

Ontario

Stokes, A.B.: The Toronto Psychiatric Hospital 1926-1966. Canadian Psychiatric Association Journal 12:521-523, 1967 ⟨II-03843⟩

1946-1979

Quebec

Goldman, D.L., Arvanitakis, K.: D. Ewen Cameron's Day Hospital and the Day Hospital Movement. Canadian Journal of Psychiatry 26:365-368, 1981 ⟨II-04639⟩

All embracing

Canada

Burgess, T.J.W.: A Historical Sketch of our Canadian Institutions for the Insane. PTRSC, Section IV, 2-122, 1898 ⟨II-00151⟩

Incarceration, P.O.W., Internment and Concentration Camps

1919-1945

Other

Christie, K.: Behind Japanese Barbed Wire -- A Canadian Nursing Sister in Hong Kong. Royal Canadian Military Institute Year Book, 11-13, 1979 ⟨II-04993⟩

Collins, R.: A Man Sent From God. Reader's Digest, August 1983. pp 144-175 ⟨II-05192⟩

Quaggin, A.: Prisoner and Doctor: Practice in a POW Camp. Canadian Family Physician 28:1431-1432, 1434, 1982 ⟨II-04982⟩

Instruments

1760-1815

Canada

Scott, J.W.: Preconfederation Medical Instruments. Canadian (Antique) Collector 13:42-45, 1978 ⟨II-00150⟩

1816-1867

Canada

Segall, H.N.: Introduction of the Stethoscope and Clinical Auscultation in Canada. JHMAS 22:414-417, 1967 ⟨II-00149⟩

1868-1918

United States

Shephard, D.A.E.: The Contributions of Alexander Graham Bell and Thomas Alva Edison to Medicine. BHM 51:610-616, 1977 ⟨II-03707⟩

Jews

1816-1867

Quebec

Ballon, H.C.: Aaron Hart David, M.D. (1812-1882). CMAJ 86:115-122, 1962 ⟨II-01783⟩

1868-1918

Manitoba

Medovy, H.: The Early Jewish Physicians in Manitoba. Historical and Scientific Society of Manitoba. Papers. Series 3, No. 29:23-39, 1972-3 ⟨II-02103⟩

Quebec

Segall, H.N.: Stories of and about Goldbloom, Goldblatt, Greenspon and Gross, "The Four G's" of the Class of the McGill Medicine Class of 1916. Journal of the Canadian Jewish Historical Society 6:17-32, 1982 ⟨II-05193⟩

Laboratories and Research Institutes

1868-1918

Manitoba

Fox, J.G.: The History of Provincial Health Laboratory Services in Manitoba. University of Manitoba Medical Journal 49:118-124, 1979 ⟨II-01799⟩

Nova Scotia

Mackenzie, D.J.: The origin and development of a medical laboratory service in Halifax. Nova Scotia Medical Bulletin 43:179-184, 1964 ⟨II-03673⟩

Ontario

Defries, R.D.: The First Forty Years 1914-1955 Connaught Medical Research Laboratories University of Toronto. Toronto, University of Toronto Press, 1968, 342 p. ⟨II-04611⟩

1919-1945

Manitoba

Mitchell, R.: The Progress of an idea: the story of the Winnipeg Clinic Research Institute. CMAJ 94:132-137, 1966 ⟨II-03650⟩

1946-1979

Ontario

Linton, R.: The Collip Medical Research Laboratory. University of Western Ontario Medical Journal 28:39-45, 1958 ⟨II-03852⟩

Libraries

1816-1867

Ontario

Anderson, H.B.: History of the Library of the Academy of Medicine, Toronto. Bulletin of the Academy of Medicine, Toronto 20:239-52, 1946 ⟨II-04032⟩

Quebec

Benjamin, M: The McGill Medical Librarians, 1829-1929. Bulletin of the Medical Library Association 50:1-16, 1962 〈II-04026〉

Wylde, C.F.: A Short History of the Medical Library of McGill University. The Canadian Journal of Medicine and Surgery 76:146-153, 1934 〈II-03463〉

1868-1918

Canada

Keys, T.: Canada's Contribution to the Medical Library Association. Bulletin of the Medical Library Association 47:419-423, 1959 〈II-00146〉

British Columbia

Gibson, W.C.: History of Medical Library Services in British Columbia. B.C. Medical Journal 3:210-213, 1961 〈II-04135〉

Ontario

Anderson, H.B.: A Brief History of the Development of the Library and the Academy Since its Inception. Bulletin of the Academy of Medicine, Toronto, May 1932, pp 34-39 〈II-00144〉

Gwyn, N.B.: Sir William Osler's Contributions to the Library of the Academy of Medicine, Toronto. Bulletin of the Academy of Medicine, Toronto 20:266-271, 1946-47 〈II-00145〉

Klotz, O.: The Library. Bulletin of the Academy of Medicine, Toronto, May 1932, pp 49-52 〈II-00147〉

Poole, M.E.M.: The Library of the Academy of Medicine, Toronto. Canadian Journal of Medicine and Surgery 76:144-146, 1934 〈II-03820〉

1919-1945

Quebec

Dumas, P.: William Osler et la Bibliotheca Osleriana. L'UMC 100:539-545, 1971 〈II-00142〉

Gray, C.: The Osler Library: a collection that represents the mind of its collector. CMAJ 119:1442-1445, 1978 〈II-00143〉

MacDermot, H.E.: The Osler Library, Montreal. CMAJ 76:1077, 1957 〈II-03679〉

Roland, C.G.: The Osler Library. JAMA 200:161-166, 1967 〈II-05021〉

1980-1989

Quebec

Kalsner, J.: The Unique Stress Library of Dr. Hans Selye. CMAJ 129:288-289, 1983 〈II-05208〉

All embracing

Ontario

Dunn, M., Baldwin, M. (edit): A Directory of Medical Archives in Ontario. Toronto, The Hannah Institute for the History of Medicine, 1983. 〈II-05280〉

Styran, R., Watson, A.: Books of Materia Medica in Toronto Libraries: The Renaissance Publications of a Traditional Character. Renaissance Reformation 6:23-9, 1969/70 〈II-05331〉

Licensure and Regulation

1500-1699

Quebec

LeBlond, S.: La Legislation Medicale a la Periode Francaise. Bulletin du College des Medecins et Chirurgiens da la Province de Quebec 9(3):50-53, 1969 〈II-02433〉

Riddell, W.R.: The First College of Surgeons in Canada. Canadian Journal of Medicine and Surgery 70:25-30, 1931 〈II-04001〉

Roy, J.E.: Medicine and the Law. In Histoire du Notariat au Canada, Vol 1, 1889. pp 8-23 〈II-00341〉

1760-1815

Ontario

Anderson, H.B.: Medical Licensure and Medical Boards in Upper Canada. CMAJ 18:209-213, 1928 〈II-01809〉

Campbell, C.T.: Medical Legislation in Ontario. Ontario Medical Journal 1:47-51, 1892 〈II-04110〉

MacNab, E.: A Legal History of Health Professions in Ontario. Toronto, Queen's Printer, 1970. 152 p. 〈II-00139〉

Riddell, W.R.: The medical profession in Ontario. A legal and historical sketch. Canadian Journal of Medicine and Surgery 30:131-153, 1911 〈II-03792〉

Riddell, W.R.: Some Early Legislation and Legislators in Upper Canada. Toronto, The Carswell Co., Limited, 1913. 39 p. 〈II-00140〉

Quebec

Gauvreau, J.: L'Enquete du Conseil Legislatif. L'UMC 60:642-50, 1931 〈II-01869〉

Gauvreau, J.: Le College des Medecins et Chirurgiens de la Province de Quebec, son evolution depuis la cession jusqu'a nos jours. L'UMC 61:513-519, 618-626, 1932 〈II-01830〉

LeBlond, S.: La Legislation Medicale a la Periode Anglaise. Bulletin du College des Medecins et Chirurgiens da la Province de Quebec 10(3):71-77, 1970 〈II-02414〉

Roy, J.E.: Licensure and Control of the Profession. In:Histoire du Notariat au Canada, Vol. II, 1900. pp 498-516 〈II-00141〉

1816-1867

Ontario

Riddell, W.R.: Examination for license to practise sixty years ago. Canada Lancet 46:735-741, 1913 〈II-03833〉

Quebec

Desjardins, E.: La Medecine au Quebec et le Choix de ses Gouverneurs. L'UMC 91:345-348, 1962 〈II-02356〉

Freedman, N.B.: History of Medical Licensure in Quebec Previous to 1847. L'Action Medicale 23:28-30, 1947 〈II-00136〉

Freedman, N.B.: The College in the Eighteen Sixties. L'Action Medicale 23:128-129, 1947 〈II-00132〉

Freedman, N.B.: The College 1850-1852. L'Action Medicale 23:109-111, 1947 〈II-00133〉

Freedman, N.B.: The College 1848-1850. L'Action Medicale 23:87-91, 1947 ⟨II-00134⟩

Freedman, N.B.: The Establishment of the College 1847. L'Action Medicale 23:69-73, 1947 ⟨II-00135⟩

LeBlond, S.: La Medecine dan la Province de Quebec anant 1847. Cahier des Dix 35:69-95, 1970 ⟨II-00137⟩

Tunis, B.R.: Medical Licensing in Lower Canada: The Dispute over Canada's First Medical Degree. CHR 55:489-504, 1974 ⟨II-00138⟩

1868-1918

Canada

Kerr, R.B.: History of the Medical Council of Canada. Ottawa, The Medical Council of Canada, 1979. 131 p. ⟨II-00131⟩

British Columbia

McDonnell, C.E.: Early medical legislation. British Columbia Medical Journal 20:44-5, 1978 ⟨II-03117⟩

1946-1979

Saskatchewan

Wolfe, S.: The Saskatchewan Medical Care Insurance Act, 1961, and the Impasse with the medical profession. Journal of Public Health 53:731-735, 1963 ⟨II-03588⟩

All embracing

Canada

Freedman, N.B.: History of Medical Licensure in Canada. L'Action Medicale 23:13-15, 1947 ⟨II-00128⟩

Literature and Medicine

1816-1867

Ontario

Scarlett, E.P.: Delta: A Problem in Authorship. CMAJ 55:299-304, 1946 ⟨II-04375⟩

1868-1918

Canada

McCrae, J.: In Flanders Fields. New York/London, G.P. Putnam's Sons, 1919. 141 p. ⟨II-00877⟩

Prescott, J.F.: The Extensive Medical Writings of Soldier-Poet John McCrae. CMAJ 122-110, 113-114, 1980 ⟨II-00876⟩

Shortt, S.E.D.: Andrew Macphail: The Ideal in Nature. In: The Search for an Ideal: Six Canadian Intellectuals and Their Convictions in an Age of Transition 1890-1930. Toronto/Buffalo, Univ. of Toronto Press, 1976. pp 13-38 ⟨II-00879⟩

Swartz, D.: Canadian Doctors Who Have Distinguished Themselves in Other Fields. Manitoba Medical Review 34:645-655, 1954 ⟨II-03845⟩

Ontario

Pierce, L.: Albert Durrant Watson (1859-1926). Toronto, 1924. 30 p. n.p. ⟨II-03616⟩

Quebec

Craig, R.H.: Reminiscences of W.H. Drummond. The Dalhousie Review 5:161-169, 1925-6 ⟨II-01940⟩

Fish, A.H.: Dr. William Henry Drummond, 1854-1907. CACHB 12:1-8, 1947 ⟨II-01886⟩

Leacock, S.: Andrew Macphail. Queen's Quarterly 45:445-463, 1938 ⟨II-02208⟩

McNally, L.B.: Dr. William Drummond: Poet - Physician to the "Habitant". CAMSI Journal 22:9-16, 1963 (Feb) ⟨II-00878⟩

1919-1945

Manitoba

Stich, K.P.: Eclampsia and the study of F.P. Grove's women. Canadian Notes and Queries, No. 22, December 1978. pp 7-8 ⟨II-00873⟩

Quebec

Dumas, P.: Un Medecin-Psychiatre Qui Avait Ete Poete, Gullaume LaHaise et Son Double, Guy Delahaye. L'UMC 100:321-326, 1971 ⟨II-02403⟩

1946-1979

Canada

Roper, G.: Robertson Davies' Fifth Business and "That Old Fantastical Duke of Dark Corners, C.G. Jung.". Journal of Canadian Fiction 1:33-39, 1972 ⟨II-05387⟩

Magic and Occult and Mystic

1868-1918

Manitoba

Rankin, L.: A Many Sided Man [T.G.Hamilton]. The Alumni Journal [University of Manitoba] 41:4-7, 1981 ⟨II-04114⟩

Ontario

Bucke, R.M.: Cosmic Consciousness. New York, E.P. Dutton and Co., Inc., 1923. 384 p. ⟨II-00872⟩

Chant, C.A.: Albert Durrant Watson. Journal of the Royal Astronomical Society of Canada 20:153-157, 1926 ⟨II-02898⟩

Lauder, B.: Two Radicals: Richard Maurice Bucke and Lawren Harris. Dalhousie Review 56:307-318, 1976-77 ⟨II-02677⟩

1919-1945

Manitoba

Campbell, D.F.: The Reality of Psychic Phenomena. University of Manitoba Medical Journal 22:12-19, 1950 ⟨II-02335⟩

Quebec

Cantero, A: Occult Healing Practices in French Canada. CMAJ 20:303-306, 1929 ⟨II-04106⟩

Medicine, General

1500-1699

Canada

Charlton, M: Medicine in Canada. Montreal Medical Journal 37:424-432, 735-738, 1908; 38:26-30, 38: 662-666, 1909 ⟨II-04100⟩

Doyle, F.P.: The French Canadian Contribution to the Health Services of Canada. Winnipeg Clinic Quarterly 20:56-62, 1967 ⟨II-04075⟩

Foucher, A.A.: A Page of History: The Origin, Evolution and Present Condition of the Practice of Medicine in Canada. Montreal Medical Journal 33:841-55, 1904 ⟨II-04046⟩

Hattie, W.H.: Pioneers of Medicine in Canada. CMAJ 14:324, 1925 ⟨II-04156⟩

Jutras, A.: La Medecine Francaise au Canada. Le Journal de l'Hotel-Dieu de Montreal 15:85-105, 1947 ⟨II-04694⟩

MacDonald, R.I.: Canadian Milestones in Clinical Medicine. Bulletin of the Medical Librarians Association 48:27-32, 1960 ⟨II-03671⟩

Panneton, P.: Les Notes Medicales dan les Ecrits d'Americ Vespuce. L'UMC 74:1388-1397, 1945 ⟨II-02345⟩

Pariseau, L.E.: Canadian Medicine and Biology During the French Regime. In: Tory, H.M. (edit): A History of Science in Canada. Toronto, The Ryerson Press, 1939, pp. 58-68. ⟨II-04914⟩

Newfoundland

Parsons, W.D.: A brief history of medicine in Newfoundland. Newfoundland Medical Association Newsletter 13:5-7, 1971 ⟨II-03785⟩

Perlin, A.B.: History and Health in Newfoundland. Canadian Journal of Public Health 61:313-316, n.d. ⟨II-03784⟩

Nova Scotia

Jost, A.C.: Notes on Some Old Time Practitioners. Nova Scotia Medical Bulletin 6:3-10, 1927 ⟨II-03975⟩

Scammmell. H.L.: A brief history of medicine in Nova Scotia. Dalhousie Medical Journal 19:33-36, 79-83, 91-96, 1965-66 ⟨II-03723⟩

Quebec

Abbott, M.E.: Historic Montreal: Metropolis of Canada and Mother of the Cities of the West. Annals of Internal Medicine 6:815-838, 1932 ⟨II-04039⟩

Birkett, H.S.: A Brief Account of the History of Medicine in the Province of Quebec from 1535 to 1838. Medical Record, July 1908, pp 1-46 ⟨II-04020⟩

Birkett, H.S.: A Short Account of the History of Medicine in Lower Canada. Annals of Medical History 1(4):315-324, 1939 ⟨II-00869⟩

Desjardins, E.: L'origine de la profession medicale au Quebec. L'UMC 103:918-30, 1112-9, 1279-92, 1974 ⟨II-05447⟩

Desjardins, E.: La profession medicale au Quebec. L'UMC 103:1279-92, 1450-8, 1974 ⟨II-05446⟩

Drummond, W.H.: Pioneers of Medicine in the Province of Quebec. Montreal Medical Journal 27:646-653, 1898 ⟨II-04080⟩

Gelfand, T.: Who Practised Medicine in New France?: A Collective Portrait. In: Roland, C.G. (ed.): Health, Disease and Medicine: Essays in Canadian History. Toronto, Hannah Institute for the History of Medicine, 1984, 16-35 ⟨II-05392⟩

LeBlond, S.: La France et la medecine canadienne. La Revue de L'Universite Laval 4:571-587, 1950 ⟨II-04666⟩

LeBlond, S.: Histoire de la Medecine au Canada Francais. Cahiers Med Lyonnais 45:2389-2396, 1969 ⟨II-02402⟩

Macbeth, R.A.: Medicine in French Canada from 1608 to 1763. In International Congress for the History of Medicine, 25th Quebec, 1976. Proceedings, Volume III, 1976. p. 931-943 ⟨II-00870⟩

Massicotte, E.Z.: Les Medecins et Chirurgiens de la Region de Montreal. L'UMC 50:483-485, 1921 ⟨II-02382⟩

Massicotte, E.Z.: Medecins et Chirurgiens Sous le Regime Francais. L'UMC 50:156, 1921 ⟨II-02384⟩

Massicotte, E.Z.: Notes pour l'Histoire de la Medecine au Canada: Les Chirurgiens de Montreal au XVIIe Siecle. L'UMC 50:266-271, 1921 ⟨II-02383⟩

Mercier, O.: Trois Siecles de Medecine au Canada Francais. L'UMC 71:801-806, 1942 ⟨II-02366⟩

Mercier, O.: Three Centuries of Medicine in French Canada. Nova Scotia Medical Bulletin 29:207-212, 1950 ⟨II-03747⟩

Morin, V.: L'evolution de la medecine au Canada francais. Cahier Des Dix 25:65-83, 1960 ⟨II-04690⟩

Nicholls, A.G.: The Romance of Medicine in New France. Dalhousie Review 7:226-234, 1927-28 ⟨II-02109⟩

Poulet, J.: L'Implanation Medicale en Nouvelle France. In International Congress for the History of Medicine, 25th, Quebec, 1976. Proceedings, Volume III, 1976. p. 1081-1093 ⟨II-00871⟩

St. Jacques, E.: Histoire Medicale de Montreal Depuis sa Fondation Jusqu'a la Fin du XIXe Siecle. L'UMC 61:256-259, 1932 ⟨II-02375⟩

Watermann, R.A.: Medizinalwesen Kanadas: in der Zeit von Nouvelle France (1600 bis 1763). R.A. Waterman, 1978. 60p. ⟨II-04983⟩

1700-1759

Canada

MacDermot, H.E.: Notes on Canadian Medical History. British Medical Journal 1:925-930, 1955 ⟨II-03691⟩

Newfoundland

MacPherson, C.: Medical History in Newfoundland. Nova Scotia Medical Bulletin 28:61-67, 1949 ⟨II-03682⟩

Quebec

Desjardins, E.: L'evolution de la medecine a Montreal: III. L'UMC 106:752, 755-58, 749-50, 1977 ⟨II-05240⟩

Desjardins, E.: L'Evolution de la medecine au Quebec. L'UMC 106:1284-315, 1977 ⟨II-05245⟩

Desjardins, E.: L'evolution de la medecine au Quebec: VIII. L'UMC 106:1537-56, 1977 ⟨II-05250⟩

1760-1815

Canada

Cleveland, D.E.H.: Canadian Medicine and its Debt to Scotland. CMAJ 52:90-95, 1945 ⟨II-04381⟩

Heagerty, J.J.: Medical Practice in Canada Under the British Regime. In: Tory, H.M. (edit): A History of

Science in Canada. Toronto, The Ryerson Press, 1939, pp. 69-86. ⟨II-04915⟩

Lefebvre, J.J., Desjardins, E.: Les medecins canadiens diplomes des universites etrangeres au XIX siecle. L'UMC 101:935-51, 1972 ⟨II-05334⟩

Malloch, A.: Medical Interchange Between the British Isles and America Before 1801. London, Royal College of Physicians, 1946, pp ix, 143 ⟨II-03681⟩

British Columbia

Brougher, J.C.: Early Medicine in the Pacific Northwest. Northwest Medicine 62:34-39, 1963 ⟨II-04019⟩

Cousland, P.A.C.: Early Medicine of Vancouver Island. CMAJ 55:393, 398, 1946 ⟨II-04089⟩

Nova Scotia

Hattie, W.H.: Note on a Medical Family [Almon]. CMAJ 20:306, 1929 ⟨II-04158⟩

Webster, C.A.: History of the early medical men of Yarmouth and conditions in the early days. Nova Scotia Medical Bulletin 16:193-198, 1937 ⟨II-03989⟩

Ontario

Anderson, H.B.: An Historical Sketch of the Medical Profession of Toronto. CMAJ 16:446-452, 1926 ⟨II-02330⟩

Canniff, W.: The Medical Profesion in Upper Canada 1783-1850. Toronto, William Briggs, 1894. 688 p. ⟨II-00868⟩

Gilder, S.S.B.: Toronto, the Meeting Place. British Medical Journal 1:1207-09, 1955 ⟨II-04131⟩

Lauriston, V.: A Centennial Chronicle of Kent Doctors. Chatham, Shepherd Printing Co. Ltd. 1967. p. 248 ⟨II-04382⟩

Lockwood, T.M.: A History of Medical Practice in and Around Port Credit (1789-1963). Ontario Medical Review 30:653-658, 1963 ⟨II-03745⟩

Starr, F.N.G.: The passing of the surgeon in Toronto. Canadian Journal of Medicine and Surgery 10:313-335, 1901 ⟨II-03719⟩

Quebec

Bernier, J.: Le corps medical quebecois a la fin du XVIIIe siecle. In: Roland, C.G. (ed.): Health, Disease and Medicine: Essays in Canadian History. Toronto, Hannah Institute for the History of Medicine, 1984, 36-64 ⟨II-05393⟩

Desjardins, E.: L'evolution de la medecine a Montreal. IV. L'UMC 106:892-900, 902, 904, 1977 ⟨II-05242⟩

Desjardins, E.: L'Evolution de la medecine a Montreal. L'UMC 106:1027-52, 1977 ⟨II-05246⟩

1816-1867

Canada

Abbey, N.D.: Personalities in Western Canadian Medicine. University of Toronto Medical Journal 29:177-180, 1952 ⟨II-04040⟩

Scarlett, E.P.: Eastern Gate and Western Cavalcade. Canadian Services Medical Journal 12:851-870, 1956 ⟨II-03711⟩

British Columbia

MacDermot, J.H.: Medical Men and Place Names of British Columbia. CMAJ 61:533-536, 1949 ⟨II-03677⟩

Monro, A.S.: The Medical History of British Columbia. CMAJ 25:336-42, 470-77; 26:88-93, 225-230, 345-348, 601-607, 725-732, 27:187-193, 1931-32 ⟨II-03288⟩

Redford, J.B.: Some pioneers in the medical history of British Columbia. CAMSI Journal 11:24-26, 1952 ⟨II-03814⟩

Manitoba

Mitchell, R.: The early doctors of Manitoba. CMAJ 33:89-94 ⟨II-03668⟩

Nova Scotia

MacKenzie, K.A.: A Century of Medicine in Nova Scotia. Nova Scotia Medical Bulletin 32:290-295, 1953 ⟨II-03697⟩

Ontario

Anderson, H.B.: The Medical Profession of Toronto. In:Middleton, J.E.: The Municipality of Toronto: A History. Toronto and New York, Dominion Publishing Co., vol II, 1923. pp 609-628 ⟨II-00865⟩

Curtis, J.D.: St. Thomas and Elgin Medical Men of the Past. St. Thomas, Ontario, 1956. 122 p. ⟨II-00866⟩

Gibson, T: Notes on the Medical History of Kingston. CMAJ 18:446-451, 1928 ⟨II-04136⟩

Holbrook, J.H.: A Century of Medical Achievement. In: Wingfield, A.H.(ed): The Hamilton Centennial, 1846-1946. The Hamilton Centennial Committee, 1946 ⟨II-03262⟩

Kaiser, T.E.: A history of the medical profession of the County of Ontario. Ontario County Medical Association, 1934 ⟨II-03106⟩

Legett, L.: History of Medicine in Guelph. Guelph, Westmount Medical Building, 1980 ⟨II-02101⟩

Small, B.: Medical Memoirs of Bytown. Montreal Medical Journal 34:549-560, 1905 ⟨II-03732⟩

Quebec

Desjardins, E.: L'evolution de la medecine interne a Montreal, le premier centenaire (1820-1920). L'UMC 106:237-58, 1977 ⟨II-05238⟩

Freedman, N.B.: Medical Practise in Montreal in the Eighteen Forties... L'Action Medicale 23:45-47, 1947 ⟨II-00867⟩

1868-1918

Canada

Chatenay, H.P., Young, M.A.R.: The Country Doctors. Red Deer, Mattrix Press, 1980, 272 p. ⟨II-04649⟩

Gibson, W.C.: Some Canadian Physicians. In: Creative Minds in Medicine. Illinois, Charles C. Thomas, Publisher 1963. pp 123-149 ⟨II-04134⟩

Gibson, W.C.: Some Canadian Contributions to Medicine. JAMA 200: 860-864, 1967 ⟨II-04132⟩

MacDermot, H.E.: One Hundred Years of Medicine in Canada, 1867-1967. Toronto, McClelland and Stewart Ltd., 1967. 224 p ⟨II-00863⟩

Parks, A.E.: The evolution of Canadian Medical practice during the last century. Modern Medicine of Canada 32:41-90, 1967 ⟨II-00864⟩

Alberta

Hardwick, E., Jameson, E., Treguillus, E.: The Science, the Art and the Spirit: Hospitals, Medicine and Nursing in Calgary. Calgary, Century Calgary Publications, 1975, 160 p. ⟨II-04469⟩

Jamieson, H.C.: A short sketch of medical progress in Alberta. CMAJ 20:188-190, 1929 ⟨II-03665⟩

Jamieson, H.C.: Early Medicine in Alberta: The First Seventy-Five Years. Alberta, Canadian Medical Association, 1947. 214 p. ⟨II-00862⟩

Johnson, G.R.: Place Names Up to 1930 Commemorating Medical Men Who Have Practised Their Profession in Alberta. Alberta Medical Bulletin 18:53-54, 1953 ⟨II-03976⟩

Robinson, D.: Early CPR Doctors of Alberta and the West. Alberta Medical Bulletin 18: August 1953 ⟨II-03798⟩

British Columbia

Banks, P.J.: Medical History of British Columbia: Some Aspects. British Columbia Medical Journal 3:399-401, 1973 ⟨II-00859⟩

Black, D.M.: Kelowna Medical History. Okanagan Historical Society Annual Report 44:26-33, 1980 ⟨II-05114⟩

Manitoba

Fahrni, G.S.: The Medical Class of 1911. University of Manitoba Medical Journal 68-72, 1980 ⟨II-03637⟩

Mitchell, R.: A Centennial Medical Calendar (Manitoba) 1867-1967. Winnipeg Clinic Quarterly 20:72-88, 1967 ⟨II-03692⟩

Newfoundland

Carson, W, Carson, S: Pioneers of Medicine in Newfoundland. CMAJ 79:581, 1958 ⟨II-04071⟩

Nova Scotia

Benvie, R.M.: West River Medical Doctors. Nova Scotia Medical Bulletin 26:79-85, 1947 ⟨II-04025⟩

Webster, C.A.: Yarmouth Doctors of the 1870's. Nova Scotia Medical Bulletin 6:5-14, 1927 ⟨II-03675⟩

Prince Edward Island

Sinnot, J.C.: A History of the Charlottetown Clinic. Charlottetown, 1975 ⟨II-05145⟩

Quebec

Desjardins, E.: L'evolution de la medecine au Quebec: VII. L'UMC 106:1416-38, 1977 ⟨II-05249⟩

Gordon, A.H.: Medicine in Montreal in the 'Nineties'. CMAJ 53:495-99, 1945 ⟨II-04376⟩

LeBlond, S.: La Medecine et les Medecins a Quebec en 1872. L'UMC 101:2720-2725, 1972 ⟨II-04665⟩

1980-1989
Manitoba

Mitchell, R.: Medicine in Manitoba: The Story of Its Beginnings. Winnipeg, Stovel-Advocate Press, Ltd., 141 p. ⟨II-00855⟩

Prince Edward Island

Lea, R.G.: History of the Practice of Medicine in Prince Edward Island. P.E.I., Prince Edward Island Medical Society. III p. ⟨II-00854⟩

All embracing
Canada

Desjardins, E.: L'Evolution Medicale au Canada. L'UMC 96:1232-1237, 1967 ⟨II-02358⟩

Foucher, A.A.: Origine -- Evolution -- Etat Actuel de la Medecine au Canada. L'UMC 33:388-408, 1904 ⟨II-02352⟩

Heagerty, J.J.: Four Centuries of Medical History in Canada; and a Sketch of the Medical History of Newfoundland. Toronto, Macmillan Co. of Canada Ltd., 1928. 374 p. Vol. II ⟨II-00852⟩

Heagerty, J.J.: The Romance of Medicine in Canada. Toronto, Ryerson Press, 1940. 113 p. ⟨II-00851⟩

Howell, W.B.: Medicine in Canada. New York, Paul B. Hoeber Inc., 1933. 137 p. ⟨II-00853⟩

Jack, D.: Rogues, Rebels, And Geniuses: The story of Canadian Medicine. Toronto, Doubleday, 1981, 662p. ⟨II-04328⟩

Jamieson, H.C.: Milestones in Canadian Medicine. CMAJ 59:279-281, 1948 ⟨II-04622⟩

Lecours, A.: La Medecine Francaise D'Hier et D'Aujourd'Hui au Canada. L'UMC 79:792-796, 1950 ⟨II-02355⟩

Roland, C.G. (edit): Health, Disease and Medicine: Essays in Canadian History. Toronto, Hannah Institute for the History of Medicine, 1984. 464 pp. ⟨II-05391⟩

Swan, R.: The history of medicine in Canada. Medical History 12:42-51, 1968 ⟨II-03733⟩

British Columbia

McKechnie, R.E.: Strong Medicine. Vancouver, J.J. Douglas Ltd., 1972, 193 p. ⟨II-04466⟩

Rose, T.F.: From Shaman to Modern Medicine. A Century of the Healing Arts in British Columbia. Vancouver, Mitchell Press Ltd., 1972. 187 p. ⟨II-00856⟩

New Brunswick

Lawrence, J.W.: The Medical Men of St. John. New Brunswick Historical Society Collections 1:273-305, 1894-97 ⟨II-05157⟩

Stewart, W.B.: Medicine in New Brunswick. New Brunswick, New Brunswick Medical Society, 1974. 413 p. ⟨II-00858⟩

North West Territories

Brett, H.B.: A Synopsis of Northern Medical History. CMAJ 100:521-525, 1969 ⟨II-04017⟩

Ontario

Bull, W.P.: From Medicine Man to Medical Man. Toronto, George J. McLeod Ltd., 1934. 457 p. ⟨II-00850⟩

Seaborn, E.: The March of Medicine in Western Ontario. Toronto, Ryerson Press, 1944. 386 p. ⟨II-00857⟩

Prince Edward Island

Lea, R.G.: History of Medicine in Prince Edward Island. Nova Scotia Medical Bulletin 52:212-4, 1973 ⟨II-05438⟩

Quebec

Abbott, M.E.: History of Medicine in the Province of Quebec. Toronto, Macmillan Co. of Canada Ltd., 1931. 97 p. ⟨II-00848⟩

Ahern, M.J., Ahern, G.: Notes Pour servir a l'Histoire de la Medecine dans le Bas-Canada Depuis la fondation de Quebec jusqu'au commencement du XIXe siecle. Quebec, 1923. 563 p. ⟨II-05261⟩

Birkett, H.S.: A Short Account of the History of Medicine in Lower Canada. Annals of Medical History, series 3 1(4):314-324, 1939 ⟨II-00849⟩

Brazeau, J.: The French-Canadian Doctor in Montreal. Thesis (M.A.), Montreal, McGill University, 1951 ⟨II-05156⟩

Desjardins, E.: Historie de la profession medicale au Quebec. L'UMC 104(7):1137-42, 1975 ⟨II-05329⟩

Desjardins, E.: Biographies de medecins du Quebec. L'UMC 107:873-8, 1978 ⟨II-05357⟩

Kourllsky, R.: La medecine canadienne-francaise et la France. La Vie Medicale au Canada Francais 1:696-704, 1972 ⟨II-02401⟩

Mental Health

1816-1867

Ontario

Greenland, C: Work as Therapy in the Treatment of Chronic Mental Illness. Canadian Psychiatric Association Journal 7:11-15, 1962 ⟨II-04190⟩

Greenland, C.: The Treatment of the Mentally Retarded in Ontario -- an Historical Note. Canadian Psychiatric Association Journal 8:328-336, 1963 ⟨II-00847⟩

1868-1918

Canada

Greenland, C: Canadian Pioneers in Mental Retardation. Rehabilation in Canada 17:3-6, 1967-68 ⟨II-04189⟩

Martin, C.F.: The Mental Hygiene Movement in Canada. The Canadian Journal of Medicine and Surgery 63:167-173, 1928 ⟨II-03683⟩

Porteous, C.A.: Some notes on the formation of the Canadian National Committee for Mental Hygiene. CMAJ 8:634-639, 1918 ⟨II-03789⟩

Russel, C.M.: The Origin, Organization and Scope of the Canadian National Committee for Mental Hygiene. CMAJ 8:538-546, 1918 ⟨II-03714⟩

British Columbia

Foulkes, R.A.: British Columbia Mental Health Services: Historical Perspective to 1961. CMAJ 85:649-655, 1961 ⟨II-00846⟩

Ontario

Greenland, C: Services for the Mentally Retarded in Ontario 1870-1930. Ontario History 54:267-274, 1962 ⟨II-04191⟩

1919-1945

Ontario

Pollock, S.J.: Social Policy for Mental Health in Ontario 1930-1967. Thesis (Ph.D.), Toronto, University of Toronto, 1978. unpublished ⟨II-05034⟩

Microbiology

1868-1918

Manitoba

Bell, L.G.: My Father -- Gordon Bell. Winnipeg Clinic Quarterly 23:77-93, 1970 ⟨II-02078⟩

Bigelow, W.A.: Dr. Frederick Todd Cadham, an appreciation. CMAJ 84:673-674, 1961 ⟨II-01891⟩

Stark, E.: The History of Medical Bacteriology in Manitoba. Canadian Journal of Public Health 39:168-170, 1948 ⟨II-03720⟩

Wilt, J.C.: The history of medical microbiology at the University of Manitoba. Manitoba Medical Review 50(3):16-21, 1970 ⟨II-03586⟩

Ontario

Farrar, C.B.: I Remember J.G. Fitzgerald. American Journal of Psychiatry 120:49-52, 1963 ⟨II-02927⟩

Military Medicine

1700-1759

Nova Scotia

Webster, J.C. (edit.): Diary of John Thomas. In: Diary of John Thomas: Journal of Louis de Courville. Nova Scotia, Public Archives of Nova Scotia, 1937. pp. 10-39 ⟨II-00844⟩

1760-1815

Canada

Hayward, P.: Surgeon Henry's Trifles: Events of a Military Life. London, Chatto and Windus, 1970. 281 p. ⟨II-00840⟩

Nadeau, G.: Un Savant Anglais a Quebec a La Fin du XVIIe Siecle le Docteur John-Mervin Nooth. L'UMC 74:49-74, 1945 ⟨II-02393⟩

Ontario

Dunlop, W.: Recollections of the American War 1812-1814. Toronto, Historical Publishing Co., 1905. 112 p. ⟨II-01846⟩

Graham, W.H.: The Tiger of Canada West. Toronto/Vancouver, Clarke, Irwin and Co. Ltd., 1962. 308 p. ⟨II-00839⟩

Klinck, C.F.: William "Tiger" Dunlop. "Blackwoodian Backwoodsman". Toronto, Ryerson Press, 1958. 185 p. ⟨II-00841⟩

Roland, C.G.: War Amputations in Upper Canada. Archivaria 10:73-84, 1980 ⟨II-00842⟩

United States

Gorssline, R.M.: Medical Notes on Burgoyne's Campaigns, 1776-77. Canadian Defence Quarterly 6:356-363, 1928-29 ⟨II-04192⟩

Morison, D.: The Doctor's Secret Journal. Mackinac Island, Mackinac Island State Park Commission, 1960. 48 p. ⟨II-00380⟩

1816-1867

Canada

Hitsman, J.M.: A Medical Officer's Winter Journey in Canada. Canadian Army Journal 12:46-64, 1958 ⟨II-04149⟩

Howell, W.B.: Walter Henry, Army Surgeon. CMAJ 36:302-310, 1937 ⟨II-02908⟩

Rae, I.: The Strange Story of Dr. James Barry. London, Longmans, Green and Co., 1958. pp 124 ⟨II-00835⟩

Rose, J.: The Perfect Gentleman. [Dr. James Barry]. London, England, Hutchinson and Co. (Publishers) Ltd., 1977. 160 p. ⟨II-00837⟩

United States

Kelly, A.D.: Variable Veracity. Ontario Medical Review 35:256-258, 1968 ⟨II-03970⟩

Other

LeBlond, S.: Ne a la Grosse-Ile. Cahier des Dix 40:113-139, 1975 ⟨II-02400⟩

McGuire, C.R.: The Canadian Connection with St. Helena. Stampex Canada Catalogue 1981. pp [6]-[13]-[16] ⟨II-03945⟩

1868-1918

Canada

Bruce, H.A.: Politics and the Canadian Army Medical Corps. Toronto, William Briggs, 1919. 321 p. ⟨II-00806⟩

Cummins, J.F.: The Organization of the Medical Services in the North West Campaign of 1885. Bulletin of the Vancouver Medical Association 20:72-78, 1943 ⟨II-04087⟩

Garner, J.: Military Medical Services in Canada. I: The Beginnings. CMAJ 112:1350-4, 1975 ⟨II-05327⟩

Lewis, D.S.: Campbell B. Keenan, D.S.O., M.D., C.M., F.R.C.S. [C], 1867 to 1953. Canadian Journal of Surgery 15:287-294, 1972 ⟨II-04292⟩

McCabe, J.P.: The Birth of the Royal Canadian Army Medical Corps. U.S. Armed Forces Medical Journal 5:1016-1024, 1954 ⟨II-03832⟩

Ower, J.J.: Pictures on Memory's Walls, Part 11 (Army Days). CACHB 19(2):35-62, 1954 ⟨II-00749⟩

Ritchie, J.B.: Early Surgeons of the North West Mounted Police, II: Doctor John George Kittson: First Surgeon. CACHB 22:130-143, 1957 ⟨II-02686⟩

Ritchie, J.B.: Early Surgeons of the North West Mounted Police: V. Doctor Richard Barrington Nevitt. CACHB 22:249-265, 1958 ⟨II-02641⟩

Ritchie, J.B.: Early Surgeons of the North-West Mounted Police (R.B. Nevitt). RCMP Quarterly 24:61-65, 1958 ⟨II-02642⟩

Alberta

Loew, F.M.: Veterinary Surgeons in the North West Mounted Police: Incident at Lethbridge, 1890. Canadian Veterinary Journal 18:233-40, 1977 ⟨II-05426⟩

Pennefather, J.P.: A Surgeon with the Alberta Field Force. Alberta History 26(4):1-14, 1978 ⟨II-02979⟩

Ritchie, J.B.: Early Surgeons of the North West Mounted Police. III Doctor George Alexander Ken-

nedy, Part 2. CACHB 22(3):201-218, 1957 ⟨II-00823⟩

Ritchie, J.B.: Early Surgeons of the North West Mounted Police. III Doctor George Alexander Kennedy. CACHB 22(2):171-181, 1957 ⟨II-00824⟩

Ritchie, J.B.: Early Surgeons of the North West Mounted Police. CACHB 21(4):93-101, 1957 ⟨II-00825⟩

Manitoba

Gorssline, R.M.: The Medical Services of the Red River Expeditions, 1870-71. Canadian Defence Quarterly 3:83-89, 1925-6 ⟨II-03680⟩

Nova Scotia

Archibald, B.O.: December 6th, 1917. Nova Scotia Medical Bulletin 29:303-305, 1950 ⟨II-04030⟩

Hayes, J.: Nova Scotia Medical Services in the Great War. In: Hunt, M.S.: Nova Scotia's Part in the Great War. Halifax, Nova Scotia Veteran Publishing Co., Ltd., 1920. pp 177-225 ⟨II-00813⟩

Saskatchewan

Fisher, A.J.: The First Canadian Army Medical Corps. CACHB 4(3):4-12, 1939 ⟨II-00812⟩

Horsey, A.J.: Some medical and surgical cases in late campaign -- North-West Rebellion. The Canada Lancet 18:223-227, 1885-6 ⟨II-00814⟩

Mitchell, R.: Medical Services in the North-West Rebellion of 1885. CMAJ 60:518-521, 1949 ⟨II-04623⟩

Ross, H.E.: A Glimpse of 1885. Saskatchewan History 21:24-29, 1968 ⟨II-03800⟩

Ryerson, G.S.: Medical Notes from the North West Field Force. The Canada Lancet 17:295-297, 1884-5 ⟨II-00826⟩

United Kingdom

Brown, T.E.: Shell Shock in the Canadian Expeditionary Force, 1914-1918: Canadian Psychiatry in the Great War. In: Roland, C.G.(ed.): Health, Disease and Medicine: Essays in Canadian History. Toronto, Hannah Institute for the History of Medicine, 1984, 308-332 ⟨II-05406⟩

Other

Adami, J.G.: War Story of the Canadian Army Medical Corps, 1914-1915. Vol. 1. The First Contingent. Toronto, Musson Book Co., Ltd., 1918. 286 p. ⟨II-00803⟩

Austin, L.J.: My Experiences as a German Prisoner. London: Andrew Melrose Ltd., 1915, 158 p. ⟨II-04458⟩

Bell, F. McK.: The First Canadians in France. The Chronicle of a military hospital in the war zone. New York, George H. Doran Co., 1917. 308 p. ⟨II-00804⟩

Boyd, W.: With a Field Ambulance at Ypres. Toronto, Musson Book Co. Ltd., 1916. 110 p. ⟨II-00805⟩

Cameron, K.: No. 1 Canadian Hospital, 1914-1919. New Brunswick, The Tribune Press, 1938 667 p. ⟨II-00808⟩

Clint, M.B.: Our Bit. Memories of War Services by a Canadian Nurse. Montreal, Royal Victoria Hospital, 1934. 177 p. ⟨II-00809⟩

Eliott, J.H.: The history of a great Canadian military hospital. CMAJ 40:396-397, 1939 ⟨II-03593⟩

Fetherstonhaugh, R.C.: No. 3 Canadian General Hospital (McGill), 1914-1919. Montreal, The Gazette Printing Co., 1928. 274 p. ⟨II-00811⟩

Gosse, N.H.: Doctor Macpherson's Modesty. Nova Scotia Medical Bulletin 28:122, 1949 ⟨II-03639⟩

Holland, C.W.: An Historical Sketch of the Dalhousie Unit. Nova Scotia Medical Bulletin 8:105-108, 1929 ⟨II-04146⟩

Keenan, C.G.: Notes of a Regimental Doctor in a Mounted Infantry Corps. Montreal Medical Journal 31:389-400, 1902 ⟨II-02317⟩

Laird, D.H.: Prisoner Five-One-Eleven. Toronto, Ontario Press, Ltd. (1917?), 115 p. ⟨II-04217⟩

Mackenzie, J.J.: Number 4 Canadian Hospital. The Letters of Professor Mackenzie, K.C. from the Salonika Front. Toronto, Macmillan Co. of Canada Ltd., 1933. 247 p. ⟨II-00816⟩

Manion, R.J.: A Surgeon in Arms. New York, D. Appleton and Co., 1918. 310 p. ⟨II-03613⟩

Nasmith, G.G.: On the Fringe of the Great Fight. Toronto, McClelland, Goodchild and Stewart Publishers, 1917. 263 p. ⟨II-00821⟩

Rae, H. [pseud]: Maple Leaves in Flanders Fields. Toronto, William Briggs, n.d. 268 p. ⟨II-02328⟩

Rheaume, P.Z.: Notes sur l'hopital general Canadien No. 6. L'UMC 49-345-348, 1920 ⟨II-02371⟩

Roland, C.G.: Battlefield Surgery and the Stretcher-bearers' Experience. In: Shephard, D.A.E.: Levesque, A.(edit): Norman Bethune: His Time and His Legacy. Ottawa, Canadian Public Health Assoc., 1982. pp 44-53 ⟨II-04926⟩

Snell, A.E.: The C.A.M.C. with the Canadian Corps during the Last Hundred Days of the Great War. Ottawa, F.A. Acland, 1924. 292 p. ⟨II-00828⟩

Vaux, R.L.: Some notes on the organization and working of a cavalry field ambulance. The Western Medical News 4(7):167-173, 191-201, 1912 ⟨II-00831⟩

1919-1945

Ontario

McCutcheon, J.W.: The Second-War Years. Ontario Medical Review 34:755-57, 1967 ⟨II-03809⟩

Other

Allan, T., Gordon, S.: The Scalpel, The Sword: The Story of Doctor Norman Bethune. New York, Prometheus Book, 1959, 320 p. ⟨II-01848⟩

Crawford, J.N.: Barbed Wire Humour [Hong Kong]. CMAJ 57:593-596, 1947 ⟨II-04085⟩

Feasby, W.R.: Official History of the Canadian Medical Services 1939-1945, Vol. 2 -- Clinical Subjects. Ottawa, Edmond Cloutier, 1953. 537 p. ⟨II-00797⟩

Feasby, W.R.: Official History of the Canadian Medical Services 1939-1945, Vol 1 -- Organization and Campaigns. Ottawa, Edmond Cloutier, 1956. 568 p. ⟨II-00796⟩

Hillsman, J.B.: Eleven Men and a Scalpel. Winnipeg, Columbia Press Ltd., 1948. 144p. ⟨II-04934⟩

Keddy, G.W.A.: Experiences in a 600 Bed Hospital in Normandy. Nova Scotia Medical Bulletin 25:131-135, 1947 ⟨II-03972⟩

MacFarlane, J.A.: Dieppe in Retrospect. Lancet 1:498-500, 1943 ⟨II-04327⟩

"Pooch" (Corrigan, C.E.): Tales of a Forgotten Theatre. Winnipeg, D. Day Publishers, 1969. 223 p. ⟨II-00799⟩

Tait, W.M.: The Evacuation from Greece. CMAJ 49:314-317, 1943 ⟨II-03757⟩

Walton, C.H.A.: A Medical Odyssey. Winnipeg, The Winnipeg Clinic, 1980 ⟨II-05075⟩

Watson, M.C.: Medical aspects of the Normandy invasion. CMAJ 53:99-111, 1945 ⟨II-03739⟩

1946-1979

Other

Hunter, K.A., Andrew, J.E.: The R.C.A.M.C. in the Korean War. Canadian Services Medical Journal 10:5-15, 1954 ⟨II-00795⟩

Mortuary Practices

1700-1759

Newfoundland

Pocius, G.L.: Eighteenth and Nineteenth Century Newfoundland Gravestones: Self-Sufficiency, Economic Specialization, and the Creation of Artifacts. Material History Bulletin 12:1-16, 1981 ⟨II-05390⟩

1868-1918

Alberta

Stanley, G.D.: A Pioneer Funeral. CACHB 11(1):13-15, 1946 ⟨II-00793⟩

Ontario

Murray, G.: In Funerals also -- Time Brings Changes. York Pioneer 73:10-17, 1978 ⟨II-03284⟩

Musculoskeletal System

1919-1945

Quebec

Demers, R.: L'evolution de la rhumatologie au Quebec. L'Union Medicale 108(7):1-10, 1979 ⟨II-02399⟩

Museums

1760-1815

Ontario

Way, B.W.: Versatile Doctors of Upper Canada. Canadian Doctor, April 1962, pp 33-37, 65 ⟨II-03987⟩

1816-1867

New Brunswick

Ingersoll, L.K.: A Man and a Museum. Museum Memo 4:2-5, 1972 ⟨II-04141⟩

Ontario

Duncan, D.: The Doctor's Home. Canadian [Antique] Collector 13:22-27, 1978 ⟨II-00791⟩

1868-1918

Ontario

Lem. C.: Bethune Memorial House. Ontario Museum Association Quarterly 7(2):5-6, 1978 〈II-00790〉

Nowell-Smith, F.M.: The History of Medicine Museum Academy of Medicine, Toronto 1907-1981. Thesis (Master of Museum Studies), Toronto, University of Toronto, 1981. 65 p. 〈II-05285〉

Quebec

Abbott, M.E.: The Osler Pathological Collection in the Medical Historical Museum of McGill University. Journal of Technical Methods and Bulletin of the International Association of Medical Museums 14:21-27, 1935 〈II-02325〉

1919-1945

Ontario

Godfrey, C.M.: The History of Medicine Museum, Academy of Medicine. Ontario Medical Review 32:868-871, 1965 〈II-04128〉

1946-1979

Manitoba

Shaw, E.C.: Make the Attempt. (This doctor-historian out-flanked the bureaucrats and enriched his area's heritage by doing it.). Canadian Doctor 45:30-32, 34-35, 1978 〈II-00789〉

Ontario

Minhinnick, J.: Macaulay House, Picton. Ontario Museum Association Quarterly 7(2):17-21, 1978 〈II-00786〉

Paterson, G.R.: A Non-Active Practice: An Active Museum. Bulletin of the Ontario College of Pharmacy pp 49-51, 1971 〈II-05081〉

Scott, J.W.: The History of Medicine Museum. In: Jarrell, R.A.; Ball, N.R.: Science, Technology, and Canadian History. Waterloo, Wilfrid Laurier Univ. Press, 1980. pp 206-207 〈II-00787〉

Senior, J.E.: A Different Museum. Ontario Museum Association Quarterly 8(2):16-17, 1979 〈II-00788〉

1980-1989

Ontario

Oliver, C.: Toronto's Medical Museum Packed with Items of Historical Significance. CMAJ 117:525-30, 1977 〈II-05248〉

All embracing

Canada

Pettigrew, E.: The Healing Archives: Exploring our Medical Past. The Review [Imperial Oil Ltd.] 66(4): 10-13, 1982 〈II-05007〉

Naval Medicine

1816-1867

North West Territories

Cyriax, R.J.: A Historic Medicine Chest. CMAJ 57:295-300, 1947 〈II-04084〉

Other

Gibb, G.D.: Report of the Sick on Board the Ship "St. George," from Liverpool, Bound for New York with 338 Steerage Passengers with cases, and Remarks on Ventilation. British American Journal of Medical and Physical Science 5:9-13, 1849 〈II-02613〉

1919-1945

Canada

Best, C.H., Solandt, D.Y.: The Activities of the RCN Medical Research Unit. CMAJ 48:96-99, 1943 〈II-04023〉

Best, C.H.: The Division of Naval Medical Research, Royal Canadian Navy. In: Selected Papers of Charles H. Best. Toronto, University of Toronto Press, 1963. pp 679-683 〈II-00785〉

Negroes

1816-1867

Ontario

Cameron, S., Falk, L.A.: Some Black Medical History: Dr. Martin R. Delany's Canadian Years as Medical Practitioner and Abolitionist (1856-1864). In International Congress for the History of Medicine, 25th, Quebec, 1976. Proceedings, Volume II, 1976. p. 537-545 〈II-00783〉

Neurology

1816-1867

Canada

Feindel, W: Highlights of Neurosurgery in Canada. JAMA 200:853-59, 1967 〈II-04055〉

1868-1918

Canada

Turnbull, F.: Neurosurgery in Canada. Surgical Neurology 2:81-4, 1974 〈II-05418〉

Quebec

Penfield, W., Francis, W.W., Russell, C.: Tributes to Colin Kerr Russel 1877-1956. CMAJ 77:715-723, 1957 〈II-02687〉

1919-1945

Canada

Feindel, W.: The Contributions of Wilder Penfield and the Montreal Neurological Institute to Canadian Neurosciences. In: Roland, C.G. (ed): Health, Disease and Medicine: Essays in Canadian History. Toronto, Hannah Institute for the History of Medicine, 1984, 347-358. 〈II-05382〉

Quebec

Lewis, J.: Something Hidden: A Biography of Wilder Penfield. Toronto, Doubleday Canada Ltd., 1981, 311 p. 〈II-04798〉

Penfield, W.: The significance of the Montreal Neurological Institute. In: Neurological Biographies and Addresses. London, Oxford University Press, 1936. pp 36-54 〈II-03823〉

Penfield, W.: No Man Alone. Boston/Toronto, Little, Brown and Co., 1977. 398 p. ⟨II-00782⟩

Saucier, J.: Montreal Neurology. CMAJ 82:892-894, 1960 ⟨II-03726⟩

All embracing
Canada

Griffin, J.D.: Trepanation Among Early Canadian Indians. Canadian Psychiatric Association Journal 21:123-125, 1976 ⟨II-04180⟩

Numismatics
1816-1867
Canada

Hart, G.D.: The Confederation Worm Token. CMAJ 97:39-40, 1967 ⟨II-04161⟩

Nursing
1500-1699
Quebec

Atherton, W.H.: The Saintly Life of Jeanne Mance: first Lay Nurse in North America. Hospital Progress 26:182-190, 192-201, 234-243, 1945 ⟨II-03627⟩

D'Allaire, M.: Jeanne-Mance a Montreal en 1642: une femme d'action qui force les evenements. Forces 23:38-46, 1973 ⟨II-04701⟩

Daveluy, M.C.: Jeanne Mance. DCB 1:483-487, 1966 ⟨II-00779⟩

Desjardins, E., Flanagan, E.C., Giroux, S.: Heritage: History of the Nursing Profession in Quebec from the Augustinians and Jeanne Mance to Medicare. Association of Nurses of the Province of Quebec, 1971. 247 p. ⟨II-05255⟩

1816-1867
Manitoba

Murphy, M: A Hundred Years in St. Boniface. Canadian Nurse 40:311-319, 1944 ⟨II-03988⟩

Quebec

Fournet, P.A.: Mere de la Nativite et les Origines des Soeurs de Misericorde, 1848-1898. Montreal, Institution des Sourds-Muets, 1898 ⟨II-02480⟩

1868-1918
Canada

Beaton-Mamak, M.: The V.O.N. (Victorian Order of Nurses): Caring Since 1898. Dimensions in Health Service 52(3):22-3, 1975 ⟨II-05330⟩

Duchaussois, P.: The Grey Nuns in the Far North (1867-1917). Toronto, McClelland and Stewart, 1919 pp. 287 ⟨II-05262⟩

Mills, T.M.: Women's Lib in the 1890's: they didn't have to fight for it. Atlantic Advocate 63:51-52, 1972 ⟨II-03712⟩

Montgomery, M.I.R.: The Legislative Healthscape of Canada: 1867-1975. In: LaSor, B.; Elliott, M.R.: Issues in Canadian Nursing. Scarborough, Prentice-Hall of Canada, Ltd., 1977. pp 128-153 ⟨II-03291⟩

Nicholson, G.W.L.: Canada's Nursing Sisters. Toronto, A.M. Hakkert Ltd., 1975. 272 p. ⟨II-00778⟩

Alberta

Cahsman, T.: Heritage of Service: The History of Nursing in Alberta. Edmonton, Alberta Association of Registered Nurses, 1966. 340 p. ⟨II-05431⟩

Cashman, A.W.: Heritage of Service. The History of Nursing in Alberta. Edmonton, The Alberta Association of Registered Nurses, 1966 ⟨II-05102⟩

Colley, K.B.: While Rivers Flow: Stories of Early Alberta. Saskatoon, The Western Producer, 1970, 148 p. ⟨II-04462⟩

Stewart, I.: These were our yesterdays. A history of district nursing in Alberta. Calgary, Irene Stewart, 1979. ⟨II-05107⟩

British Columbia

Street, M.M.: Watch-Fires on the Mountains: The Life and Writings of Ethel Jones. Toronto, University of Toronto Press, 1973. 336 p. ⟨II-04118⟩

Manitoba

Bellamy, M: Beyond the Call of Duty. Manitoba Pagaent 20(4):13-17, 1975 ⟨II-04009⟩

Johns, E.: The Winnipeg General Hospital School of Nursing, 1887-1953. Np/Nd ⟨II-00776⟩

Newfoundland

Cockerill, A: Ready Aye Ready. North/Nord May-June, 1976. pp 22-27 ⟨II-04064⟩

Ontario

Forster, J.M.: The Origin and Development of Nursing in the Ontario Hospitals and the Outlook. Ontario Journal of Neuropsychiatry 3:31-33, 1923 ⟨II-00775⟩

Riddell, D.G.: Nursing and the law: The History of Legislation in Ontario. In: Innis, M.Q.: Nursing Education in a Changing Society. Toronto, University of Toronto Press, 1970. pp 16-45 ⟨II-03653⟩

Risk, M.Mc.: A Study of the Origins and Development of Public Health Nursing in Toronto, 1890-1918. Thesis (M.Sc.), Toronto, University of Toronto, 1973 ⟨II-05143⟩

Quebec

Gordon, K.: Miss Webster of the Montreal General Hospital. CMAJ 28:552-556, 1933 ⟨II-02897⟩

MacDermot, H.E.: History of the School of Nursing of the Montreal General Hospital. Montreal, The Southam Printing Co. Ltd., 1961, 152 p. ⟨II-04471⟩

Yukon

H., R.: The Experiences of a Klondike Nurse. CMAJ 71:129-137, 1932 ⟨II-04166⟩

Mills, T.M.: Gold Rush Nurse. North/Nord 3:10-13, 1973 ⟨II-04625⟩

1919-1945
Canada

Bergstrom, I.: Mary Berglund: Backwoods Nurse. Canadian Nurse 72(9):45-49, 1976 ⟨II-00773⟩

King, M.K.: The development of university nursing education. In; Innis, M.Q.: Nursing Education in a Changing Society. Toronto, University of Toronto Press, 1970. pp 67-85 ⟨II-03652⟩

Alberta

Tunney, E.: Sisters of Service, Edson, Alberta, 1926-1976, 50 Years of Service. Edson, Sisters of Service, 1976 ⟨II-05108⟩

Wilson, B.: To Teach This Art. The History of the Schools of Nursing at the University of Alberta, 1924-1974. Edmonton, Hallamshire Publishers, 1977 ⟨II-05109⟩

Ontario

Beamish, R.M.: Fifty Years a Canadian Nurse. New York, Vantage Press, 1970 344 p. ⟨II-05012⟩

Carpenter, H.M.: The University of Toronto School of Nursing: An agent of change. In: Innis, M.Q.:Nursing Education in a Changing Society. Toronto, University of Toronto Press, 1970. pp 86-108 ⟨II-03651⟩

McNichol, V.E.: Smiling Through Tears. Bloomingdale, Ont., One M. Printing Co., 1970, 1:256 p. Bridgeport, Ont., Union Print, 1971, 2:408 p., 3:489 p., 4:494 p., 5:379 p. ⟨II-04929⟩

Spalding, J.W.: Sunrise to Sunset. Scarborough, Centennial College Press, 1978. 174 p. ⟨II-00381⟩

Quebec

Arsenault, L.: Les Fondatrices. Revue d'Histoire et de Traditions Populaires de la Gaspesie 14:88-96, 1976 ⟨II-04675⟩

Tunis, B.R.: In Caps and Gowns. Montreal, McGill University Press, 1966. 154 p. ⟨II-03120⟩

Other

Duthie, M.: Unsung Heroines: Alberta Nurses in Foreign Fields. CACHB 20:88-95, 1956 ⟨II-00774⟩

Ewen, J.: China Nurse 1932-1939. Toronto, McClelland and Stewart Ltd., 1981. 162 p. ⟨II-03850⟩

1946-1979

Ontario

Alderson, H.J.: Twenty-Five Years A-Growing (The History of the School of Nursing, McMaster University). Hamilton, McMaster University, 1976. 333 p. ⟨II-00772⟩

All embracing

Canada

Gibbon, J.M.: Three Centuries of Canadian Nursing. Toronto, Macmillan Co. of Canada Ltd., 1947. 505 p. ⟨II-01835⟩

Newfoundland

Nevitt, J.: White Caps and Black Bands: Nursing in Newfoundland to 1934. Newfoundland, Jesperson Press Printing Limited, 1978 ⟨II-00771⟩

Nutrition and Diet

1760-1815

Other

Senior, J.E.: Feeding the 19th Century Baby. Canadian Collector, May/June 1978, pages 37-41 ⟨II-04804⟩

1868-1918

Saskatchewan

Rowles, E.: Bannock, Beans and Bacon: An Investigation of Pioneer Diet. Saskatchewan History 5:1-15, 1952 ⟨II-00360⟩

Obstetrics

1760-1815

Canada

Ward, W.P.: Unwed Motherhood in Nineteenth-Century English Canada. Historical Papers, Halifax, 1981. Canadian Historical Association, pages 34-56 ⟨II-04815⟩

Ontario

Biggs, C.L.: The Case of the Missing Midwives: A History of Midwifery in Ontario from 1795-1900. Ontario History 75:21-35, 1983 ⟨II-05091⟩

1816-1867

Canada

Mitchinson, W.: Historical Attitudes Toward Women and Childbirth. Atlantis 4(2)13:34, 1979, Part II ⟨II-00770⟩

White, G.M.: The history of obstetrical and gynecological teaching in Canada. American Journal of Obstetrics and Gynecology 77:465-474, 1959 ⟨II-03582⟩

Nova Scotia

Kennedy, J.E.: Jane Soley Hamilton, Midwife. Nova Scotia Historical Review 2:6-30, 1982 ⟨II-05120⟩

Ontario

Oppenheimer, J.: Childbirth in Ontario: The Transition from Home to Hospital in the Early 20th Century. Ontario History 75:36-60, 1983 ⟨II-05092⟩

Watson, M.C.: An account of an obstetrical practice in Upper Canada. CMAJ 40:181-188, 1939 ⟨II-03591⟩

Quebec

Fuhrer, C.: The Mysteries of Montreal. [Midwifery]. Montreal, John Lovell and Son, 1881. 245 p. ⟨II-00769⟩

1868-1918

Manitoba

Black, E.F.E.: The Department of Obstetrics and Gynecology. University of Manitoba Medical Journal 51:103-112, 1981 ⟨II-04882⟩

Farrar, C.B.: Osler's Story of "The Baby on the Track". CMAJ 90:781-784, 1964 ⟨II-05281⟩

Ontario

Robinson, M.O.: Give my Heart. (The Dr. Marion Hilliard Story). New York, Doubleday and Co., Inc., 1964. 348 p. ⟨II-00768⟩

1919-1945
Canada

Coshie, W.G.: The History of the Society of Obstetricians and Gynaecologists of Canada. 1944-1966. Toronto, N.p., 1968 p.65 ⟨II-04379⟩

Manitoba

Adamson, G: Reminiscences. Winnipeg Clinic Quarterly 23:101-103, 1970 ⟨II-04036⟩

1946-1979
Quebec

Pelrine, E.W.: Morgentaler: The Doctor who couldn't turn away. Canada, Gage Publishing Ltd., 1975. 210 p. ⟨II-00763⟩

Occupational Medicine
1816-1867
Ontario

Jarvis, E.: Municipal Compensation Cases: Toronto in the 1860's. Urban History Review 3:14-22, 1976 ⟨II-04210⟩

1868-1918
Canada

Bradwin, E.: The medical system on frontier works. In The Bunkhouse Man. Toronto, Buffalo, Univ. of Toronto Press, 1972. pp 139-154 ⟨II-00760⟩

Kay, K.: Development of Industrial Hygiene in Canada. Industrial Safety Survey 22(1):1-11, 1946 ⟨II-00762⟩

1919-1945
British Columbia

Menzies, A.M.: An unusual introduction to practice. CMAJ 80:985-987, 1959 ⟨II-03769⟩

Ophthalmology
1816-1867
Canada

MacMillan, J.A.: Notes on the history of ophthalmology in Canada. American Journal of Ophthalmology 31:199-206, 1948 ⟨II-03674⟩

Ontario

Houston, P.J.F.: Early Ophthalmology in Toronto. CMAJ 24:708-710, 1931 ⟨II-00357⟩

1868-1918
Quebec

Birkett, H.S.: Buller, the Ophthalmologist, Politzer, the Otologist, and Lefferts, the Laryngologist. Transactions of the American Academy of Ophthalmology and Oto-Laryngology, pp 24-34, 1927 ⟨II-01937⟩

Desjardins, E.: L.E. Desjardins (1837-1919): Un Des Pionniers De L'Ophtalmologie Au Canada Francais. Canadian Journal of Surgery 12:165-171, 1969 ⟨II-04703⟩

Desjardins, E.: L'evolution de l'ophthalmologie au Quebec. L'UMC 105:803-12, 1976 ⟨II-05230⟩

Desjardins, E.: L'evolution de l'ophthalmologie a Montreal: III. L'UMC 105:1101-12, 1976 ⟨II-05231⟩

Desjardins, E.: L'evolution de l'ophthalmologie au Quebec: II. L'UMC 105:846, 848-9, 851, 1976 ⟨II-05237⟩

Desjardins, E.: L'evolution de l'opthalmologie au Quebec: IV. L'UMC 106:101-8, 1977 ⟨II-05239⟩

1919-1945
Canada

Cambell, M.W.: No Compromise: The Story of Colonel Baker and the CNIB. Toronto and Montreal, McClelland and Steward Ltd., 1965, 217p. ⟨II-04933⟩

1946-1979
Canada

Cass, E.: A Decade of Northern Ophthalmology. Canadian Journal of Ophthalmology 8:210-17, 1973 ⟨II-05349⟩

Orthopedics
1816-1867
Quebec

MacDermot, H.E.: George Edgeworth Fenwick (1825-1894). Canadian Journal of Surgery 11:1-4, 1968 ⟨II-04296⟩

1868-1918
Ontario

Salter, R.B.: Scientific Contributions to Orthopaedic Surgery by the Staff of the Hospital for Sick Children, Toronto 1875 to 1975. In International Congress for the History of Medicine, 25th, Quebec, 1976. Proceedings, Volume III, 1976. p. 1225-1243 ⟨II-00756⟩

1919-1945
Canada

Hazlett, J.W.: The Canadian Orthopaedic Association: A Historical Review. Canadian Journal of Surgery 13:1-4, 1970 ⟨II-04301⟩

Manitoba

Boyd, W.: Cause and Effect: the Fifth Alexander Gibson Memorial Lecture. CMAJ 92:868-874, 1965 ⟨II-03281⟩

1946-1979
Ontario

McCafffery, M.: Missionary Doctor -- In Deepest Toronto (Dr. Robert B. Salter). Canadian Family Physician 25:487-490, 1979 ⟨II-00755⟩

Otorhinolaryngology
1868-1918
Canada

Wishart, J.G.: Canadian Oto-Laryngology. Canadian Journal of Medicine and Surgery 52:127-135, 1922 ⟨II-03587⟩

Paleopathology

Pre-1500
British Columbia

Hall, R., German, T.: Dental Pathology, Attrition, and Occlusal Surface Form in a Prehistoric Sample from British Columbia. Syesis 8:275-89, 1975 ⟨II-05456⟩

1500-1699
Ontario

Harris, R.I.: Osteological Evidence of Disease Amongst the Huron Indians. University of Toronto Medical Journal 27(1):71-75, 1949 ⟨II-00754⟩

1760-1815
Alberta

Skinner, M.: The Seafort Burial Site (FcPr100), Rocky Mountain House (1835-1861): Life and Death During the Fur Trade. Western Canadian Journal of Anthropology 3:126-145, 1972-73 ⟨II-04204⟩

All embracing
Ontario

Kidd, K.E.: A Note on the Palaeopathology of Ontario. American Journal of Physical Anthropology 12:610-615, 1954 ⟨II-03960⟩

Parasitology

1868-1918
Canada

Fallis, A.M.: John L. Todd: Canada's First Professor of Parasitology. CMAJ 129:486, 488-89, 1983 ⟨II-05269⟩

Pathology

1500-1699
Quebec

Cadotte, M.: A Propos de La Premiere Autopsie au Canada: En L'Annee 1536. L'UMC 103:1791-1796, 1974 ⟨II-00343⟩

1816-1867
Quebec

LeBlond, S.: Le Meurtre de Pierre Dion. Laval Medical 21:3-10, 1956 ⟨II-01895⟩

Nadeau, G.: Un Cas d'Adipocire a Berthier en 1844. L'UMC 72:180-184, 1943 ⟨II-02344⟩

Other

Mitchell, C.A.: Walter Henry et l'Autopsie de l'Empereur Napoleon I. L'UMC 94:1651-1653, 1965 ⟨II-02394⟩

1868-1918
Alberta

Ower, J.J.: Pictures on Memory's Walls. CACHB 19(1):1-22, 1954 ⟨II-00748⟩

Quebec

Abbott, M.E.: More about Osler. Bulletin of the Institute of the History of Medicine 5:765-796, 1937 ⟨II-02635⟩

Adami, M.: J. George Adami: A Memoir. London, Constable and Co., Ltd., 1930. 179 p. ⟨II-00746⟩

MacDermot, H.E.: John McCrae's Autopsy Book. CMAJ 40:495, 1939 ⟨II-03594⟩

Rodin, A.E.: John McCrae, Poet-Pathologist. CMAJ 88:204-205, 1963 ⟨II-00753⟩

Rodin, A.E.: Osler's Museum Specimens of Heart Disease. Chest 60:587-594, 1971 ⟨II-03866⟩

Rodin, A.E.: Canada's Foremost Pathologist of the Nineteenth Century -- William Osler. CMAJ 107:890-896, 1972 ⟨II-00752⟩

Rodin, A.E.: Osler's Autopsies: Their Nature and Utilization. Medical History 17(1):37-48, 1973 ⟨II-00751⟩

Rodin, A.E.: Oslerian Pathology: an Assessment and Annotated Atlas of Museum Specimens. Kansas, Coronado Press, 1981. 250 p. ⟨II-03761⟩

1946-1979
Ontario

Shulman, M.: Coroner. Toronto/Montreal/Winnipeg/Vancouver, Fitzhenry and Whiteside, 1975. 154 p. ⟨II-00744⟩

Pediatrics

1700-1759
Quebec

Fortier, de la Broquerie: La Protection de l'enfance au Canada francais du XVIIIe siecle jusquau debut du XXe siecle. In: International Congress of the History of Medicine, 24th, Budapest, 1974. Acta. Budapest, 1976. pp 157-71 ⟨II-05243⟩

1760-1815
Quebec

Robert, G.: L'Aide a la Famille Dans la Province de Bourgogne et son Extension au Royaume de France ainsi Qu'au Canada. International Congress for the History of Medicine, Paris, 1982. Proceedings, vol. 1:56-59, 1982. ⟨II-05274⟩

1816-1867
Quebec

Ward, P.W.: The Standard of Living in Montreal, Canada, 1850-1900. International Congress for the History of Medicine, Paris, 1982. Proceedings, vol. 1:71-74, 1982. ⟨II-05273⟩

1868-1918
Canada

Chute, A.L.: Canadian Paediatric Contributions to Medical Progress. Bulletin of the Medical Library Association 48:37-43, 1960 ⟨II-04098⟩

Manitoba

Medovy, H.: Pediatrics in Manitoba: Goals and Accomplishments. The Journal-Lancet 87:34-37, 1967 ⟨II-05019⟩

Quebec

Fortier, de la Broquerie: Histoire de la pediatrie au Quebec. Vie Medicale au Canada Francais 1:400-5; 705-16; 795-810, 1972 ⟨II-05435⟩

Goldbloom, A: Pediatrics and Medical Practice. CMAJ 60:620-623, 1949 ⟨II-04113⟩

Letondal, P.: Introduction a L'Histoire de la Pediatrie au Canada Francais. In International Congress for the History of Medicine, 25th, Quebec, 1976. Proceedings, Volume II, 1976. p. 885-894 ⟨II-00742⟩

Letondal, P.: Raoul Masson (1875-1928): Pionnier de la pediatrie au Canada Francais. L'UMC 108:1-4, 1979 ⟨II-00741⟩

United Kingdom

Gray, C.: Dr. Thomas Barnardo's Orphans were Shipped 500 km to Save Body and Soul. CMAJ 121:981-982, 986-987, 1979 ⟨II-00740⟩

1919-1945

Canada

Buckley, S.: Efforts to Reduce Infant Maternity Mortality in Canada Between the Two World Wars. Atlantis 2(2):76-84, 1977 ⟨II-01823⟩

Ebbs, J.H.: The History of the Canadian Pediatric Society. CMAJ 76:662-664, 1957 ⟨II-04074⟩

Ebbs, J.H.: The Canadian Paediatric Society: its early years. CMAJ 123:1235-1237, 1980 ⟨II-02982⟩

Fortier, B.: The Canadian Pediatric Society -- La Societe canadienne de pediatrie (1922-1972). La Vie Medicale au Canada Francais 2:573-587, 670-682, 1072-1091, 1973 ⟨II-02479⟩

Strong-Boag, V.: Intruders in the Nursery: Childcare Professionals Reshape the Years One to Five, 1920-1940. In: Parr, J. (ed): Childhood and Family in Canadian History, Toronto, McClelland and Stewart, 1982. pp 160-178 ⟨II-04885⟩

Manitoba

Medovy, H.: Blue Babies and Well Water. Alumni Journal 38:4-7, 1978 ⟨II-04992⟩

Ontario

De Kiriline, L.: The Quintuplets' First Year. Toronto, The MacMillan Company of Canada Limited, 1936. 221 p. ⟨II-05001⟩

Matthews, R.M.: Permissiveness and Dr. Blatz: Where Did Society's Ideas on Child-Raising Go Wrong?. CMAJ 122:99-101, 1980 ⟨II-00739⟩

Quebec

Goldbloom, A.: Small Patients. The Autobiography of a Children's Doctor. Toronto, Longmans, Green and Co., 1959. 316 p. ⟨II-00738⟩

1946-1979

Canada

Schrire, C., Steiger, W.L.: Arctic Infanticide Revisited. Etudes/Inuit/Studies 5:111-117, 1981 ⟨II-05414⟩

Ontario

Bryans, A.M., Padfield, C.J., Partington, M.W.: Eastern Ontario Paediatric Association, the first 15 years. Ontario Medical Review 45:71-72,89, 1978 ⟨II-00737⟩

Periodicals

1760-1815

Ontario

Wallace, W.S.: The Periodical Literature of Upper Canada. CHR 12:4-22, 1931 ⟨II-01853⟩

1816-1867

Canada

Gibb, D.: The Necessity of Supporting a Medical Journal in the Dominion of Canada. Canadian Medical Journal and Monthly Record 4:317, 1867-68 ⟨II-01534⟩

MacDermot, H.E.: A Bibliography of Canadian Medical Periodicals. Montreal, Renouf Publishing Co., 1934. 21 pp ⟨II-01533⟩

MacDermot, H.E.: Early Medical Journalism in Canada. CMAJ 72:536-539, 1955 ⟨II-01532⟩

Roland, C.G.: The Natural History of 19th Century Canadian Medical Periodicals. In: International Congress for the History of Medicine, 28th, Paris, 1982. Proceedings, vol. 1:219-223, 1982 ⟨II-05279⟩

Roland, C.G., Potter, P.: An Annotated Bibliography of Canadian Medical Periodicals, 1826-1975. Toronto, The Hannah Institute for the History of Medicine, 1979. 77 pp. ⟨II-05027⟩

Ontario

Bond, C.C.J.: Alexander James Christie, Bytown Pioneer -- His Life and Times, 1787-1843. Ontario History 56(1):16-36, 1964 ⟨II-01927⟩

Roland, C.G.: Ontario Medical Periodicals as Mirrors of Change. Ontario History 72:5-15, 1980 ⟨II-00735⟩

Spurr, J.W.: Edward John Barker, M.D. Editor and Citizen. Historic Kingston 27:113-126, 1979 ⟨II-00736⟩

Quebec

Bensley, E.H.: Canadians Should Publish in Canadian Journals. CMAJ 83:1163, 1960 ⟨II-01536⟩

Desjardins, E.: La petite histoire du journalisme medical Canadien. L'UMC 101:309-14, 1972; 1190-96, 1972 ⟨II-05421⟩

Heagerty, J.J.: Centenary of first Canadian medical journal. CMAj 16:59-60, 1926 ⟨II-01535⟩

Keel, O., Keating, P.: Author du Journal de Medecine de Quebec/Quebec Medical Journal (1826-1827): Programme Scientifique et Programme de Medicalisation. In: Jarrell, R.A.; Roos, A.E. (edit): Critical Issues in the History of Canadian Science, Technology and Medicine. Thornhill and Ottawa, HSTC Publications, 1983. pp 101-134. ⟨II-05190⟩

MacDonnell, R.: The Oldest Medical Journal in Canada. Canada Medical and Surgical Journal 13:1-7, 1884 ⟨II-00732⟩

Pariseau, L.: Le Centenaire de la Fondation du "Journal de Medecine de Quebec". L'UMC 55:1-7, 1926 ⟨II-02478⟩

Saucier, J.: Petite Histoire du Journalisme Medical au Canada Francais. L'UMC 65:1039-1049, 1936 ⟨II-02376⟩

Trudel, J.J.: Quelques journaux medicaux de langue Francaise au Canada historique. Winnipeg Clinical Quarterly 20:5-8, 1967 ⟨II-02395⟩

1868-1918

Canada

Kelly, A.D.: Publish or Perish. CMAJ 97:348, 1967 ⟨II-03965⟩

MacDermot, H.E.: The Fiftieth Anniversary of the Association Journal. CMAJ 84:1-5, 1961 ⟨II-01854⟩

Routley, T.C.: Canadian Medical Association Journal. CACHB 10:10-16, 1945 ⟨II-03803⟩

Routley, T.C.: Volume one -- Number one of the Canadian Medical Association Journal. CACHB 10:10-16, 1945 ⟨II-00726⟩

S[herrington] A.: Seventy Years of Editorial Excellence. CMAJ 125:85-83, 1981 ⟨II-04640⟩

British Columbia

Seidelman, W.: Pages from the past: B.C's first medical journal. B.C. Medical Journal 18:7-9, 1976 ⟨II-01855⟩

Manitoba

Mitchell, R.: Early Medical Journals in Manitoba. Manitoba Medical Review 35:39-40, 1955 ⟨II-01538⟩

Mitchell, R.: Manitoba Medical Journals. Winnipeg Clinical Quarterly. 20:9-19, 1967 ⟨II-01537⟩

Nova Scotia

Gosse, M.E.B.: Medical Journalism in the Maritimes. Nova Scotia Medical Bulletin 32:253-259, 1953 ⟨II-01539⟩

Ontario

Defries, R.D.: A Forgotten Chapter in the Story of the Canadian Public Health Association. Canadian Journal of Public Health 50:83-85, 1959 ⟨II-04004⟩

Roland, C.G.: James Neish and the Canadian Medical Times. McGill Medical Journal 36:107-125, 1967 ⟨II-00727⟩

Quebec

Amyot, R.: Rememoration d'evenements dans le monde medical entre les 75 et 100 anniversaires de l'union medicale du Canada. L'UMC 101:2368-75, 1972 ⟨II-05353⟩

Benoit, E.T.: Mes Souvenirs de L'Union Medicale. L'UMC 61:97-109, 1932 ⟨II-02446⟩

Boissonnault, C.M.: Un Periodique oublie [L'Anti-Vaccinateur Canadien-Francais, Montreal, 1885]. La lutte contre la vaccination au XIXe sie. Laval Medical 32:178-184, 1961 ⟨II-02475⟩

Desjardins, E.: Le Premier Siecle de L'Union Medicale du Canada. L'UMC 100:2331-2333, 1971 ⟨II-02449⟩

Desjardins, E.: Le premier siecle de L'Union Medicale du Canada. L'UMC 100:2331-33, 1971 ⟨II-05342⟩

Dumas, P.: Les neuf redacteurs en chef de l'union Medicale du Canada. L'UMC 101:303-8, 1972 ⟨II-05338⟩

Fortier, A.: Bio-Bibliographie du Professor L.-E. Fortier. Ecole de Bibliothecaires, de l'Universite de Montreal, 1952. 39 p. n.p. ⟨II-02477⟩

Gauvreau, J.: "L'Union Medicale du Canada": en liaison avec le College des Medecins et Chirurgiens pendant 60 ans: 1872 a 1932. L'UMC 61:123-143, 1932 ⟨II-02451⟩

LeSage, A.: Bulletin 1872-1922: Le Cinquantenaire de L'Union Medicale du Canada. L'UMC 51:1-10, 1922 ⟨II-02448⟩

LeSage, A.: Le Programme de L'Union Medicale du Canada 1872-1932. L'UMC 61:553-562, 1932 ⟨II-02445⟩

LeSage, A.: Les Debuts de L'Union Medicale Durant L'Annee 1872. Le Dr. Rottot. L'UMC 61:78-95, 1932 ⟨II-02398⟩

LeSage, A.: 75e Anniversaire de la Fondation de "L'Union Medicale du Canada" 1872-1947. L'UMC 75:1265-1304, 1946; 76:300-327, 1947 ⟨II-02452⟩

N(icholls), A.G.: Dr. A.D. Blackader and the Journal. CMAJ 21:367, 1939 ⟨II-00724⟩

Rottot, J.P.: Retrospective; L'Union Medicale du Canada. L'UMC 101:952, 1972 ⟨II-05332⟩

Saucier, J.: Quand nos Peres Lisaient "L'Union Medicale". L'UMC 75:1341-1346, 1946 ⟨II-01856⟩

1919-1945

Canada

Bensley, E.H.: Dr. Hugh Ernest MacDermot. CMAJ 128:860-861, 1983 ⟨II-05126⟩

Alberta

MacDermot, H.E.: The Calgary Associate Clinic Historical Bulletin. CMAJ 78:792, 1958 ⟨II-01540⟩

Scarlett, E.P.: Tenth Anniversary of the Bulletin. CACHB 10:1-4, 1945 ⟨II-01541⟩

Ontario

Routley, T.C.: Adopting an Offical Journal. Ontario Medical Review 31:349-354, 1964 ⟨II-03766⟩

Quebec

Clay, C.C.: The Founding of the "McGill Medical Undergraduate Journal". McGill Medical Journal 13:457-68, 1944 ⟨II-04093⟩

Saskatchewan

Houston, C.S.: The early years of the Saskatchewan Medical Quarterly. CMAJ 118:1122,1127-1128, 1978 ⟨II-00717⟩

1946-1979

Manitoba

Blum, A.: Vaisrub: Good Language with a Light Touch. CMAJ 127:308-309, 1982 ⟨II-04917⟩

Blum, A.: Vaisrub: Good Language with a light touch. University of Manitoba Medical Journal 53:14-15, 1983 ⟨II-05135⟩

Quebec

Desjardins, E.: Le Debut de Volume 100 de L'Union Medicale du Canada. L'UMC 100:43-44, 1971 ⟨II-02444⟩

Pharmacy

1500-1699

Manitoba

McDougall, D.: The History of Pharmacy in Manitoba. Historical and Scientific Society of Manitoba. Papers. Series 3, No. 11:18-29, 1956 ⟨II-02105⟩

Quebec

Hattie, W.H.: Canada's First Apothecary. Dalhousie Review 10:376-381, 1930-31 ⟨II-02099⟩

1700-1759

Canada

Paterson, G.R.: Canadian Pharmacy in Preconfederation Medical Legislation. JAMA 200:849-852, 1967 ⟨II-00350⟩

Quebec

Giovanni, M. (Sister): The Role of Religious in Pharmacy under Canada's "Ancien Regeme". University of Toronto, 1962. Thesis, Univ of Toronto, Bachelor of Science in Pharmacy. ⟨II-00346⟩

1760-1815

British Columbia

Smith, P.H.: Pharmacy in British Columbia. Canadian Pharmaceutical Journal 91:690-692, 1958 ⟨II-00714⟩

Ontario

Dellandrea, J.: Packaging the panacea...Medicine Bottles in Upper Canada. Canadian Collector, May/June 1978, pages 54-57 ⟨II-04802⟩

Quebec

Coderre, E.: Pharmacy in Old Quebec. Canadian Pharmaceutical Journal 90:784-785, 1957 ⟨II-00713⟩

1816-1867

Canada

Saunders, W.: Pharmacy in Canada before 1871. Canadian Pharmaceutical Journal 75:10-11, 70, 1942 ⟨II-00712⟩

Newfoundland

James, J.F.: Pharmacy in Newfoundland. Canadian Pharmaceutical Journal 91:630-631, 1958 ⟨II-00711⟩

Nova Scotia

Curtis, H.: How Pharmacy Grew in the Maritimes. Canadian Pharmaceutical Journal 82:16, 35, 1949 ⟨II-00710⟩

MacDougall, D.S.: This Nova Scotia Pharmacy. Modern Pharmacy 63(2):12-13, 1948 ⟨II-03755⟩

Ontario

Paterson, G.R.: The History of Pharmacy in Ontario. Canadian Pharmaceutical Journal 100:3-8, 1967 ⟨II-05094⟩

Segal, R.L.: The Pharmacy and its Pharmacists. Bulletin of the Ontario College of Pharmacy 20:36-39, 1971 ⟨II-03730⟩

Stieb, E.W.: Tinctures, Salt-Mouths, and Carboys. Bulletin of the Ontario College of Pharmacy 20:42-43, 1971 ⟨II-03836⟩

Stokes, P.J.: The Restoration of the Niagara Apothecary. Bulletin of the Ontario College of Pharmacy 20:33-35, 1971 ⟨II-03841⟩

1868-1918

Canada

Frewin, M.: A History of the Canadian Pharmaceutical Association, Inc. Canadian Pharmaceutical Journal 90:588-616, 1957 ⟨II-00703⟩

Guest, R.G.: The Development of Patent Medicine Legislation. Applied Therapeutics 8:786-789, 1966 ⟨II-04169⟩

Kennedy, D.R.: One Hundred Years of Pharmacy Legislation. In One Hundred Years of Pharmacy in Canada 1867 - 1967. Toronto, Canadian Academy of the History of Pharmacy, 1969. pp. 25-37. ⟨II-00704⟩

Paterson, G.R., Moisley, P.T.: 50 Years of the Canadian Pharmaceutical Association. Journal of American Pharmaceutical Association 18(8):481-485, 1957 ⟨II-00707⟩

Paterson, G.R.: A Year of Pharmaceutical Legislation -- 1908. Canadian Pharmaceutical Journal 91:385, 1958 ⟨II-00705⟩

Paterson, G.R.: The Canadian Conference of Pharmaceutical Faculties. American Journal of Pharmaceutical Education 22:201-209, 1958 ⟨II-05086⟩

Paterson, G.R.: The Canadian Formulary. American Journal of Hospital Pharmacy 17:427-437, 1960 ⟨II-00706⟩

Preston, J.W.: The Canadian Pharmaceutical Association, 1907-1957. Canadian Pharmaceutical Association, 1957 ⟨II-05090⟩

Sonnedecker, G.: Pharmaceutical Education, 1867 and 1967. In One Hundred Years of Pharmacy in Canada 1867 - 1967. Toronto, Canadian Academy of the History of Pharmacy, 1969. pp. 1-10. ⟨II-00708⟩

Stieb, E.W.: One Hundred Years of Organized Pharmacy. In One Hundred Years of Pharmacy in Canada 1867 - 1967. Toronto, Canadian Academy of the History of Pharmacy, 1969. pp. 11-24. ⟨II-00709⟩

Alberta

Anderson, A.J.: The Golden Anniversary of the Alberta Pharmaceutical Association, 1911-1961. Edmonton: Alberta Pharmaceutical Association, 1961. ⟨II-05098⟩

Murray, J.R.: Pharmaceutical Education in Alberta. Canadian Pharmaceutical Journal 91:692-94, 1958 ⟨II-03748⟩

Manitoba

Johnston, J.L.: Pharmacy 100: The Centenary of Pharmacy in Manitoba. The Alumni Journal [University of Manitoba] 38:7-10, 1978 ⟨II-03978⟩

Ontario

Des Roches, B.P.: The First 100 Years of Pharmacy in Ontario. Canadian Pharmaceutical Journal 23:225-27, 1972 ⟨II-05420⟩

Jackson, S.W.: The First Pharmacy Act of Ontario. Ontario College of Pharmacy [1971?] ⟨II-05089⟩

Stieb, E.W.: Pharmaceutical Education in Ontario. I: Prelude and Beginnings. Pharmacy in History 16:64-71, 1974 ⟨II-05449⟩

1919-1945
Manitoba

Young, J.: Frontier Pharmacies of Flin Flon. Modern Pharmacy 38(3):18-20, 1953 ⟨II-00700⟩

Nova Scotia

MacKnight, J.J.: George Arnold Burbidge, Dean of Pharmacy in the Maritimes and a Founder of Canadian Pharmacy; A Biography. Toronto, Canadian Academy of the History of Pharmacy, 1976. ⟨II-05234⟩

Photography
1868-1918
Ontario

Craig, B., Dodds, G.: The Picture of Health. Archivaria 10:191-223, 1980 ⟨II-00361⟩

Physical Mecicine and Rehabilitation
1868-1918
Canada

Hussey, C.: Tait McKenzie, a Sculptor of Youth. Philadelphia, J.B. Lippincott Co., 1930. 107 p. ⟨II-00696⟩

Kozar, A.J.: R. Tait McKenzie, The Sculptor of Athletics. Knoxville, University of Tennessee Press, 1975. 118 p. ⟨II-00697⟩

Morton, D.: "Noblest and Best": Retraining Canada's War Disabled 1915-23. Journal of Canadian Studies 16:75-85, 1981 ⟨II-04881⟩

Segsworth, W.E.: Retraining Canada's Disabled Soldiers. Ottawa, J. de Labroquerie Tache, 1920. 193 p. ⟨II-00698⟩

Ontario

Leys, J.F.: A physical fitness shrine in Canada. CMAJ 82:1330-1332, 1960 ⟨II-03736⟩

United States

Ebbs, J.H.: R. Tait McKenzie: Medical Contributions. In: Davidson, S.A.; Blackstock, P. (edit) : The R. TAit McKenzie Memorial Addresses. Canadian Association for Health, Physical Education and Recreation, 1980. pp 42-44 ⟨II-00377⟩

Leys, J.F.: Theirs Be The Glory. In: Davidson, S.A.; Blackstock, P. (Edit.) the R. Tait McKenzie Memorial Addresses. Canadian Association for Health, Physical Education and Recreation, 1980. 7-14 ⟨II-00376⟩

McKenzie, R.T.: Compensations at 70. Transactions and Studies of the College of Physicians of Philadelphia 6:271-281, 1838 ⟨II-03662⟩

Wolffe, J.B.: A Man Unique in History. In: Davidson, S.A.; Blackstock, P. (edit): The R. Tait McKenzie Memorial Addresses. Canadian Association for Health, Physical Education and Recreation, 1980. pp 15-23 ⟨II-00378⟩

1919-1945
Canada

Witridge, M.E.: Some observations on the evolution of rehabilitation in Canada. Medical Services Journal, Canada 23:869-894, 1967 ⟨II-03584⟩

Physiology
1919-1945
Saskatchewan

Fiddes, J., Jaques, L.B.: Reminiscences. Saskatoon, University of Saskatchewan (Dept. of Physiology and Pharmacology), 1970. 101 p. ⟨II-00695⟩

Jaques. L.B.: The Department of Physiology, University of Saskatchewan. The Physiologist 2 (5): 12-14, 1978 ⟨II-04315⟩

Politics
1760-1815
Canada

Taylor, M.G.: The Role of the Medical Profession in the Formulation and Execution of Public Policy. Canadian Journal of Economics and Political Science 26:108-127, 1960 ⟨II-00694⟩

Quebec

Guerra, F.: Les Medecins Patriotes. In International Congress for the History of Medicine, 25th, Quebec, 1976. Proceedings, Volume II, 1976. p. 746-754 ⟨II-00692⟩

Neatby, H.: The Political Career of Adam Mabane. CHR 16:137-150, 1935 ⟨II-00693⟩

Warren, F.C., Fabre-Surveyer, E.: From Surgeon's Mate to Chief Justice -- Adam Mabane (1734-1792). PTRSC 3rd series, 24(II): 189-210, 1930 ⟨II-03131⟩

1816-1867
Nova Scotia

Tait, D.H.: Dr. Charles Tupper: A Father of Confederation. Collections of the Nova Scotia Historical Society 36:279-300, 1968 ⟨II-00689⟩

Ontario

Landon, F.: The Duncombe Uprising of 1837 and some of its consequences. PTRSC series 3, vol. 25:83-98, 1931 ⟨II-03605⟩

Read, C.: The Duncombe rising, its aftermath, anti-Americanism, and sectarianism. Histoire Sociale/Social History 9(17):47-69, 1976 ⟨II-03091⟩

Read, C.F.: The Rising in Western Upper Canada, 1837-38. Thesis (Ph.D.), University of Toronto, 1976. Microfiche #2795 ⟨II-00681⟩

Sissons, C.B.: Dr. John Rolph's own account of the Flag of Truce incident in the Rebellion of 1837. CHR 19:56-59, 1938 ⟨II-00685⟩

Stewart, I.A.: The 1841 Election of Dr. William Dunlop as Member of Parliament for Huron County. Ontario Historical Society Papers and Records 39:51-62, 1947 ⟨II-02100⟩

Quebec

Audet, L.-P.: Jean-Baptiste Meilleur etait-il un candidat valable au poste de Surintendant de l'education pour les Bas-Canada en 1842?. Cahier Des Dix 31:163-201, 1966 ⟨II-04684⟩

Bernard, J.P.: Thomas Boutillier. DCB 9:73-74, 1976 ⟨II-00670⟩

Desjardins, E.: La Profession de Foi Politique du Docteur Marc-Pascal Laterriere. L'UMC 99:1294-1300, 1970 ⟨II-02472⟩

LeBlond, S.: Le Docteur Cyrille-Hector-Octave Cote et le Mouvement Baptiste Francais au Canada. Lavale Medicale 30(5):634-641, 1960 ⟨II-02474⟩

Link, E.P.: Vermont physicians and the Canadian Rebellion of 1837. Vermont History 37(3), 1969 ⟨II-00677⟩

Major, E.J.S.: Les Medecins et les Troubles de 1837-1838. L'UMC 95:1429-131, 1966 ⟨II-02453⟩

Seguin, R-L.: Le docteur Valois, un patriote ignore. Le Bulletin des Recherches Historiques 60:86-91, 1954 ⟨II-00684⟩

1868-1918

Canada

Chrichton, A.: The Shift From Enterpreneurial to Political Power in the Canadian Health System. Social Science and Medicine 10:59-66, 1976 ⟨II-05428⟩

Godler, Z.: Doctors and the new immigrants. Canadian Ethnic Studies 9(1):6-17, 1977 ⟨II-00660⟩

British Columbia

McKelvie, B.A.: Lieutenant-Colonel Israel Wood Powell, M.D., C.M. British Columbia Historical Quarterly 11:33-54, 1947 ⟨II-05119⟩

Manitoba

Campbell, M.: Dr. J.C. Schultz. Historical and Scientific Society of Manitoba Papers, series 3, No. 20:7-12, 1965 ⟨II-02676⟩

Halpenny, J.: Sir John Christian Schultz (1840-1896). In Kelly, H.W./Burrage, W.L.: Dictionary of American Med. Biog. New York/London, D. Appleton and Co., 1928. pp 1083-1084 ⟨II-00661⟩

Scarlett, E.P.: Sir John Christian Schultz (1840-1896). CACHB 8(2):1-7, 1943 ⟨II-00664⟩

Smith. W.D.: Curtis James Bird. DCB 10:67-68, 1972 ⟨II-00665⟩

Nova Scotia

Longley, J.W.: Sir Charles Tupper. Toronto, Makers of Canada (Morang) Ltd., 1916. 304 p. ⟨II-05074⟩

McInnis, R.: Sir Charles Tupper - Nova Scotia's Father of Confederation. Dalhousie Medical Journal 20:99-106, 1967 ⟨II-03848⟩

McIntosh, A.W.: The Career of Sir Charles Tupper in Canada, 1864-1900. Thesis, University of Toronto, Ph.D., 1970, 598 p. ⟨II-04931⟩

Saunders, E.M. (Edit.): The Life and Letters of the Rt. Hon. Sir Charles Tupper, Bart., K.C.M.G., Vol. 1 and Vol. 2. New York, Frederick A. Stokes Co., 1916. 319 p. -- Vol II 298 p. ⟨II-00663⟩

Simpson, J.H.L.: The life of Sir Charles Tupper. CMAJ 40:606-610, 1939 ⟨II-03470⟩

Tupper, C.: Recollections of Sixty Years. Cassell and Company, Ltd, London, New York, Toronto and Melbourne, 1914, 414 p. ⟨II-04636⟩

Ontario

Ross, A.M.: Recollections and Experiences of an Abolitionist, From 1855 to 1865. Toronto, Rowsell and Hutchison, 1876. 203 p. ⟨II-00662⟩

1919-1945

Ontario

Repka, W.: Howard Lowrie M.D.: Physician Humanitarian. Toronto, Progress Books, 1977 104p. ⟨II-04310⟩

Routley, T.C.: A Breach of Contract. Ontario Medical Review 34:165-68, 176, 1967 ⟨II-03802⟩

Quebec

Desjardins, E.: Les Revendications des Medecins en L'an 1935. L'UMC 99:2077-2081, 1970 ⟨II-02471⟩

MacLeod, W., Park, L., Ryerson, S.: Bethune: The Montreal Years. Toronto, James Lorimer and Company, 1978, 167 p. ⟨II-04930⟩

Saskatchewan

Tyre, R.: Douglas in Saskatchewan: The Story of a Socialist Experiment. Vancouver, Mitchell Press, 1962. 212 p. ⟨II-00659⟩

Other

Tse-Tung, M.: In Memory of Norman Bethune. China's Medicine 5:325-333, 1967 ⟨II-00658⟩

1946-1979

Ontario

Shulman, M.: Member of the legislature. Toronto/Montreal/Winnipeg/Vancouver, Fitzhenry and Whiteside, 1979. 226 p. ⟨II-00653⟩

Saskatchewan

Brand, L.M.: Saskatchewan Graffiti or Where were you in '62? (Memories of pre-medicare trench warfare -- how one group of doctors fought against socialized medicine.). Canadian Doctor 45:95, 97-98, 1979 ⟨II-00652⟩

Eager, E.: Wheat, Medicare and Gerrymander in the Saskatchewan Election of 1971. Lakehead University Review 5:7-16, 1972 ⟨II-04811⟩

Taylor, Lord.: Saskatchewan adventure: a personal record. Part I, background to the story. CMAJ 110:720,723,725,727, 1974 ⟨II-00654⟩

Taylor, Lord.: Saskatchewan adventure: a personal record. Part II, making contact. CMAJ 110:829,831-836, 1974 ⟨II-00655⟩

Preventive Medicine
1946-1979
Quebec

Reid, D.: De la medecine traditionnelle a la medecine preventive: analyse des reformes de sante au Quebec. L'UMC 109:774-777, 1980 ⟨II-04682⟩

Primitive and Amerindian Medicine
Pre-1500
British Columbia

Cybulski, J.S.: Modified Human Bones and Skulls from Prince Rupert Harbour, British Columbia. Canadian Journal of Archaeology 2:15-31, 1978 ⟨II-02627⟩

1500-1699
Canada

Abler, T.S.: Iroquois Cannibalism: Fact not Fiction. Ethnohistory 27:309-316, 1980 ⟨II-05364⟩

Blanchard, D.: Who or What's a Witch? Iroquois Persons of Power. American Indian Quarterly 6:218-237, 1982 ⟨II-05266⟩

Chechire, N., Waldron, T., Quinn, A., Quinn, D.: Frobisher's Eskimos in England. Archivaria 10:23-50, 1980 ⟨II-00646⟩

Fenton, W.N.: Contacts between Iroquois herbalism and colonial medicine. Annual Report Smithsonian Institution, 1941-42, pp 502-528 ⟨II-00609⟩

Lafleche, G.: Le chamanisme des Amerindiens et des missionnaires de la Nouvelle-France. Studies in Religion/Sciences Religieuses 9:137-160, 1980 ⟨II-04219⟩

Orr, R.B.: Practice of Medicine and Surgery by the Canadian tribes in Champlain's time. Annual Archaeological Report, 1915. pp. 35-37 ⟨II-00650⟩

Wallace, A.F.C.: Dreams and the Wishes of the Soul: A Type of Psychoanalytic Theory among the Seventeenth Century Iroquois. American Anthropologist 60:234-247, 1958 ⟨II-00651⟩

Quebec

Jury, E.M.: Carigouan. DCB 1:164-165, 1966 ⟨II-00648⟩

Jury, E.M.: Tehorenhaegnon. DCB 1:634-635, 1966 ⟨II-00647⟩

Monet, J.: Etienne Pigarouich. DCB 1-548-549, 1966 ⟨II-00649⟩

1760-1815
Newfoundland

Pearson, A.A.: John and William Hunter: Patrons of the Arts. In International Congress for the History of Medicine, 25th, Quebec, 1976. Proceedings, Volume III, 1976. p. 1053-1062 ⟨II-00645⟩

1868-1918
Canada

Graham-Cumming, G: Health of the Original Canadians, 1867-1967. Medical Services Journal of Canada 23:115-166, 1967 ⟨II-04186⟩

Parker, S.: Eskimo Psychopathology in the Context of Eskimo Personality and Culture. American Anthropologist, 64:76-96, 1962 ⟨II-03783⟩

Romaniuk, A.: Increase in Natural Fertility During the Early Stages of Modernization: Canadian Indians Case Study. Demography 18:157-172, 1981 ⟨II-04912⟩

Alberta

Denny, C.: Blackfoot Magic. The Beaver 275(2):14-15, 1944 ⟨II-03310⟩

Luxton, E.G.: Stony Indian Medicine. In: Foster, J.E. (edit): The Developing West, Alberta, Univ. of Alberta Press, 1983. pp 101-121. ⟨II-05050⟩

British Columbia

Boas, F.: Current Beliefs of the Kwakiutl Indians. Journal American Folk-lore 45(176):177-260, 1932 ⟨II-00638⟩

Edwards, G.T.: Bella Coola Indian and European Medicines. The Beaver 311(3):4-11, 1980 ⟨II-03619⟩

Kidd, H.M.: John Antle. CMAJ 65: 484-489, 1951 ⟨II-04631⟩

Sapir, E.: A Girl's Puberty Ceremony among the Nootka Indians. PTRSC, section II:67-80, 1913 ⟨II-00644⟩

Nova Scotia

Wallis, W.D.: Medicines used by the Micmac Indians. American Anthropologist 24:24-30, 1922 ⟨II-00639⟩

United States

Ritzenthaler, R.E.: Chippewa Preoccupation with Health; Change in a Traditional Attitude Resulting from Modern Health Problems. Bulletin of the Public Museum of the City of Milwaukee 19:175-258, 1953 ⟨II-02691⟩

1919-1945
Canada

Hallowell, A.I.: The role of conjuring in Saulteaux Society, Vol. 2. New York, Octagon Books, 1971. 96 p. ⟨II-00642⟩

Landes, R.: Ojibwa religion and the Midewiwin. Madison/Milwaukee/London, University of Wisconsin Press, 1968. 250 p. ⟨II-00643⟩

Manitoba

Hallowell, A.I.: The Passing of the Midewiwin in the Lake Winnipeg Region. American Anthropologist 38:33-51, 1936 ⟨II-00640⟩

Hallowell, A.I.: The social function of anxiety in a primitive society. American Sociological Review 6:869-881, 1941 ⟨II-00641⟩

North West Territories

Casteel, R.W.: A Sample of Northern North American Hunter -- Gatherers and the Malthusian Thesis: An Explicitly Quantified Approach. In: Browman, D.L. (edit): Early Native Americans. Paris/New York, Mouton Publishers, 1980. pp 301-319 ⟨II-05188⟩

1946-1979
Canada

Coodin, F.J.: Some observations on Eskimo health. The Journal-Lancet 87(2):51-55, 1967 ⟨II-00632⟩

Wenzel, G.W.: Inuit Health and the Health Care System: Change and Status Quo. Etudes/Inuit/Studies, 5:7-15, 1981 ⟨II-05413⟩

British Columbia

Banfill, B.J.: With the Indians of the Pacific. Toronto, The Ryerson Press, 1966, 176 p. ⟨II-04624⟩

Edwards, G.T.: Oolachen Time in Bella Coola. The Beaver, 309(2):32-37, 1978 〈II-00633〉

New Brunswick

Lacey, L.: Micmac Indian Medicine: A Traditional Way of Health. Antigonish, N.S., Formac Limited, 1977. 74 p. 〈II-00635〉

Ontario

Weaver, S.M.: Medicine and politics among the Grand River Iroquois: A study of the Non-Conservatives. Publications in Ethnology 4:1-182, 1972 〈II-00636〉

Quebec

Normandeau, L., Legare, J.: La Mortalite infantile des Inuit du Nouveau-Quebec. Canadian Review of Sociology and Anthropology 16:260-275, 1979 〈II-05117〉

Saskatchewan

Fieber, F.: Natural Medicines of the Cree Indians. The Beaver, 309(4):57-59, 1979 〈II-00634〉

1980-1989
Canada

Weslager, C.A.: Cures Among the Delawares in Canada. In: Magic Medicines of the Indians. Somerset, N.J., Middle Atlantic Press 〈II-00629〉

British Columbia

Jilek, W.G.: Indian Healing: Shamanic Ceremonialism in the Pacific Northwest Today. Hancock House, 1982. 〈II-05412〉

All embracing
Canada

Ackerknecht, E.H.: Medicine and Disease Among Eskimos. Ciba Symposia 10:916-921, 1948 〈II-00603〉

Bailey, A.G.: Disease and Treatment. In: The Conflict of European and Eastern Algonkian Cultures 1504-1700. Toronto/Buffalo, University of Toronto Press, 1969. pp 76-83 〈II-05365〉

Beaugrand-Champagne, A.: Les Maladies et la Medecine des Anciens Iroquois. Cahier des Dix 9:227-242, 1944 〈II-04691〉

Brown, W.C.: Disease Among the Aborigines of America and Their Knowledge of Treatment. Canadian Journal of Medicine and Surgery 51:155-58, 1922 〈II-04016〉

Bryce, P.H.: The history of the American Indians in relation to health. Ontario Historical Society Papers and Records 12:128-141, 1914 〈II-00605〉

Fortuine, R.: The Health of the Eskimos, as Portrayed in the Earliest Written Accounts. BHM 45:97-114, 1971 〈II-00610〉

Gariepy, P.U.: La Chirurgie Chez Les Indiens du Nord-Amerique. L'UMC 66:526-534, 1937 〈II-02439〉

Hrdlicka, A.: Disease, Medicine and Surgery Among the American Aborigines. JAMA 99:1661-1666, 1932 〈II-02960〉

Hutchens, A.R.: Indian Herbalogy of North America. Windsor, Merco, 1969. 382 p. 〈II-05258〉

Jackson, W.S.T.: Medicine among the North American Indians. CACHB 20(2):39-44, 1955 〈II-00613〉

Kinietz, W.V.: Indians of the Great Lakes -- Huron: Shamans and Medical Practice. Michigan University Museum of Anthropology Occasional Contributions, 10:131-160, 1940 〈II-00615〉

Margetts, E.L.: Indian and Eskimo medicine, with notes on the early history of psychiatry among French and British colonists. In Howells, John G.,ed. World History of Psychiatry. New York, Brunner/Mazel, Publisher, 1975. pp 400-431 〈II-00619〉

McCardle, B.: Bibliography of the History of Canadian Indian and Inuit Health. Edmonton, Treaty and Aboriginal Rights Research of the Indian Association of Alberta, 1981 89 p. 〈II-04641〉

Mechling, W.H.: Medical Practices. Anthropologica 8:239-263, 1959 〈II-00620〉

Mitchell, R.: North American Indian Medicine. Manitoba Medical Review 36:242-244, 1956 〈II-00621〉

Morgan, M.V.: Indian Medicine. The Beaver 264(2):38, 1933 〈II-03307〉

Murphy, H.H.: Indian Medicine. CMAJ 17:725-27, 1927 〈II-03752〉

Prud'Homme, L-A: Forts en Medicine et Jongleurs. PTRSC 30[1]:7-10, 1936 〈II-04696〉

Ross, J.F.W.: The Indian and the Indian Medicine Man. Canadian Practitioner and Review, May 1903 〈II-00623〉

Sersha, T.M.: The Use of Plant Medicines by the Dakota Indians. Thesis (M.A.) Manitoba, University of Manitoba, 1973. 〈II-05022〉

Stone, E.: Medicine Among the Iroquois. Annals of Medical History 6:529-539, 1934 〈II-03842〉

Trigger, B.G.: The Individual and Society: Theories About Illness. In: The Huron Farmers of the North. New York/Chicago, Holt, Rinehart and Winston, 1969. pp 113-120 〈II-02628〉

Vogel, V.J.: American Indian Medicine. Norman, University of Oklahoma Press, 1970 〈II-00628〉

Weiner, M.A.: Earth Medicine -- Earth Food. Plant Remedies, Drugs, and Natural Foods of the North American Indians. New York, Collier Books, 1972. 230 p. 〈II-05259〉

Young, T.K.: Sweat Baths and the Indians. CMAJ 119:406, 408-09, 1978 〈II-05254〉

Youngken, H.W.: The drugs of the North American Indian. American Journal of Pharmacy 96:485-502, 1924 〈II-00630〉

Youngken, H.W.: The drugs of the North American Indian (II). American Journal of Pharmacy 97:257-271, 1925 〈II-00631〉

Alberta

Dempsey, H.A.: A Blackfoot winter count. Calgary, Glenbow-Alberta Inst 1965. 20 p. 〈II-00608〉

Johnson, G.R.: Ground Medicine. CACHB 17(2):37-39, 1952 〈II-00614〉

Johnston, A.: Uses of Native Plants by the Blackfoot Indians. Alberta Historical Review 8(4):8-13, 1960 〈II-02971〉

MacLean, J.: The Medicine Stone. The Beaver 258:116-7, 1927 ⟨II-03251⟩

MacLean, J.: Blackfoot Medical Priesthood. Alberta Historical Review 9(2):1-7, 1961 ⟨II-02970⟩

Schaeffer, C.E.: Blackfoot shaking tent. Calgary, Glenbow-Alberta Inst 1969. 39 p. ⟨II-00624⟩

British Columbia

Barbeau, M.: Medicine-men on the North Pacific Coast. National Museum of Canada Bulletin 152:1-95, 1973. (Anthropological Series 42) ⟨II-00604⟩

Darby, G.E.: Indian medicine in British Columbia. CMAJ 28:433-438, 1933 ⟨II-03088⟩

Fiddes, G.W.J.: He Took Down His Shingle (A Backward Look at the Indian Medicine Man). Canadian Journal of Public Health 56:400-401, 1965 ⟨II-04053⟩

Gunn, S.W.A.: Kwatkiutl House and Totem Poles. British Columbia, Whiterocks Publications, 1966. 24 p. ⟨II-00612⟩

Gunn, S.W.A.: Medecine Totemique et Chamanisme Chez Les Indiens du Nord-Quest Americain. Bull d'abonnement a la revue 5:97-105, 1978 ⟨II-02470⟩

Gunn, S.W.A.: Traditional Medicine among Native Indians of Western Canada. Dialogue 68:6-7, 1979 ⟨II-00611⟩

Honigmann, J.J.: Witchcraft Among Kaska Indians. In: Walker, D.E.(edit): Systems of North American Witchcraft and Sorcery. Moscow, Idaho, Univ. of Idaho, 1970. pp 221-238 ⟨II-05361⟩

Kautz, S.: Trephining. Snaug. 3(2):16-19, 1975 ⟨II-03992⟩

Kidd, G.E.: Trepanation Among the Early Indians of British Columbia. CMAJ 55:513-516, 1946 ⟨II-03951⟩

Large, R.G.: Drums and Scalpel. Vancouver, Mitchell Press Limited, 1968. 145 p. ⟨II-00373⟩

Leechman, D.: Trephined Skulls from British Columbia. PTRSC 38:99-102, 1944 ⟨II-03869⟩

MacDermot, J.H.: Food and Medicinal Plants used by the Indians of British Columbia. CMAJ 61:177-183, 1949 ⟨II-00616⟩

Miles, J.E.: The Psychiatric Aspects of the Traditional Medicine of the British Columbia Coast Indians. Canadian Psychiatric Association Journal 12:429-431, 1967 ⟨II-04786⟩

Watkins, D.: The Practice of Medicine Among the Indians. Okanagan Historical Society Report 34:30-32, 1970 ⟨II-03609⟩

New Brunswick

MacDonald, E.: Indian Medicine in New Brunswick. CMAJ 80:220-224, 1959 ⟨II-00618⟩

Stewart, W.B.: Indian Medicine in New Brunswick. In International Congress for the History of Medicine, 25th Quebec, 1976. Proceedings, Volume III, 1976. p. 1320-1326 ⟨II-00625⟩

Van Wart, A.F.: The Indians of the Maritime Provinces, their diseases and native cures. CMAJ 59:573-577, 1948 ⟨II-00626⟩

Newfoundland

Peacock, F.W.: Some Eskimo Remedies and Experiences of an Amateur Doctor among the Labrador Eskimo. CMAJ 56:328-330, 1947 ⟨II-00622⟩

Nova Scotia

Chandler, R.F., Hooper, S.N., Freeman, L.: Herbal Remedies of the Maritime Indians. Journal of Ethnopharmacology 1(1):49-68, 1979 ⟨II-00606⟩

Ontario

Dailey, R.C.: The Midewiwin, Ontario's First Medical Society. Ontario History 50:133-138, 1958 ⟨II-00607⟩

Daniels, P.: "A Certaine Kind of Herbe": Smoking Pipes of the Ontario Iroquois. Rotunda 13(2):4-9, 1980 ⟨II-05367⟩

Paper, J.: From shaman to mystic in Ojibwa religion. Studies in Religion/Sciences Religieuses 9:185-199, 1980 ⟨II-04201⟩

Parker, A.C.: Indian Medicine and Medicine Men. Thirty-Sixth Annual Archaeological Report (Toronto), 1928. pp 9-17 ⟨II-04820⟩

Shimony, A.: Iroquois Witchcraft at Six Nations. In: Walker, D.E.(edit): Systems of North American Witchcraft and Sorcery. Moscow, Idaho, Univ. of Idaho, 1970. pp 239-265 ⟨II-05362⟩

Young, T.K.: Changing Patterns of Health and Sickness among the Cree-Ojibwa of Northwestern Ontario. Medical Anthropology 3:191-223, 1979 ⟨II-04212⟩

Printing and Bibliography
1816-1867
Canada

Roland, C.G., Potter, P.: An Annotated Bibliography of Canadian Medical Periodicals 1826-1975. Toronto, The Hannah Institute for the History of Medicine, 1979. 77 p. ⟨II-05027⟩

Ontario

Hill, H.P.: The Bytown Gazette: A Pioneer Newspaper. Ontario Historical Society Papers and Records 27:407-423, 1931 ⟨II-00529⟩

1868-1918
Canada

Roland, C.G.: Some Addena to Abbott's Classified Bibliography of Sir William Osler. BHM 38:78-79, 1964 ⟨II-01860⟩

Routley, T.C.: The Murray Brothers. CMAJ 78:449-450, 1958 ⟨II-01791⟩

1919-1945
Canada

Dumas, P.: William Osler et la Bibliotheca Osleriana. L'UMC 100:539-545, 1971 ⟨II-00528⟩

All embracing
Canada

Roland, C.G.: The Possible Consequences of a Bibliography of Canadian Medical Periodicals. In: Jarrell,

R.A., Ball, N.R.: Science, Technology and Canadian History. Kingston, Wilfrid Laurier Univ. Press, 1980. pp 208-211 ⟨II-00375⟩

Professionalization

1500-1699

Nova Scotia

Campbell, D.A.: The Growth and Organization of the Medical Profession in Nova Scotia. Canadian Journal of Medicine and Surgery 18:351-364, 1905 ⟨II-04103⟩

1760-1815

Ontario

Price, M.J.: The Professionalization of Medicine in Ontario During the 19th Century. Thesis (M.A.), Hamilton, McMaster University, 1977 ⟨II-05155⟩

Quebec

Bernier, J: Francois Blanchet et le Mouvement Reformiste en Medecine au Debut du XIXe Siecle. Revue d'Histoire de l'Amerique Francaise 34:223-244, 1980 ⟨II-04685⟩

Tunis, B.R.: Issues in the Professionalization of Medicine, Lower Canada, 1788-1847. Newsletter, Canadian Society for the History of Medicine, 6:17-20, 1981 ⟨II-04800⟩

1816-1867

Ontario

Gidney, R.D., Millar, W.P.J.: The Origins of Organized Medicine in Ontario, 1850-1869. In: Roland, C.G. (ed.): Health, Disease and Medicine: Essays in Canadian History. Toronto, Hannah Institute for the History of Medicine. 1984, 65-95 ⟨II-05394⟩

Quebec

Bernier, J.: Vers un Nouvel Ordre Medical: Les Origines de la Corporation des Medecins et Chirurgiens du Quebec. Recherches Sociopolitiques 22:307-330, 1981 ⟨II-05271⟩

1868-1918

Canada

Barr, J.W.: Medical Council of Canada. II: More About the Origins of the Council. CMAJ 111:267, 1974 ⟨II-05448⟩

Neatby, H.: The Medical Profession in the North-West Territories. CACHB 14:61-77, 1950 ⟨II-03787⟩

British Columbia

Andrews, M.W.: Medical Services in Vancouver, 1886-1920: A Study in the Interplay of Attitudes, Medical Knowledge, and Administrative Structures. Thesis (Ph.D.), British Columbia, University of British Columbia, 1979. ⟨II-05159⟩

Nova Scotia

Howell, C.D.: Reform and the Monopolistic Impulse: the Professionalization of Medicine in the Maritimes. Acadiensis 9:3-22, 1981 ⟨II-04913⟩

Howell, C.D.: Elite Doctors and the Development of Scientific Medicine: The Halifax Medical Establishment and 19th Century Medical Professionalism. In: Roland, C.G.(ed.): Health, Disease and Medicine: Essays in Canadian History. Toronto, Hannah Institute for the History of Medicine, 1984, 105-122 ⟨II-05396⟩

Ontario

Kutcher, S.P.: Toronto's Metaphysicians: the social gospel and medical professionalization in Victorian Toronto. Journal of the History of Canadian Science, Technology and Medicine 5(1):41-51, 1981 ⟨II-03261⟩

McCaughey, D.: Professional Militancy: The Medical Defence Association vs. the College of Physicians and Surgeons of Ontario, 1891-1902. In: Roland, C.G. (ed.): Health, Disease and Medicine: Essays in Canadian History. Toronto, Hannah Institute for the History of Medicine, 1984, 96-104 ⟨II-05395⟩

Quebec

Bernier, J.: Les Praticiens de la Sante au Quebec, 1871-1921: Quelques Donnees Statistiques. Recherches Sociographiques 20:41-58, 1979 ⟨II-04683⟩

Bernier, J.: L'integration du corps medical quebecois a la fin du XIXe siecle. Historical Reflections 10:91-113, 1983 ⟨II-05206⟩

1919-1945

Quebec

Dussault, G.: Les Medecins du Quebec (1940-1970). Recherches Sociographiques 16:69-84, 1975 ⟨II-04688⟩

All embracing

Canada

Shortt, S.E.D.: Medical Professionalization: Pitfalls and Promise in the Historography. Journal of the History of Canadian Science, Technology and Medicine 5:210-219, 1981 ⟨II-04637⟩

Psychiatry

1760-1815

Quebec

Dumas, C.: Considerations historiques sur la psychiatrie au Quebec. L'UMC 101:2636-40, 1972 ⟨II-05339⟩

Harvey, F: Preliminaires a une Sociologie Historique des Maladies Mentales au Quebec. Recherches Sociographiques 16:113-118, 1975 ⟨II-04687⟩

1816-1867

Canada

Appleton, V.E.: Psychiatry in Canada a Century Ago. Canadian Psychiatric Association Journal 12(4):345-361, 1967 ⟨II-00601⟩

Beahre, R.: Victorian Psychiatry and Canadian Motherhood. Canadian Women's Studies 2:44-46, 1980 ⟨II-04646⟩

Greenland, C.: Work as Therapy in the Treatment of Chronic Mental Illness. Canadian Psychiatric Association Journal 7:11-15, 1962 ⟨II-00525⟩

Greenland, C.: Three pioneers of Canadian psychiatry. JAMA 200:833-842, 1967 ⟨II-00526⟩

Griffin, J.D.: Planning Psychiatric Services. Medical Services Journal of Canada 23:1245-1260, 1967 ⟨II-04187⟩

McNeel, B.H., Lewis, C.H.: Care of the Mentally Ill in Ontario: History of Treatment. Canadian Hospital 37(2):34-36, 102, 1960. 37(3):45, 106-107, 1960 ⟨II-03772⟩

Manitoba

Goldring, P.: The Doctor's Office, Walls, and North-West Bastion at Lower Fort Garry. Manuscript Report Number 51, National Historic Sites Service, 1971. pp 71 ⟨II-00602⟩

Matas, J.: The Story of Psychiatry in Manitoba. Manitoba Medical Review 41:360-364, 1961 ⟨II-00527⟩

Ontario

Baehre, R.: From Pauper Lunatics to Bucke: Studies in the Management of Lunacy in 19th Century Ontario. Thesis (Ph.M.), Waterloo, University of Waterloo, 1976, unpublished. ⟨II-05033⟩

Frankenburg, F.: The 1978 Ontario Mental Health Act in Historical Context. HSTC Bulletin 6:172-177, 1982 ⟨II-04990⟩

Quebec

Wahl, P., Greenland, C.: Du Suicide: F.A.H. LaRue, MD (1833-1881). Canadian Psychiatric Association Journal 15.95-97, 1970 ⟨II-03304⟩

1868-1918

Canada

Brown, T.E.: Dr. Ernest Jones, Psychoanalysis, and the Canadian Medical Profession, 1908-1913. In: Shortt, S.E.D.: Medicine in Canadian Society: Historical Perspectives. Montreal, McGill-Queen's University Press, 1981. pp 315-360. ⟨II-04879⟩

Desjardins, E., Dumas, C.: Le Complexe Medical de Louis Riel. L'UMC 99:1870-1878, 1970 ⟨II-02348⟩

Lowy, F.H.: Clarence B. Farrar 1874-1970 and the History of Psychiatry in Canada. Canadian Psychiatric Association Journal 20:1-2, 1975 ⟨II-05322⟩

Mundie, G.S.: The Problem of the Mentally Defective in the Province of Quebec. CMAJ 10:63-69, 1920 ⟨II-00597⟩

Manitoba

Anderson, F.W.: Louis Riel's Insanity Reconsidered. Saskatchewan History 3:104-110, 1950 ⟨II-00582⟩

Clarke, C.K.: A Critical Study of the Case of Louis Riel. Queen's Quarterly 12:379-388, 1904-05; 13:14-26, 1905-06 ⟨II-02336⟩

Desjardins, E., Dumas, C.: Le Complexe Medical de Louis Riel. L'UMC 99:1656-1661, 1870-1878, 1970 ⟨II-02469⟩

Greenland, C., Griffin, J.D.: William Henry Jackson (1861-1952): Reil's secretary (another case of involun-

tary commitment). Canadian Psychiatric Association Journal 23:469-477, 1978 ⟨II-00591⟩

Ontario

Clarke, C.K.: The Story of the Toronto General Hospital Psychiatric Clinic. Canadian Journal of Mental Hygiene 1:30, 1919 ⟨II-04465⟩

Greenland, C.: Ernest Jones in Toronto 1908-13: A Fragment of Biography. Canadian Psychiatric Association Journal 6:132-139, 1961 ⟨II-02319⟩

Greenland, C.: Richard Maurice Bucke, M.D., 1837-1902 (A Pioneer of Scientific Psychiatry). CMAJ 91:385-391, 1964 ⟨II-01932⟩

Greenland, C.: Charles Kirk Clarke, A Pioneer of Canadian Psychiatry. Toronto, Clarke Institute of Psychiatry, 1966. 31 p. ⟨II-00592⟩

Greenland, C.: Ernest Jones in Toronto 1908-13, part II. Canadian Psychiatric Association Journal 11:512-519, 1966 ⟨II-02320⟩

Greenland, C.: Richard Maurice Bucke, M.D. 1837-1902: The Evolution of a Mystic. Canadian Psychiatric Association Journal 11:146-154, 1966 ⟨II-01935⟩

Horne, J.: R.M. Bucke: Pioneer Psychiatrist, Practical Mystic. Ontario History 59:197-208, 1967 ⟨II-01824⟩

Jameson, M.A. (Edit): Richard Maurice Bucke. London, Ontario, University of Western Ontario, 1978. 126 p. ⟨II-00593⟩

Lozynsky, A.: Richard Maurice Bucke, Medical Mystic. Detroit, Wayne State University Press, 1977. 203 p. ⟨II-00594⟩

Mitchinson, W.: Gynecological Operations on the Insane. Archivaria 10:125-144, 1980 ⟨II-00595⟩

Shortt, S.E.D.: R.M. Bucke: Vital Force, Evolution and Somatic Psychiatry, 1862-1902. In: 27th International Congress of the History of Medicine, p.149-153, 1980 ⟨II-04207⟩

Shortt, S.E.D.: The Influence of French Biomedical Theory on Nineteenth-Century Canadian Neuropsychiatry: Bichat and Comte in the Work of R.M. Bucke. International Congress for the History of Medicine, Paris, 1982. Proceedings, vol. 1:309-312, 1982. ⟨II-05272⟩

Stevenson, G.H.: The Life and Work of Richard Maurice Bucke, (an appraisal). American Journal of Psychiatry 93:1127-1150, 1937 ⟨II-01930⟩

Willer, B., Miller, G.: Classification, Cause and Symptoms of Mental Illness 1890-1900 in Ontario. Canadian Psychiatric Association Journal 22:231-235, 1977 ⟨II-04794⟩

Willer, B., Miller, G: Prognosis and Outcome of Mental Illness 1890-1900 in Ontario. Canadian Psychiatric Association Journal 22:235-8, 1977 ⟨II-04795⟩

Quebec

Greenland, C.: L'Affaire Shortis and the Valleyfield Murders. Canadian Psychiatric Association Journal 7:261-271, 1962 ⟨II-00588⟩

1919-1945

Canada

Blain, D., Griffin, J.D.: Canadian Psychiatrists in Publicatins of APA, 1948-1958: Source Materials. Canadian Psychiatric Association Journal 20:543-7, 1975 ⟨II-05291⟩

Roberts, C.A.: Thirty-five years of psychiatry in Canada, 1943-1978. Psychiatric Journal of the University of Ottawa 4(1):35-38, 1979 ⟨II-00579⟩

Silverman, B.: The Early Development of Child Psychiatry in Canada. Canadian Psychiatric Association Journal 6:239-240, 1961 ⟨II-04819⟩

Ontario

Greenland, C (edit): Ontario Neuro-Psychiatric Association: Recollections from the First Fifty Years. Ontario Psychiatric Association, 1970. ⟨II-04188⟩

Other

Van Nostrand, F.H.: Three years of neuropsychiatry in the Canadian army (overseas). CMAJ 49:295-301, 367-373, 1943 ⟨II-03743⟩

1946-1979

Canada

D'Arcy, C.: The Manufacture and Obsolescence of Madness: Age, Social Policy and Psychiatric Morbidity in a Prairie Province. Social Science and Medicine 10:5-13, 1976 ⟨II-05429⟩

Dickson, I.: The Canadian Psychiatric Association 1951-1958. Canadian Journal of Psychiatry 25:86-97, 1980 ⟨II-00577⟩

Sourkes, T.L.: Twenty-Five Years of Biochemical Psychiatry. Canadian Psychiatric Association Journal 15:625-29, ⟨II-05337⟩

Ontario

Kajander, R.E.: 26 Years of Psychiatric Practice in Thunder Bay. Ontario Medical Review 50(1):13-16, 1983 ⟨II-05048⟩

Liptzin, B.: The Effects of National Health Insurance on Canadian Psychiatry: The Ontario Experience. American Journal of Psychiatry 134:248-252, 1977 ⟨II-00578⟩

Quebec

Martel, P.G.: Joliette: dix ans d'evolution psychiatrique. Laval Medical 42:1-3, 1971 ⟨II-05419⟩

Other

Senex (N. Howard-Jones): Fifteen Words that Saved Humanity. WHO Dialogue 73:7-8, 1979 ⟨II-00580⟩

All embracing

Canada

Littmann, S.K.: History and the Psychiatrist. Canadian Psychiatric Association Journal 23:430-31, 1978 ⟨II-05358⟩

[Roland, C.G.]: Canada's Psychiatrists and their History. CMAJ 89:520-521, 1963 ⟨II-00576⟩

Psychology

1816-1867

Canada

Myers, C.R.: Notes on the History of Psychology in Canada. Canadian Psychologist 6:4-19, 1965 ⟨II-03751⟩

1868-1918

Alberta

Arvidson, R.M., Nelson, T.M.: Sixty Years of Psychology at the University of Alberta. Canadian Psychologist 9:500-4, 1968 ⟨II-05459⟩

Ontario

Greenland, C.: Mary Edwards Merrill, 1858-1880: "The Psychic". Ontario History 68:81-92, 1976 ⟨II-00575⟩

Public Health

1500-1699

Canada

Bryce, P.H.: The Story of Public Health in Canada. In: Ravenel, M.P.: A Half Century of Public Health. New York, American Public Health Association, 1921. pp 56-65 ⟨II-04999⟩

Nova Scotia

Campbell, P.S., Scammell, H.L.: The Development of Public Health in Nova Scotia. Canadian Public Health Journal 30:226-238, 1939 ⟨II-04104⟩

Quebec

Gregoire, J.: The Ministry of Health of the Province of Quebec. Canadian Journal of Public Health 50:411-420, 1959 ⟨II-00574⟩

1700-1759

Canada

MacDermot, H.E.: Pioneering in Public Health. CMAJ 99:267-273, 1968 ⟨II-03686⟩

1760-1815

Canada

Amyot, G.F.: Some Historical Highlights of Public Health in Canada. Canadian Journal of Public Health 58:337-341, 1967 ⟨II-04033⟩

McCullough, J.W.S.: Early History of Public Health in Upper and Lower Canada. National Hygiene and Public Welfare 58:17-31, 1922 ⟨II-00572⟩

New Brunswick

Melanson, J.A.: The New Brunswick Department of Health and Social Services. Canadian Journal of Public Health 49:370-381, 1958 ⟨II-00573⟩

Nova Scotia

Robertson, J.S.: The Nova Scotia Department of Public Health. Canadian Journal of Public Health 50:270-283, 1959 ⟨II-03796⟩

Ontario

Brandon, K.F.: Public Health in Upper Canada. Public Health Education Journal 25:461-5, 1934 ⟨II-05137⟩

1816-1867

Canada

Bilson, G.: Science, Technology and 100 Years of Canadian Quarantine. in: Jarrell, R.A.; Roos, A.E. (edit): Critical Issues in the History of Canadian Science, Technology and Medicine. Thornhill and Ottawa, HSTC Publications, 1983. pp 89-100 ⟨II-05195⟩

Bryce, P.H.: History of Public Health in Canada. Canadian Therapeutist and Sanitary Engineer 1:287-291, 1910 ⟨II-05013⟩

Newfoundland

Baker, M.: The Development of the Office of a Permanent Medical Health Officer for St. John's, Newfoundland, 1826-1905. HSTC Bulletin 7:98-105, 1983 ⟨II-05189⟩

Miller, L.A.: The Newfoundland Department of Health. Canadian Journal of Public Health 50:228-239, 1959 ⟨II-00570⟩

Ontario

MacDougall, H.: Epidemics and the Environment: The Early Development of Public Health Activity in Toronto, 1832-1872. In: Jarrell, R.A.; Roos, A.E. (edit): Critical Issues in the History of Canadian Science, Technology and Medicine. Thornhill and Ottawa, HSTC Publications, 1983. pp 135-151 ⟨II-05194⟩

Quebec

Farley, M., Keel, O., Limoges, C.: Les Commencements de L'Administration Montrealaise de la Sante Publique (1865-1885). HSTC Bulletin 6:85-109, 1982 ⟨II-04911⟩

1868-1918

Canada

Cooper, I.: Canadian Town Planning, 1900-1930: A Historical Bibliography. Volume III, Public Health. Toronto, University of Toronto (Centre for Urban and Community Studies), 1978. 23 p. ⟨II-00560⟩

Defries, R.D.: September 22, 1910 -- The Birthdate of the Canadian Public Health Association. Canadian Journal of Public Health 50:120-122, 1959 ⟨II-04082⟩

Gough, A.F.: Public Health in Canada, 1867-1967. Medical Services Journal of Canada 23:32-41, 1967 ⟨II-03954⟩

Porter, G.D.: Pioneers in Public Health. Canadian Journal of Public Health 40:84-86, 1949 ⟨II-00566⟩

Alberta

Somerville, A.: The Alberta Department of Public Health. Canadian Journal of Public Health 50:6-19, 1959 ⟨II-00568⟩

British Columbia

Amyot, G.F.: The British Columbia Department of Health and Welfare. Canadian Journal of Public Health 49:503-515, 1958 ⟨II-04034⟩

Manitoba

Elliott, M.R., Defries, R.D.: The Manitoba Department of Health and Public Welfare. Canadian Journal of Public Health 49:458-69, 1958 ⟨II-04059⟩

Mitchell, R.: The Development of Public Health in Manitoba. Canadian Public Health Journal 26:62-69, 1935 ⟨II-03693⟩

Nova Scotia

Boyer, B.F.: Dr. William Harop Hattie, an appreciation. CMAJ 26:121-122, 1932 ⟨II-03125⟩

Ontario

Bator, P.A.: Saving Lives on the Wholesale Plan, Public Health Reform in the City of Toronto, 1900-1930. Ph. D. Thesis, University of Toronto, 1979. pp 12-111 ⟨II-03258⟩

Bator, P.A.: The Struggle to Raise the Lower Classes: Public Health Reform and the Problem of Poverty in Toronto, 1910-1921. Journal of Canadian Studies 14:43-49, 1979 ⟨II-05210⟩

Defries, R.D.: Postgraduate Teaching in Public Health in the University of Toronto, 1913-1955. Canadian Journal of Public Health 48:285-294, 1957 ⟨II-00562⟩

Defries, R.D.: Dr. Edward Playter -- A Vision Fulfilled. Canadian Journal of Public Health 50:368-377, 1959 ⟨II-02679⟩

Gagan, R.R.: Disease, Mortality and Public Health, Hamilton, Ontario, 1900-1914. Thesis, McMaster University, School of Graduate Studies, Master of Arts, April 1981, 225 p. ⟨II-04932⟩

Holbrook, J.H.: The Story of the Hamilton Health Association. Canadian Journal of Public Health 15:158-164, 219-221, 1924 ⟨II-00564⟩

MacDougall, H.: Researching Public Health Services in Ontario, 1882-1930. Archivaria 10:157-172, 1980 ⟨II-00565⟩

MacDougall, H.: Public Health in Toronto's Municipal Politics: The Canniff Years, 1883-1890. BHM 55:186-202, 1981 ⟨II-04638⟩

MacDougall, H.: "Enlightening the Public": The Views and Values of the Association of Executive Health Officers of Ontario, 1886-1903. In: Roland, C.G.(ed.): Health, Disease and Medicine: Essays in Canadian History. Toronto, Hannah Institute for the History of Medicine, 1984, 436-464 ⟨II-05411⟩

McCullough, J.W.S.: 1910-1920, A Review of Ten Years' Progress. The Provincial Board of Health, Ontario, [1920], pp. 1-48 ⟨II-03835⟩

Oliver, E.B.: Department of Health. Thunder Bay Historical Society Annual 5:29-33, 1914 ⟨II-03828⟩

Phair, J.T., Defries, R.D.: The Ontario Department of Health. Canadian Journal of Public Health 50:183-196, 1959 ⟨II-03819⟩

Powell, M.: Public Health Litigation in Ontario, 1884-1920. In: Roland, C.G.(ed.): Health, Disease and Medicine: Essays in Canadian History. Toronto, Hannah Institute for the History of Medicine, 1984, 412-435 ⟨II-05410⟩

Sandomirsky, J.R.: Toronto's Public Health Photography. Archivaria 10:145-155, 1980 ⟨II-00567⟩

Quebec

Copp, T.: Public Health. In: The Condition of the Working Class in Montreal, 1897-1929: The Anatomy of Poverty. Toronto, McClelland and Stewart, 1974. pp 88-105. ⟨II-00561⟩

Sexton, A.M.: Wyatt Galt Johnston and the Founding of the Laboratory Section. American Journal of Public Health 40:160-164, 1950 ⟨II-02668⟩

Tetrault, M.: L'etat de sante des Montrealais, 1880-1914. Thesis (M.A.), Montreal, 1979 ⟨II-05142⟩

Saskatchewan

Roth, F.B., Defries, R.D.: The Saskatchewan Department of Public Health. Canadian Journal of Public Health 49:276-285, 1958 ⟨II-03801⟩

Seymour, M.M.: Public Health Work in Saskatchewan. CMAJ 15:271-278, 1925 ⟨II-03731⟩

1919-1945

Canada

McGinnis, J.P.D.: Whose Responsibility? Public Health in Canada, 1919-1945. In: Staum, M.S., Larsen, D.E. (edit.): Doctors, Patients, and Society. Power and Authority in Medical Care. Waterloo, Wilfrid Laurier Univ. Press, 1981. pp 205-229 ⟨II-05026⟩

Alberta

Collins, P.V.: The Public Health Policies of the United Farmers of Alberta Government, 1921-1935. Thesis, M.A., University of Western Ontario, London, 1969. 143 pages ⟨II-04817⟩

British Columbia

Sutherland, N.: Social Policy, 'Deviant' Children, and the Public Health Apparatus in British Columbia Between the Wars. Journal of Educational Thought 14:80-91, 1980 ⟨II-04877⟩

1946-1979

Canada

Davey, E.L.: Two Decades of Public Service Health. Medical Services Journal,Canada 23:965-983, 1967 ⟨II-04083⟩

Dearing, W.P.: Public Health Across the Border. Canadian Journal of Public Health 43:368-377, 1952 ⟨II-00558⟩

Horowics, J.H.: The Development of Health Services in Canada During the Last Twenty Years. Canadian Journal of Public Health, 57:123-125, 1966 ⟨II-04145⟩

All embracing

Canada

Defries, R.D. (edit.): The Development of Public Health in Canada. Canadian Public Health Association, 1940. pp. 184 ⟨II-00557⟩

Quackery

1500-1699

Quebec

Ahern, M.J.: Quelques Charlatans du Regime Francais Dans la Province de Quebec. Le Bulletin Medical de Quebec 10:345-358, 1908-09 ⟨II-02468⟩

1700-1759

Quebec

Riddell, W.R.: An Eighteenth Century Quack in French Canada. New York Medical Journal 102:881-882, 1915 ⟨II-04474⟩

1816-1867

Quebec

Stanley, G.D.: Who was Stephen Ayres?. CACHB 17:54-56, 1952 ⟨II-00556⟩

1868-1918

Canada

Kelley, T.P., Jr.: The fabulous Kelley: Canada's King of the Medicine Men. Don Mills, Paper Jacks, 1975. 149 p. ⟨II-00115⟩

Ontario

Riddell, W.R.: Was the handsome "Doctor" of Carleton Place a faker?. Offprint, (n.p., n.d.) pp. 3. ⟨II-00555⟩

1919-1945

Ontario

Beach, R.: The Hands of Dr. Locke. New York, Farrar and Rinehart, 1932. 56 p. ⟨II-00553⟩

Carter, J.S.: Doctor M.W. Locke and the Williamsburg Scene. Toronto, LIfe Portrayal Series, 1933. 138 p. ⟨II-00554⟩

Kiely, E.B.: Dr. M.W. Locke Heals with his Hands. 1937 n.p., no pagination (first published as a series of articles in the Montreal Daily Herald ⟨II-01898⟩

MacDonald, J.: Dr. Locke, Healer of Men. Toronto, Maclean Publishing Co., 1933. 83 p. ⟨II-01899⟩

Race

1816-1867

Ontario

Falk, L.A., Cameron, S.: Some Black Medical History: Dr. Martin R. Delany's Canadian Years as Medical Practitioner and Abolitionist (1856-1864). Based on a presentation to the 25th International Congress of the History of Medicine, August 24, 1976, at Laval University, Quebec, Canada ⟨II-01896⟩

Radiology

1868-1918

Canada

Brecher, R.: The Rays: A History of Radiology in the United States and Canada. Baltimore, The William and Wilkins Company, 1969. 484 p. ⟨II-00550⟩

Lipinski, J.K.: Original Publications in Diagnostic Radiology by Canadian Physicians 1896-1920. CSHM Newsletter, Spring 1983. pp 8-12 ⟨II-05112⟩

Lipinski, J.K.: Some Observations on Early Diagnostic Radiology in Canada. CMAJ 129:766, 768, 1983. ⟨II-05270⟩

Manitoba

Tait, R.: The First Western Canadian X-Ray Specialist. University of Manitoba Medical Journal 45:57-59, 1975 ⟨II-00552⟩

Nova Scotia

Shephard, D.A.E.: Alexander Graham Bell, Doctor of Medicine. New England Journal of Medicine 288:166-69, 1973 ⟨II-03868⟩

Ontario

Robertson, J.K.: An experiment in medical education. The British Journal of Radiology 27:593-603, 1954 ⟨II-03797⟩

Quebec

Belisle, L-P: Histoire de la Radiologie au Canada Francais. L'UMC 88:40-52, 1959 ⟨II-02467⟩

Bonenfant, J-L: Comment les chanoines de Quebec sont devenus transparents au XIXe siecle. CSHM Newsletter, Spring 1983, pp 1-7 ⟨II-05111⟩

MacDermot, H.E.: The earliest clinical applications of the X-rays. CMAJ 28:321-22, 1933 ⟨II-03143⟩

Robertson, P.: The All-Penetrating "X". Archivaria 10-258-260, 1980 ⟨II-00551⟩

Roland, C.G.: Priority of Clinical X-Ray Reports: A Classic Dethroned?. Canadian Journal of Surgery 5: 247-251, 1962 ⟨II-04626⟩

Saskatchewan

Becker, A.: Radiological Pioneers in Saskatoon. Saskatchewan History 36:31-37, 1983 ⟨II-05196⟩

1919-1945

North West Territories

Camsell, C.: Discovery and Development of Radium at Great Bear Lake. Franklin Institute Journal 233:545-557, 1922 ⟨II-00549⟩

Ontario

Cosbie, W.G.: The Gordon Richards Memorial Lecture: Gordon Richards and the Ontario Cancer Foundation. Journal of the Canadian Association of Radiologists 9:1-7, 1958 ⟨II-02616⟩

Red Cross

1868-1918

Canada

Porter, McK.: To All Men. The Story of the Canadian Red Cross. Toronto, McClelland and Stewart Ltd., 1960. 146 p. ⟨II-00548⟩

Ontario

Watson, E.H.A.: History Ontario Red Cross 1914-1946. Toronto, Ontario Division Headquarters, 91 p. ⟨II-04987⟩

Prince Edward Island

Daley, H.: "Volunteers in Action" The Prince Edward Island Division Canadian Red Cross Society 1907-1979. np, nd ⟨II-05124⟩

Religion and Medicine

1500-1699

Canada

Calverley, R.K.: St. Rene: The Patron Saint of Anaesthetists and a Patron Saint of Canada. Canadian Anaesthetist's Society Journal 27:74-77, 1980 ⟨II-02464⟩

Ontario

Prieur, G.O.: Rene Goupil, Surgeon: The First of the Jesuit Martyrs. CACHB 12:25-31, 1947 ⟨II-02191⟩

Prieur, G.O.: Francois Gendron: The First Physician of Old Huronia. CACHB 21(1):1-7, 1956 ⟨II-00547⟩

Quebec

Champault, M.P.: Les Gendron "medecins des rois et des pauvres". PTRSC section I:35-130, 1912 ⟨II-02440⟩

D'Allaire, M.: Origine Sociale des Religieuses de L'Hopital-General de Quebec. Revue d'Histoire de l'Amerique Francaise 23:559-581, 1969-70 ⟨II-04693⟩

Jones, G.C.: The knights of the order of St. John of Jerusalem in Canada under the French regime. CMAJ 31:431-432, 1934 ⟨II-03664⟩

1760-1815

Ontario

Graham, E.: Medicine Man to Missionary. Missionaries as agents of change among the Indians of Southern Ontario, 1784-1867. Toronto, Peter Martin Associates Ltd., 1975. 125 p. ⟨II-00352⟩

1816-1867

Manitoba

Barclay, R.G.: Grey Nuns Voyage to Red River. The Beaver 297(3):15-23, 1966 ⟨II-03314⟩

Ontario

McKillop, A.B.: Dr. Bovell's Quadrilateral Mind. In: A Disciplined Intelligence. Montreal, McGill-Queen's University Press, 1979, pp 73-91 ⟨II-03283⟩

1868-1918

Ontario

Bucke, R.M.: Man's Moral Nature. New York, G.P. Putnam's Sons, 1879. 200 p. ⟨II-00543⟩

Quebec

Desjardins, E.: Le Remede Magique d'un Medecin Theosophe. L'UMC 98:444-446, 1969 ⟨II-02350⟩

Desjardins, E.: Histoire de la Profession Medicale au Quebec:XI la Mission de Dom Smeulders. L'UMC 104:810-819, 1975 ⟨II-00544⟩

Thomas, D.: The Making of a Saint. Quest 11(8):21-30, 1982 ⟨II-04997⟩

United Kingdom

Gwyn, N.B.: The Letters of a Devoted Father to an unresponsive Son. BHM 7:335-351, 1939 ⟨II-03953⟩

Other

Bensley, E.H.: Dr. Minnie Gomery. CMAJ 96:1294, 1967 ⟨II-02612⟩

Hensman, B.: The Kilborn Family: A Record of a Canadian Family's Service to Medical Work and Education in China and Hong Kong. CMAJ 97:471-483, 1967 ⟨II-02316⟩

New, P.K., Cheung, Y.: Medical Missionary Work of a Canadian Protestant Mission in China, 1902-1937. CSHM Newsletter, Spring 1982, pages 11-16 ⟨II-04883⟩

Smith, J.F.: LIfe's Waking Part. Toronto, Thomas Nelson and Sons, Ltd., 1937. 345 p. ⟨II-02313⟩

Smith, W.E.: A Canadian Doctor in West China: Forty Years under Three Flags. Toronto, Ryerson Press, 1939. 2768 p. ⟨II-00545⟩

1919-1945

Manitoba

Reimber, M.: Cornelius W. Wiebe: A Beloved Physician. Winnipeg, Hyperion Press Limited, 1983 ⟨II-05077⟩

Other

Archibald, F.E.: Salute to Sid: The Story of Dr. Sidney Gilchrist. Windsor, Lancelot Press, 1970, 127 p. ⟨II-04116⟩

Murray, F.J.: At the Foot of Dragon Hill. New York, E.P. Dutton and Co., 1975. 240 p. ⟨II-04115⟩

Penfield, W.: China Mission Accomplished. CMAJ 97:468-470, 1967 ⟨II-03822⟩

Research
1816-1867

Nova Scotia

Campbell, D.A.: Abraham Gesner (1797-1864). In: Kelly, H.W.;Burrage, W.L.: Dictionary of American Medical Biography, New York and London, D. Appleton and Co., 1928. pp 462-463 ⟨II-00540⟩

1868-1918

Canada

Ferguson, J.K.W.: Canadian Milestones in Medical Research. Bulletin of the Medical Library Association 48:21-26, 1960 ⟨II-04054⟩

1919-1945

Canada

Farquharson, R.F.: The Medical Research Council of Canada. CMAJ 85:1194-1204, 1961 ⟨II-04057⟩

Quebec

Selye, H: The Stress of My Life: A Scientist's Memories. Toronto, McClelland and Stewart, 1977. 272 p. ⟨II-04117⟩

Respiratory System
1919-1945

Quebec

White, J.J.: Edward Archibald and William Rienhoff, Jr.: Fathers of the Modern Pneumonectomy -- An Historial Footnote. Surgery 68:397-402, 1970 ⟨II-05424⟩

Resuscitation
1868-1918

United States

Henderson, A.F.: Resuscitation Experiments and Breathing Apparatus of Alexander Graham Bell. Chest 62:311-316, 1972 ⟨II-03867⟩

1946-1979

Quebec

McKendry, J.B.R.: Closed Chest Cardiac Massage: An Early Case Report. CMAJ 87:305-30, 1962 ⟨II-01788⟩

Rural Health and Pioneer Practice
1500-1699

Manitoba

Adamson, J.D.: Pioneer Medicine in Manitoba. Journal-Lancet 70:49-50, 1950 ⟨II-04035⟩

Nova Scotia

MacKenzie, K.A.: The First Physicians in Nova Scotia. CMAJ 68:610-612, 1953 ⟨II-03696⟩

Quebec

Abbott, M.E.: Mr. E.Z. Massicotte on the Physicians and Surgeons of the XVIIth and XVIIIth Centuries in the District of Montreal. CMAJ 13:197-199, 1923 ⟨II-02959⟩

LeBlond, S.: Le Medecin Autrefois, au Canada (1534-1847). Laval Medicale 12:695-709, 1947 ⟨II-04667⟩

1700-1759

Ontario

Anderson, F.J.: Medicine at Fort Detroit in the Colony of New France, 1701-1760. JHMAS 1:208-228, 1946 ⟨II-05127⟩

Quebec

Gelfand, T.: Medicine in New France: Les Francais Look at Les Canadiens during the seven years war. In: 27th International Congress of the History of Medicine, p.511-516, 1980 ⟨II-04208⟩

LeBlond, S.: Medecins et Chirurgiens en France et en Nouvelle-France. Canadian Society for the History of Medicine Newsletter, 5:3-12, 1981 ⟨II-04672⟩

1760-1815

Alberta

Stanley, G.D.: The medical annals of Alberta. CACHB 8(4):17-22, 1944 ⟨II-00538⟩

New Brunswick

Gibbon, A.D.: Some Medical Highlights of Early Saint John. CMAJ 76:896-899, 1957 ⟨II-01794⟩

Ontario

Colgate, W.: Dr. Robert Kerr: An Early Practitioner of Upper Canada. CMAJ 64:542-546, 1951 ⟨II-01838⟩

Holling, S.A., Senior, J., Clarkson, B., Smith, D.A.: Medicine for Heroes: a Neglected Part of Pioneer Life. Mississauga, Mississauga South Historical Society, 1981. 93 p. ⟨II-04783⟩

McGhie, A.G.: Historical notes on medical personalities in the Hamilton area. McGregor Clinic Bulletin 23(2):1-9, 1962 ⟨II-00537⟩

Purdon, A.L.: Early Medical Practice in the Niagara Peninsula. In: Villages in the Niagara Peninsula. Proceeding, Second Annual Niagara Peninsula History Conference, Brock University, April 1980, pp. 103-112. ⟨II-04916⟩

Quebec

Belanger, L.F.: A Canadian physician in the 18th Century. University of Ottawa Medical Journal 14(4):13-15, 1972 ⟨II-02892⟩

Clouston, H.R.: Pioneer Medicine in the Chateauguay Valley. CMAJ 49:426-430, 1943 ⟨II-04326⟩

1816-1867

Canada

Mercer, W.: Edinburgh and Canadian Medicine: The First Alexander Gibson Memorial Lecure, part I. CMAJ 84:1241-1257, 1313-1317, 1961 ⟨II-01782⟩

Alberta

Jamieson, H.C.: The early medical history of Edmonton. CMAJ 29:431-437, 1933 ⟨II-03144⟩

Stanley, G.D.: Medical Pioneering in Alberta. Alberta Historical Review 1:1-6, 1953 ⟨II-02978⟩

British Columbia

Helmcken, J.S.: Some experiences in pioneer days. Western Canada Medical Journal 1:440-444, 1907 ⟨II-00531⟩

Hopwood, V.: William Fraser Tolmie: Natural Scientist and Patriot. British Columbia Studies 5:45-51, 1970 ⟨II-03250⟩

Johansen, D.O.: William Fraser Tolmie of Hudson's Bay Co. 1833-1870. The Beaver 268(2):29-32, 1937 ⟨II-03302⟩

Kidd, H.M: The William Osler Medal Essay: Pioneer Doctor John Sebastian Helmcken. BHM 21:419-461, 1947 ⟨II-02610⟩

Large, R.G.: Drums and Scalpel. From Native Healers to Physicians on the North Pacific Coast. Vancouver, Mitchell Press Limited, 1968. 145 p. ⟨II-00532⟩

McDonnell, C.E.: B.C. Medical History. British Columbia Medical Journal 19:348-9, 1977 ⟨II-03148⟩

Manitoba

Mitchell, R.: Early Doctors of Red River and Manitoba. Historical and Scientific Society of Manitoba. Papers. Series 3, No. 4:37 -47, 1947-8 ⟨II-02106⟩

New Brunswick

Oborne, H.G.: Samuel Tilley Gove 1813-1897: The Chronicle of a Canadian Doctor of a Century Ago. CACHB 12(2):31-38, 1947 ⟨II-00533⟩

Nova Scotia

Morse, F.W.: A Country Doctor's Life, 1855-1898. Nova Scotia Medical Bulletin 46:169-175, 1967 ⟨II-03278⟩

Reid, J.W.: Presidential Address. CMAJ 70:335-338, 1954 ⟨II-03815⟩

Ontario

Bond, C.C.J.: Alexander James Christie, Bytown Pioneer, His Life and Times, 1787-1843. Ontario History 56:17-36, 1964 ⟨II-00523⟩

Elliott, J.H.: John Gilchrist, J.P., L.M.B.U.C., M.P.: A Pioneer New England Physician in Canada. BHM 7:737-750, 1939 ⟨II-02911⟩

Roland, C.G.: Diary of a Canadian Country Physician: Jonathan Woolverton (1811-1883). Medical History 14:168-180, 1971 ⟨II-04889⟩

Spack, V.M.: The Story of a Pioneer Doctor -- Harmaunus Smith. Wentworth Bygones 5:40-43, 1964 ⟨II-01811⟩

Quebec

Ballon, H.C.: Aaron Hart David, M.D. (1812-1882). CMAJ 86:115-112, 1962 ⟨II-01873⟩

Cadotte, M.: Les Memoires de Philippe Aubert de Gaspe et les Medecins. L'UMC 105:1250-1268, 1976 ⟨II-00524⟩

1868-1918

Alberta

Baker, J.O.: A Medical Man from Glengarry and Stormont -- Part I History. CACHB 18(1):7-16, 1953 ⟨II-00484⟩

Baker, J.O.: A Medical Man from Glengarry and Stormont -- Part II Reflections. CACHB 18(2):1-12, 1953 ⟨II-00485⟩

Coulson, F.S.: "The First Surgeon in the West" -- Frank Hamilton Mewburn (1858-1929). CACHB 10(2):120-125, 1945 ⟨II-00486⟩

Jamieson, H.C.: The Early Doctors of Southern Alberta. CMAJ 38:391-397, 1938 ⟨II-03596⟩

Jamieson, H.C.: Southern Alberta Medicine in the Eighties. CMAJ 54:391-396, 1946 ⟨II-04377⟩

Ritchie, J.B.: Doctor John George Kittson: First Surgeon. CACHB 22(1):130-144, 1957 ⟨II-00497⟩

S., G.D.: Edward Hector Rouleau. CACHB 5:4-10, 1940 ⟨II-03813⟩

S., G.D.: Unforgettable Incidents. CACHB 7:12-14, 1942 ⟨II-03717⟩

Scarlett, E.P.: Medical Sources of Alberta Place-Names. CACHB 20:70-72, 1955 ⟨II-03709⟩

Stanley, G.D.: A Brief Summary of Medical Beginnings. CACHB 2(3):9-12, 1937 ⟨II-00504⟩

Stanley, G.D.: Dr. Robert George Brett (1851-1929). CACHB 4(1):5-12, 1939 ⟨II-00506⟩

Stanley, G.D.: Unforgettable incidents in pioneer practice. CACHB 7:8-10, 1942 ⟨II-00518⟩

Stanley, G.D.: Early days at High River, Alberta. CACHB 8(3):13-14, 1943 ⟨II-00512⟩

Stanley, G.D.: Medical Pioneering in Alberta: Unforgettable Incidents in Pioneer Practice. CACHB 7(4):9-10, 1943 ⟨II-00511⟩

Stanley, G.D.: Unforgettable Incidents. CACHB 9:54-56, 1944 ⟨II-03718⟩

Stanley, G.D.: How to make a successful start. CACHB 9(4):76-78, 1945 ⟨II-00513⟩

Stanley, G.D.: Medical Pioneering in Alberta. CACHB 10(1):74-78, 1945 ⟨II-00514⟩

Stanley, G.D.: Unforgettable incidents in private practice. CACHB 10(3):147-148, 1945 ⟨II-00508⟩

Stanley, G.D.: Unforgettable Incidents. CACHB 15:13-14, 1950 ⟨II-03721⟩

Stanley, G.D.: Medical Pioneering in Alberta. CACHB 17(4):75-78, 1953 ⟨II-00503⟩

Troy, M.T.: Early Medicine and Surgery in Calgary. Canadian Journal of Surgery 19:449-453, 1976 ⟨II-04329⟩

British Columbia

Green, D.: Dr. William John Knox 1878-1967: beloved Doctor of the Okanagan. Okanagan Historical Society Report 33:8-18, 1969 ⟨II-03622⟩

McDonnell, C.E.: Medical care on Burrard Inlet 1877-1882. British Columbia Medical Journal 19:394-5, 1977 ⟨II-03149⟩

McDonnell, C.E.: Some early Practitioners. British Columbia Medical Journal 19:446-7, 1977 ⟨II-03257⟩

McDonnell, C.E.: Vancouver's early years. British Columbia Medical Journal 20:78-9, 1978 ⟨II-03116⟩

Norris, J: The Country Doctor in British Columbia: 1887-1975. An Historical Profile. B.C. Studies 49:15-39,1981 ⟨II-04070⟩

Truax, W.: Reminiscences of a Country Doctor. CMAJ 60:411-415, 1949 ⟨II-00521⟩

Manitoba

Best, B.D.: Reminiscences. Winnipeg Clinic Quarterly 23:99-101, 1970 ⟨II-04024⟩

Hershfield, C.S.: Medical Memories. Winnipeg, [n.p.] 1973, 85 p. ⟨II-05083⟩

Kippen, D: [Reminiscences]. Winnipeg Clinic Quarterly 23:94-96, 1970 ⟨II-03956⟩

Martin, R.: Medicine, Then and Now. Manitoba Medical Review 30:645-47, 1950 ⟨II-03771⟩

Mitchell, R.: Iceland's Gift to Canadian Medicne. CMAJ 4:145-151, 1961 ⟨II-01792⟩

O'Donnell, J.H.: Manitoba as I saw it from 1869 to Date, with Flash-Lights on the First Riel Rebellion. Winnipeg, Clark Brothers and Co., 1909, 158 p. ⟨II-05084⟩

Pennefather, J.D.: Thirteen Years on the Prairies: From Winnipeg to Cold Lake, Fifteen Hundred Miles. London, Kegan Paul, Trench, Trubner and Co. Ltd, 1892. 127 p. ⟨II-05085⟩

Peterkin, A., Shaw, M.: Mrs. Doctor: reminiscences of Manitoba doctors' wives. Winnipeg, Manitoba, The Prairie Publishing Company,1978. 168 p. ⟨II-00496⟩

Ryan, G: [Reminiscences]. Winnipeg Clinic Quarterly 23:97-99, 1970 ⟨II-04121⟩

Stewart, B.: [Reminiscences]. Winnipeg Clinic Quarterly 23:110-113, 1970 ⟨II-03986⟩

Thorlakson, T.K.: A Patient and His Pioneer Doctors. Winnipeg Clinic Quarterly 20:33-47, 1967. ⟨II-05080⟩

Walton, C.: [Reminiscences]. Winnipeg Clinic Quarterly 23:103-110, 1970 ⟨II-03740⟩

Newfoundland

Duncan, N.: Dr. Grenfell's Parish: the deep sea fisherman. New York/Chicago/Toronto, Fleming H. Revell Co., 1905. 155 p. ⟨II-00487⟩

Grenfell, W.T.: A Labrador Doctor (The Autobiography of Wilfred Thomason Grenfell). Boston/New York, Houghton Mifflin Co., 1919. 441 p. ⟨II-00490⟩

Thomas, G.W.: Wilfred T. Grenfell, (1865-1941) [sic]. Founder of the International Grenfell Association. Canadian Journal of Surgery 9:125-130, 1966 ⟨II-02198⟩

Nova Scotia

Smith, J.W.: Fifty Years of General Practice. Nova Scotia Medical Bulletin 27:93-96, 1948 ⟨II-03729⟩

Young, M.R.: Then and Now. Nova Scotia Medical Journal 16:560-565, 1937 ⟨II-03465⟩

Ontario

Claxton, B.: Dr. Thomas Simpson (1833-1918; McGill, Med. 1854). Canadian Services Medical Journal 13:420-438, 1957 ⟨II-01947⟩

Hunter, J: Half a Century in Medicine -- 1875-1925. Canadian Journal of Medicine and Surgery 64:71-74, 1928 ⟨II-04142⟩

Oborne, H.G.: Samuel Tilley Gove 1813-1897: The Chronicle of a Canadian Doctor of a Century Ago. CACHB 12:31-38, 1947 ⟨II-02192⟩

Oille, J.A.: My experiences in medicine. CMAJ 91:855-860, 1964 ⟨II-02314⟩

Ramsay, G.: Towards Hudson Bay. CMAJ 58:614-616, 1948 ⟨II-03816⟩

Stanley, G.D.: Dr. Hugh Lang of Granton: A Family Physician on the Old Ontario Strand. CACHB 16(1):82-87, 1951 ⟨II-00499⟩

Quebec

Gervais-Roy, C.: Un Medecin de Campagne d'autrois. Revue d'Ethnologie du Quebec 7:85-102, 1981 ⟨II-04947⟩

Morphy, A.G.: Old Times in Medicine. CMAJ 63:507-511, 1950 ⟨II-03749⟩

Saskatchewan

Boyd, A.J.: Pioneer Health: Analysis of a Survey of the Health of Saskatchewan Residents 1878 to 1914. Saskatchewan, Occupational Health Reports, No. 2, June 1971, 97 p. ⟨II-04616⟩

Houston, C.J., Houston, C.S.: Pioneer of Vision: The Reminiscences of T.A. Patrick, M.D. Saskatoon, Western Producer Prairie Books, 1980. 149 p. ⟨II-00493⟩

MacLean, H.: A Pioneer Prairie Doctor. Saskatchewan History 15:58-66, 1962 ⟨II-00494⟩

Neatby, L.H.: Chronicle of a Pioneer Prairie Family. Saskatoon, Western Producer Prairie Books, 1979. 93 p. ⟨II-00495⟩

Ritchie, J.B.: George Alexander Kennedy, M.D. 1858-1913. CMAJ I:279-286, 1958 ⟨II-01784⟩

Thomson, C.A.: Doc Shadd. Saskatchewan History 30:41-55, 1977 ⟨II-00519⟩

Thomson, C.A.: Saskatchewan's black pioneer doctor Alfred Schmitz Shadd. Canadian Family Physician 23:1343-1351, 1977 ⟨II-02071⟩

Thomson, W.A.: Incidents in early practice in the west. CACHB 10(1):79-82, 1945 ⟨II-00520⟩

Yukon

Barrett, W.T.: Reminiscences of Early Klondyke Days. University of Manitoba Medical Journal 49:141-146, 1979 ⟨II-01779⟩

1919-1945

Alberta

Hepburn, H.H.: The Evolution of Medical Practice During one Man's Lifetime. Alberta Medical Bulletin 24(3):127-132, 1959 ⟨II-00475⟩

Jackson, M.P.: On the Last Frontier: Pioneering in the Peace River Block. Letters of Mary Percy Jackson. London, The Sheldon Press, 1933. 118 p. ⟨II-00476⟩

Keywan, Z.: Mary Percy Jackson: pioneer doctor. The Beaver, pp. 41-48, Winter 1977 ⟨II-00477⟩

Parsons, W.B.: Medicine in the Thirties. Canadian Doctor 46:69-73, 1980 ⟨II-02326⟩

Manitoba

Peikoff, S.S.: Yesterday's Doctor: An Autobiography. Winnipeg, The Prairie Publishing Co., 1980. 145 p. ⟨II-00480⟩

Waugh, F.P.: Symposim on Manitoban Memories. Winnipeg Clinic Quarterly 22:116-120, 1970 ⟨II-02906⟩

Quebec

Dumas, A.: La Medecine et Mon Temps. Recherches Sociographiques 16:21-41, 1975 ⟨II-04689⟩

1946-1979

Alberta

Gibson, M.: One Man's Medicine. Toronto, Collins Publishers, 1981. 218 p. ⟨II-05047⟩

Quebec

Trent, B.: Northwoods Doctor. Philadelphia/New York, J.B. Lippincott Co., 320 p. ⟨II-00474⟩

All embracing

New Brunswick

Stewart, W.B.: Early Medicine and Surgery in New Brunswick. Canadian Journal of Surgery 22:183-190, 1979 ⟨II-04330⟩

Sanitation

1760-1815

Nova Scotia

Hanson, L.H. Jr.: The Excavation of the Engineer's Latrine at Louisbourg. Manuscript Report Number 55, National Historic Sites Service, 1968. pp. 63 ⟨II-00472⟩

Ontario

Wilson, R.: A Retrospect. A Short Review of the Steps taken in Sanitation to transform the Town of Muddy York into the Queen City of the West. Department of Public Health, City of Toronto. 37 p. ⟨II-00473⟩

1816-1867

Ontario

Ball, N., Desson, K.: The Pump-house Parthenon. Canadian Heritage, pp 16-21, Dec 1983-Jan 1984 ⟨II-05356⟩

Jones, E., McCalla, D.: Toronto Waterworks, 1840-77: Continuity and Change in Nineteenth- Century Toronto Politics. CHR 60(3):300-323, 1979 ⟨II-00358⟩

1868-1918

British Columbia

Cain, L.P.: Water and sanitation services in Vancouver: an historical perspective. British Columbia Studies, No. 30, pp 27-43, 1976 ⟨II-03254⟩

Ontario

Taylor, J.H.: Fire, Disease and Water in Ottawa: an Introduction. Urban History Review 7(1):1-37, 1979 ⟨II-03289⟩

Warfe, C.: Search for Pure Water in Ottawa: 1910-1915. Urban History Review 8:90-112, 1979 ⟨II-04211⟩

Science

1816-1867

Nova Scotia

Johnson, G.R.: Abraham Gesner - 1797-1864: A Forgotten Physician-Inventor. CACHB 13(2):30-34, 1948 ⟨II-00471⟩

MacKenzie, K.A.: Abraham Gesner, M.D., Surgeon Geologist, 1797-1864. CMAJ 59:384-387, 1948 ⟨II-04617⟩

Sex Behavior

1816-1867

Ontario

Mitchinson, W.: Medical Attitudes Towards Female Sexuality in Late Nineteenth Century English Canada. Department of History, University of Windsor, 1979. 32 p. n.p. ⟨II-00470⟩

1868-1918

Canada

Bliss, M.: Pure Books on Avoided Subjects: Pre-Freudian Sexual Ideals in Canada. Canadian Historical Association: Historical Papers, 1970. pp 89-108. ⟨II-00469⟩

Manitoba

Cooper, J.: Red Lights of Winnipeg. Historical and Scientific Society of Manitoba. Papers. Series 3. No. 27:61-74, 1970-71 ⟨II-02104⟩

Social Medicine

1760-1815

Quebec

Gilbert, M.R.: La Nouvelle Morale Sociale et L'Etat Surveillant. In International Congress for the History of Medicine, 25th, Quebec, 1976. Proceedings, volume I, 1976. p.171-192 ⟨II-00468⟩

1816-1867

Canada

Rosen, G.: The Idea of Social Medicine in America. CMAJ 61:316-323, 1949 ⟨II-04621⟩

1919-1945

Quebec

Park, L.: The Bethune Health Group. In: Shephard, D.A.E.; Levesque, A.(edit): Norman Bethune: His Times and His Legacy. Ottawa, Ontario, Canadian Public Health Association, 1982. pp 138-144. ⟨II-04920⟩

Social Welfare

1500-1699

Quebec

Reid, A.G.: The first poor-relief system of Canada. CHR 27:424-431, 1946 ⟨II-00467⟩

1700-1759

Nova Scotia

Williams, R.: Poor Relief and Medicine in Nova Scotia, 1749-1783. Collections of the Nova Scotia Historical Society, 24:33-56, 1938 ⟨II-03099⟩

1760-1815

New Brunswick

Greenhous, B.: Paupers and Poorhouses: the development of Poor Relief in early New Brunswick. Histoire Sociale/Social History 1:103-128, 1968 ⟨II-03306⟩

Nova Scotia

Martell, J.S.: Nova Scotia's Contribution to the Canadian Relief Fund in the War of 1812. CHR 23:297-302, 1943 ⟨II-00466⟩

Ontario

Baehre, R.: Paupers and Poor Relief in Upper Canada. Historical Papers, 1981. pages 57-80 ⟨II-04814⟩
Splane, R.B.: Social Welfare in Ontario 1791-1893: A Study of Public Welfare Administration. Toronto, University of Toronto Press, 1965. 305 p. ⟨II-02692⟩

1816-1867

Canada

Rooke, R.P., Schnell, R.L.: Childhood and Charity in Nineteenth-Century British North America. Social History 15:157-179, 1982 ⟨II-04928⟩

New Brunswick

Whalen, J.M.: The nineteenth-century Almshouse System in Saint John County. Histoire Sociale/Social History 7:5-27, 1971 ⟨II-03089⟩

Nova Scotia

Hart, G.E.: The Halifax Poor Man's Friend Society, 1820-27, An Early Social Experiment. CHR 34:109-123, 1953 ⟨II-01861⟩

Ontario

Angus, M.S.: Health, Emigration and Welfare in Kingston, 1820-1840. In: Oliver Mowat's Ontario, edited by D. Swainson, pp. 120-35. Toronto, MacMillan, 1972 ⟨II-05140⟩
Johnson, J.K.: The Chelsea Pensioners in Upper Canada. Ontario History 53:272-289, 1961 ⟨II-00464⟩
Langmuir, J.W.: Asylums, Prisons and Public Charities of Ontario and their Systems of Management. Can. Mon. 5:239-47, 1880 ⟨II-05160⟩

Quebec

Bradbury, B.: The Fragmented Family: Family Strategies in the Face of Death, Illness, and Poverty, Montreal, 1860-1885. In: Parr, J.(ed): Childhood and Family in Canadian History, Toronto, McClelland and Stewart, 1982. pp 109-128 ⟨II-04886⟩

1868-1918

Canada

Hareven, T.K.: An ambiguous alliance: some aspects of American influences on Canadian Social Welfare. Histoire Sociale/Social History 3:82-98, 1969 ⟨II-03305⟩

Manitoba

McArton, D.: 75 Years in Winnipeg's Social History. Canadian Welfare 25:11-19, 1949 ⟨II-03663⟩
Thompson, J.H.: The Beginning of our Regeneration: The Great War and Western Canadian Reform Movements. Canadian Historical Association: Historical Papers, pp 227-245, 1972 ⟨II-00463⟩

Ontario

Piva, M.J.: The Workmen's Compensation Movement in Ontario. Ontario History 67:39-56, 1975 ⟨II-04875⟩
Rutman, L.: In the Children's Aid: J.J. Kelso and Child Welfare in Ontario. Toronto, University of Toronto Press, 1982. 356 p. ⟨II-04918⟩
Smellie, T.S.T.: The origin and history of the Fort William Relief Society. Thunder Bay Historical Society Annual 3:17-19, 1912-13 ⟨II-03728⟩

1919-1945

Nova Scotia

Forbes, E.R.: Prohibition and the Social Gospel in Nova Scotia. Acadiensis 1:11-36, 1971 ⟨II-00461⟩

Ontario

Routley, T.C.: Medical Welfare plan is born. Ontario Medical Review 33:864-68, 1966 ⟨II-03807⟩

Routley, T.C.: Managing Medical Relief. Ontario Medical Review 34:30-34, 1967 ⟨II-03806⟩

Quebec

Copp, T.: The Health of the People: Montreal in the Depression Years. In: Shephard, D.A.E.; Levesque, A. (edit): Norman Bethune: His Times and His Legacy. Ottawa, Canadian Public Health Assoc., 1982, pp 129- 137 ⟨II-04919⟩

Societies, Academies, Foundations
1760-1815
Quebec

Gauvreau, J.: Le College des Medecins et Chirurgiens de la Province de Quebec: Avant-Propos. L'UMC 60:334-340, 1931 ⟨II-02380⟩

Gauvreau, J.: Le College des Medecins et Chirurgiens de la Province de Quebec: 1760-1847 Vue D'Ensemble sur Cette Epoque. L'UMC 60:426-431, 1931 ⟨II-02381⟩

1816-1867
Canada

Jacques, A.: How it all began. CMAJ 97:934-937, 1967 ⟨II-00459⟩

Kelly, A.D.: Origin and Organization of the CMA. CMAJ 107:559-561, 1972 ⟨II-03971⟩

Primrose, A.: The Canadian Medical Association. CMAJ 27:194-199, 1932 ⟨II-03086⟩

Nova Scotia

Hattie, W.H.: The First Minute Book [Medical Society of Nova Scotia]. Nova Scotia Medical Bulletin 8:155-161, 1929 ⟨II-04159⟩

MacKenzie, K.A.: Founders of the Medical Society of Nova Scotia. Nova Scotia Medical Bulletin 32:240-245, 1953 ⟨II-03688⟩

Scammell, H.L.: A Century in Retrospect. CMAJ 69:349-352, 1953 ⟨II-03722⟩

Stewart, C.B.: Highlights of the Past Anniversaries. Nova Scotia Medical Bulletin 32:246-252, 1953 ⟨II-03837⟩

Walker, S.L.: The Medical Society of Nova Scotia. Nova Scotia Medical Bulletin 8:191-96, 1929 ⟨II-03741⟩

Ontario

Gladstone, R.M.: The Academy of Medicine, Toronto. University of Toronto Medical Journal 37:92-94, 1960 ⟨II-04130⟩

Quebec

Desjardins, E.: Les societes de chirurgie du Quebec. L'UMC 103:1749-54, 1973 ⟨II-05444⟩

Gauthier, C.A.: Histoire de la Societe Medicale de Quebec. Laval Medical 8:60-121, 1943 ⟨II-04668⟩

Gauvreau, J.: Le Bureau Medicale de Montreal/the Montreal Medical Board 1839-1847. L'UMC 61:42-55 ⟨II-02378⟩

Gauvreau, J.: La Societe Medicale de Quebec 1826. L'UMC 60:880-884, 1931 ⟨II-02379⟩

Gauvreau, J.: Une Page D'Histoire: Le College des Medecins et Chirurgiens de la Province de Quebec. L'UMC 67:53-63, 1938 ⟨II-02374⟩

LeBlond, S.: Joseph Painchaud. L'UMC 82:1-6, 1953 ⟨II-00454⟩

McKee, S.H.: Abstracts from the Early Records of the Montreal Medico-Chirurgical Society. CMAJ 16:839-844, 1926 ⟨II-01805⟩

1868-1918
Canada

Desjardins, E.: Et Avant L'Acfas, Il Y Eut La Spaslac. L'UMC 100:1402-1406, 1971 ⟨II-02462⟩

Kelly, A.D.: The Secretarial Succession in the Canadian Medical Association. CMAJ 81:583-86, 1959 ⟨II-03964⟩

Kelly, A.D.: The Crest and Seal of the Canadian Medical Association. CMAJ 85:1016, 1961 ⟨II-01790⟩

Kelly, A.D.: Our Oldest Affiliate [Canadian Medical Protective Association]. CMAJ 98:369-370, 1968 ⟨II-03966⟩

King, F.E.: The Past and the Future of Canadian Voluntary Tuberculosis Associations. Canadian Journal of Public Health 59:123-125, 1968 ⟨II-03957⟩

MacDermot, H.E.: Seventy-Five Years of the Association. CMAJ 47:69-72, 1942 ⟨II-03853⟩

Proctor, H.A.: Historical Sketches of the Defence Medical Association of Canada and of the Canadian Forces Medical Services. Medical Services Journal pp 305-309, 1965 ⟨II-03818⟩

Wherrett, G.J.: The Diamond Jubilee of the Canadian Tuberculosis Association. CMAJ 84:99-101, 1961 ⟨II-03460⟩

Alberta

Fish, A.H.: The meeting of the Canadian Medical Association, August 12th and 13th, 1889, Banff, Alberta. CACHB 8(3):10-12, 1943 ⟨II-00453⟩

Learmonth, G.E.: The Fiftieth Anniversary of the Alberta Medical Association. Alberta Medical Bulletin 20:50-57, 1955 ⟨II-03738⟩

MacDermot, H.E.: The Annual Meeting at Banff, in 1889. CMAJ, 54:496-498, 1946 ⟨II-04378⟩

Scarlett, E.P.: A Walled Stead. Alberta Medical Bulletin 21:3-9, 1956 ⟨II-03710⟩

British Columbia

Kidd, G.E.: History of the Vancouver Medical Association. Bulletin of the History of Medicine 19:50-52, 1945; 23:5-8, 1946-47; 23:101-102, 1946-47; 23:148-150; 195-196; 233-235; 264-67; 290-96, 1946-47; 24:7-10, 1947-48 ⟨II-03963⟩

McDonnell, C.E.: Early VMA activities -- The founding of the BCMA. British Columbia Medical Journal 20:182-4, 1978 ⟨II-03113⟩

McDonnell, C.E.: The founding of the VMA [Vancouver Medical Association]. British Columbia Medical Journal 20:144-6, 1978 ⟨II-03114⟩

McDonnell, C.E.: The VMA and the government. British Columbia Medical Journal 20:246-8, 1978 ⟨II-03318⟩

Manitoba

Mitchell, R.: An Abortive Attempt. How a Meeting of Medical Men Met in 1883 Hoping to Establish a Medical Association in Winnipeg. Manitoba Medical Review 50:17, 1970 ⟨II-05423⟩

Pope, E.: The profession in Winnipeg. Western Canada Medical Journal 2:121-128, 1908 ⟨II-00455⟩

New Brunswick

Jennings, F.C.: The New Brunswick Medical Society. CMAJ 81:400-402, 1959 ⟨II-03980⟩

Newfoundland

Kingsmill, D.P.: The International Grenfell Association. McGill Medical Journal 25:121-127, 1956 ⟨II-03958⟩

North West Territories

Stanley, G.D.: The North-West Territories Medical Association. CACHB 16(2):38-39, 1951 ⟨II-00458⟩

Nova Scotia

Kendall, A.S.: Cape Breton Medical Society. Nova Scotia Medical Bulletin 8:109-113, 1929 ⟨II-03973⟩

W., S.L.: The Medical Society of Nova Scotia 1869 to 1916. Nova Scotia Medical Bulletin 8:423-427, 1929 ⟨II-04164⟩

Ontario

Elliott, J.H.: The Early Records of the University of Toronto Medical Society. University of Toronto Medical Journal 9:225-229, 1932 ⟨II-04061⟩

Ferguson, J.: History of the Ontario Medical Association, 1880-1930. Toronto, Murray Printing Co. Ltd., 1930. 142 p. ⟨II-00452⟩

Fielden, E.C.: The Academy on its Fiftieth Anniversary. Bulletin of the Academy of Medicine, Toronto 30:33-46, 1956 ⟨II-04052⟩

Gallie, W.E.: The Opening of Osler Hall. Bulletin of the Academy of Medicine, Toronto 25:41-46, 1951 ⟨II-04066⟩

Linell, E.A.: The Academy of Medicine of Toronto 1907-1957. CMAJ 76:437-442, 1957 ⟨II-03735⟩

Routley, T.C.: Affiliation with CMA. Ontario Medical Review 30:785-787, 801, 1963 ⟨II-03763⟩

Routley, T.C.: Introduction (Routley's History of the OMA). Ontario Medical Review 30:593-94, 1963 ⟨II-03762⟩

Routley, T.C.: Some Early Achievements. Ontario Medical Review 30:725-729, 1963 ⟨II-03811⟩

Routley, T.C.: The Formative Years. Ontario Medical Review 30:659-662, 1963 ⟨II-03812⟩

Routley, T.C.: Membership Becomes Continuous. Ontario Medical Review 31:208-211, 231, 1964 ⟨II-03765⟩

Routley, T.C.: The War Years. Ontario Medical Review 31:27-30, 1964 ⟨II-03759⟩

Ryerson, E.S.: Events Leading to the Formation of an Academy. Bulletin of the Academy of Medicine [Toronto] 5:26-33, 1932 ⟨II-00457⟩

Sawyer, G.: The First 100 Years: A History of the Ontario Medical Association. Toronto, Ontario Medical Association, 1980. 337 p. ⟨II-01810⟩

Quebec

Cohen, J.J.: British Medicine in Greater Britain: the BMA Montreal Meeting, 1897. McGill Medical Journal 36:159-168, 1967 ⟨II-04090⟩

Desjardins, E.: Le Centenaire de la Societe Medicale de Montreal. L'UMC 100:1188-1194, 1971 ⟨II-02461⟩

LeBlond, S.: Une Conference Inedite du Docteur Joseph Painchaud. Laval Medical 39:355-360, 1968 ⟨II-04661⟩

Scriver, W de M.: Nothing new under the sun [Montreal Medico-Chirurgical Society]. CMAJ 80:299-303, 1959 ⟨II-03724⟩

1919-1945

Canada

Berube, B.: How did the CMA Survive. CMAJ 127:530-532, 1982 ⟨II-04984⟩

Fortier, de la Broquerie: La Societe canadienne de Pediatrie (1922-1972). Vie Medicale au Canada Francais 2:573-4, 1973 ⟨II-05436⟩

Gridgeman, N.T.: Biological Sciences at the National Research Council of Canada: The Early Years to 1952. Waterloo, Wilfrid Laurier University Press, 1979. 153 p. ⟨II-00448⟩

MacDermot, H.E.: History of the Canadian Medical Association, Vol. II. Toronto, Murray Printing and Gravure Ltd., 1958. 153 p. ⟨II-00449⟩

Nova Scotia

Walker, S.L.: Medical Society Rennaisance. Nova Scotia Medical Bulletin 8:570-79, 1929 ⟨II-03742⟩

Ontario

Kelly, A.D.: Dr. Kelly Takes Over. Ontario Medical Review 34:532-33, 536, 1967 ⟨II-03764⟩

Kelly, A.D.: Effort to Control Cancer. Ontario Medical Review 34:585-86, 609, 1967 ⟨II-03758⟩

Routley, T.C.: Setting up the districts. Ontario Medical Review 31:95-99, 1964 ⟨II-03810⟩

Routley, T.C.: The Bid to Rout Routley. Ontario Medical Review 31:285-287, 290, 1964 ⟨II-03767⟩

Routley, T.C.: Dr. Kelly Joins the Staff. Ontario Medical Review 34:237-241, 1967 ⟨II-03779⟩

Routley, T.C.: Dr. Routley Resigns. Ontario Medical Review 34:387-392, 1967 ⟨II-03780⟩

Routley, T.C.: Routley's History of the O.M.A. : Conclusion. Ontario Medical Review 34:453-456, 1967 ⟨II-01797⟩

Routley, T.C.: The Reluctant Contractors. Ontario Medical Review 34:91-98, 1967 ⟨II-03781⟩

Quebec

Etziony, M.B.: History of the Montreal Clinical Society, 1923-1963. n.p., - n.d., 50 p. ⟨II-05008⟩

Lee, E.J.: History of the Osler Society of McGill. McGill Medical Journal 34:146-148, 1965 ⟨II-03737⟩

Leger, J.: L'association des medecins de langue francaise du Canada et L'Union Medicale du Canada. L'UMC 101:2376-2377, 1972 ⟨II-02460⟩

Tidmarsh, C.J.: The History of the Osler Society. McGill Medical Journal 25:176-78, 1956 ⟨II-03870⟩

1946-1979

Canada

Dickson, I.: The Canadian Psychiatric Association, 1951-1958. Canadian Journal of Psychiatry 25:86-97, 1980 ⟨II-00446⟩

Melville, K.I.: A progress report on the Canadian Society of Chemotherapy. International Journal of Clinical Pharmacology 1:373-375, 1968 ⟨II-03109⟩

Ontario

Dunham, H.S.: The London Meeting [of the O.M.A.]. Ontario Medical Review 35:310-11, 1968 ⟨II-04077⟩

Dunham, H.S.: The Ottawa Meeting [of the O.M.A.]. Ontario Medical Review 35:361-62, 1968 ⟨II-04076⟩

Dunham, H.S.: Voices for the G.P. Ontario Medical Review 35:259-60, 1968 ⟨II-04079⟩

Kelly, A.D.: Dr. Dunham Appointed. Ontario Medical Review 35:86-88, 1968 ⟨II-03768⟩

Other

Howard-Jones, N.: What was WHO -- Thirty Years Ago?. Dialogue 59:28-34, 1979 ⟨II-00447⟩

Specialization and Practice Organisation
1500-1699

Quebec

Massicotte, E.Z.: Document pour l'histoire de la medecine en Canada. L'UMC 49:375-376, 1920 ⟨II-02385⟩

1868-1918

Canada

Campbell, A.D.: Consultations then and now. CMAJ 89:1030-1032, 1963 ⟨II-04102⟩

British Columbia

Burris, H.L.: Medical Saga: The Burris Clinic and Early Pioneers. Vancouver, Mitchell Press Limited, 1967. 248 p. ⟨II-00368⟩

United States

Hewitt, R.M., Eckman, J.R., Miller, R.D.: The Mayo Clinic and the Canadians. CMAJ 91:1161-1172, 1964 ⟨II-04151⟩

1919-1945

Canada

Lewis, D.S.: The Royal College of Physicians and Surgeons of Canada 1920-1960. Montreal, McGill University Press, 1962. 241 p. ⟨II-00441⟩

Routley, T.C.: The Founding of the Royal College of Physicians and Surgeons of Canada. CMAJ, 73:104-106, 1955 ⟨II-04648⟩

Alberta

Stanley, G.D.: Daniel Stewart Macnab, October 28, 1879 - February 2, 1951. CACHB 16(1):10-20, 1951 ⟨II-00445⟩

Ontario

Lockwood, A.L.: Founder's Philosophy Still Pervades Toronto's Earliest Medical Clinic. Canadian Doctor 29(3):34-37, 1963 ⟨II-03760⟩

McGhie, A.G.: The development of group practice. McGregor Clinic Bulletin 23(2):17-23, 1962 ⟨II-00442⟩

Sport Medicine
1816-1867

Canada

Gear, J.L.: Factors Influencing the Development of Government Sponsored Physical Fitness Programmes in Canada from 1850 to 1972. Canadian Journal of the History of Sport and Physical Education 3:1-25, 1972 ⟨II-04810⟩

Quebec

Metcalfe, A.: The evolution of organized physical recreation in Montreal, 1840-1895. Histoire Sociale/Social History II(21):144-166, 1978 ⟨II-03090⟩

1868-1918

Alberta

Coulson, F.S.: Frank Hamilton Mewburn (1858-1929). CACHB 10:120-125, 1945 ⟨II-01909⟩

Quebec

Howell, W.B.: F.J. Shepherd: His Life and Times. Toronto and Vancouver, J.M. Dent and Sons Ltd., 1934. 251 p. ⟨II-01821⟩

State Medicine
1760-1815

Canada

Stieb, E.W.: Three centennials: a retrospective view of Canada's pure food and drug legislative. In International Congress for the History of Medicine, 25th, Quebec, 1976. Proceedings, Volume 111, 1976. p. 1327.1340 ⟨II-00440⟩

Quebec

Roland, C.G.: Dr. James Bowman vs Canada: A Struggle to Obtain Payment for Government Service. In International Congress for the History of Medicine, 25th, Quebec, 1976. Proceedings, Volume III, 1976. p. 1158-1170 ⟨II-00439⟩

1816-1867

Canada

Crichton, A.: Medicine and the State in Canada. In: Staum, M.S.; Larsen, D.E. (edit.): Doctors, Patients, and Society, Power and Authority in Medical Care. Waterloo, Wilfrid Laurier Univ. Press, 1981. pp 231-252 ⟨II-05025⟩

Defries, R.D.: The Federal and Provincial Health Services in Canada. Toronto, Canadian Public Health Association, 1959. 147 p. ⟨II-05128⟩

1868-1918
Canada

Bilson, G.: "Muscles and Health": Health and the Canadian Immigrant, 1867-1906. In: Roland, C.G.(ed.): Health, Disease and Medicine: Essays in Canadian History. Toronto, Hannah Institute for the History of Medicine, 1984, 398-411 ⟨II-05409⟩

Liston, A.: To Cure the Sick and Protect the Healthy. In International Congress for the History of Medicine, 25th, Quebec, 1976. Proceedings, Volume 1, 1976. p. 217-228 ⟨II-00437⟩

Morrell, C.A.: Government Control of Food and Drugs. Canadian Pharmacy Journal 90:342-344, 1957 ⟨II-00438⟩

Pugsley, L.I.: The Administration and Development of Federal Statutes on Foods and Drugs in Canada. Medical Services Journal, Canada 23:387-449, 1967 ⟨II-03817⟩

1919-1945
British Columbia

Richmond, G.: Prison Doctor. Surrey, Nunaga Publishing, 1975. 186 p. ⟨II-04223⟩

Saskatchewan

Acker, M.S.: The Saskatchewan Story: A Review and Prospect. Part I: Saskatchewan's Health Services In Perspective. Journal of Public Health 53:717-20, 1967 ⟨II-04037⟩

Sigerist, H.E.: Saskatchewan Health Services Survey Commission. In: Roemer, M.I. (edit). Henry E. Sigerist on the Sociology of Medicine. New York, M.D. Publications, Inc. pp 209-228. ⟨II-00435⟩

1946-1979
Saskatchewan

Badgley, R.F.: The Public and Medical Care in Saskatchewan. Journal of Public Health 53:720-724, 1963 ⟨II-04043⟩

Badgley, R.F., Wolfe, S.: Doctors' Strike (Medical Care and Conflict in Saskatchewan). Toronto, Macmillan of Canada Ltd., 1967. 201 p. ⟨II-00431⟩

MacTaggart, K.: The First Decade. Ottawa, Canadian Medical Association, 1973. 132 p. ⟨II-00432⟩

Tollefson, E.A.: Bitter Medicine. The Saskatchewan Medicare Feud. Saskatoon, Modern Press. 236 p. ⟨II-00433⟩

All embracing
Canada

Lynch, M.J., Raphael, S.S.: Medicine and the State. Illinois, Charles C. Thomas, Publisher, 1963. 449 p. ⟨II-00430⟩

Statistics and Demography
1500-1699
Canada

Goudreault, L.: Naissance de la Statistique Alieniste au Canada Jusqu'en 1867. In International Congress for the History of Medicine, 25th Quebec, 1976. Proceedings, Volume 11, 1976. p. 706-726 ⟨II-00429⟩

Ontario

Dickinson, J.A.: The Pre-contact Huron Population. A Reappraisal. Ontario History 72:173-179, 1980 ⟨II-01800⟩

Starna, W.A.: Mohawk Iroquois Populations: A Revision. Ethnohistory 27:371-382, 1980 ⟨II-05363⟩

Quebec

Desjardins, B, Beauchamp, P, Legare, J: Automatic Family Reconstitution: the French-Canadian Seventeenth- Century Experience. Journal of Family History 2:56-76, 1977 ⟨II-04790⟩

1700-1759
Quebec

Henripin, J.: From Acceptance of Nature to Control: The Demography of the French Canadians Since the Seventeenth Century. Canadian Journal of Economics and Political Science 23(1):10-19, 1957 ⟨II-02984⟩

1760-1815
Canada

Crosby, A.W.: Virgin Soil Epidemics as a Factor in the Aboriginal Depopulation in America. William and Mary Quarterly 33:289-299, 1976 ⟨II-03263⟩

Quebec

Landry, Y.: Mortalite, nuptialite et canadianisation des troupes francaises de la guerre de Sept Ans. Histoire Social/Social History 12:299-315, 1979 ⟨II-04663⟩

1816-1867
Canada

Gee, E.M.T.: Early Canadian Fertility Transition: a Components Analysis of Census Data. Canadian Studies in Population 6:23-32, 1979 ⟨II-04812⟩

British Columbia

Marshall, J.T.: A Century of Population Growth in British Columbia. Canadian Journal of Public Health 50:64-70, 1959 ⟨II-03770⟩

1868-1918
Ontario

Emery, G.: Ontario's Civil Registration of Vital Statistics, 1869-1926: The Evolution of an Administrative System. Canadian Historical Review 64:468-493, 1983 ⟨II-05416⟩

McKinnon, N.E.: Mortality Reductions in Ontario, 1900-1942. Canadian Journal of Public Health 35:481-4, 1944 ⟨II-04456⟩

McKinnon, N.E.: Mortality Reductions in Ontario 1900-1942 III. The Age Groups of 50 and Over. Canadian Journal of Public Health 36:368-73, 1945 ⟨II-04452⟩

McKinnon, N.E.: Mortality Reductions in Ontario, 1900-1942 II. Canadian Journal of Public Health 36:285-298, 1945 ⟨II-04453⟩

Quebec

Philippe, P., Gomila, J.: Inbreeding Effects in a French Canadian Isolate. Evolution of Inbreeding. Zeitschrift Fur Morphologie und Anthropologie 64:54-9, 1972 〈II-05333〉

1946-1979
Quebec

Wilkins, R.: L'Inegalite Sociale face a la Mortalite a Montreal, 1975-1977. Cahiers quebecois de demographie 9:157-184, 1980 〈II-04946〉

All embracing
Canada

Martin, C.: The European Impact on the Culture of a Northeastern Algonquian Tribe: an ecological interpretation. William and Mary Quarterly 31:3-26, 1974 〈II-03259〉

Surgery

1500-1699
Canada

Macbeth, R.A.: Canadian Surgery During the French Regime, 1608 to 1763. Canadian Journal of Surgery 20:71-82, 1977 〈II-04332〉

Mitchell, R.: Early northern surgeons. The Beaver 284(4):22-24, 1954 〈II-03309〉

Quebec

Caron, W.M.: The Early Surgeons of Quebec. Canadian Journal of Surgery 8:239-253, 1965 〈II-04302〉

Desjardins, E.: Les Origines de la Chirurgie au Canada. L'UMC 94:1445-1448, 1965 〈II-00340〉

Massicotte, E.Z.: Les Chirurgiens de Montreal au XVIIe Siecle. L'UMC 46:310-315, 1917 〈II-02435〉

Panneton, P.: Comment le premier Chirurgien a pratiquer en Quebec faillit contracter une maladie cordiere et definitive. L'UMC 76:41-45, 1947 〈II-02434〉

1700-1759
Quebec

Gaumond, E.: Une Operation Chirurgicale a l'Hotel-Dieu de Quebec en 1700. Canadian Journal of Surgery 2:323-328, 1959 〈II-04699〉

1760-1815
Ontario

Gordon, S.D.: Contributions of Surgeons to the Development of Upper Canada. Bulletin of the Medical Library Association 48:33-36, 1960 〈II-00428〉

Quebec

Blanchet, J., Fremont, C.J.: L'evolution de la chirurgie au Quebec. L'UMC 106(3):358-3, 1977 〈II-05236〉

Desjardins, E.: l'evolution de la chirurgie a Montreal: II. L'UMC 105(10)1564, 1566, 1568, 1976 〈II-05232〉

1816-1867
Quebec

Desjardins, E.: L'evolution de la chirurgie a Montreal (1843-1949). L'UMC 105:1398-410, 1976 〈II-05286〉

Desjardins, E.: L'Evolution de la chirurgie au Quebec. L'UMC 106:1198-211, 1977 〈II-05247〉

Elliott, J.M.: The Early English Surgeons of Quebec. Laval Medical 30:78-84, 1960 〈II-04062〉

1868-1918
Canada

Connor, J.T.H.: Joseph Lister's System of Wound Management and the Canadian Medical Practitioner, 1867-1900. Thesis (M.A.), London, University of Western Ontario, 1980. 177 p. 〈II-05415〉

Alberta

Campbell, P.M.: Frank Hamilton Mewburn. CACHB 15(4):61-69, 1951 〈II-00422〉

Macbeth, R.A.: Alexander Russell Munroe: 1879-1965. Canadian Journal of Surgery 10:3-10, 1967 〈II-03279〉

Rawlinson, H.E.: Frank Hamilton Mewburn, OBE, MD, CM, LLD, LT.-Col., CAMC, Professor of Surgery, University of Alberta, Pioneer Surgeon. Canadian Journal of Surgery 2:1-5, 1958 〈II-03632〉

British Columbia

Jamieson, J.E.: Okanagan's First Amputation. Okanagan Historical Society Annual Report 36:139-140, 1972 〈II-05115〉

Manitoba

Elkin, SJ: Hospital Practice in the Early Nineties. Manitoba Medical Review 46:466-67, 1966 〈II-04063〉

Ferguson, C.C.: One Hundred Years of Surgery 1883-1983. Winnipeg, Peguis Publishers Limited, 1983. 〈II-05097〉

Mitchell, R.: Manitoba Surgical Pioneers James Kerr (1849-1911) and H.H. Chown (1859-1944). Canadian Journal of Surgery 3:281-285, 1960 〈II-03715〉

Nova Scotia

Scammell, H.L.: John Stewart. Canadian Journal of Surgery 4:263-267, 1960-61 〈II-04309〉

Ontario

Bruce, H.A.: Varied Operations. Toronto, Longmans, Green and Co., 1958. 366 p. 〈II-00421〉

Gallie, W.E.: George Armstrong Peters: (As I remember him). Canadian Journal of Surgery 2:119-122, 1959 〈II-02682〉

Groves, A.: All in a day's work. (Leaves from a doctor's case-book). Toronto, Macmillan Co. of Canada Ltd., 1934. 181 p. 〈II-00423〉

Harris, C.W.: Abraham Groves of Fergus: The First Elective Appendectomy?. Canadian Journal of Surgery 4:405-410, 1961 〈II-00424〉

Janes, R.M.: Dr. Clarence Leslie Starr. Canadian Journal of Surgery 3:109-111, 1959-60 〈II-04307〉

Olmsted, A.I.: Ingersoll Olmsted (1864-1937). Canadian Journal of Surgery 3:1-4, 1959-60 〈II-04305〉

Stanley, G.D.: Dr. Abraham Groves 1847-1935: A Great Crusader of Canadian Medicine. CACHB 13(1):4-10, 1948 〈II-00426〉

Quebec

Blackader, A.D.: Dr. Francis J. Shepherd. CMAJ 20:210-211, 1929 ⟨II-01943⟩

Desjardins, E.: B.G. Bourgeois (1877-1943). Canadian Journal of Surgery 9:1-5, 1966 ⟨II-04297⟩

Desjardins, E.: L'Ecole D'Amedee Marien Et Ses Eleves Rheaume Et Pare. Canadian Journal of Surgery 9:325-331, 1966 ⟨II-04702⟩

Desjardins, E.: Trois etapes de la chirurgie: 1872, 1972 et 2002. L'UMC 101:2337-46, 1972 ⟨II-05340⟩

MacDermot, H.E.: Francis J. Shepherd, M.D. LL.D. (Harvard, Mcgill, Queen's), Hon. F.R.C.S. Eng., Hon. F.A.C.S. Canadian Journal of Surgery 1:5-7, 1957-8 ⟨II-04312⟩

MacDermot, H.E.: History of Canadian Surgery: George Edgeworth Fenwick (1825-1894). Canadian Journal of Surgery 11:1-4, 1968 ⟨II-02920⟩

Penfield, W.: Edward Archibald: 1872-1945. CMAJ I:167-174, 1958 ⟨II-01785⟩

1919-1945

Manitoba

Fahrni, G.S.: Prairie Surgeon. Winnipeg, Queenston House Publishing, Inc., 1976. 138 p. ⟨II-00413⟩

Nova Scotia

Morton, C.S.: John George MacDougall, MD, CM(McGill), FACS, FRCS(C). Nova Scotia Medical Bulletin 29:185-194, 1950 ⟨II-03293⟩

Ontario

Jones, W.A.: Lorimer John Austin, MA, MB, M.Ch, FRCS(C), FACS, 1880-1945. Canadian Journal of Surgery 5:1-5, 1962 ⟨II-03948⟩

Kelly, A.D.: Dr. Ernest Clifford Janes, an appreciation. CMAJ 95:1163-1164, 1966 ⟨II-02648⟩

Murray, G.: Medicine in the Making. Toronto, Ryerson Press, 1960. 235 p. ⟨II-00415⟩

Murray, G.: Quest in Medicine. Toronto, Ryerson Press, 1963. 185 p. ⟨II-00416⟩

Quebec

Allan, T.: The Scalpel, The Sword. (The Story of Dr. Norman Bethune). Boston, Little, Brown and Co., 1952. 336 p. ⟨II-00411⟩

All embracing

British Columbia

Wride, R.J.: 'Surgery in British Columbia'. American Surgeon 38:471-6, 1972 ⟨II-05425⟩

Newfoundland

Thomas, G.W.: Surgery in the Sub-Arctic: A Thoracic Surgeon's Odyssey. Journal of Thoracic and Cardiovascular Surgery 70:203-13, 1975 ⟨II-05324⟩

Quebec

Desjardins, E., Lapointe-Manseau, L.: Les chirurgiens de Ville-Marie. L'UMC 102:1934-42, 1973 ⟨II-05389⟩

Symbolism and Heraldry
1816-1867

Quebec

Hanaway, J: The Coats-of-Arms of McGill University and the Faculty of Medicine. McGill Medical Journal 29:78-87, 1960 ⟨II-04165⟩

1946-1979

Canada

Kelly, A.D.: The Mace [Canadian Medical Association]. CMAJ 96:1540-41, 1967 ⟨II-03974⟩

Therapeutic Cults excluding Homeopathy
1946-1979

Ontario

Lee, H.K.: Honoring the Founder in His Country: Conception and Struggle for Canada's Memorial College. Chiropractic History 1:43-46, 1981 ⟨II-04888⟩

Therapeutics
1760-1815

Ontario

Gibson, T.: News notes illustrative of the practice of medicine in Upper Canada, in the early years of the nineteenth century. CMAJ 22:699-700, 1930 ⟨II-03110⟩

1868-1918

Manitoba

Mitchell, R.: Acorus Calamus. The Beaver 298(4):24-26, 1968 ⟨II-03313⟩

Quebec

Hundahl, S.: Acupuncture and Osler. JAMA 240:737, 1978 ⟨II-05253⟩

Thibault, M.: Histoire de la Radiotherapie a l'hotel de Quebec. Vie Medicale au Canada Francais 2:955-6, 1973 ⟨II-05434⟩

1919-1945

Other

Evans, EH: Thoughts on Therapy after Twenty-Five Years in General Practice. Applied Therapeutics, 725-726, 730-734, 1961 ⟨II-04058⟩

All embracing

Canada

Heizer, R.T.: The Use of the Enema Among the Aboriginal American Indians. Ciba Symposia 5:1686-1693, 1944 ⟨II-04153⟩

Transport of Sick and Wounded
1868-1918

Other

Noyes, F.W.: Stretcher-Bearers...at the Double. Toronto, The Hunter-Rose Company, Limited (printers), 311 p. ⟨II-00408⟩

1946-1979
Saskatchewan

Roemer, M.I.: The Saskatchewan Air Ambulance Service: Medical and Public Health Aspects. CMAJ 75:529-533, 1956 ⟨II-00407⟩

Travel and Exploration
1500-1699
Canada

Desjardins, E.: Les Observations Medicales de Jacques Cartier et de Samuel de Champlain. L'UMC 99:677-681, 1970 ⟨II-02459⟩

Little, S.W.: Physicians to the Company of Adventurers. CAMSI Journal 17:7, 9-10,13-14, 1958 (Apr) ⟨II-00405⟩

Lonjias, H.T.: Physicians as Explorers in the New World. Ciba Symposia 2:643-652, 1940 ⟨II-03955⟩

Poynter, F.N.L.(edit): The Journal of James Yonge (1647-1721). Hamden, Connecticut, Archon Books, 1963 ⟨II-02905⟩

1760-1815
Canada

Stewart, D.A.: Sir John Richardson: Surgeon, Physician, Sailor, Explorer, Naturalist, Scholar. CMAJ 24:292-297, 1931 ⟨II-00351⟩

Manitoba

Stewart, D.A.: An Obstetrician-Adventurer to the Hudson's Bay in 1812 -- Dr. Thomas McKeevor. CMAJ 18:738-740, 1928 ⟨II-01806⟩

1816-1867
Canada

Ballon, H.C.: Sir James Hector, MD 1834-1907. CMAJ 87:66-74, 1962 ⟨II-02607⟩

Fortune, R.: Doctors Afield: John Rae, Surgeon to the Hudson's Bay Company. New England Journal of Medicine 268:37-39, 1963 ⟨II-01786⟩

Hamilton, Z.W.: Admiralty Documents concerning Dr. John Rae. CACHB 9(1):32-35, 1944 ⟨II-00394⟩

Johnson, G.R.: Sir John Richardson (1787-1865). CACHB 7(1):1-10, 1942 ⟨II-00395⟩

Mitchell, R.: Physician, fur trader and explorer. The Beaver 267(2):16-20 ⟨II-03299⟩

Mitchell, R.: Dr. John Rae, Arctic Explorer, and his search for Franklin. CMAJ 28:85-90, 1933 ⟨II-03092⟩

Mitchell, R.: Sir James Hector. CMAJ 66:497-499, 1952 ⟨II-02608⟩

Richards, R.L.: Rae of the Arctic. Medical History 19(2):176-193, 1975 ⟨II-00400⟩

Smith, W.G.: Immigration, Past and Future. Canadian Journal of Mental Hygiene, 1:47-57,130-140, 1919-20. ⟨II-04799⟩

Swinton, W.E.: Physicians as Explorers: Richard King: Arugmentative Cassandra in the Search for Franklin. CMAJ 117:1330,1333,1336,1341, 1977 ⟨II-02671⟩

Swinton, W.E.: Physicians as Explorers: Robert McCormich: Travels by Open Boat in Arctic Canada. CMAJ 117:1205-1208, 1977 ⟨II-03266⟩

Swinton, W.E.: Sir John Richardson: Immense journeys in Rupert's Land. CMAJ 117:1095-1100, 1977 ⟨II-04478⟩

Alberta

Stanley, G.D.: Medical Pioneers in Alberta. Alberta Medical Bulletin 19:40-43, 1954 ⟨II-03844⟩

British Columbia

Harvey, A.G.: Meredith Gairdner: Doctor of Medicine. British Columbia Historical Quarterly 9:89-111, 1945 ⟨II-02938⟩

Smith, D.B. (Edit.): The Reminiscences of Doctor John Sebastian Helmcken. British Columbia, University of British Columbia Press, 1975. 373 p. ⟨II-00401⟩

North West Territories

Donaldson, B.: Rae's wintering home. CACHB 20(4):95-99, 1956 ⟨II-00393⟩

United States

Thorington, J.M.: Four Physicians-Explorers of the Fur Trade Days. Annals of Medical History, ser. 3, 4:294-301, 1942 ⟨II-04910⟩

1868-1918
Canada

Millman, T.: Impressions of the West in the Early 'Seventies, from the Diary of the Assistant Surgeon of the B.N.A. Boundary Survey,. Women's Canadian Historical Society of Toronto 26: 15-56, 1927-1928 ⟨II-04627⟩

Alberta

Dempsey, H.A. (Editor): A winter at Fort MacLeod (R.B. Nevitt). Alberta, Glenbow-Alberta Institute, 1974. 134 p. ⟨II-00390⟩

1919-1945
North West Territories

Copland, D: Livingstone of the Arctic. Ottawa, D. Copland, 1967. 183 p. ⟨II-04119⟩

Tropical Medicine
1919-1945
Other

McK, N.: Alexander Francis Mahaffy, CMG, BA, MB, DPH; an appreciation. CMAJ 88:906-907, 1963 ⟨II-03624⟩

Urology
1919-1945
Ontario

Willinsky, A.I.: A Doctor's Memoirs. Toronto, Macmillan Co. of Canada Ltd., 1960. 183 p. ⟨II-00389⟩

Veterinary Medicine
1816-1867
New Brunswick

Barker, C.A.V.: M.A. Cuming, v.s. (Edin.), M.R.C.V.S.: A Biography and the Inducement to Settle in New Brunswick in 1852. The Canadian Veterinary Journal 17:123-135, 1976 ⟨II-05384⟩

Ontario

Barker, C.A.V.: The Ontario Veterinary College: Temperance Street Era. The Canadian Veterinary Journal 16:319-328, 1975 ⟨II-05383⟩

1868-1918
Canada

Saunders, L.Z.: Some Pioneers in Comparative Medicine. Canadian Veterinary Journal 14:27-35, 1973 ⟨II-00388⟩

Ontario

Barker, C.A.V.: John G. Rutherford and the Controversial Standards of Education at the Ontario Veterinary College from 1864 to 1920. The Canadian Veterinary Journal 18:327-340, 1977 ⟨II-05385⟩

Evans, A.M., Barker, C.A.V.: Century One: A History of the Ontario Veterinary Association 1874-1974. Guelph, A.M. Evans, C.A.V. Barker, 1976. 516 p. ⟨II-05386⟩

Quebec

Murphy, D.A.: Osler, Now a Veterinarian!. CMAJ 83:32-35, 1960 ⟨II-02331⟩

War
1868-1918
Nova Scotia

Metson, G.: The Halifax explosion, December 6, 1917. Toronto/Montreal/New York, McGraw-Hill Ryerson Limited, 1978. 173 p. ⟨II-00386⟩

Other

Nasmith, G.G.: On the Fringe of the Great Fight. Toronto, McClelland, Goodchild and Stewart, 1917. 263 p. ⟨II-01543⟩

Ryerson, G.S.: Looking backward. Toronto, The Ryerson Press, 1924. 264 p. ⟨II-00387⟩

1919-1945
Other

Russell, R.: The Spanish Civil War: Reminiscences of a Veteran of the Mackenzie- Papineau Battalion. In: Shephard, D.A.E. Levesque, A.(edit): Norman Bethune: His Times and His Legacy. Ottawa, Canadian Public Health Association, 1982. pp 170-76 ⟨II-04921⟩

All embracing
Canada

Nadeau, G.: Indian Scalping: Technique in Different Tribes. BHM 10:178-194, 1941 ⟨II-00385⟩

Women in Medicine
1500-1699
Canada

Douglas, J.: The Status of Women in New England and New France. Queen's Quarterly 19:359-374, 1911-12 ⟨II-02337⟩

1816-1867
Canada

Hacker, C.: The Indomitable Lady Doctors. Toronto, Clarke, Irwin and Co. Ltd., 1974. 259 p. ⟨II-00384⟩

Roberts, W.: Six New Women: A Guide to the Mental Map of Women Reformers in Toronto. Atlantis 3:145-164, 1977-8 ⟨II-02065⟩

1868-1918
Canada

Buckley, S.: Ladies or Midwives? Efforts to Reduce Infant and Maternal Mortality. In: Kealey, L.(edit): A Not Unreasonable Claim. Toronto, The Women's Press, 1979. pp 131-149 ⟨II-03151⟩

Kelly, K: Medicine...The Distaff Side. Canadian Doctor, May 1961. pp 24-39 ⟨II-03961⟩

Lovejoy, E.P.: Canada. In: Women Doctors of the World. New York, The MacMillan Company, 1957. pp 111-118 ⟨II-05014⟩

Percival, E.: Women in Medicine. CMAJ 23:436-438, 1930 ⟨II-03146⟩

Alberta

Buck, R.M.: The Doctor Rode Side-Saddle. McClelland and Steward Ltd., 1974, 175 p. ⟨II-04467⟩

Manitoba

Douglass, M.E.: A Pioneer Woman Doctor of Western Canada (C. Ross). Mantoba Medical Review 27:255-256, 1947 ⟨II-02673⟩

Thomas, L.B.: Some Manitoba Women who did First Things. Historical and Scientific Society of Manitoba. Papers. Series 3, No. 4:13-25, 1947-8 ⟨II-02107⟩

Nova Scotia

N., R.: Dr. Jane L. Heartz Bell. CMAJ 90:946, 1964 ⟨II-02077⟩

Nichols, R.B.: Early Women Doctors of Nova Scotia. Nova Scotia Medical Bulletin 29:14-21, 1950 ⟨II-03826⟩

Ontario

Godfrey, C.M.: The Origins of Medical Education of Women in Ontario. Medical History 17:89-94, 1973 ⟨II-00379⟩

Ray, J.: Emily Stowe. Fitzhenry and Whiteside Ltd., 1978. 63 p. ⟨II-03641⟩

Squair, J.: Admission of Women to the University of Toronto. Part 1. University of Toronto Monthly 24:209-212, 1924 ⟨II-03640⟩

Strong-Boag, V.: Canada's Women Doctors: Feminism Constrained. In: Kealy, L. (edit.): A Not Unreasonable Claim. Toronto, The Women's Press, 1979. pp 109-129 ⟨II-03150⟩

Strong-Boag, V. (edit.): A Woman with a Purpose: The Diaries of Elizabeth Smith 1872-1884. Toronto/Buffalo/London, University of Toronto Press, 1980. 298 pp ⟨II-02689⟩

Thompson, J.E.: The Influence of Dr. Emily Howard Stowe on the Woman Suffrage Movement in Canada. Ontario History 54:253-266, 1962 ⟨II-01819⟩

Quebec

Scriver, J.B.: McGill's First Women Medical Students. McGill Medical Journal 16:237-43, 1947 ⟨II-02327⟩

Saskatchewan

Buck, R.M.: The Mathesons of Saskatchewan Diocese. Saskatchewan History 13:41-62, 1960 ⟨II-03846⟩

United States

Angel, B., Angel, M.: Charlotte Whitehead Ross. Winnipeg, Pegius Publishers Limited, 1982. ⟨II-05076⟩

1919-1945

Canada

Archer, C.: Woman takes man's job. Canadian Doctor 47 (1): 55-6, 1981 ⟨II-04214⟩

Ontario

McConnachie, K.: Methodology in the Study of Women in History: a Case study of Helen MacMurchy, M.D. Ontario History 75-61-70, 1983 ⟨II-05095⟩

Robinson, M.O.: Give My Heart; the Dr. Marion Hilliard Story. New York, Doubleday and Co., Inc., 1964. 348 p. ⟨II-01843⟩

AUTHOR LISTING

A

A., F.M.: Dr. William Oliver Rose. CMAJ 34:595-596, 1936 ⟨I-03449⟩

A., G.H.: Canada's First Hospital Celebrates its Tercentenary 300th Anniversary at Hotel Dieu, Quebec. Canadian Hospital 16:9-11, 1939 ⟨II-04041⟩

Abbey, N.D.: Personalities in Western Canadian Medicine. University of Toronto Medical Journal 29:177-180, 1952 ⟨II-04040⟩

Abbott, M.E.: An Historical Sketch of the Medical Faculty of McGill University. Montreal Medical Journal 31:561-672, 1902 ⟨II-04213⟩

Abbott, M.E.: McGill's Heroic Past 1821-1921. Montreal, McGill University, 1921. 30 p. ⟨II-04120⟩

Abbott, M.E.: Mr. E.Z. Massicotte on the Physicians and Surgeons of the XVIIth and XVIIIth Centuries in the District of Montreal. CMAJ 13:197-199, 1923 ⟨II-02959⟩

Abbott, M.E.: Sir William Osler Memorial Volume. Montreal, International Association of Medical Museums, Bull No. IX, 1926. 634 p. ⟨I-01250⟩

Abbott, M.E.: An early Canadian biologist -- Michel Sarrazin (1659-1735) his life and times. CMAJ 19:600-607, 1928 ⟨I-01982⟩

Abbott, M.E.: An Early Canadian Biologist -- Michel Sarrazin (1659-1735) His Life and Times. CMAJ 19:600-607, 1928 ⟨II-02064⟩

Abbott, M.E.: Andrew Fernando Holmes (1797-1860). In Kelly HW, Burrage WL: Dictionary of American Medical Biography. New York and London, D. Appleton and Co., 1928. pp. 581-582. ⟨I-01360⟩

Abbott, M.E.: History of Medicine in the Province of Quebec. Toronto, Macmillan Co. of Canada Ltd., 1931. 97 p. ⟨II-00848⟩

Abbott, M.E.: Historic Montreal: Metropolis of Canada and Mother of the Cities of the West. Annals of Internal Medicine 6:815-838, 1932 ⟨II-04039⟩

Abbott, M.E.: The Faculty of Medicine of McGill University. Surgery, Gynecology and Obstetrics 60:242-253, 1935 ⟨II-04038⟩

Abbott, M.E.: The Osler Pathological Collection in the Medical Historical Museum of McGill University. Journal of Technical Methods and Bulletin of the International Association of Medical Museums 14:21-27, 1935 ⟨II-02325⟩

Abbott, M.E.: More about Osler. Bulletin of the Institute of the History of Medicine 5:765-796, 1937 ⟨I-02534⟩

Abbott, M.E. (Edit.): Classified And Annotated Bibliography of Sir William Osler's Publications. Montreal, Medical Museum, McGill University, 1939. 163 p. ⟨I-01256⟩

Abelmann, W.H.: In Memoriam -- Elors Bajusz 1926-1973. Recent Advances in Studies in Cardiac Structure and Metabolism 6:5-20, 1975 ⟨I-05381⟩

Abler, T.S.: Iroquois Cannibalism: Fact not Fiction. Ethnohistory 27:309-316, 1980 ⟨II-05364⟩

Acker, M.S.: The Saskatchewan Story: A Review and Prospect. Part I: Saskatchewan's Health Services In Perspective. Journal of Public Health 53:717-20, 1967 ⟨II-04037⟩

Ackerknecht, E.H.: Medicine and Disease Among Eskimos. Ciba Symposia 10:916-921, 1948 ⟨II-00603⟩

Adami, J.G.: An Epizootic of Rabies; and a Personal Experience of M. Pasteur's Treatment. British Medical Journal 2:808-810, 1889 ⟨I-03413⟩

Adami, J.G.: War Story of the Canadian Army Medical Corps, 1914-1915. Vol. 1. The First Contingent. Toronto, Musson Book Co., Ltd., 1918. 286 p. ⟨II-00803⟩

Adami, M.: J. George Adami: A Memoir. London, Constable and Co., Ltd., 1930. 179 p. ⟨I-00028⟩

Adamson, G: Reminiscences. Winnipeg Clinic Quarterly 23:101-103, 1970 ⟨II-04036⟩

Adamson, J.D.: Dr. A.T. Mathers -- The Retiring Dean. University of Manitoba Medical Journal 21:4-7, 1950 ⟨I-01583⟩

Adamson, J.D.: Pioneer Medicine in Manitoba. Journal-Lancet 70:49-50, 1950 ⟨II-04035⟩

Agnew, G.H.: Canadian Hospitals, 1920 to 1970, a Dramatic Half Century. Toronto, University of Toronto Press, 1974. 276 p. ⟨II-00169⟩

Ahern, M.J.: Quelques Charlatans du Regime Francais Dans la Province de Quebec. Le Bulletin Medical de Quebec 10:345-358, 1908-09 ⟨II-02468⟩

Ahern, M.J., Ahern, G.: Notes Pour servir a l'Histoire de la Medecine dans le Bas-Canada Depuis la fondation de Quebec jusqu'au commencement du XIXe siecle. Quebec, 1923. 563 p. ⟨II-05261⟩

Ahern, M.J., Ahern, G.: Jean Francois Gaultier (1708-1756). In Kelly HW, Burrage WL: Dictionary of American Medical Biography. New York and London, D. Appleton and Co., 1928. pp. 457-458. ⟨I-01396⟩

Aikenhead, D.C.: William Webster, MD, Anesthetist: an appreciation. Anesthesia and Analgesia 16:312-317, 1937 ⟨I-02733⟩

Alderson, H.J.: Twenty-Five Years A-Growing (The History of the School of Nursing, McMaster University). Hamilton, McMaster University, 1976. 333 p. ⟨II-00772⟩

Aldren, B.: Life in Upper Canada in 1837. CMAJ 20:65-67, 1929 ⟨II-00356⟩

Aldwinckle, J.: Oshawa General Hospital "Heart-beat of the Community". Oshawa, Oshawa General Hospital, 1975, 263 p. ⟨II-04606⟩

Alexander, E.: Kenneth George McKenzie, Canada's First Neurosurgeon. Journal of Neurosurgery 41:1-9, 1974 ⟨I-05371⟩

Allaire, M d': L'hopital-general de Quebec 1692-1764. Montreal, Fides [1971]. 251 p. ⟨II-05354⟩

Allan, F.N.: Diabetes Before and After Insulin. Medical History 16:266-73, 1972 ⟨II-05437⟩

Allan, F.N.: The Discovery of Insulin. New England Journal of Medicine 297:283-4, 1977 ⟨II-05241⟩

Allan, T.: The Scalpel, The Sword. (The Story of Dr. Norman Bethune). Boston, Little, Brown and Co., 1952. 336 p. ⟨II-00411⟩

Allard, S.: L'Hotel-Dieu de Montreal: Trois Siecles de Devouement et de Progres. L'UMC 70:1271-1272, 1941 ⟨II-02363⟩

Allodi, F., Kedward, H.B.: The Evolution of the Mental Hospital in Canada. Canadian Journal of Public Health 68:219-24, 1977 ⟨II-05251⟩

Amyot, G.F.: The British Columbia Department of Health and Welfare. Canadian Journal of Public Health 49:503-515, 1958 ⟨II-04034⟩

Amyot, G.F.: Some Historical Highlights of Public Health in Canada. Canadian Journal of Public Health 58:337-341, 1967 ⟨II-04033⟩

Amyot, R.: Donation Marion, 1897-1971. L'UMC 100:1197-1198, 1971 ⟨I-01298⟩

Amyot, R.: Rememoration d'evenements dans le monde medical entre les 75 et 100 anniversaires de l'union medicale du Canada. L'UMC 101:2368-75, 1972 ⟨II-05353⟩

Anderson, A.J.: The Golden Anniversary of the Alberta Pharmaceutical Association, 1911-1961. Edmonton: Alberta Pharmaceutical Association, 1961. ⟨II-05098⟩

Anderson, A.L.: The School of Medical Sciences and the Medical College of the University of Saskatchewan. CACHB 17:1-9, 1952 ⟨II-00265⟩

Anderson, F.J.: Medicine at Fort Detroit in the Colony of New France, 1701-1760. JHMAS 1:208-228, 1946 ⟨II-05127⟩

Anderson, F.W.: Louis Riel's insanity reconsidered. Saskatchewan History 3:104-110, 1950 ⟨II-02624⟩

Anderson, H.B.: John L. Davison, M.D. CMAJ 7:549-551, 1917 ⟨I-01511⟩

Anderson, H.B.: The Medical Profession of Toronto. In: Middleton, J.E.: The Municipality of Toronto: A History. Toronto and New York, Dominion Publishing Co., vol II, 1923. pp 609-628 ⟨II-00865⟩

Anderson, H.B.: George Sterling Ryerson. CMAJ 15:971, 1925 ⟨I-01183⟩

Anderson, H.B.: An Historical Sketch of the Medical Profession of Toronto. CMAJ 16:446-452, 1926 ⟨II-02330⟩

Anderson, H.B.: Medical Licensure and Medical Boards in Upper Canada. CMAJ 18:209-213, 1928 ⟨II-01809⟩

Anderson, H.B.: A Brief History of the Development of the Library and the Academy Since its Inception. Bulletin of the Academy of Medicine, Toronto, May 1932, pp 34-39 ⟨II-00144⟩

Anderson, H.B.: Dr. James Algernon Temple. CMAJ 26:258, 1932 ⟨I-03042⟩

Anderson, H.B.: Frederick William Marlow, MD, CM. CMAJ 35:463, 1936 ⟨I-02869⟩

Anderson, H.B.: History of the Library of the Academy of Medicine, Toronto. Bulletin of the Academy of Medicine, Toronto 20:239-52, 1946 ⟨II-04032⟩

Anderson, J.F.C.: Dr. James George Keber Lindsay. CMAJ 55:416, 1946 ⟨I-03084⟩

Anderson, J.R.: Dr. H.B. Longmore. CMAJ 67:71, 1952 ⟨I-04539⟩

Anderson, W.G.: Dr. Richard Parsons. CMAJ 52:111, 1945 ⟨I-04359⟩

Anderson, W.J.: The Life of F.M., H.R.H. Edward, Duke of Kent. Ottawa/Toronto, Hunter, Rose and Co., 1870. 241 p. ⟨II-00114⟩

Andison, A.W.: Elinor Black. CMAJ 126:869, 1982 ⟨I-04769⟩

Andrews, M.W.: Epidemic and Public Health: Influenza in Vancouver, 1918-1919. B.C. Studies 34:1-24, 1977 ⟨II-04031⟩

Andrews, M.W.: Medical Attendance in Vancouver, 1886-1920. B.C. Studies 40:32-56, 1978-1979 ⟨I-03552⟩

Andrews, M.W.: Medical Services in Vancouver, 1886-1920: A Study in the Interplay of Attitudes, Medical Knowledge, and Administrative Structures. Thesis (Ph.D.), British Columbia, University of British Columbia, 1979. ⟨II-05159⟩

Andrews, M.W.: The Course of Medical Opinion on State Health Insurance in British Columbia, 1919-1939. Social History 16:129-41, 1983 ⟨II-05276⟩

Angel, B., Angel, M.: Charlotte Whitehead Ross. Winnipeg, Pegius Publishers Limited, 1982. ⟨I-05053⟩

Angus, M.S.: Lord Sydenham's one hundred and fifteen days in Kingston. Historic Kingston 15:36-49, 1967 ⟨II-03252⟩

Angus, M.S.: Health, Emigration and Welfare in Kingston, 1820-1840. In: Oliver Mowat's Ontario, edited by D. Swainson, pp. 120-35. Toronto, MacMillan, 1972 ⟨II-05140⟩

Angus, M.S.: Kingston General Hospital: A Social and Institutional History. Montreal/London, McGill-Queen's University Press, 1973. 205 p. ⟨II-00182⟩

Angus, M.S.: James Sampson. DCB 9:699-701, 1976 ⟨I-01113⟩

Angus, M.S.: Harriet (Cartwright) Dobbs. DCB 11:265-66, 1982 ⟨I-04860⟩

Angus, M.S.: Horatio Yates. DCB 11:940-41, 1982 ⟨I-04859⟩

Angus, M.S.: John Robinson Dickson. DCB 11:263-264, 1982 ⟨I-04864⟩

Appleton, V.E.: Psychiatry in Canada a Century Ago. Canadian Psychiatric Association Journal 12(4):345-361, 1967 ⟨II-00601⟩

Archambault, P.-R.: L'Evolution d'un Hopital [l'hopital du Sacre-Couer, Montreal]. L'UMC 89:1076-1079, 1960 ⟨II-04662⟩

Archer, C.: Woman takes man's job. Canadian Doctor 47(1): 55-6, 1981 ⟨II-04214⟩

Archer, C.I.: Cannibalism in the Early History of the Northwest Coast: Enduring Myths and Neglected Realities. CHR 71:453-479, 1980 ⟨II-02943⟩

Archibald, A.: Master Surgeons of America: James Bell. Surgery, Gynecology and Obstetrics 37:93-96, 1923 ⟨I-04288⟩

Archibald, B.O.: December 6th, 1917. Nova Scotia Medical Bulletin 29:303-305, 1950 ⟨II-04030⟩

Archibald, E.: Dr. George Eli Armstrong. CMAJ 29:103-104, 1933 ⟨I-03075⟩

Archibald, E.: Dr. Francis Alexander Carron Scrimger. CMAJ 36:323, 1937 ⟨I-03435⟩

Archibald, F.E.: Salute to Sid: The Story of Dr. Sidney Gilchrist. Windsor, Lancelot Press, 1970. 127 pp. ⟨I-03936⟩

Argue, J.F.: Dr. Robert Henry Wynyard Powell. CMAJ 32:590, 1935 ⟨I-01034⟩

Armour, R.G.: Dr. Henry Seaton Hutchison. CMAJ 30:337, 1934 ⟨I-03537⟩

Armstrong, F.H.: Lucius James O'Brien. DCB 9:606-607, 1976 ⟨I-01263⟩

Arsenault, L.: Les Fondatrices. Revue d'Histoire et de Traditions Populaires de la Gaspesie 14:88-96, 1976 ⟨II-04675⟩

Arvidson, R.M., Nelson, T.M.: Sixty Years of Psychology at the University of Alberta. Canadian Psychologist 9:500-4, 1968 ⟨II-05459⟩

Atherton, A.B.: William Bayard (1814-1907). In Kelly HW, Burrage WL: Dictionary of American Medical Biography. New York and London, D. Appleton and Co., 1928. pp. 76-77 ⟨I-00980⟩

Atherton, W.H.: The Saintly Life of Jeanne Mance: first Lay Nurse in North America. Hospital Progress 26:182-190, 192-201, 234-243, 1945 ⟨I-03427⟩

A[tlee], H.B.: Harry Goudge Grant. Nova Scotia Medical Bulletin 33:168-170, 1954 ⟨I-02157⟩

Atlee, H.B.: Dalhousie Medical School 1907-1957. Dalhousie Medical Journal 11(1):21-33, 1958 ⟨II-00266⟩

Atwater, E.C.: The protracted labor and brief life of a country medical school: the Auburn Medical Institution, 1825. JHMAS 34:334-352,1979 ⟨I-01202⟩

Audet, L.-P.: Index Analytique du Memorial de l'Education dans le Bas-Canada du Dr. Jean-Baptiste Meilleur. PTRSC. Series 4, 2:49-62, 1964 ⟨I-04949⟩

Audet, L.-P.: Jean-Baptiste Meilleur etait-il un candidat valable au poste de Surintendant de l'Education pour les Bas-Canada en 1842?. Cahier Des Dix 31:163-201, 1966 ⟨I-04656⟩

Audet, L.-P.: Hector Peltier. DCB 10:588-589, 1972 ⟨I-01239⟩

Audet, L.-P.: Louis Giard. DCB 11:345-46. 1982 ⟨I-04845⟩

Austin, L.J.: My Experiences as a German Prisoner. London: Andrew Melrose Ltd., 1915, 158 p. ⟨II-04458⟩

B

B., A.A.: Dr. Atholl Munro McNabb: an appreciation. CMAJ 86:1042-1043, 1962 ⟨I-02543⟩

B., B.: Hans Selye. CMAJ 123:316, 1980 ⟨I-02853⟩

B., B.: John Wendell MacLeod. CMAJ 123:557, 1980 ⟨I-01584⟩

B., H.E.: Hospital for the Insane, London, Ontario. Canadian Journal of Medicine and Surgery 4:44-48, 1898 ⟨II-04029⟩

B., H.J.: Dr. William Boyd. Bulletin Academy of Medicine, Toronto 52(8):110-115, 1979 ⟨I-00937⟩

B, J.N.E.: Dr. Nelson Beemer. Canadian Journal of Medicine and Surgery 76:133-135, 1934 ⟨I-03887⟩

B., J.W.: Dr. John Angus Davies. CMAJ 90:1479, 1964 ⟨I-05229⟩

Badgley, R.F.: The Public and Medical Care in Saskatchewan. Journal of Public Health 53:720-724, 1963 ⟨II-04043⟩

Badgley, R.F., Wolfe, S.: Doctors' Strike (Medical Care and Conflict in Saskatchewan). Toronto, Macmillan of Canada Ltd., 1967. 201 p. ⟨II-00431⟩

Badgley, R.F., Wolfe, S: The Doctors' Right to Strike. In: Torrey, E.F. (edit): Ethical Issues in Medicine: The Role of Physician in Today's Society. Boston, Little, Brown and Company, 1968 pp 301-321 ⟨II-04028⟩

Baehre, R.: From Pauper Lunatics to Bucke: Studies in the Management of Lunacy in 19th Century Ontario. Thesis (Ph.M.), Waterloo, University of Waterloo, 1976, unpublished. ⟨II-05033⟩

Baehre, R.: Paupers and Poor Relief in Upper Canada. Historical Papers, 1981. pages 57-80 ⟨II-04814⟩

Bagnall, J.S.: Dental Education in Canada. Journal of the Canadian Dental Association 18:310-314, 1952 ⟨II-05204⟩

Bailey, A.A.: Dr. Donald C. Balfour, an appreciation. CMAJ 89:831-382, 1963 ⟨I-03903⟩

Bailey, A.A.: Dr. Jessie A. McGeachy. CMAJ 94:923, 1966 ⟨I-03210⟩

Bailey, A.G.: Disease and Treatment. In: The Conflict of European and Eastern Algonkian Cultures 1504-1700. Toronto/Buffalo, University of Toronto Press, 1969. pp 76-83 ⟨II-05365⟩

Bailey, T.M.: For the Public Good. Hamilton, The Planned Parenthood Society of Hamilton, 1974 37 p. ⟨II-05000⟩

Bain, I.: The Development of Family Planning in Canada. Canadian Journal of Public Health 55:334-340, 1964 ⟨II-04796⟩

Baird, G: 999 Queen: A Collective Failure of Imagination. City Magazine [Toronto 2(3and4):34-59, 1976 ⟨II-03952⟩

Baker, J.: Tributes from the United States [W.C. MacKenzie]. Canadian Journal of Surgery 22,307-308, 1979 ⟨I-04287⟩

Baker, J.O.: A Medical Man from Glengarry and Stormont -- Part I History. CACHB 18(1):7-16, 1953 ⟨II-00484⟩

Baker, J.O.: A Medical Man from Glengarry and Stormont -- Part II Reflections. CACHB 18(2):1-12, 1953 ⟨II-00485⟩

Baker, M.: Thomas Howley. DCB 11:429-30, 1982 ⟨I-04847⟩

Baker, M.: The Development of the Office of a Permanent Medical Health Officer for St. John's, Newfoundland, 1826-1905. HSTC Bulletin 7:98-105, 1983 ⟨II-05189⟩

Baldwin, R.M., Baldwin, J.: The Baldwins and The Great Experiment. Longmans, 1969, 269 p. ⟨I-04516⟩

Ball, N., Desson, K.: The Pump-house Parthenon. Canadian Heritage, pp 16-21, Dec 1983-Jan 1984 ⟨II-05356⟩

Ballon, H.C.: Aaron Hart David, M.D. (1812-1882). CMAJ 86:115-122, 1962 ⟨I-01574⟩

Ballon, H.C.: Sir James Hector, M.D. 1834-1907. CMAJ 87:66-74, 1962 ⟨I-02484⟩

Ballon, H.C., Ballon, S.C.: Hiram Nahum Vineberg 1857-1945. Canadian Jewish Historical Society Journal 3:1-9, 1979 ⟨I-02865⟩

Baltzen, D.M.: Dr. William Alexander Cluff. CMAJ 44:431-432, 1941 ⟨I-03350⟩

Banfill, B.J.: With the Indians of the Pacific. Toronto, The Ryerson Press, 1966, 176 p. ⟨II-04624⟩

Banks, P.J.: Medical History of British Columbia: Some Aspects. British Columbia Medical Journal 3:399-401, 1973 ⟨II-00859⟩

Banting, F.G.: Diabetes and Insulin. Stockholm, P.A. Norstedt and Fils, 1925. pp 1-20 ⟨II-00099⟩

Banting, F.G.: The History of Insulin. Edinburgh Medical Journal 36:1-18, 1929 ⟨II-00098⟩

Barbeau, M.: Medicine-men on the North Pacific Coast. National Museum of Canada Bulletin 152:1-95, 1973. (Anthropological Series 42) ⟨II-00604⟩

Barclay, R.G.: Grey Nuns Voyage to Red River. The Beaver 297(3):15-23, 1966 ⟨II-03314⟩

Bardeen, C.R.: John Bruce MacCallum (1876-1906). In Kelly HW, Burrage WL: Dictionary of American Medical Biography. New York and London, D. Appleton and Co., 1928. pp. 769-770 ⟨I-01434⟩

Baril, G., Boucher, R.: Resultats de Quelques Recherches Bibliographiques: Sur la Tuberculose des Indiens du Canada avant la Penetrasion Europeenne. L'UMC 55:519-521, 1926 ⟨II-02447⟩

Barker, C.A.V.: The Ontario Veterinary College: Temperance Street Era. The Canadian Veterinary Journal 16:319-328, 1975 ⟨II-05383⟩

Barker, C.A.V.: M.A. Cuming, vs. (Edin.), M.R.C.V.S.: A Biography and the Inducement to Settle in New Brunswick in 1852. The Canadian Veterinary Journal 17:123-135, 1976 ⟨II-05384⟩

Barker, C.A.V.: John G. Rutherford and the Controversial Standards of Education at the Ontario Veterinary College from 1864 to 1920. The Canadian Veterinary Journal 18:327-340, 1977 ⟨II-05385⟩

Barker, L.F.: Dr. Campbell Meyers. CMAJ 17:968, 1927 ⟨II-00583⟩

Barlow, W.L.: Dr. George Eli Armstrong, an appreciation. CMAJ 29:104, 1933 ⟨I-01487⟩

Barootes, E.W.: Dr. Norman Bethune: Inspiration for a Modern China. CMAJ 122:1176-1184, 1980 ⟨I-00953⟩

Barr, J.W.: Medical Council of Canada. II: More About the Origins of the Council. CMAJ 111:267, 1974 ⟨II-05448⟩

Barr, M.L., Rossiter,R.J.: James Bertram Collip 1892-1965. Biographical Memoirs of Fellows of the Royal Society 19:235-267, 1973 ⟨I-02008⟩

Barr, M.L.: James Bertram Collip (1892-1965); A Canadian Pioneer in Endocrinology. In International Congress for the History of Medicine, 25th, Quebec, 1976. Proceedings, volume 11, 1976. p. 469-476 ⟨II-00256⟩

Barr, M.L.: A Century of Medicine at Western. London, Ontario, University of Western Ontario, 1977. 672 p. ⟨II-00267⟩

Barr, M.L.: Archibald Bruce Macallum, 1885-1976. PTRSC series IV, 15:99-100, 1977 ⟨I-03036⟩

Barrett, W.T.: Reminiscences of Early Klondyke Days. University of Manitoba Medical Journal 49:141-146, 1979 ⟨I-01570⟩

Barrt, M.L.: George Herbert Stevenson 1894-1976. PTRSC series 4, 15:114-116, 1977 ⟨I-01646⟩

Barry, J.L., Carr, D.H., Buck, R.C.: Dr. Henry Alan Lawson Skinner. CMAJ 96:1182, 1967 ⟨I-01686⟩

Bastenie, P.A.: L'isolement de l'insuline. Bulletin Academie Royale Medicine Belgique 11:321-8, 1971 ⟨II-05458⟩

Bastin, C.H.: Dr. D.L. Beckingsale. CMAJ 20:571, 1929 ⟨I-03499⟩

Bastin, C.H.: Dr. Duncan Bell-Irving. CMAJ 20:451, 1929 ⟨I-03509⟩

Bastin, C.H.: Dr. Henry Mortimer Cunningham. CMAJ 23:726, 1930 ⟨I-03024⟩

Bastin, C.H.: Dr. Edward Charles Arthur. CMAJ 27:332, 1932 ⟨I-03057⟩

Bates, D.G.: Dr. J.W. Crane -- A Biography. University of Western Ontario Medical Journal 28:125-130, 1958 ⟨I-02016⟩

Bateson, U.E.: Dr. F.R. Eccles. CMAJ 14:764, 1924 ⟨I-02777⟩

Bator, P.A.: Saving Lives on the Wholesale Plan, Public Health Reform in the City of Toronto, 1900-1930. Ph. D. Thesis, University of Toronto, 1979. pp 12-111 ⟨II-03258⟩

Bator, P.A.: The Struggle to Raise the Lower Classes: Public Health Reform and the Problem of Poverty in Toronto, 1910-1921. Journal of Canadian Studies 14:43-49, 1979 ⟨II-05210⟩

Baxter, J.B.M.: Colonel Murray MacLaren. CMAJ 48:180-181, 1943 ⟨I-01751⟩

Bayard, W.: History of the General Public Hospital in the City of Saint John, N.B. Saint John, N.B., s.n. 1896 ⟨II-00183⟩

Bayne, J.R.D.: A Defence of Dr. James Douglas. CMAJ 51:277-278, 1944 ⟨I-04441⟩

Bayne, J.R.D., Nadero, B.: A Defence of Dr. James Douglas. CMAJ 51:277-278, 1944 ⟨II-04472⟩

Bayne, J.R.D.: The Lot of Few Men [Murdo Morrison, the Megantic Outlaw]. CMAJ 66:178-180, 1952 ⟨II-04628⟩

Bazin, A.T.: Francis J. Shepherd. McGill News 36:25, 55, 57-59, 1955 ⟨I-01693⟩

Beach, R.: The Hands of Dr. Locke. New York, Farrar and Rinehart, 1932. 56 p. ⟨I-01304⟩

Beahre, R.: Victorian Psychiatry and Canadian Motherhood. Canadian Women's Studies 2:44-46, 1980 ⟨II-04646⟩

Beamish, R.E.: Dr. Albert Clifford Abbott: Pioneer Surgeon of Western Canada. CMAJ 128:862, 864, 1983 ⟨I-05072⟩

Beamish, R.E.: Dr. Albert Clifford Abbott: Pioneer Experimental Surgeon of Western Canada. University of Manitoba Medical Journal 53:84-88, 1983 ⟨I-05288⟩

Beamish, R.M.: Fifty Years a Canadian Nurse. New York, Vantage Press, 1970 344 p. ⟨II-05012⟩

Beaton-Mamak, M.: The Lonely Legend of Norman Bethune. Dimensions in Health Service 51:14-6, 1974 ⟨I-05372⟩

Beaton-Mamak, M.: The V.O.N. (Victorian Order of Nurses): Caring Since 1898. Dimensions in Health Service 52(3):22-3, 1975 ⟨II-05330⟩

Beatty, J.D.: History of Medical Education in Toronto. University of Toronto Medical Journal 47:152-57, 1970 ⟨II-05158⟩

Beaugrand-Champagne, A: Les Maladies et la Medecine des Anciens Iroquois. Cahier des Dix 9:227-242, 1944 ⟨II-04691⟩

Beaumier-Paquet, M.: Une page memorable do la medecine a Quebec. Quebec, Editions Garneau, 1976. 121 p. ⟨II-04942⟩

Beck, J.M.: George Murray. DCB 11:633, 1982 ⟨I-04854⟩

Becker, A.: Radiological Pioneers in Saskatoon. Saskatchewan History 36:31-37, 1983 ⟨II-05196⟩

Becker, W.J.: Biography: Dr. William Boyd. University of Manitoba Medical Journal 39:41-45, 1967 ⟨I-02057⟩

Bedwell, S.F.: D'Anville's Doom. A Neurological Vignette from Historic Halifax. The Canadian Journal of Neurological Sciences 7:1-8, 1980 ⟨II-00345⟩

Beeuwkes, A.M.: The Prevalence of Scurvy Among Voyageurs to America -- 1493-1600. Journal of American Dietetic Association 24:300-303, 1948 ⟨II-04027⟩

Belanger, H.: Martin Descouts. DCB 3:182, 1974 ⟨I-01014⟩

Belanger, L.F.: Un Ancetre de la Medecine Trifluvienne: Pierre de Sales La Terriere (1743-1815). L'UMC 69:860-863, 1940 ⟨I-02240⟩

Belanger, L.F.: A Canadian physician in the 18th century. University of Ottawa Medical Journal 14(4):13-15, 1972 ⟨I-02700⟩

Belanger, L.F.: On a Nickle and a Prayer. A Personal Outlook on the Early Days of the Medical School. Ottawa, University of Ottawa Press, 1978. ⟨II-00240⟩

Belisle, L-P: Histoire de la Radiologie au Canada Francais. L'UMC 88:40-52, 1959 ⟨II-02467⟩

Bell, F. McK.: The First Canadians in France. The Chronicle of a military hospital in the war zone. New York, George H. Doran Co., 1917. 308 p. ⟨II-00804⟩

Bell, L.G.: Doctor Donald McEachern. University of Manitoba Medical Journal 23:64-65, 1951 ⟨I-03211⟩

Bell, L.G.: Dr. Clifford Gilmour. CMAJ, 67:483, 1952 ⟨I-04554⟩

Bell, L.G.: Dr. Alvin Mathers: an appreciation. CMAJ 82:336, 339, 1960 ⟨I-03430⟩

Bell, L.G.: My Father -- Gordon Bell. Winnipeg Clinic Quarterly 23:77-93, 1970 ⟨I-02047⟩

Bellamy, M: Beyond the Call of Duty. Manitoba Pageant 20(4):13-17, 1975 ⟨II-04009⟩

Bender, L.P.: Old and New, Canada 1753-1844: Historic Scenes and Social pictures, or The Life of Joseph-Francois Perrault. Montreal, Dawson Brothers, Publishers, 1882, 291 p. ⟨I-04438⟩

Benjamin, M: The McGill Medical Librarians, 1829-1929. Bulletin of the Medical Library Association 50:1-16, 1962 ⟨II-04026⟩

Bennett, E.M.G.: Louis Hebert. DCB 1:367-368, 1966 ⟨I-01366⟩

Benoit, E.T.: Mes Souvenirs de L'Union Medicale. L'UMC 61:97-109, 1932 ⟨II-02446⟩

Bensley, E.H.: Bishop's Medical College. CMAJ 72:463-465, 1955 ⟨II-00268⟩

Bensley, E.H.: Sculduggery in the Dead House. CACHB 22:245-248, 1958 ⟨II-00033⟩

Bensley, E.H.: Alexis St. Martin. CMAJ 80:907-909, 1959 ⟨I-01971⟩

Bensley, E.H.: Canadians Should Publish in Canadian Journals. CMAJ 83:1163, 1960 ⟨II-01536⟩

Bensley, E.H.: Dr. William James Deadman. CMAJ 92:1138-1139, 1965 ⟨I-01465⟩

Bensley, E.H.: Dr. Minnie Gomery. CMAJ 96:1294,1967 ⟨I-02493⟩

Bensley, E.H.: The Caldwell - O'Sullivan Duel: A Prelude to the Founding of the Montreal General Hospital. CMAJ 100:1092-1095, 1969 ⟨II-00184⟩

Bensley, E.H.: Alexis St. Martin and Dr. Bunting. BHM 44:101-8, 1970 ⟨II-05388⟩

Bensley, E.H.: The Beginning of Teaching at McGill University. McGill Journal of Education 6:23-24, 1971 ⟨II-01542⟩

Bensley, E.H.: McGill University's Most Infamous Medical Graduate. CMAJ 109:1024, 1973 ⟨I-05377⟩

Bensley, E.H.: Archibald Hall. DCB 9:357-358, 1976 ⟨I-01345⟩

Bensley, E.H.: Pages of History. (Montreal, Montreal General Hospital), 1981. 40 p. ⟨II-04216⟩

Bensley, E.H.: James Grant: ship's surgeon on the ill-fated Empress of Ireland. CMAJ 126:318-9, 1982 ⟨I-04757⟩

Bensley, E.H.: Robert Palmer Howard. DCB 11:428-29, 1982 ⟨I-04846⟩

Bensley, E.H.: Dr. Hugh Ernest MacDermot. CMAJ 128:860-861, 1983 ⟨I-05071⟩

Benvie, R.M.: West River Medical Doctors. Nova Scotia Medical Bulletin 26:79-85, 1947 ⟨II-04025⟩

Bergstrom, I.: Mary Berglund: Backwoods Nurse. Canadian Nurse 72(9):45-49, 1976 ⟨II-00773⟩

Beriner, J.: Trois siecles de charite a l'Hotel-Dieu de Montreal. Montreal, Therien, 1949 ⟨II-05149⟩

Bernard, J.P.: Thomas Boutillier. DCB 9:73-74, 1976 ⟨II-00670⟩

Bernier, J.: L'Histoire de la Medecine Quebecoise aux XVIIIe et XIXe siecles: Problems et Sources. Department d'Histoire, Universite Laval, 1978. 13 p. n.p. ⟨II-02424⟩

Bernier, J.: Les Praticiens de la Sante au Quebec, 1871-1921: Quelques Donnees Statistiques. Recherches Sociographiques 20:41-58, 1979 ⟨II-04683⟩

Bernier, J.: Francois Blanchet et le Mouvement Reformiste en Medecine au Debut du XIXe Siecle. Revue d'histoire de l'amerique Francaise 34:223-244, 1980 ⟨I-04657⟩

Bernier, J.: Vers un Nouvel Ordre Medical: Les Origines de la Corporation des Medecins et Chirurgiens du Quebec. Recherches Sociopolitiques 22:307-330, 1981 ⟨II-05271⟩

Bernier, J.: Pierre Beaubien. DCB 11:57-58, 1982 ⟨I-04843⟩

Bernier, J.: L'integration du corps medical quebecois a la fin du XIXe siecle. Historical Reflections 10:91-113, 1983 ⟨II-05206⟩

Bernier, J.: Philippe-Louis-Francois Badelard. DCB 5:46-47, 1983 ⟨I-05317⟩

Bernier, J.: Le corps medical quebecois a la fin du XVIIIe siecle. In: Roland, C.G. (ed.): Health, Disease and Medicine: Essays in Canadian History. Toronto, Hannah Institute for the History of Medicine, 1984, 36-64 ⟨II-05393⟩

Berry, E.G.: Whitman's Canadian Friend. Dalhousie Review 24:77-82, 1944-45 ⟨I-02024⟩

Berry, J.N.: Sir Frederick Banting's Dream. Canadian Notes and Queries 23:7, 1980 ⟨I-00961⟩

Berube, B.: Dr. F.N.G. Starr: in memory of the medical statesman. CMAJ 127:417, 419-421, 1982 ⟨I-04890⟩

Berube, B.: How did the CMA Survive. CMAJ 127:530-532, 1982 ⟨II-04984⟩

Besnard, J.: Les diverses professions de Robert Giffard. Nova Fancia 4:322-329, 1929 ⟨I-04937⟩

Best, B.D.: Dr. John D. McQueen. CMAJ 60:102, 1949 ⟨I-04504⟩

Best, B.D.: Reminiscences. Winnipeg Clinic Quarterly 23:99-101, 1970 ⟨II-04024⟩

Best, C.H.: Sir Frederick Banting. University of Toronto Quarterly 10:249-254, 1940-41 ⟨I-04367⟩

Best, C.H., Solandt, D.Y.: The Activities of the RCN Medical Research Unit. CMAJ 48:96-99, 1943 ⟨II-04023⟩

Best, C.H.: The First Clinical Use Of Insulin. Diabetes 5:65-67, 1956 ⟨II-00103⟩

Best, C.H.: A Canadian Trail of Medical Research. Journal of Endocrinology 19:1-17, 1959 ⟨II-00101⟩

Best, C.H.: Diabetes since Nineteen Hundred and Twenty. CMAJ 82(21):1061-1066, 1960. ⟨II-00102⟩

Best, C.H.: Forty Years of Interest in Insulin. British Medical Bulletin 16(3):179-182, 1960 ⟨II-00100⟩

Best, C.H.: The Internal Secretion of the Pancreas. CMAJ 87:1046-1051, 1962 ⟨II-04022⟩

Best, C.H.: The Division of Naval Medical Research, Royal Canadian Navy. In: Selected Papers of Charles H. Best. Toronto, University of Toronto Press, 1963. pp 679-683 ⟨II-00785⟩

Best, C.H.: Impact of Insulin on Metabolic Pathway. Recollections of 1921. Israel Journal of Medical Sciences 8:181-85, 1972 ⟨II-05352⟩

Best, C.H.: Nineteen Hundred Twenty-One in Toronto. Diabetes 21:385-95, 1972 ⟨II-05351⟩

Bigelow, W.A.: Dr. Frederick Todd Cadham, an appreciation. CMAJ 84:673-674, 1961 ⟨I-01481⟩

Bigelow, W.A.: Forceps, Fin, and Feather. Manitoba, D.W. Friesen and Sons Ltd., 1969. 116 p. ⟨I-00940⟩

Bigelow, W.G.: 150 Years 1829-1979: Toronto General Hospital. N.p. / n.d. ⟨II-00185⟩

Biggs, C.L.: The Case of the Missing Midwives: A History of Midwifery in Ontario from 1795-1900. Ontario History 75:21-35, 1983 ⟨II-05091⟩

Bilas, I.: Pierre-Etienne Fortin. DCB 11:320-21, 1982 ⟨I-04837⟩

Bilson, G.: Cholera!. Canadian Historical Magazine 1(2):41-55, 1973 ⟨II-03107⟩

Bilson, G.: Two Cholera Ships in Halifax. Dalhousie Review 53:449-459, 1973 ⟨II-00082⟩

Bilson, G.: The Cholera Epidemic in Saint John, N.B., 1854. Acadiensis 4:85-99, 1974-5 ⟨II-00080⟩

Bilson, G.: Cholera in Upper Canada, 1832. Ontario History 67:15-30, 1975 ⟨II-00081⟩

Bilson, G.: Canadian Doctors and the Cholera. Historical Papers, CHA, 1977. pp 104-119. ⟨II-00079⟩

Bilson, G.: The first epidemic of Asiatic Cholera in Lower Canada, 1832. Medical History 21:411-433, 1977 ⟨II-00083⟩

Bilson, G.: Science, Technology and 100 Years of Canadian Quarantine. in: Jarrell, R.A.; Roos, A.E. (edit): Critical Issues in the History of Canadian Science, Technology and Medicine. Thornhill and Ottawa, HSTC Publications, 1983. pp 89-100 ⟨II-05195⟩

Bilson, G.: "Muscles and Health": Health and the Canadian Immigrant, 1867-1906. In: Roland, C.G.(ed.): Health, Disease and Medicine: Essays in Canadian Medicine. Toronto, Hannah Institute for the History of Medicine, 1984, 398-411 ⟨II-05409⟩

Birkett, H.S.: A Brief Account of the History of Medicine in the Province of Quebec from 1535 to 1838. Medical Record, July 1908, pp 1-46 ⟨II-04020⟩

Birkett, H.S.: Buller, the Ophthalmologist, Politzer, the Otologist, and Lefferts, the Laryngologist. Transactions of the American Academy of Ophthalmology and Oto- Laryngology, pp 24-34, 1927 ⟨I-01714⟩

Birkett, H.S.: Dr. Ernest Hamilton White. CMAJ 29:218, 1933 ⟨I-01722⟩

Birkett, H.S.: A Short Account of the History of Medicine in Lower Canada. Annals of Medical History, series 3 1(4):314-324, 1939 ⟨II-00849⟩

Biron, H.: Antoine Chaudillon. DCB 2:140-141, 1969 ⟨I-01017⟩

Biron, H.: Pierre Baudeau. DCB 2:47-48, 1969 ⟨I-00993⟩

Birt, A.R.: The Canadian Dermatological Association: First 50 Years. International Journal of Dermatology 16:289-295, 1977 ⟨II-00071⟩

Black, D.M.: Tularaemia in British Columbia. CMAJ 78:16-18, 1958 ⟨II-04021⟩

Black, D.M.: Kelowna Medical History. Okanagan Historical Society Annual Report 44:26-33, 1980 ⟨II-05114⟩

B[lack], E.F.E.: Dr. Frederick Gallagher McGuinness: an appreciation. CMAJ 99:145, 1968 ⟨I-03206⟩

Black, E.F.E.: Thinking Back. CMAJ 105:143-144, 1971 ⟨I-03884⟩

Black, E.F.E.: Not So Long Ago. University of Manitoba Medical Journal 45:54-56, 1975 ⟨II-00242⟩

Black, E.F.E.: The Department of Obstetrics and Gynecology. University of Manitoba Medical Journal 51:103-112, 1981 ⟨II-04882⟩

Blackader, A.D.: Dr. Francis J. Shepherd. CMAJ 20:210-211, 1929 〈I-01677〉

Blain, D., Griffin, J.D.: Canadian Psychiatrists in Publicatins of APA, 1948-1958: Source Materials. Canadian Psychiatric Association Journal 20:543-7, 1975 〈II-05291〉

Blais, J.M.: Un geant canadien celebre: Edouard Beaupre (1881-1904). Neuro-Chirurgie 19(2):23-34, 1973 〈I-05295〉

Blais, M.C.: Yves Phlem. DCB 3:518-520, 1974 〈II-00113〉

Blakeley, P.R.: George Moir Johnston. DCB 10:382-383, 1972 〈I-01330〉

Blakeley, P.R.: Leonard Lockman. DCB 3:405, 1974 〈I-01317〉

Blakeley, P.R.: And Having a Love for People. Nova Scotia Historical Quarterly 5:167-175, 1975 〈II-04013〉

Blakeley, P.R.: Frederick William Morris. DCB 9:573-574, 1976 〈I-01453〉

Blakeney, A.E.: Press Coverage of the Medicare Dispute in Saskatchewan: I. Queen's Quarterly 70:352-361, 1963-64 〈II-02322〉

Blanchard, D.: Who or What's a Witch? Iroquois Persons of Power. American Indian Quarterly 6:218-237, 1982 〈II-05266〉

Blanchard, R.J.: James Wilford Good, M.B, L.R.C.P. (Edin), F.A.C.S. CMAJ 16:1283, 1926 〈I-01614〉

Blanchet, J., Fremont, C.J.: L'evolution de la chirurgie au Quebec. L'UMC 106(3):358-3, 1977 〈II-05236〉

Blatz, W.E., Chant, N., et al: Collected Studies on the Dionne Quintuplets. Toronto, The University of Toronto Press, 1937. Discontinuous pagination. 〈II-01545〉

Blatz, W.E.: The Five Sisters: A Study of Child Psychology. Toronto, McClelland and Stewart Ltd., 1938. 209 p. 〈II-01544〉

Blishen, B.R.: Doctors and Doctrines. Toronto, University of Toronto Press, 1969. 202 p. 〈II-00246〉

Bliss, M.: Pure Books on Avoided Subjects: Pre-Freudian Sexual Ideals in Canada. Canadian Historical Association: Historical Papers, 1970. pp 89-108. 〈II-00469〉

Bliss, M.: The Discovery of Insulin. Toronto, McClelland and Stewart Limited, 1982. 304 p. 〈II-05020〉

Bliss, M.: The Aetiology of the Discovery of Insulin. In: Roland, C.G. (ed.): Health, Disease and Medicine: Essays in Canadian History. Toronto, Hannah Institute for the History of Medicine, 1984, 333-346 〈II-05405〉

Blogg, H.: James Bovell (1817-1880). In Kelly HW, Burrage WL: Dictionary of American Medical Biography. New York and London, D. Appleton and Co., 1928. pp.126-127. 〈I-00012〉

Blum, A.: Vaisrub: Good Language with a Light Touch. CMAJ 127:307-308, 1982 〈I-04903〉

Blum, A.: Remembering Sam Vaisrub. University of Manitoba Medical Journal 53:17-19, 1983 〈I-05132〉

[Blum, A.]: Samuel Vaisrub, M.D., Clinician, Editor, 'Amateur'. University of Manitoba Medical Journal 53:16-17, 1983 〈I-05131〉

Blum, A.: Vaisrub: Good Language with a Light Touch. University of Manitoba Medical Journal 53:14-15, 1983 〈I-05133〉

Boas, F.: Current Beliefs of the Kwakiutl Indians. Journal American Folk-lore 45(176):177-260, 1932 〈II-00638〉

Boissonnault, C.M.: Histoire de la Faculte de Medecine de Laval. Quebec, Les Presses Universitaires Laval, 1953. 438 p. 〈II-02427〉

Boissonnault, C.M.: Un Periodique oublie [L'Anti-Vaccinateur Canadien-Francais, Montreal, 1885]. La lutte contre la vaccination au XIXe sie. Laval Medical 32:178-184, 1961 〈II-02475〉

Boissonnault, C.M.: Jean Demosny. DCB 1:255-256, 1966 〈I-01006〉

Boissonnault, C.M.: Michel Gamelain de la Fontaine. DCB 1:320-321, 1966 〈I-01398〉

Boissonnault, C.M.: Antoine Forestier. DCB 2:226, 1969 〈I-01020〉

Boissonnault, C.M.: Jean Martinet de Fonblanche. DCB 2:465-566, 1969 〈I-01022〉

Boissonnault, C.M.: Joseph Painchaud. DCB 10:563-564, 1972 〈I-01237〉

Boissonnault, C.M.: Charles-Jacques Fremont. DCB 9:286-287, 1976 〈I-02232〉

Boissonnault, C.M.: Joseph Morrin. DCB 9:572-573, 1976 〈I-01451〉

Boivin, B.: Jean-Francois Gaultier. DCB 3:241, 675-681, 1974 〈II-00348〉

Bond, C.C.J.: Alexander James Christie, Bytown Pioneer -- His Life and Times, 1787-1843. Ontario History 56(1):16-36, 1964 〈I-01704〉

Bond, C.C.J.: Edward van Cortlandt. DCB 10:691-692, 1972 〈I-01189〉

Bonenfant, J-L: Comment les chanoines de Quebec sont devenus transparents au XIXe siecle. CSHM Newsletter, Spring 1983, pp 1-7 〈II-05111〉

Bothwell, R.S.: The Health of the Common People. In: English, J. and J.O. Stubbs, (eds.), Mackenzie King: Widening the Debate. The Macmillan Company of Canada Ltd., pp 191-220 〈II-04200〉

Bothwell, R.S., English, J.R.: Pragmatic Physicians: Canadian Medicine and Health Care Insurance 1910-1945. Univ of Western Ontario Med J 46(3):14-17, 1976 〈II-00252〉

Botterell, E.H.: Dr. Kenneth George McKenzie. CMAJ 91:880-881, 1964 〈I-03200〉

Boucot, K.R.: R. Tait McKenzie: A Biographical Sketch. Archives of Environmental Health 14:652-656, 1967 〈I-03219〉

Bouvier, L.F.: The Spacing of Births Among French-Canadian families: An Historical Approach. Canadian Review of Social Anthropology 5(1):17-26, 1968 〈II-05455〉

Bowden, B., Hall, R.: The Impact of Death: An Historical and Archival Reconnaissance into Victorian Ontario. Archivaria 14:93-105, 1982 〈II-05264〉

Bowman, F.B.: Donald C. Balfour. CMAJ 89:361, 1963 〈I-03901〉

Boyd, A.J.: Pioneer Health: Analysis of a Survey of the Health of Saskatchewan Residents 1878 to 1914. Saskatchewan, Occupational Health Reports, No. 2, June 1971, 97 p. ⟨II-04616⟩

Boyd, W.: With A Field Ambulance at Ypres. Toronto, Musson Book Co. Ltd., 1916. 110 p. ⟨I-00936⟩

Boyd, W.: Dr. Sara Meltzer. CMAJ 47:600, 1942 ⟨I-04279⟩

Boyd, W.: George Lyman Duff: In Memoriam. CMAJ 78:962-963, 1958 ⟨I-01581⟩

Boyd, W.: Cause and Effect: The Fifth Alexander Gibson Memorial Lecture. CMAJ 92:868-874, 1965 ⟨I-03186⟩

Boyer, B.F.: Dr. William Harop Hattie, an appreciation. CMAJ 26:121-122, 1932 ⟨II-03125⟩

Boyle, D.: Notes on the Life of Dr. Joseph Workman. Toronto, Arbuthnot Bros. and Co., 1894. pp 8 ⟨I-02720⟩

Bradbury, B.: The Fragmented Family: Family Strategies in the Face of Death, Illness, and Poverty, Montreal, 1860-1885. In: Parr, J.(ed): Childhood and Family in Canadian History, Toronto, McClelland and Stewart, 1982. pp 109-128 ⟨II-04886⟩

Bradwin, E.: The medical system on frontier works. In The Bunkhouse Man. Toronto, Buffalo, Univ. of Toronto Press, 1972. pp 139-154 ⟨II-00760⟩

Braithwaite, M.: Sick Kids: The Story of the Hospital for Sick Children in Toronto. Toronto, McClelland and Stewart Ltd., 1974. 204 p. ⟨II-00173⟩

Brand, L.M.: Saskatchewan Graffiti or Where were you in '62? (Memories of pre-medicare trench warfare — how one group of doctors fought against socialized medicine.) Canadian Doctor 45:95, 97-98, 1979 ⟨II-00652⟩

Brandon, K.F.: Public Health in Upper Canada. Public Health Education Journal 25:461-5, 1934 ⟨II-05137⟩

Brandson, B.J.: Dr. Jasper Halpenny: an appreciation. CMAJ 24:324, 1931 ⟨I-03068⟩

Brasset, E.A.: A Doctor's Pilgrimage: an autobiography. Philadelphia, J.B. Lippincott Co., 1951. 256 p. ⟨I-04828⟩

Brazeau, J.: The French-Canadian Doctor in Montreal. Thesis (M.A.), Montreal, McGill University, 1951 ⟨II-05156⟩

Brecher, R.: The Rays: A History of Radiology in the United States and Canada. Baltimore, The William and Wilkins Company, 1969. 484 p. ⟨II-00550⟩

Bredin, T.F.: Henry Septimus Beddome. DCB 11:63-64, 1982 ⟨I-04844⟩

Brett, H.B.: A Synopsis of Northern Medical History. CMAJ 100:521-525, 1969 ⟨II-04017⟩

Brien, W.P.: Dr. Norman Arnold McCormick. CMAJ 98:64, 1968 ⟨I-01762⟩

Brink, G.C.: How Pasteurization of Milk Came to Ontario. CMAJ 91:972-973, 1964 ⟨II-04018⟩

Brodie, F.: Col. William Belfry Hendry, DSO, VD, MB, FRCS(C), FCOG. CMAJ 40:524+526, 1939 ⟨I-01735⟩

Brougher, J.C.: Early Medicine in the Pacific Northwest. Northwest Medicine 62:34-39, 1963 ⟨II-04019⟩

Browarny, L.: A Friend in Need. St. John Ambulance in Calgary. Calgary, Century Calgary Publications, 1975 ⟨II-05099⟩

Brown, A.: Dr. David Edwin Robertson, an appreciation. CMAJ 50:391, 1944 ⟨I-02500⟩

Brown, A., Drake, T.G.H., Ebbs, J.H.: Dr. Fred F. Tisdall. CMAJ 61:86, 1949 ⟨I-04502⟩

Brown, A.: Frederick F. Tisdall, MD, MB(Tor), MRCS (Eng), LRCP (Lond) FRCP(C). CMAJ 64:263-265, 1951 ⟨I-02701⟩

Brown, C.P.: Leprosy in Canada. Canadian Journal of Public Health 43:252-58, 1952 ⟨II-04015⟩

Brown, C.P.: The Quarantine Service of Canada. Canadian Journal of Public Health 46:449-453, 1955 ⟨II-00228⟩

Brown, J.: R. Tait McKenzie, on the Centennial of His Birth. Archives Environmental Health 14:651, 1967 ⟨I-03217⟩

Brown, J.N.E.: The Hospitals of Toronto. In: Middleton, J.E.: The Municipality of Toronto: A History. Toronto and New York, Dominion Publishing Co., vol II, 1923. pp 631-651. ⟨II-00187⟩

Brown, J.R., McLean, D.M.: Smallpox -- a Retrospect. CMAJ 87:765-67, 1962 ⟨II-04014⟩

Brown, T.E.: Dr. Ernest Jones, Psychoanalysis, and the Canadian Medical Profession, 1908-1913. In: Shortt, S.E.D.: Medicine in Canadian Society: Historical Perspectives. Montreal, McGill-Queen's University Press, 1981. pp 315-360. ⟨II-04879⟩

Brown, T.E.: Architecture as Therapy. Archivaria 10:99-124, 1980 ⟨II-00161⟩

Brown, T.E.: Shell Shock in the Canadian Expeditionary Force, 1914-1918: Canadian Psychiatry in the Great War. In: Roland, C.G. (ed.): Health, Disease and Medicine: Essays in Canadian History. Toronto, Hannah Institute for the History of Medicine, 1984, 308-332 ⟨II-05406⟩

Brown, W.C.: Disease Among the Aborigines of America and Their Knowledge of Treatment. Canadian Journal of Medicine and Surgery 51:155-58, 1922 ⟨II-04016⟩

Bruce, H.A.: Politics and the Canadian Army Medical Corps. Toronto, William Briggs, 1919. 321 p. ⟨II-00806⟩

Bruce, H.A.: Varied Operations. Toronto, Longmans, Green and Co., 1958. 366 p. ⟨II-00421⟩

Bruce, H.A.: Memories of a Fellow of the Royal College of Surgeons of 1896. CMAJ 84:762, 733, 1961 ⟨I-03885⟩

Bryans, A.M., Padfield, C.J., Partington, M.W.: Eastern Ontario Paediatric Association, the first 15 years. Ontario Medical Review 45:71-72,89, 1978 ⟨II-00737⟩

Bryce, P.H.: History of Public Health in Canada. Canadian Therapeutist and Sanitary Engineer 1:287-291, 1910 ⟨II-05013⟩

Bryce, P.H.: The history of the American Indians in relation to health. Ontario Historical Society Papers and Records 12:128-141, 1914 ⟨II-00605⟩

Bryce, P.H.: The Story of Public Health in Canada. In: Ravenel, M.P.: A Half Century of Public Health. New York, American Public Health Association, 1921. pp 56-65 ⟨II-04999⟩

Buck, R.M.: The Mathesons of Saskatchewan Diocese. Saskatchewan History 13:41-62, 1960 ⟨I-03560⟩

Buck, R.M.: The Doctor Rode Side-Saddle. McClelland and Steward Ltd., 1974, 175 p. ⟨I-04426⟩

Bucke, R.M.: Man's Moral Nature. New York, G.P. Putnam's Sons, 1879. 200 p. ⟨II-00543⟩

Bucke, R.M.: Cosmic Consciousness. New York, E.P. Dutton and Co., Inc., 1923. 384 p. ⟨II-00872⟩

Buckley, S.: Efforts to Reduce Infant Maternity Mortality in Canada Between the Two World Wars. Atlantis 2(2):76-84, 1977 ⟨II-01823⟩

Buckley, S.: Ladies or Midwives? Efforts to Reduce Infant and Maternal Mortality. In: Kealey, L.(edit): A Not Unreasonable Claim. Toronto, The Women's Press, 1979. pp 131-149 ⟨II-03151⟩

Buehrle, R.: The Roots of our Medical School. University of Toronto Medical Journal 44:219-24, 1967 ⟨II-05350⟩

Buffam, F.: Robert Tait McKenzie. McGill Medical Journal 37:225-232, 1968 ⟨I-03199⟩

Buffam, G.B.B.: James Boyd Roberts. CMAJ 123:695, 1980 ⟨I-01579⟩

Bull, W.P.: From Medicine Man to Medical Man. Toronto, George J. McLeod Ltd., 1934. 457 p. ⟨II-00850⟩

Bumsted, J.M.: Lord Selkirk's Highland Regiment and the Kildonan Settlers. The Beaver, pp. 16-21, Autumn 1978 ⟨II-00339⟩

Bunn, J.: Smallpox Epidemic of 1869-70. Alberta Historical Review 11(2):13-19, 1963 ⟨II-02969⟩

Burgess, H.: Health by remote control. The Beaver 301(4):50-55, 1970 ⟨II-03308⟩

Burgess, T.J.W.: A Historical Sketch of our Canadian Institutions for the Insane. PTRSC, Section IV, 2-122, 1898 ⟨II-00151⟩

Burgess, T.J.W.: Abstract of a Historical Sketch of Canadian Institutions for the Insane. American Journal of Insanity 55:667-711, 1899 ⟨II-00162⟩

Burrage, W.L.: Robert Nelson (1793-1844). In Kelly HW, Burrage WL: Dictionary of American Medical Biography. New York and London, D. Appleton and Co., 1928. p. 900 ⟨I-01275⟩

Burris, H.L.: Medical Saga: The Burris Clinic and Early Pioneers. Vancouver, Mitchell Press Limited, 1967. 248 p. ⟨II-00368⟩

C

C., A.W.: Charles Best: The Codiscoverer of Insulin. CMAJ 118:167-168, 1978 ⟨II-02079⟩

C., C.J.: Major-General John Taylor Fotheringham, CMG, MD. CMAJ 43:87-88, 1940 ⟨I-01216⟩

C., G.C.: Dr. Willmot E.L. Sparks, an appreciation. CMAJ 89-99, 1963 ⟨I-01658⟩

C.J.J.: Dr. James H. Burns. Canadian Journal of Medicine and Surgery 3:47-48, 1898 ⟨I-01548⟩

C., R.: Dr. Jonathan C. Meakins. CMAJ 81:857, 1959 ⟨I-01755⟩

C., R.A., H., R.C.A.: Memory and Appreciation: John William Lovett Doust 1914-1980. Canadian Journal of Psychiatry 25:683, 1980 ⟨I-02880⟩

C, W.G.: Dr. Norman Strahan Shenstone. CMAJ 102:1112-1113, 1970 ⟨I-01675⟩

Cadotte, M.: A Propos de La Premiere Autopsie au Canada: En L'Annee 1536. L'UMC 103:1791-1796, 1974 ⟨II-00343⟩

Cadotte, M.: Le Docteur Adrien Duchesne, Le Premier Expert Medico-Legal de La Nouvelle-France (1639). L'UMC 104:276-278, 1975 ⟨I-01008⟩

Cadotte, M.: Les Memoires de Philippe Aubert de Gaspe et Les Medecins. L'UMC 105:1250-1268, 1976 ⟨I-02259⟩

Cadotte, M., Lessard, R.: Jean-Baptiste Rieutord. DCB 5:712-713, 1983 ⟨I-05305⟩

Cahsman, T.: Heritage of Service: The History of Nursing in Alberta. Edmonton, Alberta Association of Registered Nurses, 1966. 340 p. ⟨II-05431⟩

Cain, L.P.: Water and sanitation services in Vancouver: an historical perspective. British Columbia Studies, No. 30, pp 27-43, 1976 ⟨II-03254⟩

Caissie, F.: Joseph-Godric Blanchet. DCB 11:85-86, 1982 ⟨I-04861⟩

Calverley, R.K.: St. Rene: The Patron Saint of Anaesthetists and a Patron Saint of Canada. Canadian Anaesthetist's Society Journal 27:74-77, 1980 ⟨II-02464⟩

Cambell, M.W.: No Compromise: The Story of Colonel Baker and the CNIB. Toronto and Montreal, McClelland and Steward Ltd., 1965, 217p. ⟨II-04933⟩

Cameron, A.T.: Dr. Thorsten Ingvaldsen. CMAJ 23:116-117, 1930 ⟨I-03021⟩

Cameron, A.T.: The late Professor Swale Vincent. CMAJ 30:335, 1934 ⟨I-03535⟩

Cameron, G.D.W.: The First Donald Fraser Memorial Lecture. Canadian Journal of Public Health 51:341-348, 1960 ⟨I-02800⟩

Cameron, I.: One Hundred Years of Dalhousie. Dalhousie Medical Journal 21:5-9, 1967 ⟨II-04109⟩

Cameron, I.H.: Richard Barrington Nevitt, an appreciation. CMAJ 19:382-383, 1928 ⟨I-03503⟩

Cameron, I.H.: Dr. Adam Henry Wright. CMAJ 23:725-726, 1930 ⟨I-01149⟩

Cameron, J.S.: Dr. John Burritt Mann. CMAJ 16:333, 1926 ⟨I-01599⟩

Cameron, K.: No. 1 Canadian Hospital, 1914-1919. New Brunswick, The Tribune Press, 1938 667 p. ⟨II-00808⟩

Cameron, M.: Captain B.W. Wheeler, MBE, M.D., FRCP(C), Late Indian Medical Service. Alberta Medical Bulletin 29:57-58, 1964 ⟨I-05187⟩

Cameron, M.H.V.: Dr. Gideon Silverthorn. CMAJ 17:129, 1927 ⟨I-01688⟩

Cameron, M.H.V.: Allan Roy Dafoe, OBE, MB. CMAJ 49:149, 1943 ⟨I-01514⟩

Cameron, M.H.V.: William Thomas Aikins (1827-1895). CMAJ 64:161-163, 1951 ⟨I-01068⟩

Cameron, M.H.V.: Jefferson Medical College in 1850 [for Canadian students]. CMAJ 66:73-75, + 82, 1952 ⟨II-04630⟩

Cameron, M.H.V.: Medical Education in Toronto. CACHB 17:71-74, 1953 ⟨II-00297⟩

Cameron, S., Falk, L.A.: Some Black Medical History: Dr. Martin R. Delany's Canadian Years as Medical Practitioner and Abolitionist (1856-1864). In International Congress for the History of Medicine, 25th, Quebec, 1976. Proceedings, Volume II, 1976. p. 537-545 ⟨II-00783⟩

Campbell, A.D.: The Late Dr. J.R. Goodall. CMAJ 58:304, 1948 ⟨I-02152⟩

Campbell, A.D.: Consultations then and now. CMAJ 89:1030-1032, 1963 ⟨II-04102⟩

Campbell, C.T.: Medical Legislation in Ontario. Ontario Medical Journal 1:47-51, 1892 ⟨II-04110⟩

Campbell, D.A.: The Growth and Organization of the Medical Profession in Nova Scotia. Canadian Journal of Medicine and Surgery 18:351-364, 1905 ⟨II-04103⟩

Campbell, D.A.: Abraham Gesnr (1797-1864). In: Kelly, H.W.;Burrage, W.L.: Dictionary of American Medical Biography, New York and London, D. Appleton and Co., 1928. pp 462-463 ⟨II-00540⟩

Campbell, D.A.: Alexander Macdonald (1784-1859). In Kelly HW, Burrage WL: Dictionary of American Medical Biography. New York and London, D. Appleton and Co., 1928. pp. 780-781. ⟨I-01452⟩

Campbell, D.A.: Charles Cogswell (1813-1892). In Kelly HW, Burrage WL: Dictionary of American Medical Biography. New York and London, D. Appleton and Co., 1928. p. 243. ⟨I-00923⟩

Campbell, D.A.: Daniel McNeil Parker (1822-1907). In Kelly HW, Burrage WL: Dictionary of American Medical Biography. New York and London, D. Appleton and Co., 1928. pp. 937-938. ⟨I-01242⟩

Campbell, D.A.: Edward Farrell (1843-1901). In Kelly HW, Burrage WL: Dictionary of American Medical Biography. New York and London, D. Appleton and Co., 1928. p. 399. ⟨I-01211⟩

Campbell, D.A.: Henry Greggs Farish (1770?-1856). In Kelly HW, Burrage WL: Dictionary of American Medical Biography. New York and London, D. Appleton and Co., 1928. p. 395. ⟨I-01209⟩

Campbell, D.A.: John Bernard Gilpin (1810-1892). In Kelly, H.W., Burrage, W.L.: Dictionary of American Med Biog. New York/London, D. Appleton and Co., 1928, p. 470. ⟨II-00044⟩

Campbell, D.A.: John Somers (1840-1898). In Kelly HW, Burrage WL: Dictionary of American Medical Biography. New York and London, D. Appleton and Co., 1928. p. 1142 ⟨I-01099⟩

Campbell, D.A.: Rufus Smith Black (1812-1893). In Kelly HW, Burrage WL: Dictionary of American Medical Biography. New York and London, D. Appleton and Co., 1928. pp. 102-103 ⟨I-00979⟩

Campbell, D.A.: William Johnston Almon (1816-1901). In Kelly HW, Burrage WL: Dictionary of American Medical Biography. New York, London, D. Appleton and Co., 1928. p. 22. ⟨I-00029⟩

Campbell, D.A.: William B. Slayter (1841-1898). In Kelly HW,Burrage WL: Dictionary of American Medical Biography. New York and London, D. Appleton and Co., 1928. p. 1120 ⟨I-01098⟩

Campbell, D.A.: William Scott Muir (1853-1902). In Kelly HW, Burrage WL: Dictionary of American Medical Biography. New York and London, D. Appleton and Co., 1928. pp. 883-884. ⟨I-01446⟩

Campbell, D.F.: The Reality of Psychic Phenomena. University of Manitoba Medical Journal 22:12-19, 1950 ⟨II-02335⟩

Campbell, M.: Dr. J.C. Schultz. Historical and Scientific Society of Manitoba Papers, series 3, No. 20:7-12, 1965 ⟨I-02579⟩

Campbell, M.F.: Holbrook of the San. Toronto, The Ryerson Press, 1953. 212 p. ⟨I-03419⟩

Campbell, P.M.: Leverett George DeVeber. CMAJ 15:971, 1925 ⟨I-01504⟩

Campbell, P.M.: Frank Hamilton Mewburn. CACHB 15(4):61-69, 1951 ⟨II-00422⟩

Campbell, P.S., Scammell, H.L.: The Development of Public Health in Nova Scotia. Canadian Public Health Journal 30:226-238, 1939 ⟨II-04104⟩

Campbell, W.R.: Anabasis. CMAJ 87:1055-1061, 1962 ⟨II-04105⟩

Campbell, W.R.: Andrew Almon Fletcher. CMAJ 92:145-146, 1965 ⟨I-02790⟩

Campbell, W.R.: Walter R. Campbell 1890-1981. PTRSC series 4, 19:69-71, 1981 ⟨I-04956⟩

C[ampbell], W.W.: William Henry Drummond. PTRSC 3d. Series, vol. 1, viii-ix, 1907 ⟨I-01197⟩

Camsell, C.: Discovery and Development of Radium at Great Bear Lake. Franklin Institute Journal 233:545-557, 1922 ⟨II-00549⟩

Canniff, W.: The Medical Profesion in Upper Canada 1783-1850. Toronto, William Briggs, 1894. 688 p. ⟨II-00868⟩

Canniff, W.: John Rolph (1793-1870). In Kelly HW, Burrage WL: Dictionary of American Medical Biography. New York and London, D. Appleton and Co., 1928. pp. 1055-1056. ⟨I-01135⟩

Canniff, W.: William Rees. In Kelly HW, Burrage WL: Dictionary of American Medical Biography. New York and London, D. Appleton and Co., 1928. pp. 1020-1021 ⟨I-01225⟩

Cant, D: The Cottage Hospital System in Newfoundland. Newfoundland Medical Association Newsletter 13:19-20, 23, 1971 ⟨II-04107⟩

Cantero, A: Occult Healing Practices in French Canada. CMAJ 20:303-306, 1929 ⟨II-04106⟩

Capacchione, L. (trans.), Endicott, J. (trans.), Perly, C. (trans.): Bethune: His Story in Pictures. Toronto, N.C. Press Ltd., 1975. 77 p. ⟨I-00970⟩

Caron, W.M.: The Early Surgeons of Quebec. Canadian Journal of Surgery 8:239-253, 1965 ⟨II-04302⟩

Carpenter, H.M.: The University of Toronto School of Nursing: An agent of change. In: Innis, M.Q.:Nursing Education in a Changing Society. Toronto, University of Toronto Press, 1970. pp 86-108 ⟨II-03651⟩

Carpenter, P.: E. Kirk Lion. CMAJ 123:1265, 1980 ⟨I-02884⟩

Carpenter, P.: Gordon Samuel Fahrni. CMAJ 123:1060, 1980 ⟨I-02773⟩

Carr, F.H.: The early days of insulin manufacture. The Diabetic Journal 4:355-357, 1946 ⟨II-00233⟩

Carson, W, Carson, S: Pioneers of Medicine in Newfoundland. CMAJ 79:581, 1958 ⟨II-04071⟩

Carswell, S.: The Story of Lions Gate Hospital: The Realization of a Pioneer Settlement's Dream, 1908-1980. West Vancouver, Carswell, 1980. ⟨II-05125⟩

Carter, J.S.: Doctor M.W. Locke and the Williamsburg Scene. Toronto, Life Portrayal Series, 1933. 138 p. ⟨I-01303⟩

Carter-Edwards, D.: The Brick Barracks at Fort Malden. Research Bulletin 100:1-34, 1978. Ottawa, Parks Canada ⟨II-00163⟩

Casgrain, H.R.: Histoire de l'Hotel-Dieu de Quebec. Montreal, Beauchemin, 1894 ⟨II-02436⟩

Casgrain, H.R.: L'Hotel-Dieu de Quebec. Montreal, C.O. Beauchemin and Fils, 1896, 592 p. ⟨II-04704⟩

Cash, P., Pine, C.: John Jeffries and the Struggle Against Smallpox in Boston (1775-1776) and Nova Scotia (1776-1779). Bulletin of the History of Medicine 57:93-97, 1983 ⟨II-05113⟩

Cashman, A.W.: Heritage of Service. The History of Nursing in Alberta. Edmonton, The Alberta Association of Registered Nurses, 1966 ⟨II-05102⟩

Cashman, J.: The Gentleman from Chicago. New York/Evanston/San Francisco/London, Harper and Row, Publishers, 1973. 310 p. ⟨I-00907⟩

Cass, E.: A Decade of Northern Ophthalmology. Canadian Journal of Ophthalmology 8:210-17, 1973 ⟨II-05349⟩

Casselman, J.I.: Venereal Disease in Ontario and Canada, 1900-1930. Thesis (M.A.), Kingston, Queen's University, 1981 ⟨II-04978⟩

Casson, A.J.: The doctor as an artist. Northward Journal No.'s 14 and 15:21-24, 1979 ⟨I-03188⟩

Casteel, R.W.: A Sample of Northern North American Hunter -- Gatherers and the Malthusian Thesis: An Explicitly Quantified Approach. In: Browman, D.L. (edit): Early Native Americans. Paris/New York, Mouton Publishers, 1980. pp 301-319 ⟨II-05188⟩

Cauchon, R.: L'hopital St-Francois d'Assis: Souvenirs Personnels et Petite Histoire (1914-1954). [Np, nd, ca 1982] ⟨II-04941⟩

Caulfield, A.H.W.: Dr. Leonard Milton Murray. CMAJ 25:503, 1931 ⟨I-03159⟩

Cauvreau, J.: Le Docteur Laurent Catellier: Ex-Doyen de l'Universite-Laval, Quebec 1839-1918. L'UMC 47:86, 1918 ⟨I-00913⟩

Cecil, R.L.: Dr. J. Wallace Graham: an appreciation. CMAJ 88:107, 1963 ⟨I-02163⟩

Chabot, R., Monet, J., Roby, Y.: Robert Nelson. DCB 10:544-547, 1972 ⟨I-01270⟩

Chabot, R.: Michel-Francois Valois. DCB 9:802-803, 1976 ⟨I-01192⟩

Chaisson, A.F.: Dr. William Paine -- Loyalist. CMAJ 69:446-447, 1953 ⟨I-02286⟩

Chalifoux, J.P.: Robert Lea MacDonnell. DCB 10:470-471, 1972 ⟨I-01437⟩

Champault, M.P.: Les Gendron "medecins des rois et des pauvres". PTRSC section I:35-130, 1912 ⟨II-02440⟩

Chandler, R.F., Hooper, S.N., Freeman, L.: Herbal Remedies of the Maritime Indians. Journal of Ethnopharmacology 1(1):49-68, 1979 ⟨II-00606⟩

Chant, C.A.: Albert Durrant Watson. Journal of the Royal Astronomical Society of Canada 20:153-157, 1926 ⟨I-02706⟩

Chapman, J.K.: The mid-nineteenth-century temperance movement in New Brunswick and Maine. CHR 35:43-60, 1954 ⟨II-00075⟩

Chapman, M.: Infanticide and Fertility Among Eskimos: A Computer Simulation. American Journal of Physical Anthropology 53:317-327, 1980 ⟨II-04202⟩

Chapman, T.L.: Drug Use in Western Canada. Alberta History 24(4):18-27, 1976 ⟨II-00107⟩

Chapman, T.L.: Early Eugenics Movement in Western Canada. Alberta History 25(4):9-17, 1977 ⟨II-02980⟩

Charles, C.A.: The Medical Profession and Health Insurance: an Ontario Case Study. Social Science and Medicine 10:33-38, 1976 ⟨II-05123⟩

Charlton, M: Medicine in Canada. Montreal Medical Journal 37:424-432, 735-738, 1908; 38:26-30, 38:662-666, 1909 ⟨II-04100⟩

Charlton, M.: Louis Hebert. Johns Hopkins Hospital Bulletin 25:158-160, 1914 ⟨I-04652⟩

Charlton, M.: Christopher Widmer. Annals of Medical History 4:346-350, 1922 ⟨I-04899⟩

Charlton, M.: Louis Hebert (-1627). In Kelly HW, Burrage WL: Dictionary of American Medical Biography. New York and London, D. Appleton and Co., 1928. pp. 549-551. ⟨I-01367⟩

Chase, L.A.: Dr. George Jamieson Whetham. CMAJ 24:476, 1931 ⟨I-03067⟩

Chase, L.A.: Dr. Murdoch Angus MacKay. CMAJ 31:107-108, 1934 ⟨I-03526⟩

Chase, L.A.: The Trend of Diabetes in Saskatchewan 1905 to 1934. CMAJ 36:366-369, 1937 ⟨II-04099⟩

Chase, L.A.: Dr. Neil John MacLean. CMAJ 56:115, 1947 ⟨I-03406⟩

Chatenay, H.P.: Echoes of Silence. The Chronicles of William Graham Mainprize, M.D., 1911-1974. Edmonton, H.P. Chatenay, 1978. ⟨I-05061⟩

Chatenay, H.P., Young, M.A.R.: The Country Doctors. Red Deer, Mattrix Press, 1980, 272 p. ⟨II-04649⟩

Chechire, N., Waldron, T., Quinn, A., Quinn, D.: Frobisher's Eskimos in England. Archivaria 10:23-50, 1980 ⟨II-00646⟩

Chevrier, G.R.: Dr. Thomas Gibson. CMAJ 45:193, 1941 ⟨I-03518⟩

Cheymol, J.: A propos de la decouverte de l'insuline par Banting et Best, il y a cinquante ans. Bulletin de l'Academie Nationale de Medecine 155:836-52, 1971 ⟨II-05348⟩

Chih-cheng, C. (adapted): Norman Bethune in China. Peking, Foreign Languages Press, 1975. 114 p. ⟨I-00954⟩

Chipman, W.W.: William Gardner, M.D. CMAJ 16:1284, 1926 ⟨I-01612⟩

Chown, B.: Dr. T. Glendenning Hamilton, (an appreciation). CMAJ 32:710-711, 1935 ⟨I-01343⟩

Chown, B: The Story of the Winnipeg Rh Laboratory. Journal-Lancet 87:38-40, 1967 ⟨II-04097⟩

Chown, H.H.: Dr. Robert Johnstone Blanchard. CMAJ 19:500, 1928 ⟨I-03505⟩

Chrichton, A.: The Shift From Enterpreneurial to Political Power in the Canadian Health System. Social Science and Medicine 10:59-66, 1976 ⟨II-05428⟩

Christie, K.: Behind Japanese Barbed Wire -- A Canadian Nursing Sister in Hong Kong. Royal Canadian Military Institute Year Book, 11-13, 1979 ⟨II-04993⟩

Chute, A.L.: Canadian Paediatric Contributions to Medical Progress. Bulletin of the Medical Library Association 48:37-43, 1960 ⟨II-04098⟩

Chute, A.L.: Dr. George A. McNaughton. CMAJ 96:381, 1967 ⟨I-02544⟩

Clare. H.: Accomplishments of the Past, and Hopes for the Future. Ontario Journal of Neuro-Psychiatry 1:11-18, 1921 ⟨II-04464⟩

Clark, D.: A psycho-medical history of Louis Riel. American Journal of Insanity 44:33-51, 1887 ⟨II-02620⟩

Clarke, C.K.: A Critical Study of the Case of Louis Riel. Queen's Quarterly 12:379-388, 1904-05; 13:14-26, 1905-06 ⟨II-02336⟩

Clarke, C.K.: A History of the Toronto General Hospital. Toronto, William Briggs, 1913. 147 p. ⟨II-00188⟩

Clarke, C.K.: The Story of the Toronto General Hospital Psychiatric Clinic. Canadian Journal of Mental Hygiene 1:30, 1919 ⟨II-04465⟩

Clarke, I.H.: Public Provisions for the Mentally Ill in Alberta, 1907-1936. Thesis (M.A.) Calgary, University of Calgary, 1973. ⟨II-05023⟩

Clarkson, F.A.: Dr. Thomas Chisholm, M.P. 1842-1931. CMAJ 29:82-86, 1933 ⟨I-03009⟩

Clarkson, F.A.: Dr. Bertram Spencer, MB, MRCS. CACHB 7(3):1-5, 1942 ⟨I-01102⟩

Clarkson, F.A.: Jabez Henry Elliott. CMAJ 50:264-267, 1944 ⟨I-02778⟩

Clarkson, F.A.: Jabez Henry Elliott: 1873-1942. Bulletin of the Academy of Medicine [Toronto] 17:95-100, 1944 ⟨I-04420⟩

Clarkson, F.A.: The Medical Faculty of the University of Toronto. CACHB 13:21-30, 1948 ⟨II-00300⟩

Clarkson, F.A.: The Canadian Album -- Men of Canada. CACHB 14:17-25, 1949 ⟨II-00210⟩

Clarkson, F.A.: Douglass Stanley: An Appreciation. CACHB 19(1):27-30, 1954 ⟨I-01086⟩

Clarkson, F.A.: Dr. Daniel Clark: A Physician of old Ontario. CACHB 22:157-170, 1957 ⟨I-01524⟩

Claxton, B.: Dr. Thomas Simpson (1833-1918; McGill, Med. 1854). Canadian Services Medical Journal 13:420-438, 1957 ⟨I-01681⟩

Clay, C.C.: The Founding of the "McGill Medical Undergraduate Journal". McGill Medical Journal 13:457-68, 1944 ⟨II-04093⟩

Clegg, H.: Dr. T. Clarence Routley, an appreciation. CMAJ 88:1046, 1963 ⟨I-01673⟩

Cleghorn, R.A.: D. Ewan Cameron, M.D., F.R.C.P. (C). CMAJ 97:984-985, 1967 ⟨I-01701⟩

Cleveland, D.E.H.: Canadian Medicine and its Debt to Scotland. CMAJ 52:90-95, 1945 ⟨II-04381⟩

Cleveland, D.E.H.: The Edinburgh Tradition in Canadian Medical Education. Bulletin of the Vancouver Medical Association 28:216-220, 1952 ⟨II-04094⟩

Cleveland, D.E.H.: The Canadian Dermatological Association -- First 25 Years. CMAJ çé:863-865, 1956 ⟨II-04095⟩

Clint, M.B.: Our Bit. Memories of War Services by a Canadian Nurse. Montreal, Royal Victoria Hospital, 1934. 177 p. ⟨II-00809⟩

Clouston, H.R.: Pioneer Medicine in the Chateauguay Valley. CMAJ 49:426-430, 1943 ⟨II-04326⟩

Cochran, A.W.: Notes on the Measures Adopted by Government, between 1775 and 1786, to check the St. Paul's Disease. Transactions of the Literary and Historical Society of Quebec 4:139-152, 1841 ⟨II-00119⟩

Cockerill, A: Ready Aye Ready. North/Nord May-June, 1976. pp 22-27 ⟨II-04064⟩

Coderre, E.: Pharmacy in Old Quebec. Canadian Pharmaceutical Journal 90:784-785, 1957 ⟨II-00713⟩

Cohen, J.J.: British Medicine in Greater Britain: the BMA Montreal Meeting, 1897. McGill Medical Journal 36:159-168, 1967 ⟨II-04090⟩

Colbeck, W.K.: The First Record of an Anesthetic in Ontario. CMAJ 32:84-85, 1935 ⟨II-04091⟩

Cole, D.: Sigismund Bacstrom's northwest coast drawings and an account of his curious career. British Columbia Studies, 46:61-86, 1980 ⟨I-03166⟩

Colgate, W.: Dr. Robert Kerr: An Early Practitioner of Upper Canada. CMAJ 64:542-546, 1951 ⟨II-01838⟩

Collard, E.: Flowers to heal and comfort: Mrs. Traill's Books for Collectors. Canadian Collector, May/June 1978. pages 32-36 ⟨II-04805⟩

Colley, K.B.: While Rivers Flow: Stories of Early Alberta. Saskatoon, The Western Producer, 1970, 148 p. ⟨II-04462⟩

Collier, H.B.: Ralph Faust Shaner 1893-1976. PTRSC series 4, 16:113-114, 1978 ⟨I-04957⟩

Collins, P.V.: The Public Health Policies of the United Farmers of Alberta Government, 1921-1935. Thesis, M.A., University of Western Ontario, London, 1969. 143 pages ⟨II-04817⟩

Collins, R.: A Man Sent From God. Reader's Digest, August 1983. pp 144-175. ⟨I-05172⟩

Collip, J.B.: Reminiscences on the Discovery of Insulin. CMAJ 87:1045, 1962 ⟨II-04092⟩

Collip, J.B.: Professor E.G.D. Murray, an appreciation. CMAJ 92:95-97, 1965 ⟨I-03215⟩

Comrie, J.D.: The part played by Scotland in early Canadian medical development. CMAJ 23:841-844, 1930 ⟨II-03147⟩

Condon, A.G.: John Caleff. DCB 5:134-135, 1983 ⟨I-05315⟩

Connell, J.C.: Dr. A.R.B. Williamson. CMAJ 20:213-214, 1929 ⟨I-02729⟩

Connell, W.T.: The Medical Faculty -- Queen's University. CACHB 13:45-50, 1948 ⟨II-00301⟩

Connor, J.T.H.: Joseph Lister's System of Wound Management and the Canadian Medical Practitioner, 1867-1900. Thesis (M.A.), London, University of Western Ontario, 1980. 177 p. 〈II-05415〉

Connor, J.T.H.: Preservatives of Health: Mineral Water Spas of Nineteenth Century Ontario. Ontario History 75:135-152, 1983 〈II-05207〉

Connor, J.T.H.: To be Rendered Unconscious of Torture: Anesthesia and Canada, 1847-1920. Thesis (M. Phil.), Waterloo, University of Waterloo, 1983 〈II-05079〉

Coodin, F.J.: Some observations on Eskimo health. The Journal-Lancet 87(2):51-55, 1967 〈II-00632〉

Cooke, A.: Richard King. DCB 10:406-408, 1972 〈I-01321〉

Cooke, R.: A Thumb-Nail Sketch of Dr. Thomas Beath. University of Manitoba Medical Journal 26:13, 1954 〈I-03891〉

Cooper, I.: Canadian Town Planning, 1900-1930: A Historical Bibliography. Volume III, Public Health. Toronto, University of Toronto (Centre for Urban and Community Studies), 1978. 23 p. 〈II-00560〉

Cooper, J.: Red Lights of Winnipeg. Historical and Scientific Society of Manitoba. Papers. Series 3. No. 27:61-74, 1970-71 〈II-02104〉

Cooper, R.C.: Dr. William Burton Tufts. CMAJ 127:309, 1982 〈I-04901〉

Copeman, W.S.C.: Dr. Wallace Graham: an appreciation. CMAJ 88:168, 1963 〈I-02161〉

Copland, D.: Livingstone of the Arctic. Ottawa, D. Copland, 1967. 183 p 〈I-03940〉

Copland, D: Livingstone of the Arctic. Ottawa, D. Copland, 1967. 183 p. 〈II-04119〉

Copp, T.: Public Health. In: The Condition of the Working Class in Montreal, 1897-1929: The Anatomy of Poverty. Toronto, McClelland and Stewart, 1974. pp 88-105. 〈II-00561〉

Copp, T.: The Health of the People: Montreal in the Depression Years. In: Shephard, D.A.E.; Levesque, A. (edit): Norman Bethune: His Times and His Legacy. Ottawa, Canadian Public Health Assoc., 1982, pp 129- 137 〈II-04919〉

Corrigan, S.H.: Anson Buck, MD, MRCS (Eng.) 1833-1919. CMAJ 34:564-569, 1936 〈I-01706〉

Corrigan, S.H.: Doctor Clarkson Freeman 1827-1895: a sketch. CMAJ 23:438-440, 1938 〈I-03030〉

Cosbie, W.G.: The Gordon Richards Memorial Lecture: Gordon Richards and the Ontario Cancer Foundation. Journal of the Canadian Association of Radiologists 9:1-7, 1958 〈I-02498〉

Cosbie, W.G.: Frederick Marlow (1877-1936) and the Development of the Modern Treatment of Carcinoma of the Cervix. Canadian Journal of Surgery 5:357-365, 1962 〈I-03429〉

Cosbie, W.G.: William Rawlins Beaumont. DCB 10:38-39, 1972 〈I-00014〉

Cosbie, W.G.: The Toronto General Hospital 1819-1965: A Chronicle. Toronto, Macmillan of Canada Ltd., 1975. 373 p. 〈II-00189〉

Cosbie, W.G.: The History of the Society of Obstetricians and Gynaecologists of Canada. 1944-1966. Toronto, N.p., 1968 p.65 〈II-04379〉

Couch, J.H.: History of fractures in Canada. CMAJ 45:174-177, 1941 〈II-03669〉

Coulson, F.: Michel Sarrazin (1659-1734). CACHB 7(2):1-6, 1942 〈I-01118〉

Coulson, F.S.: Frank Hamilton Mewburn (1858-1929). CACHB 10:120-125, 1945 〈I-01733〉

Cousland, P.A.C.: Early Medicine of Vancouver Island. CMAJ 55:393, 398, 1946 〈II-04089〉

Cox, M.A.: Dr. George Alfred McNaughton. CMAJ 96:380, 1967 〈I-02304〉

Coyne, J.H.: Richard Maurice Bucke--A Sketch. PTRSC Section 2, 159-196, 1906 〈I-00004〉

Coyne, J.H.: Richard Maurice Bucke. Toronto, Henry S. Saunders, 1923. 77 p. 〈I-01165〉

Craig, B., Dodds, G.: The Picture of Health. Archivaria 10:191-223, 1980 〈II-00361〉

Craig, B.: Smallpox in Ontario: Public and Professional Perceptions of Disease, 1884-1885. In Roland, C.G. (ed.): Health, Disease and Medicine: Essays in Canadian History. Toronto, Hannah Institute for the History of Medicine, 1984, 215-249 〈II-05401〉

Craig, G.M.: Two Contrasting Upper Canadian Figures: John Rolph and John Strachan. PTRSC IV, 12:237-248, 1974 〈I-01405〉

Craig, G.M.: John Rolph. DCB 9:683-690, 1976 〈I-01132〉

Craig, G.M.: Michael Barrett. DCB 11:53-54, 1982 〈I-04842〉

Craig, H.: The Loyal and Patriotic Society of Upper Canada and its Still-Born Child: The "Upper Canada Preserved" Medal. Ontario History 52:31-52, 1960 〈II-00190〉

Craig, R.H.: Reminiscences of W.H. Drummond. The Dalhousie Review 5:161-169, 1925-6 〈I-01694〉

Crane, J.W.: The University of Western Ontario, London, Ontario. CACHB 13:1-3, 1948 〈II-00270〉

Crawford, J.N.: Barbed Wire Humour [Hong Kong]. CMAJ 57:593-596, 1947 〈II-04085〉

Crete-Begin, L.: Charles-Christophe Malhiot. DCB 10:490-491, 1972 〈I-01438〉

Crichton, A.: Medicine and the State in Canada. In: Staum, M.S.; Larsen, D.E. (edit.): Doctors, Patients, and Society, Power and Authority in Medical Care. Waterloo, Wilfrid Laurier Univ. Press, 1981. pp 231-252 〈II-05025〉

Cronin, F.: Elixir or not, Ginseng is a Lucrative Cash Crop. Canadian Geographic 102(6): 60-63, 1982 〈II-04994〉

Cronin, G.: End of an Era; The story of Scarborough General Hospital. Toronto, Women's Auxiliary Scarborough General Hospital, [1974], 40 p. 〈II-04607〉

Crosby, A.W.: Virgin Soil Epidemics as a Factor in the Aboriginal Depopulation in America. William and Mary Quarterly 33:289-299, 1976 〈II-03263〉

Cross, M.S.: Charles Duncombe. DCB 9:228-232, 1976 〈I-00884〉

Cruikshank, J.: Becoming a Woman in Athapaskan Society: Changing Traditions on the Upper Yukon River. Western Canadian Journal of Anthropology 5(2):1-14, 1975 ⟨II-04206⟩

Crummey, J.M.: The daybooks of Robert MacLellan: a comparative study of a Nova Scotia family practice during World War 1. CMAJ 120:492-494, 497, 1979 ⟨II-00251⟩

Cullen, T.S.: The House Surgeons of the Toronto General Hospital 1890, 1891. Canadian Journal of Medicine and Surgery 52:66-70, 1922 ⟨II-04086⟩

Cummins, J.F.: The Organization of the Medical Services in the North West Campaign of 1885. Bulletin of the Vancouver Medical Association 20:72-78, 1943 ⟨II-04087⟩

Currie, A.: Dr. Ernest Hamilton White. CMAJ 29:218, 1933 ⟨I-01720⟩

Currie, M.G.: A Pioneer Woman in Canadian Medicine. Nova Scotia Medical Bulletin 33:266-267, 1954 ⟨I-03930⟩

Curtis, H.: How Pharmacy Grew in the Maritimes. Canadian Pharmaceutical Journal 82:16, 35, 1949 ⟨II-00710⟩

Curtis, J.D.: St. Thomas and Elgin Medical Men of the Past. St. Thomas, Ontario, 1956. 122 p. ⟨II-00866⟩

Curtis, J.F.: The First Medical School in Upper Canada. Ontario Medical Review 34:449-452, 1967 ⟨II-01798⟩

Cushing, H.: The Life of Sir William Osler. Oxford, Claredon Press, 1925; 2 Vols., 685 p., 728 p. ⟨I-01257⟩

Cushing, H.B.: Dr. A. MacKenzie Forbes. CMAJ 21:109, 1929 ⟨I-02793⟩

Cushing, J.E., Casey, T., Robertson, M.: A Chronicle of Irish Emigration to Saint John, New Brunswick, 1847. New Brunswick, The New Brunswick Museum, 1979. 77 p. ⟨II-00066⟩

Cybulski, J.S.: Modified Human Bones and Skulls from Prince Rupert Harbour, British Columbia. Canadian Journal of Archaeology 2:15-31, 1978 ⟨II-02627⟩

Cyriax, R.J.: A Historic Medicine Chest. CMAJ 57:295-300, 1947 ⟨II-04084⟩

D

D., D.M.: Dr. Jonathan C. Meakins. CMAJ 81:857, 1959 ⟨I-01756⟩

D., E.F.: The Best Biography. The Medical Post, pp 8, 24, 35 (Sept. 7); 20, 22 (Sept. 21); 22-23 (October 5), 1971 ⟨I-03886⟩

D., J.F.: Dr. Anna Marion Hilliard. CMAJ 79:295, 1958 ⟨I-04896⟩

D., J.K.M.: Dr. Joseph Bulmer Thackeray. CMAJ, 72:713-4, 1955 ⟨I-04576⟩

D., W.A.: Dr. Vaughan Elderkin Black. CMAJ 35:698, 1936 ⟨I-02874⟩

D., W.J.: Dr. Frederick Bruce Mowbray. CMAJ 25:749, 1931 ⟨I-03152⟩

Dade, C.: Notes on the Cholera Seasons of 1832 and 1834. Canadian Journal of Industry, Science, and Art, No. 37:17-28, 1862 ⟨II-04801⟩

Dailey, R.C.: The Midewiwin, Ontario's First Medical Society. Ontario History 50:133-138, 1958 ⟨II-00607⟩

Dale, J.: 100 Years of Dental Education in Canada: 1875-1975. Ontario Dentist 53(6):33-39, 1976 ⟨II-05457⟩

Daley, H.: "Volunteers in Action" The Prince Edward Island Division Canadian Red Cross Society 1907-1979. np, nd ⟨II-05124⟩

D'Allaire, M.: Origine Sociale des Religieuses de L'Hopital-General de Quebec. Revue d'Histoire de l'Amerique Francaise 23:559-581, 1969-70 ⟨II-04693⟩

D'Allaire, M.: Jeanne-Mance a Montreal en 1642: une femme d'action qui force les evenements. Forces 23:38-46, 1973 ⟨I-04658⟩

Damude, E.F.: The First Ten Years. Toronto, The Physicians' Services Incorporated Foundation, 1980. 139 p. ⟨II-02909⟩

Daniels, P.: "A Certaine Kind of Herbe": Smoking Pipes of the Ontario Iroquois. Rotunda 13(2):4-9, 1980 ⟨II-05367⟩

Darby, G.E.: Indian medicine in British Columbia. CMAJ 28:433-438, 1933 ⟨II-03088⟩

D'Arcy, C.: The Manufacture and Obsolescence of Madness: Age, Social Policy and Psychiatric Morbidity in a Prairie Province. Social Science and Medicine 10:5-13, 1976 ⟨II-05429⟩

Dauphinee, J.A.: Ray Fletcher Farquharson, 1897-1965. PTRSC series 4, 4:83-9, 1966 ⟨I-04774⟩

Daveluy, M.C.: Jeanne Mance. DCB 1-483-487, 1966 ⟨II-00779⟩

Davey, E.L.: Two Decades of Public Service Health. Medical Services Journal, Canada 23:965-983, 1967 ⟨II-04083⟩

David, A.H.: Reminiscences Connected with the Medical Profession in Montreal During the Last Fifty Years. The Canada Medical Record 11:1-8, 1882 ⟨II-00307⟩

Davidson, A.L.: Pharmacopoeial Drug Control in Canada. Canadian Pharmaceutical J 78:53, 73-74, 1945 ⟨II-00261⟩

Davies, J.W.: A Historical Note on the Reverend John Clinch, First Canadian Vaccinator. CMAJ 102(9):957-61, 1970 ⟨I-05292⟩

Davis, D.J.: John Rochfort. DCB 9:681-682, 1976 ⟨I-01226⟩

Davison, J.L.: Dr. Ross as a Man. Canada Lancet 45:331-334, 1912 ⟨I-01146⟩

Day, O.J.: Dr. Robert Francis Rorke. CMAJ 60:203-4, 1949 ⟨I-04493⟩

Deadman, W.J.: James Franklin McLay. CMAJ 26:379, 1932 ⟨I-03062⟩

Deadman, W.J.: Frederick Samuel Lampson Ford, CMG, MD. CMAJ 52:109, 1945 ⟨I-02125⟩

Deadman, W.J.: Douglas Gordon McIlwraith, M.B. CMAJ 58:414, 1948 ⟨I-04510⟩

Deane, R.B.: Frank Hamilton Mewburn. CMAJ 20:306-308, 1929 ⟨I-03453⟩

Deane, R.B.: Augustus L. Jukes: A Pioneer Surgeon. CACHB 2(4):1-4, 1938 ⟨I-01334⟩

Dearing, W.P.: Public Health Across the Border. Canadian Journal of Public Health 43:368-377, 1952 ⟨II-00558⟩

Death, J.: My Cholera Experiences. St. John, N.B., Sun, 1892 ⟨II-00084⟩

Dechene, L., Robert, J.-C.: Le cholera de 1832 dans le Bas-Canada: Mesure des inegalites devant la mort. In: The Great Mortalities: Methodological Studies of Demographic Cries in the Past, edited by H. Charbonneau and A. Larose, pp. 229-56. Liege: Ondina, 1979. ⟨II-05139⟩

Defries, R.D.: Dr. John Gerald FitzGerald. CMAJ 43:190-192, 1940 ⟨I-03362⟩

Defries, R.D.: Dr. Thomas Fraser. CMAJ, 71:401, 1954 ⟨I-04567⟩

Defries, R.D.: Postgraduate Teaching in Public Health in the University of Toronto, 1913-1955. Canadian Journal of Public Health 48:285-294, 1957 ⟨II-00562⟩

Defries, R.D.: A Forgotten Chapter in the Story of the Canadian Public Health Association. Canadian Journal of Public Health 50:83-85, 1959 ⟨II-04004⟩

Defries, R.D.: Dr. Edward Playter - A Vision Fulfilled. Canadian Journal Public Health 50:368-377, 1959 ⟨I-02582⟩

Defries, R.D.: September 22, 1910 -- The Birthdate of the Canadian Public Health Association. Canadian Journal of Public Health 50:120-122, 1959 ⟨II-04082⟩

Defries, R.D.: The Federal and Provincial Health Services in Canada. Toronto, Canadian Public Health Association, 1959. 147 p. ⟨II-05128⟩

Defries, R.D.: The First Forty Years 1914-1955 Connaught Medical Research Laboratories University of Toronto. Toronto, University of Toronto Press, 1968, 342 p. ⟨II-04611⟩

Defries, R.D. (edit.): The Development of Public Health in Canada. Canadian Public Health Association, 1940. pp. 184 ⟨II-00557⟩

De Gaspe, P.A.: Memoires. Montreal, Bibliotheque Canadienne-Francaise, 1971. 435 p. ⟨I-00891⟩

De Kiriline, L.: The Quintuplets' First Year. Toronto, The MacMillan Company of Canada Limited, 1936. 221 p. ⟨II-05001⟩

Delage, C.F.: Arthur Vallee (1882-1939). PTRSC 33:155-157, 1939 ⟨I-03577⟩

Delaney, R.J.: Dr. Robert Meredith Janes: an appreciation. CMAJ 95:1400, 1966 ⟨I-01745⟩

Delaney, R.J.: Dr. Robert Meredith Janes (1894-1966): Professor of Surgery, University of Toronto (1947-1957). Canadian Journal of Surgery 12:1-11, 1969 ⟨I-02551⟩

DeLarue, N.C.: Lung Cancer in Historical Perspective: Lessons from the Past, Implications of Present Experience, Challenges for the Future. Canadian Journal of Surgery 23:549-557, 1980 ⟨II-04331⟩

Delarue, N.C.: Dr. J.R. Frank Mills. CMAJ 125:112, 1981 ⟨I-04557⟩

Dellandrea, J.: Packaging the panacea...Medicine Bottles in Upper Canada. Canadian Collector, May/June 1978, pages 54-57 ⟨II-04802⟩

Delva, P.: Norman Bethune: L'influence de l'hopital du Sacre-Coeur. In: Shephard, D.A.E.; Levesque, A.(edit.): Norman Bethune: His Times and His Legacy. Ottawa, Canadian Public Health Assoc., 1982. pp 85-91 ⟨II-04948⟩

Demers, R.: L'evolution de la rhumatologie au Quebec. L'Union Medicale 108(7):1-10, 1979 ⟨II-02399⟩

Dempsey, H.A.: A Blackfoot winter count. Calgary, Glenbow-Alberta Inst 1965. 20 p. ⟨II-00608⟩

Dempsey, H.A. (Editor): A winter at Fort MacLeod (R.B. Nevitt). Alberta, Glenbow-Alberta Institute, 1974. 134 p. ⟨II-00390⟩

Denholm, K.A.: History of Parry Sound General Hospital. Margaret Higham, 1973, 44 p. ⟨II-04470⟩

Denis, R.: Leon Longtin, M.D., F.R.C.P.(C), 1907-1979. Canadian Anaesthetists Society Journal 27:181-182, 1980 ⟨I-01053⟩

Denny, C.: Blackfoot Magic. The Beaver 275(2):14-15, 1944 ⟨II-03310⟩

De Santana, H.: Danby: Images of Sport. Toronto, Amerley House Limited, 1978. 64 p. ⟨I-01280⟩

Desilets, A.: Luc-Hyacinthe Masson. DCB 10:499-500, 1972 ⟨I-01439⟩

Desilets, A.: Sir Etienne-Paschal Tache. DCB 9:774-779, 1976 ⟨I-02251⟩

Desjardins, B, Beauchamp, P, Legare, J: Automatic Family Reconstitution: the French-Canadian Seventeenth- Century Experience. Journal of Family History 2:56-76, 1977 ⟨II-04790⟩

Desjardins, E.: Donald A. Hingston, 1868-1950. L'UMC 80:3-5, 1951 ⟨I-02527⟩

Desjardins, E.: Sir William Hales Hingston (1829-1907). Canadian Journal of Surgery 2:225-232, 1958-9 ⟨I-04236⟩

Desjardins, E.: La Medecine au Quebec et le Choix de ses Gouverneurs. L'UMC 91:345-348, 1962 ⟨II-02356⟩

Desjardins, E.: Les Origines de la Chirurgie au Canada. L'UMC 94:1445-1448, 1965 ⟨II-00340⟩

Desjardins, E.: B.G. Bourgeois (1877-1943). Canadian Journal of Surgery 9:1-5, 1966 ⟨I-04230⟩

Desjardins, E.: Dr. Gerard Casgrain. CMAJ 95:738, 1966 ⟨I-01560⟩

Desjardins, E.: L'Ecole de Medecine et de Chirurgie de Montreal: Ses Doyens. L'UMC 95:967-977, 1966 ⟨II-02389⟩

Desjardins, E.: L'Ecole D'Amedee Marien Et Ses Eleves Rheaume Et Pare. Canadian Journal of Surgery 9:325-331, 1966 ⟨I-04659⟩

Desjardins, E.: L'Evolution Medicale au Canada. L'UMC 96:1232-1237, 1967 ⟨II-02358⟩

Desjardins, E.: Dr. Charles-Edouard Hebert. CMAJ 98:796-797, 1968 ⟨I-02492⟩

Desjardins, E.: L'Hopital General des Freres Charon a Ville-Marie. L'UMC 98:2108-2112, 1969 ⟨II-02372⟩

Desjardins, E.: L'Odyssee du Sieur Timothee Sylvain, Medecin de Montreal. L'UMC 98:91-94, 1969 ⟨I-02245⟩

Desjardins, E.: L.E. Desjardins (1837-1919): Un Des Pionniers De L'Opthalmologie Au Canada Francais. Canadian Journal of Surgery 12:165-171, 1969 ⟨I-04660⟩

Desjardins, E.: L.E. Desjardins (1837-1919): Un Des Pionniers De L'Ophtalmologie Au Canada Francais. Canadian Journal of Surgery 12:165-171, 1969 ⟨II-04703⟩

Desjardins, E.: La Medecine a Forfait aux Debuts de Ville-Marie. L'UMC 98:239-242, 1969 ⟨II-02454⟩

Desjardins, E.: Le Destin Tragique de Manuscript Historique de Labrie. L'UMC 98:1119-1125, 1969 ⟨I-01772⟩

Desjardins, E: Le Docteur Pierre La Terriere et ses Traverses. L'UMC 98:797-801, 1969 ⟨I-02239⟩

Desjardins, E.: Le Docteur Jean Saucier. CMAJ 100:446-447, 1969 ⟨I-05043⟩

Desjardins, E.: Le Remede Magique d'un Medecin Theosophe. L'UMC 98:444-446, 1969 ⟨II-02350⟩

Desjardins, E.: Deux Medecins Montrealais du XIX Siecle Adeptes de la Pensee Ecologique. L'UMC 99:487-492, 1970 ⟨I-01348⟩

Desjardins, E.: La Grande Epidemie de "Picote Noire". L'UMC 99:1470-1477, 1970 ⟨II-02406⟩

Desjardins, E.: La Profession de foi Politique du Docteur Marc-Pascal Laterriere. L'UMC 99:1294-3000, 1970 ⟨I-02243⟩

Desjardins, E., Dumas, C.: Le Complexe Medical de Louis Riel. L'UMC 99:1870-1878, 1970 ⟨II-02348⟩

Desjardins, E.: Les Honoraries Medicaux D'Antan. L'UMC 99:897-902, 1970 ⟨II-02437⟩

Desjardins, E.: Les Observations Medicales de Jacques Cartier et de Samuel de Champlain. L'UMC 99:677-681, 1970 ⟨II-02351⟩

Desjardins, E.: Les Revendications des Medecins en L'an 1935. L'UMC 99:2077-2081, 1970 ⟨II-02471⟩

Desjardins, E.: Montreal aux Prises en 1847 Avec les Victimes de la Faim. L'UMC 99:305-313, 1970 ⟨II-02357⟩

Desjardins, E.: Et Avant L'Acfas, Il Y Eut La Spaslac. L'UMC 100:1402-1406, 1971 ⟨I-01234⟩

Desjardins, E., Flanagan, E.C., Giroux, S.: Heritage: History of the Nursing Profession in Quebec from the Augustinians and Jeanne Mance to Medicare. Association of Nurses of the Province of Quebec, 1971. 247 p. ⟨II-05255⟩

Desjardins, E.: L'Enseignement Medicale a Montreal au Milieu du XIX Siecle. L'UMC 100:305-309, 1971 ⟨II-02428⟩

Desjardins, E.: L'Epidemie de Cholera de 1832. L'UMC 100:2395-2401, 1971 ⟨II-02410⟩

Desjardins, E.: L'Hotel-Dieu, St. Patrick's Hospital et St. Lawrence School of Medicine. L'UMC 100:1794-1799, 1971 ⟨II-02418⟩

Desjardins, E.: Le Cas D'Alexis Saint-Martin. L'UMC 100:964-968, 1971 ⟨II-00359⟩

Desjardins, E.: Le Centenaire de la Societe Medicale de Montreal. L'UMC 100:1188-1194, 1971 ⟨II-02461⟩

Desjardins, E.: Le Debut de Volume 100 de L'Union Medicale du Canada. L'UMC 100:43-44, 1971 ⟨II-02444⟩

Desjardins, E.: Le premier siecle de L'Union Medicale du Canada. L'UMC 100:2331-33, 1971 ⟨II-05342⟩

Desjardins, E.: Un Duel Resulta D'Une Polemique Autour de L'Hotel-Dieu et du Montreal General Hospital. L'UMC 100:530-535, 1971 ⟨II-02359⟩

Desjardins, E.: La petite histoire du journalisme medical Canadien. L'UMC 101:309-14, 1972; 1190-96, 1972 ⟨II-05421⟩

Desjardins, E.: Trois etapes de la chirurgie: 1872, 1972 et 2002. L'UMC 101:2337-46, 1972 ⟨II-05340⟩

Desjardins, E.: Un precurseur de la recherche medicale au XIX siecle: le docteur Joseph-Alexandre Crevier. L'UMC 101:708-11, 1972 ⟨I-05376⟩

Desjardins, E.: L'Hopital de Jeanne Mance: 1642-1673. L'UMC 102:1136-42, 1973 ⟨II-05346⟩

Desjardins, E.: L'hopital de la Misericorde de Montreal. L'UMC 102:400-05, 1973 ⟨II-05347⟩

Desjardins, E.: L'Universite Laval de Quebec. L'UMC 102:630-35, 1973 ⟨II-05345⟩

Desjardins, E.: La medecine populaire au Canada francais. L'UMC 101:1595-601, 1972;102:154-59, 1973 ⟨II-05344⟩

Desjardins, E.: Le mal de la Baie Saint-Paul. L'UMC 102:2148-52, 1973 ⟨II-05445⟩

Desjardins, E.: Le role social du premier hopital de Montreal. L'UMC 102:1041-42, 1973 ⟨II-05341⟩

Desjardins, E., Lapointe-Manseau, L.: Les chirurgiens de Ville-Marie. L'UMC 102:1934-42, 1973 ⟨II-05389⟩

Desjardins, E.: Les societes de chirurgie du Quebec. L'UMC 103:1749-54, 1973 ⟨II-05444⟩

Desjardins, E.: L'origine de la profession medicale au Quebec. L'UMC 103:918-30, 1112-9, 1279-92, 1974 ⟨II-05447⟩

Desjardins, E.: La profession medicale au Quebec. L'UMC 103:1279-92, 1450-8, 1974 ⟨II-05446⟩

Desjardins, E.: La vieille Ecole de Medecine Victoria. L'UMC 103:117-25, 1974 ⟨II-05453⟩

Desjardins, E.: Histoire de la Profession Medicale au Quebec:XI la Mission de Dom Smeulders. L'UMC 104:810-819, 1975 ⟨II-00544⟩

Desjardins, E.: Historie de la profession medicale au Quebec. L'UMC 104(7):1137-42, 1975 ⟨II-05329⟩

Desjardins, E.: Francis Badgley. DCB 9:16-17, 1976 ⟨I-00986⟩

Desjardins, E.: L'evolution de l'ophthalmologie au Quebec. L'UMC 105:803-12, 1976 ⟨II-05230⟩

Desjardins, E.: L'evolution de l'ophthalmologie a Montreal: III. L'UMC 105:1101-12, 1976 ⟨II-05231⟩

Desjardins, E.: l'evolution de la chirurgie a Montreal: II. L'UMC 105(10)1564, 1566, 1568, 1976 ⟨II-05232⟩

Desjardins, E.: L'evolution de l'ophthalmologie au Quebec: II. L'UMC 105:846, 848-9, 851, 1976 ⟨II-05237⟩

Desjardins, E.: L'evolution de la chirurgie a Montreal (1843-1949). L'UMC 105:1398-410, 1976 ⟨II-05286⟩

Desjardins, E.: Les conseillers en droit canonique de l'Ecole de Medecine Victoria. L'UMC 105:626-30, 1976 ⟨II-05233⟩

Desjardins, E.: L'evolution de la medecine interne a Montreal, le premier centenaire (1820-1920). L'UMC 106:237-58, 1977 ⟨II-05238⟩

Desjardins, E.: L'evolution de l'opthalmologie au Quebec: IV. L'UMC 106:101-8, 1977 ⟨II-05239⟩

Desjardins, E.: L'evolution de la medecine a Montreal: III. L'UMC 106:752, 755-58, 749-50, 1977 ⟨II-05240⟩

Desjardins, E.: L'evolution de la medecine a Montreal. IV. L'UMC 106:892-900, 902, 904, 1977 ⟨II-05242⟩

Desjardins, E.: L'Evolution de la medecine au Quebec. L'UMC 106:1284-315, 1977 ⟨II-05245⟩

Desjardins, E.: L'Evolution de la medecine a Montreal. L'UMC 106:1027-52, 1977 ⟨II-05246⟩

Desjardins, E.: L'Evolution de la chirurgie au Quebec. L'UMC 106:1198-211, 1977 ⟨II-05247⟩

Desjardins, E.: L'evolution de la medecine au Quebec: VII. L'UMC 106:1416-38, 1977 ⟨II-05249⟩

Desjardins, E.: L'evolution de la medecine au Quebec: VIII. L'UMC 106:1537-56, 1977 ⟨II-05250⟩

Desjardins, E.: Biographies de medecins du Quebec. L'UMC 107:873-8, 1978 ⟨II-05357⟩

Desjardins, E.: Joseph Emery-Coderre. DCB 11:302-303, 1982 ⟨I-04869⟩

Desjardins, E.: Jacques Denechaud. DCB 5:248-249, 1983 ⟨I-05312⟩

Desloges, A.H., Ranger, J.A.: Historique de la Lutte Antivenerienne dans la Province de Quebec. L'UMC 61:235-242, 1932 ⟨II-02442⟩

Des Roches, B.P.: The First 100 Years of Pharmacy in Ontario. Canadian Pharmaceutical Journal 23:225-27, 1972 ⟨II-05420⟩

Dewar, G.F.: Dr. Stephen Rice Jenkins: an appreciation. CMAJ 21:620-621, 1929 ⟨I-02275⟩

Dickinson, J.A.: The Pre-contact Huron Population. A Reappraisal. Ontario History 72:173-179, 1980 ⟨II-01800⟩

Dickson, I.: The Canadian Psychiatric Association, 1951-1958. Canadian Journal of Psychiatry 25:86-97, 1980 ⟨II-00446⟩

Dionne, L.: Hommage Au Docteur Jacques Turcot. Canadian Journal of Surgery 20:567, 1977 ⟨I-04289⟩

Dittrick, H.: The Old Days in Toronto. CACHB 7(4):6-9, 1943 ⟨II-00271⟩

Dittrick, H.: Our family doctor, the Mayor. CACHB 10:160-163, 1946 ⟨I-01266⟩

Dodd, D.: The Hamilton Birth Control Clinic of the 1930's. Ontario History 75:71-86, 1983 ⟨II-05093⟩

Dolgoy, M: The First Ten Years of the College of General Practice (Alberta Division). Canadian Family Physician 15:71-76, 1969 ⟨II-04081⟩

Dollar, H.: Dr. Lillias Cringan McIntyre. CMAJ 97:760, 1967 ⟨I-02849⟩

Dolman, C.E.: The Reverend James Bovell, M.D. 1817-1880. In: G.F.G. Stanley(edit.): Pioneers of Canadian Science Toronto, University of Toronto Press, 1966 ⟨I-02496⟩

Dolman, C.E.: James Bovell. DCB 10:83-85, 1972 ⟨I-00011⟩

Dolman, C.E.: The Donald T. Fraser Memorial Lecture, 1973. Landmarks and Pioneers in the Control of Diptheria. Canadian Journal of Public Health 64:317-36, 1973 ⟨II-05443⟩

Donaldson, B.: Dr. Manchester of New Westminster. CACHB 20:81-88, 1956 ⟨I-03428⟩

Donaldson, B.: L'Hotel Dieu de Quebec. CACHB 21:57-62, 1956 ⟨II-00198⟩

Donaldson, B.: Rae's wintering home. CACHB 20(4):95-99, 1956 ⟨II-00393⟩

Donaldson, B.: Hotel Dieu de Montreal. CACHB 21:112-122, 1957 ⟨II-00197⟩

Dorward, C.: Below the Flight Path. A History of the Royal Alexandra Hospital and School of Nursing. Edmonton, Royal Alexandra Hospital, 1968. ⟨II-05103⟩

Douglas, J.: Journals and Reminiscences of James Douglas, M.D. New York, 1910. 254 p. ⟨II-04222⟩

Douglas, J.: The Status of Women in New England and New France. Queen's Quarterly 19:359-374, 1911-12 ⟨II-02337⟩

Douglass, M.E.: A pioneer woman doctor of Western Canada (C.Ross). Manitoba Medical Review 27:255-256, 1947 ⟨I-02577⟩

Douville, R.: Jacques Dugay. DCB 2:202-203, 1969 ⟨I-01019⟩

Douville, R.: Andre Arnoux. DCB 3:18-20, 1974 ⟨I-00031⟩

Douville, R.: Charles Alavoine. DCB 3:7-8, 1974 ⟨I-00032⟩

Doyle, F.P.: The French Canadian Contribution to the Health Services of Canada. Winnipeg Clinic Quarterly 20:56-62, 1967 ⟨II-04075⟩

Drake, D.: A Systematic Treatise, historical, etiological and practical, on the Principal Diseases of the Interior Valley of North America, as they appear in the Caucasian, African, Indian, and Esquimaux Varieties of its Population. Cincinnati, Winthrop B. Smith and Co., Publishers, 1850, 878 p. ⟨II-00231⟩

Draper, H.H.: The Aboriginal Eskimo Diet in Modern Perspective. American Anthropologist 79:309-316, 1977 ⟨II-04998⟩

Drolet, A.: Adrien Du Chesne. DCB 1:287, 1966 ⟨I-01007⟩

Drolet, A.: Florent Bonnemere. DCB 1:107-108, 1966 ⟨I-00998⟩

Drolet, A.: Louis Chartier. DCB 1:201, 1966 ⟨I-00932⟩

Drolet, A.: Louis Maheut. DCB 1:479-480, 1966 ⟨I-01456⟩

Drolet, A.: Quelques remedes indigenes a travers la correspondance de Mere Sainte- Helene. Cahiers Histoire 22:30-7, 1970 ⟨II-05454⟩

Drummond, W.H.: Pioneers of Medicine in the Province of Quebec. Montreal Medical Journal 27:646-653, 1898 ⟨II-04080⟩

Dube, J.E.: Dr. David James Evans, an appreciation. CMAJ 19:501-502, 1928 ⟨I-03496⟩

Dube, J.E.: Le Passe -- Leur Evolution -- Le Present. L'UMC 61:144-234, 1932 ⟨II-02373⟩

Dube, J.E.: 1636-1936: Celebration, A L'Hotel-Dieu de Montreal, du Tricentenaire de la Fondation de L'Institut des Religieuses Hospitalieres de Saint-Joseph, a la Fleche, France. L'UMC 65:547-556, 1936 ⟨II-02361⟩

Dubin, I.N.: A Letter From John McCrae to Maude Abbott: January 9, 1918. Perspectives in Biology and Medicine 24:667-669, 1981 ⟨I-04193⟩

Duchaussois, P.: The Grey Nuns in the Far North (1867-1917). Toronto, McClelland and Stewart, 1919 pp. 287 ⟨II-05262⟩

Duchesne, R.: Problemes d'histoire des sciences au Canada francais. Institut d'histoire et de sociopolitique des sciences/Universite de Montreal, 1978. 13 p. ⟨II-02404⟩

Duclos, L.: Agathe Veronneau. DCB 3:643, 1974 ⟨I-01194⟩

Duff, G.L.: William Boyd: a Biographical Sketch. Laboratory Investigation 5:389-395, 1956 ⟨I-04758⟩

Dufour, P., Hamelin, J.: Pierre de Sales Laterriere. DCB 5:735-738, 1983 ⟨I-05298⟩

Dufresne, R.: L'Ecole de Medecine et de Chirurgie de Montreal (1843-1891). L'UMC 75:1314-1325, 1946 ⟨II-02390⟩

Dufresne, R.R.: Leon Gerin-Lajoie. CMAJ 80:398, 1959 ⟨I-02248⟩

Dulong, G.: Medecine Populaire au Canada Francais. In International Conress for the History of Medicine, 25th, Quebec, 1976. Proceedings, volume II, 1976. p. 625-633 ⟨II-00223⟩

Dumas, A.: La Medecine et Mon Temps. Recherches Sociographiques 16:21-41, 1975 ⟨II-04689⟩

Dumas, C.: Considerations historiques sur la psychiatrie au Quebec. L'UMC 101:2636-40, 1972 ⟨II-05339⟩

Dumas, P.: Un Medecin-Psychiatre Qui Avait Ete Poete, Gullaume LaHaise et Son Double, Guy Delahaye. L'UMC 100:321-326, 1971 ⟨I-02230⟩

Dumas, P.: William Osler et la Bibliotheca Osleriana. L'UMC 100:539-545, 1971 ⟨II-00142⟩

Dumas, P.: Les neuf redacteurs en chef de l'union Medicale du Canada. L'UMC 101:303-8, 1972 ⟨II-05338⟩

Dumas, P.: Jean-Baptiste Meilleur, medecin, chimiste, publiciste et educateur. L'UMC 102:406-13, 1973 ⟨I-05375⟩

Duncan, D.: The Doctor's Home. Canadian [Antique] Collector 13:22-27, 1978 ßii-00791⟩

Duncan, K.: Irish Famine, Immigration and the Social Structure of Canada West. Canadian Review of Sociology and Anthropology 2:19-40, 1964-5 ⟨II-00221⟩

Duncan, L.M.C.: Gordon L. Anderson. CMAJ 125:1059, 1981 ⟨I-04650⟩

Duncan, N.: Dr. Grenfell's Parish: the deep sea fisherman. New York/Chicago/Toronto, Fleming H. Revell Co., 1905. 155 p. ⟨II-00487⟩

Dunham, H.S.: Model Hospital By-Laws. Ontario Medical Review 35:417-18, 1968 ⟨II-04078⟩

Dunham, H.S.: P.S.I. is born. Ontario Medical Review 35:151-52, 1968 ⟨II-03808⟩

Dunham, H.S.: The London Meeting [of the O.M.A.]. Ontario Medical Review 35:310-11, 1968 ⟨II-04077⟩

Dunham, H.S.: The Ottawa Meeting [of the O.M.A.]. Ontario Medical Review 35:361-62, 1968 ⟨II-04076⟩

Dunham, H.S.: Voices for the G.P. Ontario Medical Review 35:259-60, 1968 ⟨II-04079⟩

Dunlop, A.: Dunlop of that Ilk. Glasgow, Kerr and Richardson, Ltd., 1898, 150 p. ⟨I-04436⟩

Dunlop, W.: Recollections of the American War 1812-1814. Toronto, Historical Publishing Co., 1905. 112 p. ⟨I-01176⟩

Dunn, M.: The Medical Archives Inventory Project. In: Jarrell, R.A.; Ball, N.R.: Science, Technology, and Canadian History. Waterloo, Wilfrid Laurier Univ. Press, 1980. pp 202-205 ⟨II-00203⟩

Dunn, M., Baldwin, M. (edit): A Directory of Medical Archives in Ontario. Toronto, The Hannah Institute for the History of Medicine, 1983. ⟨II-05280⟩

Dupuis, N.F.: A sketch of the history of the medical college at Kingston during the first 25 years of its existence. Kingston, s.n. 1879? ⟨II-00310⟩

Durley, M.S.: Dr. Edmund Bailey O'Callaghan, His Early Years in Medicine, Montreal 1823-1828. Canadian Catholic Historical Association 47:23-40, 1980 ⟨I-04558⟩

Dussault, G.: Les Medecins du Quebec (1940-1970). Recherches Sociographiques 16:69-84, 1975 ⟨II-04688⟩

Duthie, M.: Unsung Heroines: Alberta Nurses in Foreign Fields. CACHB 20:88-95, 1956 ⟨II-00774⟩

DuVernet, S.: The Muskoka Tree: Poems of Pride for Norman Bethune. Bracebridge, Herald-Gazette Press, 1976, 73 p. ⟨I-04440⟩

Dyster, B.: William Charles Gwynne. DCB 10:325-326, 1972 ⟨I-01387⟩

E

E., G.B.: Dr. J. Christopher Colbeck. CMAJ 91:403, 1964 ⟨I-02040⟩

E., H.S.: Dr. Hugh Pius O'Neill. CMAJ 95:1331, 1966 ⟨I-02291⟩

Eager, E.: Wheat, Medicare and Gerrymander in the Saskatchewan Election of 1971. Lakehead University Review 5:7-16, 1972 ⟨II-04811⟩

Eaton, R.D.: Taeniasis in Southern Alberta, 1894-1900. CMAJ 115(10):976, 979, 981; 1976 ⟨II-05252⟩

Ebbs, J.H.: The History of the Canadian Pediatric Society. CMAJ 76:662-664, 1957 ⟨II-04074⟩

Ebbs, J.H.: R. Tait McKenzie: Medical Contributions. In: Davidson, S.A.; Blackstock, P. (edit) : The R. TAit McKenzie Memorial Addresses. Canadian Association for Health, Physical Education and Recreation, 1980. pp 42-44 ⟨II-00377⟩

Ebbs, J.H.: The Canadian Paediatric Society: its early years. CMAJ 123:1235-1237, 1980 ⟨II-02982⟩

Edgar, P.: Sir Andrew Macphail 1864-1938. PTRSC 33:147-149, 1939 ⟨I-03573⟩

Edgar, P.: Sir Andrew Macphail. Queen's Quarterly 54:8-22, 1947 ⟨I-02128⟩

Editorial: Doctor Joseph Workman. Canadian Practitioner 14:14, 1889 ⟨I-04422⟩

Editorial: T.C. Routley. CMAJ 88:816, 1963 ⟨I-02600⟩

Edmison, J.H., Baragar, C.A.: Charles Perry Templeton, CBE, DSO, VD, MD, CM. CMAJ 21:238, 1929 ⟨I-02699⟩

Edward, M.L.: Reflections of Dr. Mary Lee Edward. N,p., 1977. ⟨I-05379⟩

Edwards, G.T.: Oolachen Time in Bella Coola. The Beaver, 309(2):32-37, 1978 ⟨II-00633⟩

Edwards, G.T.: Indian Spaghetti. The Beaver, Autumn 1979. pp. 4-11. ⟨II-00219⟩

Edwards, G.T.: Bella Coola Indian and European Medicines. The Beaver 311(3):4-11, 1980 ⟨II-03619⟩

Eisen, D.: Diary of a Medical Student. Canadian Jewish Congress, 1974. 133 p. ⟨II-05010⟩

Elliott, J.H.: The history of a great Canadian military hospital. CMAJ 40:396-397, 1939 ⟨II-03593⟩

Elkin, SJ: Hospital Practice in the Early Nineties. Manitoba Medical Review 46:466-67, 1966 ⟨II-04063⟩

Elliot, A.J.: Dr. Walter Walker Wright. CMAJ 98:1157-1158, 1968 ⟨I-01723⟩

Elliot, G.R.F.: (Wallace Wilson). British Columbia Medical Journal 8:233, 1966 ⟨I-03401⟩

Elliott, H.: Dr. O.W. Stewart. CMAJ, 63:618, 1950 ⟨I-04513⟩

Elliott, J.H.: Albert Durrant Watson, M.D. CMAJ 16:991-992, 1926 ⟨I-01954⟩

Elliott, J.H.: The Early Records of the University of Toronto Medical Society. University of Toronto Medical Journal 9:225-229, 1932 ⟨II-04061⟩

Elliott, J.H.: William Tempest, MB, LMB, UC 1819-1871. Ontario Medical Association Bulletin 5:37-47, 1938 ⟨I-04762⟩

Elliott, J.H.: Colonel Alexander John Mackenzie, BA, LLB, MB, FACP, VD. CMAJ 40:409, 1939 ⟨I-02842⟩

Elliott, J.H.: John Gilchrist: A pioneer New England Physician in Canada. BHM 7:737-750, 1939 ⟨I-02775⟩

Elliott, J.H., Revell, D.G.: Medical Pioneering in Alberta (James Delamere Lafferty). CACHB 6(1):11-12, 1941 ⟨I-01306⟩

Elliott, J.H.: Osler's Class at the Toronto School of Medicine. CMAJ 47:161-165, 1942 ⟨II-00272⟩

Elliott, J.H.: Rolph Bidwell Lesslie, MA, MD. CMAJ 49:527-529, 1943 ⟨I-03037⟩

Elliott, J.M.: The Early English Surgeons of Quebec. Laval Medical 30:78-84, 1960 ⟨II-04062⟩

Elliott, M.R., Defries, R.D.: The Manitoba Department of Health and Public Welfare. Canadian Journal of Public Health 49:458-69, 1958 ⟨II-04059⟩

Emery, G.: Ontario's Civil Registration of Vital Statistics, 1869-1926: The Evolution of an Administrative System. Canadian Historical Review 64:468-493, 1983 ⟨II-05416⟩

England, F.R.: Dr. James Perrigo. CMAJ 18:757, 1928 ⟨I-02586⟩

Entin, M.A.: Dr. William Vernon Cone: an appreciation. McGill Medical Journal 29:63-69, 1960 ⟨I-02012⟩

E.R.: Dr. William Osler Abbott. CMAJ 49:447, 1943 ⟨I-04264⟩

Erb, T.: The Founding of the Medical School at Queen's. CAMSI Journal 24:39-40, 1965 (Apr) ⟨II-00311⟩

Erichsen-Brown, C.: Use of Plants for the past 500 years. Aurora, Breezy Creeks Press, 1979. 510 p. ⟨II-00051⟩

Ettinger, G.H.: Queen's University. CAMSI Journal 14:11-12, 1955 (Feb) ⟨II-00312⟩

Ettinger, G.H.: The Origins of Support for Medical Research in Canada. CMAJ 78:471-474, 1958 ⟨II-04060⟩

Etziony, M.B.: History of the Montreal Clinical Society, 1923-1963. n.p., - n.d., 50 p. ⟨II-05008⟩

Evans, A.M., Barker, C.A.V.: Century One: A History of the Ontario Veterinary Association 1874-1974. Guelph, A.M. Evans, C.A.V. Barker, 1976. 516 p. ⟨II-05386⟩

Evans, EH: Thoughts on Therapy after Twenty-Five Years in General Practice. Applied Therapeutics, 725-726, 730-734, 1961 ⟨II-04058⟩

Everett, H.S.: Dr. John Calef, Physician, Naval and Military Surgeon and Statesman. CMAJ 72:390-391, 1955 ⟨I-01547⟩

Everett, H.S.: The First Case of Pernicious Anaemia Successfully Treated in Canada. CMAJ 75:449-450, 1956 ⟨II-01793⟩

Ewen, J.: China Nurse 1932-1939. Toronto, McClelland and Stewart Ltd., 1981. 162 p. ⟨II-03850⟩

Ewing, M.: Influence of the Edinburgh Medical School on the Early Development of McGill University. Canadian Journal of Surgery 18:287-296, 1975 ⟨II-04333⟩

F

F., E.M., S., W.R.: Dr. P.A. Creelman, an appreciation. CMAJ 76:998, 1957 ⟨I-04733⟩

F., R.: Dr. Charles C. Stewart. CMAJ 78:551-552, 1958 ⟨I-01655⟩

F., T.L.: Dr. John Fenton Argue, an appreciation. CMAJ 75:456, 1956 ⟨I-04736⟩

F.A.C.: Dr. George Joshua Gillam. CMAJ 46:200, 1942 ⟨I-04274⟩

Fahrni, G.: Dr. Gordon Fahrni: reminiscing on 70 years of medicine. CMAJ 125:94-97, 1981 ⟨I-04555⟩

Fahrni, G.S.: (Wallace Wilson). British Columbia Medical Journal 8:231, 1966 ⟨I-03403⟩

Fahrni, G.S.: Prairie Surgeon. Winnipeg, Queenston House Publishing, Inc., 1976. 138 p. ⟨II-00413⟩

Fahrni, G.S.: The Medical Class of 1911. University of Manitoba Medical Journal 68-72, 1980 ⟨II-03637⟩

Falconer, J.W.: Dr. John Stewart. CMAJ 30:224, 1934 ⟨I-01717⟩

Falconer, R.A.: Charles Kirk Clarke, M.B., M.D., LL.D. CMAJ 14:349, 1924 ⟨I-02994⟩

Falk, L.A., Cameron, S.: Some Black Medical History: Dr. Martin R. Delany's Canadian Years as Medical Practitioner and Abolitionist (1856-1864). Based on a presentation to the 25th International Congress of the History of Medicine, August 24, 1976, at Laval University, Quebec, Canada ⟨II-01896⟩

Fallis, A.M.: John L. Todd: Canada's First Professor of Parasitology. CMAJ 129:486, 488-89, 1983 ⟨I-05213⟩

Farish, G.W.T.: A medical biography of the Bond-Farish family. CMAJ 23:696-698, 1930 ⟨I-03169⟩

Farley, M., Keel, O., Limoges, C.: Les Commencements de L'Administration Montrealaise de la Sante Publique (1865-1885). HSTC Bulletin 6:85-109, 1982 ⟨II-04911⟩

Farmer, G.R.D.: Dr. William James Deadman. CMAJ 92:1322, 1965 ⟨I-01466⟩

Farmer, M.H.: The ledger of an early doctor of Barton and Ancaster, 1798-1801. Wentworth Bygones 8:34-38, 1969 ⟨I-02987⟩

Farquharson, R.F.: Dr. John Hepburn, an appreciation. CMAJ 74:943, 1956 ⟨I-04727⟩

Farquharson, R.F.: The Medical Research Council of Canada. CMAJ 85:1194-1204, 1961 ⟨II-04057⟩

Farrar, C.B.: Dr. Charles D. Parfitt M.D. CMAJ 66:294, 1952 ⟨I-04548⟩

Farrar, C.B.: Dr. Norman B. Gwyn. CMAJ 66:401-2, 1952 ⟨I-04542⟩

F[arrar], C.B.: I Remember C.K. Clarke, 1857-1957. American Journal of Psychiatry 114:368-370, 1957 ⟨I-02007⟩

Farrar, C.B.: The Early Days of Treatment of Mental Patients in Canada. CAMSI Journal 21:13-15, 1962 (Feb) ⟨II-00168⟩

F[arrar], C.B.: I. Remember J.G. Fitzgerald. American Journal of Psychiatry 120:49-52, 1963 ⟨I-02791⟩

Farrar, C.B.: Osler's Story of "The Baby on the Track". CMAJ 90:781-784, 1964 ⟨II-05281⟩

Farrar, C.B.: Trevor Owen, M.B., FRCP (Lond), FRCP (C), an appreciation. CMAJ 93:1375-1376, 1965 ⟨I-02287⟩

Fauteux, A.E., Massicotte, E.Z., Bertrand, C. (editors): Annales De L'Hotel-Dieu de Montreal. Montreal, L'Imprimerie Des Editeurs Limitee, 1921, 252 p. ⟨II-04706⟩

Favreau, J.C.: Dr. J. Edouard Samson, an appreciation. CMAJ 89:832, 1963 ⟨I-01991⟩

Feasby, W.R.: Official History of the Canadian Medical Services 1939-1945, Vol. 2 -- Clinical Subjects. Ottawa, Edmond Cloutier, 1953. 537 p. ⟨II-00797⟩

Feasby, W.R.: Official History of the Canadian Medical Services 1939-1945, Vol 1 -- Organization and Campaigns. Ottawa, Edmond Cloutier, 1956. 568 p. ⟨II-00796⟩

Feasby, W.R.: The Discovery of Insulin. JHMAS 13:68-84, 1958 ⟨II-00104⟩

Feasby, W.R.: Professor William Boyd. Medical Post, Aug 16, Aug 30, Sept 13, 1966 ⟨I-02059⟩

Feindel, W: Highlights of Neurosurgery in Canada. JAMA 200:853-59, 1967 ⟨II-04055⟩

Feindel, W.: Wilder Penfield (1891-1976): The Man and His Work. Neurosurgery 1:93-100, 1977 ⟨I-01228⟩

Feindel, W.: The Contributions of Wilder Penfield and the Montreal Neurological Institute to Canadian Neurosciences. In: Roland, C.G. (ed): Health, Disease and Medicine: Essays in Canadian History. Toronto, Hannah Institute for the History of Medicine, 1984, 347-358. ⟨I-05369⟩

Fenton, W.N.: Contacts between Iroquois herbalism and colonial medicine. Annual Report Smithsonian Institution, 1941-42, pp 502-528 ⟨II-00609⟩

Ferguson, A.H.: Apneumatosis. Manitoba, Northwest and B.C. Lancet 1:163-165, 1888 ⟨I-01332⟩

Ferguson, C.C.: One Hundred Years of Surgery 1883-1983. Winnipeg, Peguis Publishers Limited ⟨II-05097⟩

Ferguson, J.: History of the Ontario Medical Association, 1880-1930. Toronto, Murray Printing Co. Ltd., 1930. 142 p. ⟨II-00452⟩

Ferguson, J.K.W.: Canadian Milestones in Medical Research. Bulletin of the Medical Library Association 48:21-26, 1960 ⟨II-04054⟩

Ferguson, J.K.W.: Dr. H. Ward Smith, an appreciation. CMAJ 97:552-553, 1967 ⟨I-01674⟩

Ferguson, R.G.: Dr. William Hall. CMAJ 30:578, 1934 ⟨I-03539⟩

Ferguson, R.G.: Dr. D.A. Stewart. CMAJ 36:435, 1937 ⟨I-03441⟩

Fetherstonhaugh, R.C.: No. 3 Canadian General Hospital (McGill), 1914-1919. Montreal, The Gazette Printing Co., 1928. 274 p. ⟨II-00811⟩

Fiddes, G.W.J.: He Took Down His Shingle (A Backward Look at the Indian Medicine Man). Canadian Journal of Public Health 56:400-401, 1965 ⟨II-04053⟩

Fiddes, J., Jaques, L.B.: Reminiscences. Saskatoon, University of Saskatchewan (Dept. of Physiology and Pharmacology), 1970. 101 p. ⟨II-00695⟩

Fieber, F.: Natural Medicines of the Cree Indians. The Beaver, 309(4):57-59, 1979 ⟨II-00634⟩

Fielden, E.C.: The Academy on its Fiftieth Anniversary. Bulletin of the Academy of Medicine, Toronto 30:33-46, 1956 ⟨II-04052⟩

Finley, F.G.: Col. James Alexander Hutchison, MD: an appreciation. CMAJ 21:237, 1929 ⟨I-01740⟩

Firth, D.C.: A Tale of Two Cities: Montreal and the Smallpox Epidemic of 1885. Thesis (M.A.), Ottawa, University of Ottawa, 1983. ⟨II-05417⟩

Fiset, P-A.: Une Correspondance Medicale Historique: Blake a Davidson. Laval Medical 23:419-448, 1957 ⟨II-02425⟩

Fish, A.H.: The meeting of the Canadian Medical Association, August 12th and 13th, 1889, Banff, Alberta. CACHB 8(3):10-12, 1943 ⟨II-00453⟩

Fish, A.H.: Dr. William Henry Drummond 1854-1907. CACHB 12:1-8, 1947 ⟨I-01196⟩

Fish, A.H.: Doctor Park of Cochrane. CACHB 13:55-61, 1948 ⟨I-01230⟩

Fish, F.G.: The Vancouver General Hospital and its Forebears. Canadian Hospital 23:34-37, 1946 ⟨II-04051⟩

Fish, F.H.: Dr. Norman Bethune 1889-1939. CACHB 10(4):151-159, 1946 ⟨I-00946⟩

Fish, F.H.: Medical Education in Canada. CACHB 17:45-54, 1952 ⟨II-00245⟩

Fisher, A.J.: The First Canadian Army Medical Corps. CACHB 4(3):4-12, 1939 ⟨II-00812⟩

Fisher, A.W.: Dr. Donald Blair Fraser, An Ontario Physician. CACHB 13(2):35-38, 1948 ⟨I-01215⟩

Fisher, T.L.: Health Insurance and Associated Medical Services Incorporated. CMAJ 40:284-289, 1939 ⟨II-03592⟩

Fishman, N.: Harold Benge Atlee. CMAJ 121:1439, 1441, 1979 ⟨I-00017⟩

Fishman, N.: John Bell, MD - Teacher to William Osler. CMAJ: 1981, 125:1042-44 ⟨I-04766⟩

Fisk, G.H.: Malaria and the Anopheles Mosquito in Canada. CMAJ :679-683, 1931 ⟨II-01839⟩

Fitz, R.: The Surprising Career of Peter la Terriere, Bachelor in Medicine. Annals of Medical History 3rd series, 3:265-282, 395-417, 1941 ⟨I-01974⟩

Fitzgerald, J.G.: Doctor Peter H. Bryce. Canadian Public Health Journal 23:88-91, 1932 ⟨I-05297⟩

Flanagan, T.E.: Louis Riel: A Case Study in Involuntary Psychiatric Confinement. Canadian Psychiatric Association Journal 23:463-8, 1978 ⟨II-05256⟩

Fleming, G.: Dr. Charles John Collwell Oliver Hastings. CMAJ 24:473, 1931 ⟨I-03044⟩

Fleming, M.W.: The Halifax Visiting Dispensary -- 100 Years Old. Nova Scotia Medical Bulletin 36:106-09, 1957 ⟨II-04050⟩

Fletcher, A.: Dr. Wallace Graham: an appreciation. CMAJ 88:222-223, 1963 ⟨I-02140⟩

Fletcher, A.A.: Early Clinical Experiences with Insulin. CMAJ 87:1052-1055, 1962 ⟨II-04049⟩

Foerster, D.K.: Alexander McPhedran. University of Toronto Medical Journal 28:244-248, 1951 ⟨I-02302⟩

Foley, A.R.: Half a Century of Diptheria Prevalence in Quebec. Canadian Public Health Journal 33:198-204, 1942 ⟨II-04047⟩

Fontaine, R.: Professor Wilfrid Derome. CMAJ 26:122, 1932 ⟨I-01035⟩

Foran, J.K.: Jeanne Mance or "The Angel of the Colony" Foundress of the Hotel Dieu Hospital, Montreal, Pioneer Nurse of North America 1642-1673. Montreal, The Herald Press, Ltd., 1931, 192 p. ⟨I-04427⟩

Forbes, E.R.: Prohibition and the Social Gospel in Nova Scotia. Acadiensis 1:11-36, 1971 ⟨II-00461⟩

Ford, F.S.L.: William Dunlop. Toronto, Murray Printing Co., 1931. 57 p. ⟨I-01960⟩

Ford, F.S.L.: William Dunlop, 1792-1848. CMAJ 25:210-19, 1931 ⟨I-03153⟩

Ford, F.S.L.: William Dunlop. Toronto, Albert Britnel Book Shop, 1934. 60 p. ⟨I-00888⟩

Forgues, L.C.: Dr. Jessie A. McGeachy. CMAJ 94:923-924, 1966 ⟨I-03209⟩

Forsey, R.R.: J. Frederick Burgess. CMAJ 68:625, 1953 ⟨I-04529⟩

Forsey, R.R.: History of the Canadian Dermatological Association. Archives of Dermatology 91:486-492, 1965 ⟨II-04048⟩

Forster, J.M.: The Origin and Development of Nursing in the Ontario Hospitals and the Outlook. Ontario Journal of Neuropsychiatry 3:31-33, 1923 ⟨II-00775⟩

Fortier, A.: Bio-Bibliographie du Professor L.-E. Fortier. Ecole de Bibliothecaires, de l'Universite de Montreal, 1952. 39 p. n.p. ⟨II-02477⟩

Fortier, A.: Histoire de la profession dentaire dans la metropole. Journal of the Canadian Dental Association 18:384-387, 1952 ⟨II-05198⟩

Fortier, B.: The Canadian Pediatric Society -- La Societe canadienne de pediatrie (1922-1972). La Vie Medicale au Canada Francais 2:573-587, 670-682, 1072-1091, 1973 ⟨II-02479⟩

Fortier, de la Broquerie: Histoire de la pediatrie au Quebec. Vie Medicale au Canada Francais 1:400-5; 705-16; 795-810, 1972 ⟨II-05435⟩

Fortier, de la Broquerie: La Societe canadienne de Pediatrie (1922-1972). Vie Medicale au Canada Francais 2:573-4, 1973 ⟨II-05436⟩

Fortier, de la Broquerie: La Protection de l'enfance au Canada francais du XVIIIe siecle jusquau debut du XXe siecle. In: International Congress of the History of Medicine, 24th, Budapest, 1974. Acta. Budapest, 1976. pp 157-71 ⟨II-05243⟩

Fortier, L.E.: "Hotel-Dieu de Montreal". La Revue Medicale du Canada 6:350-354, 1902 ⟨II-02421⟩

Fortin-Morisset, C.: Catherine Jeremie. DCB 3:314-315, 1974 ⟨I-01011⟩

Fortin-Morisset, C.: Hubert-Joseph de la Croix. DCB 3:334, 1974 ⟨I-01316⟩

Fortuine, R.: Doctors Afield: John Rae, Surgeon to the Hudson's Bay Company. New England Journal of Medicine 268:37-39, 1963 ⟨I-01577⟩

Fortuine, R.: The Health of the Eskimos, as Portrayed in the Earliest Written Accounts. BHM 45:97-114, 1971 ⟨II-00610⟩

Fortune, R.: Doctors Afield: John Rae, Surgeon to the Hudson's Bay Company. New England Journal of Medicine 268:37-39, 1963 ⟨II-01786⟩

Fotheringham, J.T.: Frederick LeMaitre Grasett. CMAJ 22:596, 1930 ⟨I-03012⟩

Foucher, A.A.: A Page of History: The Origin, Evolution and Present Condition of the Practice of Medicine in Canada. Montreal Medical Journal 33:841-55, 1904 ⟨II-04046⟩

Foucher, A.A.: Origine -- Evolution -- Etat Actuel de la Medecine au Canada. L'UMC 33:388-408, 1904 ⟨II-02352⟩

Foulkes, R.A.: British Columbia Mental Health Services: Historical Perspective to 1961. CMAJ 85:649-655, 1961 ⟨II-00846⟩

Foulkes, R.G.: Medics in the North. Medical Services Journal, Canada 18:523-550, 1962 ⟨II-04045⟩

Fournet, P.A.: Mere de la Nativite et les Origines des Soeurs de Misericorde, 1848-1898. Montreal, Institution des Sourds-Muets, 1898 ⟨II-02480⟩

Fox, J.G.: The History of Provincial Health Laboratory Services in Manitoba. University of Manitoba Medical Journal 49:118-124, 1979 ⟨II-01799⟩

Francis, D.: The Development of the Lunatic Asylum in the Maritime Provinces. Acadiensis 6:23-38, 1976-77 ⟨II-01528⟩

Francis, W.W.: Colin Russel, the Man. CMAJ 77:716-718, 1957 ⟨I-04714⟩

Francis, W.W.: Repair of Cleft Palate by Philibert Roux in 1819. A Translation of John Stephenson's De Velosynthesi. JHMAS 18:209-219, 1963 ⟨II-00094⟩

Frankenburg, F.: The 1978 Ontario Mental Health Act in Historical Context. HSTC Bulletin 6:172-177, 1982 ⟨II-04990⟩

Fraser, D.T.: John Gerald Fitzgerald (1882-1940). PTRSC 35:113-115, 1941 ⟨I-03572⟩

Fraser, H.A., Schwartz, H.W., Bethune, C.M., Atlee, H.B.: In Memoriam: Frank Roy David, MD, CM(Dal), FACS. Nova Scotia Medical Bulletin 27:237-240, 1948 ⟨I-01464⟩

Fraser-Harris, D.F.: Dr. John Stewart. CMAJ 30:223-224, 1934 ⟨I-01716⟩

Freedman, N.B.: History of Medical Licensure in Canada. L'Action Medicale 23:13-15, 1947 ⟨II-00128⟩

Freedman, N.B.: History of Medical Licensure in Quebec Previous to 1847. L'Action Medicale 23:28-30, 1947 ⟨II-00136⟩

Freedman, N.B.: Medical Practise in Montreal in the Eighteen Forties... L'Action Medicale 23:45-47, 1947 ⟨II-00867⟩

Freedman, N.B.: The College in the Eighteen Sixties. L'Action Medicale 23:128-129, 1947 ⟨II-00132⟩

Freedman, N.B.: The College 1850-1852. L'Action Medicale 23:109-111, 1947 ⟨II-00133⟩

Freedman, N.B.: The College 1848-1850. L'Action Medicale 23:87-91, 1947 ⟨II-00134⟩

Freedman, N.B.: The Establishment of the College 1847. L'Action Medicale 23:69-73, 1947 ⟨II-00135⟩

Frewin, M.: A History of the Canadian Pharmaceutical Association, Inc. Canadian Pharmaceutical Journal 90:588-616, 1957 ⟨II-00703⟩

Fryer, H.: Pioneer Doctor (A.M. Carlisle). Heritage 7:21-24, 1979 ⟨I-00906⟩

Fuhrer, C.: The Mysteries of Montreal. [Midwifery]. Montreal, John Lovell and Son, 1881. 245 p. ⟨II-00769⟩

Fulton, J.F.: John George Adami (1862-1926). In Kelly HW, Burrage WL: Dictionary of American Medical Biography. New York and London, D. Appleton and Co., 1928. p.3. ⟨I-00022⟩

F(ulton), J.F.: T. Archibald Malloch. JHMAS 8:449, 1953 ⟨I-01296⟩

Fulton, J.F.: William Willoughby Francis, 1878-1959. JHMAS 15:1-6, 1960 ⟨I-02798⟩

G

G., A.: Alexander Thomas Cameron. CMAJ 57:504-5, 1947 ⟨I-04401⟩

G., A.R., J., C.W.L.: Dr. J. Earle Hiltz. CMAJ 100:1065, 1969 ⟨I-05037⟩

G., D.C., E., G.R.F.: John Ferguson McCreary: A Man for all Seasons. CMAJ 122:123-124, 1980 ⟨I-01279⟩

G., H.B.: Beverly Charles Leech. Canadian Anaesthetist's Society Journal 7:351-352, 1960 ⟨I-03238⟩

G., H.B.: Doctor David Dawson Freeze. Canadian Anaesthetist's Society Journal 9:560, 1962 ⟨I-02826⟩

G., K.L.: Dr. W.J. Fischer, MA. CMAJ 10:1144, 1920 ⟨I-02818⟩

G., M.H.: The History of Dental Journalism in Canada. Journal of the Canadian Dental Association 18:335-38, 1952 ⟨II-05201⟩

G., N.B.: Dr. Robert Hyndman Mullin. CMAJ 14:889, 1924 ⟨I-02993⟩

Gagan, R.R.: Disease, Mortality and Public Health, Hamilton, Ontario, 1900-1914. Thesis, McMaster University, School of Graduate Studies, Master of Arts, April, 1981. 225 pages ⟨I-04894⟩

Gagnon, J.P.: Marc-Pascal de Sales Laterriere. DCB 10:431-432, 1972 ⟨I-02253⟩

Galarneay, C.: Jacques Dorion. DCB 10:236, 1972 ⟨I-01204⟩

Galbraith, W.S.: Frank Hamilton Mewburn. CMAJ 20:329, 1929 ⟨I-03454⟩

Gale, G.L., DeLarue, N.D.: Surgical History of Pulmonary Tuberculosis: The Rise and Fall of Various Technical Procedures. Canadian Journal of Surgery 12:381-388, 1969 ⟨II-04303⟩

Gale, G.L.: The Changing Years. The Story of Toronto Hospital and the Fight against Tuberculosis. Toronto, West Park Hospital, 1979. 134 p. ⟨II-00174⟩

Gale, G.L.: Tuberculosis in Canada: a Century of Progress. CMAJ 126:526, 528-529, 1982 ⟨II-04822⟩

Gallie, W.E.: Dr. Edward Archibald. CMAJ 54:197, 1946 ⟨I-04348⟩

Gallie, W.E.: The Opening of Osler Hall. Bulletin of the Academy of Medicine, Toronto 25:41-46, 1951 ⟨II-04066⟩

Gallie, W.E.: George Armstrong Peters: (As I remember him). Canadian Journal of Surgery 2:119-122, 1959 ⟨I-02585⟩

Galloway, H.P.H.: Dr. William Webster, an appreciation. CMAJ 31:691, 1934 ⟨I-01719⟩

Gariepy, P.U.: La Chirurgie Chez Les Indiens du Nord-Amerique. L'UMC 66:526-534, 1937 ⟨II-02439⟩

Garland, M.A., Talman, J.J.: Pioneer Drinking Habits and the Rise of the Temperance Agitation in Upper Canada Prior to 1840. Ontario Historical Society 27:341-364, 1931 ⟨II-04065⟩

Garner, J.: Military Medical Services in Canada. I: The Beginnings. CMAJ 112:1350-4, 1975 ⟨II-05327⟩

Gaspe, P.A. de: Memoires. Montreal, Bibliotheque Canadienne-Francaise, 1971. 435 p. ⟨I-01026⟩

Gass, C.L.: Dr. R.D. Roach. CMAJ 67:484, 1952 ⟨I-04533⟩

Gass, C.L.: John Stewart Memorial Lecture. Nova Scotia Medical Bulletin 41:188-196,1962 ⟨I-01637⟩

Gaucher, D.: La Formation des Hygienistes a L'Universite de Montreal, 1910-1975: De La Sante Publique a La Medecine Preventive. Recherches Sociographiques 20:59-85, 1979 ⟨II-04686⟩

Gaumond, E.: La Syphilis au Canada Francais Hier et Aujourd'hui. Laval Medical 7:25-65, 1942 ⟨II-02405⟩

Gaumond, E: La Petite Verole. Laval Medical 18:3-13, 1953 ⟨II-04067⟩

Gaumond, E.: Une Operation Chirurgicale a l'Hotel-Dieu de Quebec en 1700. Canadian Journal of Surgery 2:323-328, 1959 ⟨II-04699⟩

Gauthier, C.A.: Histoire de la Societe Medicale de Quebec. Laval Medical 8:60-121, 1943 ⟨II-04668⟩

Gauvreau, J.: Le Bureau Medicale de Montreal/the Montreal Medical Board 1839-1847. L'UMC 61:42-55 ⟨II-02378⟩

Gauvreau, J.: L'Ecole de Medecine et de Chirurgie de Montreal Fondee en 1843: Le Docteur Thomas Arnoldi, son Premier President. L'UMC 60:818-827, 1931 ⟨I-01773⟩

Gauvreau, J.: L'Enquete du Conseil Legislatif. L'UMC 60:642-50, 1931 ⟨II-01869⟩

Gauvreau, J.: La Societe Medicale de Quebec 1826. L'UMC 60:880-884, 1931 ⟨II-02379⟩

Gauvreau, J.: Le College des Medecins et Chirurgiens de la Province de Quebec: Avant-Propos. L'UMC 60:334-340, 1931 ⟨II-02380⟩

Gauvreau, J.: Le College des Medecins et Chirurgiens de la Province de Quebec: 1760-1847 Vue D'Ensemble sur Cette Epoque. L'UMC 60:426-431, 1931 ⟨II-02381⟩

Gauvreau, J.: Le Mal de la Baie Saint-Paul. L'UMC 60:494-500, 1931 ⟨II-01870⟩

Gauvreau, J.: Montreal Medical Institution Fondee en 1824 Par Les Medecins du Montreal General Hospital. L'UMC 60:732-736, 1931 ⟨II-01868⟩

Gauvreau, J.: "L'Union Medicale du Canada": en liaison avec le College des Medecins et Chirurgiens pendant 60 ans: 1872 a 1932. L'UMC 61:123-143, 1932 ⟨II-02451⟩

Gauvreau, J.: Dr. Daniel Arnoldi (1774-1849). CMAJ 27:79-82, 1932 ⟨I-03040⟩

Gauvreau, J.: Le College des Medecins et Chirurgiens de la Province de Quebec, son evolution depuis la cession jusqu'a nos jours. L'UMC 61:513-519, 618-626, 1932 ⟨II-01830⟩

Gauvreau, J.: Une Page D'Histoire: Le College des Medecins et Chirurgiens de la Province de Quebec. L'UMC 67:53-63, 1938 ⟨II-02374⟩

Gear, H.: Dr. Thomas Clarence Routley, an appreciation. CMAJ 88:953, 1963 ⟨I-02599⟩

Gear, J.L.: Factors Influencing the Development of Government Sponsored Physical Fitness Programmes in Canada from 1850 to 1972. Canadian Journal of the History of Sport and Physical Education 3:1-25, 1972 ⟨II-04810⟩

Gee, E.M.T.: Early Canadian Fertility Transition: a Components Analysis of Census Data. Canadian Studies in Population 6:23-32, 1979 ⟨II-04812⟩

Geikie, W.B.: An Historical Sketch of Canadian Medical Education. Canada Lancet 34:225-287, 1901 ⟨II-04140⟩

Geikie, W.B.: Sketch of the Beginning of Medical Education in York, or as it is now called, Toronto. Canada Lancet 38:579-583, 1905 ⟨II-04139⟩

Gelber, S.M.: The First Decade: Ten Years of Hospital Insurance. Medical Services Journal of Canada 2:1134-1143, 1967 ⟨II-04138⟩

Gelfand, T.: Medicine in New France: Les Francais Look at Les Canadiens during the seven years war. In: 27th International Congress of the History of Medicine, p.511-516, 1980 ⟨II-04208⟩

Gelfand, T.: Report on the Status of History of Medicine in Canadian Universities. In: Jarrell, R.A.; Ball, N.R.: Science, Technology, and Canadian History. Waterloo, Wilfrid Laurier Univ. Press, 1980. pp 199-200 ⟨II-00204⟩

Gelfand, T.: Who Practised Medicine in New France?: A Collective Portrait. In: Roland, C.G. (ed.): Health, Disease and Medicine: Essays in Canadian History. Toronto, Hannah Institute for the History of Medicine, 1984, 16-35 ⟨II-05392⟩

Gemmell, J.P.: "Good -- Doctor" Dr. J. Wilford Good, Dean of Manitoba Medical College, 1887-1898. University of Manitoba Medical Journal 51:98-103, 1981 ⟨II-04873⟩

Geoffrion, P.: Evolution de l'enseignement a la Faculte de Chirurgie Dentaire de l'Universite de Montreal. Journal of the Canadian Dental Association 18:379-381, 1952 ⟨II-05199⟩

Gerard, C: The History of Hotel-Dieu de Saint Joseph in Montreal, Quebec, Canada. Hospital Progress 23:68-71, 108-12, 165-69, 178-81, 1942 ⟨II-04137⟩

Gerber, E.W.: Robert Tait McKenzie 1867-1938. In: Innovators and Institutions in Physical Education Philadelphia, Lea and Febiger, 1971, 339-347 ⟨I-04518⟩

Gerin-Lajoie, L.: Dr. Louis de Lotbiniere Harwood. CMAJ 31:106, 1934 ⟨I-01730⟩

Gerrard, J.W.: Dr. Alvin E. Buckwold. CMAJ 93:1044, 1965 ⟨I-01713⟩

Gervais-Roy, C.: Un Medecin de Campagne d'autrois. Revue d'Ethnologie du Quebec 7:85-102, 1981 ⟨II-04947⟩

Gibb, D.: The Necessity of Supporting a Medical Journal in the Dominion of Canada. Canadian Medical Journal and Monthly Record 4:317, 1867-68 ⟨II-01534⟩

Gibb, G.D.: Report of the Sick on Board the Ship "St. George," from Liverpool, Bound for New York with 338 Steerage Passengers with cases, and Remarks on Ventilation. British American Journal of Medical and Physical Science 5:9-13, 1849 ⟨II-02613⟩

Gibbon, A.D.: The Kent Marine Hospital. New Brunswick Historical Society Collection 14:1-19, 1955 ⟨II-04069⟩

Gibbon, A.D.: Some Medical Highlights of Early Saint John. CMAJ 76:896-899, 1957 ⟨II-01794⟩

Gibbon, A.D.: Robert Bayard. DCB 9:35, 1976 ⟨I-00982⟩

Gibbon, J.M.: Three Centuries of Canadian Nursing. Toronto, Macmillan Co. of Canada Ltd., 1947. 505 p. ⟨II-01835⟩

Gibson, D.: Involuntary Sterilization of the Mentally Retarded: A Western Canadian Phenomenon. Canadian Psychiatric Association Journal 19:59-63, 1974 ⟨II-05366⟩

Gibson, M.: One Man's Medicine. Toronto, Collins Publishers, 1981. 218 p. ⟨II-05047⟩

Gibson, T.: Notes on the Medical History of Kingston. CMAJ 18:331-334, 416-451, 1928 ⟨II-01808⟩

Gibson, T: Notes on the Medical History of Kingston. CMAJ 18:446-451, 1928 ⟨II-04136⟩

Gibson, T.: News notes illustrative of the practice of medicine in Upper Canada, in the early years of the nineteenth century. CMAJ 22:699-700, 1930 ⟨II-03110⟩

Gibson, T.: A Short Account of the Early History of the Kingston General Hospital. Kingston, Hanson and Edgar, 1935 ⟨II-05148⟩

Gibson, T.: A Sketch of the Career of Doctor John Robinson Dickson. CMAJ 38:493-494, 1938 ⟨I-03370⟩

Gibson, T.: The Astonishing Career of John Palmer Litchfield. CMAJ 70:326-330, 1954 ⟨I-03229⟩

Gibson, W.C.: History of Medical Library Services in British Columbia. B.C. Medical Journal 3:210-213, 1961 ⟨II-04135⟩

Gibson, W.C.: Merchant Princes and Medicine. CMAJ 86:659-661, 1962 ⟨II-01789⟩

Gibson, W.C.: Some Canadian Physicians. In: Creative Minds in Medicine. Illinois, Charles C. Thomas, Publisher 1963. pp 123-149 ⟨II-04134⟩

Gibson, W.C.: Dr. Reuben Rabinovitch, an appreciation. CMAJ 93:988, 1965 ⟨I-02696⟩

Gibson, W.C.: (Wallace Wilson). British Columbia Medical Journal 8:234, 1966 ⟨I-03400⟩

Gibson, W.C.: Frank Fairchild Wesbrook (1868-1918). A Pioneer Medical Educator in Minnesota and British Columbia. JHMAS 22:357-379, 1967 ⟨I-01161⟩

Gibson, WC: President Wesbrook -- His University, His Profession and the Community. British Columbia Medical Journal 9:10-20, 1967 ⟨I-03932⟩

Gibson, W.C.: Some Canadian Contributions to Medicine. JAMA 200: 860-864, 1967 ⟨II-04132⟩

Gibson, W.C.: History of the Health Sciences for Undergraduates. Journal of Medical Education 47:910-11, 1972 ⟨II-05336⟩

Gibson, W.C.: Wesbrook and His University. Vancouver, Library of the University of British Columbia, 1973. 204 p. ⟨I-01162⟩

Gibson, W.C.: Pioneer Physician and Scientific Translator: Dr. Iser Steiman. Canadian Family Physician 28:549-50, 1982 ⟨I-04773⟩

Gidney, R.D., Millar, W.P.J.: The Origins of Organized Medicine in Ontario, 1850-1869. In: Roland, C.G. (ed.): Health, Disease and Medicine: Essays in Canadian History. Toronto, Hannah Institute for the History of Medicine. 1984, 65-95 ⟨II-05394⟩

Gielow, V.: Daniel David Palmer: Rediscovering the Frontier Years, 1845-1887. Chiropractic History 1:11-14, 1981 ⟨I-04840⟩

Gilbert, M.R.: La Nouvelle Morale Sociale et L'Etat Surveillant. In International Congress for the History of Medicine, 25th, Quebec, 1976. Proceedings, volume I, 1976. p.171-192 ⟨II-00468⟩

Gilder, S.S.B.: Toronto, the Meeting Place. British Medical Journal 1:1207-09, 1955 ⟨II-04131⟩

Gilder, S.S.B.: Dr. T. Clarence Routley, an appreciation. CMAJ 88:1131, 1963 ⟨I-02598⟩

Gillespie, R.: The unforgettable Doctor (William Gillespie, Kitchener). Kitchener-Waterloo Academy of Medicine, K-W Hospital, Kitchener, Ontario, 11 p. Unpublished ⟨I-01372⟩

Giovanni, M. (Sister): The Role of Religious in Pharmacy under Canada's "Ancien Regeme". University of Toronto, 1962. Thesis, Univ of Toronto, Bachelor of Science in Pharmacy. ⟨II-00346⟩

Giroux, S.: Le cholera a Quebec. National Gallery of Canada Bulletin 20:3-12, 1972 ⟨II-02409⟩

Gladstone, R.M.: The Academy of Medicine, Toronto. University of Toronto Medical Journal 37:92-94, 1960 ⟨II-04130⟩

[Godden, J.]: A Nosegay for Donald C. Graham. CMAJ 94:298, 1966 ⟨I-02115⟩

Godfrey, C.M.: The History of Medicine Museum, Academy of Medicine. Ontario Medical Review 32:868-871, 1965 ⟨II-04128⟩

Godfrey, C.M.: Trinity Medical School. Applied Therapeutics 8:1024-1028, 1966 ⟨II-04127⟩

Godfrey, C.M.: King's College: Upper Canada's First Medical School. Ontario Medical Review 33:19-22, 26, 1967 ⟨II-04129⟩

Godfrey, C.M.: The cholera epidemics in Upper Canada 1832-1866. Toronto and Montreal, Seccombe House, 1968. pp.72 ⟨II-00086⟩

Godfrey, C.M.: The Origins of Medical Education of Women in Ontario. Medical History 17:89-94, 1973 ⟨II-00379⟩

Godfrey, C.M.: Elam Stimson. DCB 9:748-749, 1976 ⟨I-01103⟩

Godfrey, C.M.: Theophilus Mack. DCB 11:558-559, 1982 ⟨I-04850⟩

Godler, Z.: Doctors and the new immigrants. Canadian Ethnic Studies 9(1):6-17, 1977 ⟨II-00660⟩

Goldbloom, A: Pediatrics and Medical Practice. CMAJ 60:620-623, 1949 ⟨I-03933⟩

Goldbloom, A.: Small Patients. The Autobiography of a children's doctor. Toronto, Longmans, Green and Co., 1959. 316 p. ⟨I-01369⟩

Goldie, W.: Dr. Alexander McPhedran. CMAJ 32:222, 1935 ⟨I-01283⟩

Goldman, D.L., Arvanitakis, K.: D. Ewen Cameron's Day Hospital and the Day Hospital Movement. Canadian Journal of Psychiatry 26:365-368, 1981 ⟨II-04639⟩

Goldring, P.: The Doctor's Office, Walls, and North-West Bastion at Lower Fort Garry. Manuscript Report Number 51, National Historic Sites Service, 1971. pp 71 ⟨II-00602⟩

Goodman, H: Inoculation in North America Prior to 1846. The Merck Report 58:15-21, 1949 ⟨II-04126⟩

Gordon, A.H.: Dr. Andrew Armour Robertson. CMAJ 15:556, 1925 ⟨I-01588⟩

Gordon, A.H.: Dr. D.A. Stewart. CMAJ 435-436, 1937 ⟨I-03440⟩

Gordon, A.H.: Dr. Henri A. Lafleur. CMAJ 41:96, 1939 ⟨I-03393⟩

Gordon, A.H.: Dr. Frederick Gault Finley. CMAJ 43:193, 1940 ⟨I-01048⟩

Gordon, A.H.: Typhoid Fever from the Inside. CMAJ 48:358-362, 1943 ⟨II-04124⟩

Gordon, A.H.: Medicine in Montreal in the 'Nineties'. CMAJ 53:495-99, 1945 ⟨II-04376⟩

Gordon, A.H.: Doctor F.H. Mackay: an appreciation. CMAJ 58:393-394, 1948 ⟨I-03220⟩

Gordon, K.: Miss Webster of the Montreal General Hospital. CMAJ 28:552-556, 1933 ⟨I-02705⟩

Gordon, R.A.: A Report on Canadian Anesthesia and the Canadian Anesthetists Society. Canadian Anesthetists' Society Journal 3:182-86, 1956 ⟨II-04122⟩

Gordon, R.A.: A Capsule History of Anesthesia in Canada. Canadian Anesthetists' Society Journal 25:75-83, 1978 ⟨II-04125⟩

Gordon, S.D.: Contributions of Surgeons to the Development of Upper Canada. Bulletin of the Medical Library Association 48:33-36, 1960 ⟨II-00428⟩

Gorssline, R.M.: The Medical Services of the Red River Expeditions, 1870-71. Canadian Defence Quarterly 3:83-89, 1925-6 ⟨II-03680⟩

Gorssline, R.M.: Medical Notes on Burgoyne's Campaigns, 1776-77. Canadian Defence Quarterly 6:356-363, 1928-29 ⟨II-04192⟩

Gosse, M.E.B.: Medical Journalism in the Maritimes. Nova Scotia Medical Bulletin 32:253-259, 1953 ⟨II-01539⟩

Gosse, N.H.: Edward Vincent Hogan, CBE, MD, CM, FACS, FRCS(C). CMAJ 28:342, 1933 ⟨I-03054⟩

Gosse, N.H.: Doctor Macpherson's Modesty. Nova Scotia Medical Bulletin 28:122, 1949 ⟨II-03639⟩

Gosselin, A.: Un Historien Canadien Oublie: le Dr. Jacques Labrie (1784-1831). PTRSC Volume 11, section I, 33-64, 1893 ⟨I-02255⟩

Goudreault, L.: Naissance de la Statistique Alieniste au Canada Jusqu'en 1867. In International Congress for the History of Medicine, 25th Quebec, 1976. Proceedings, Volume 11, 1976. p. 706-726 ⟨II-00429⟩

Gough, A.F.: Public Health in Canada, 1867-1967. Medical Services Journal of Canada 23:32-41, 1967 ⟨II-03954⟩

Gouin, J.: Antonio Pelletier, La vie et l'oeuvre d'un medecin et poete meconnu (1876-117). Montreal, Editions du Jour, 1975. 202 p. ⟨I-05211⟩

Goupil, G: Hans Selye: La Sagesse du Stress. Nouvelle Optique, 1981, 169 p. ⟨I-04196⟩

Goyer, G.: Charles-Marie Labillois. DCB 9:438-439, 1976 ⟨I-01309⟩

Graham, D.: John Beresford Leathes, 1864-1956. PTRSC Series 3, 52:89-90, 1958 ⟨I-04777⟩

G[raham], D.: Dr. John A. Oillie, an appreciation. CMAJ 87:881-882, 1962 ⟨I-02293⟩

Graham, E.: Medicine Man to Missionary. Missionaries as agents of change among the Indians of Southern Ontario, 1784-1867. Toronto, Peter Martin Associates Ltd., 1975. 125 p. ⟨II-00352⟩

Graham, E.A.: Dr. Edward Archibald. CMAJ 54: 197-8, 1946 ⟨I-04347⟩

Graham, J.E.: A Brief History of the Recent Outbreak of Smallpox in Toronto. Dominion Medical Monthly 1:123-129, 1893 ⟨II-04185⟩

Graham, J.H.: A proud Scottish Canadian. CMAJ 120:988, 1979 ⟨I-01415⟩

Graham, R.R.: Frederic Newton Gisborne Starr, CBE, MB, MD, CM, FRGS. CMAJ 30:694-695, 1923 ⟨I-01636⟩

Graham, W.H.: The Tiger of Canada West. Toronto/Vancouver, Clarke, Irwin and Co. Ltd., 1962. 308 p. ⟨II-00839⟩

Graham-Cumming, G: Health of the Original Canadians, 1867-1967. Medical Services Journal of Canada 23:115-166, 1967 ⟨II-04186⟩

Grant, D.M.: We Shall Conquer Yet. Nova Scotia Historical Quarterly 3:243-51, 1972 ⟨II-04012⟩

Grant, H.D.: Greetings from the Medical Faculty of Dalhousie University. Nova Scotia Medical Bulletin 32:270-273, 1953 ⟨II-04184⟩

Grant, M.H.L.: Historical Background of the Nova Scotia Hospital, Dartmouth and the Victoria General Hospital, Halifax. Nova Scotia Medical Bulletin 16:250-58, 314-319, 383-392, 1937 ⟨II-04181⟩

Grant, M.H.L.: Historical Sketches of Hospitals and Alms Houses in Halifax, Nova Scotia, 1749-1859. Nova Scotia Medical Bulletin 27:229-38, 294-304, 491-512, 1938 ⟨II-05147⟩

Graves, H.B.: The B.C. Division of the Canadian Anesthetists Society, 1945-1964. B.C. Medical Journal 6:478-481, 1964 ⟨II-04182⟩

Gray, C.: The Osler Library: a collection that represents the mind of its collector. CMAJ 119:1442-1445, 1978 ⟨II-00143⟩

Gray, C.: Dr. Thomas Barnardo's Orphans were Shipped 500 km to Save Body and Soul. CMAJ 121:981-982, 986-987, 1979 ⟨II-00740⟩

Gray, C.: Elizabeth Catharine Bagshaw. CMAJ 124:211, 1981 ⟨I-03241⟩

Gray, C.: Glenn Ivan Sawyer. CMAJ 124:514, 1981 ⟨I-03164⟩

Gray, C.: Harold Rocke Robertson. CMAJ 125:916, 1981 ⟨I-04418⟩

Gray, C.: Lloyd Carl Grisdale. CMAJ 125:1360, 1981 ⟨I-04716⟩

Gray, C.: Eric MacLean Found. CMAJ 127:322, 1982 ⟨I-04902⟩

Gray, C.: Gerald Halpenny. CMAJ 127:157, 1982 ⟨I-04909⟩

Gray, C.: Harry Duncan Roberts. CMAJ 126:710, 1982 ⟨I-04778⟩

Gray, C.: Jacques Genest. CMAJ 126:1216, 1982 ⟨I-04831⟩

Gray, C.: Robert Alexander Mustard. CMAJ 127:1216, 1982 ⟨I-04961⟩

Gray, C.: Robert Orville Jones. CMAJ 127:528, 1982 ⟨I-04958⟩

Gray, C.: A. Ross Tilley. CMAJ 129:154, 1983 ⟨I-05216⟩

Gray, C.: Edwin Clarence McCoy. CMAJ 129:1139, 1983 ⟨I-05319⟩

Gray, C.: Harry Bain. CMAJ 129-614, 1983 ⟨I-05184⟩

Gray, C.: Harry Medovy. CMAJ 129:375, 1983 ⟨I-05215⟩

Gray, C.: Norman Charles Delarue. CMAJ 128:185, 1983 ⟨I-05046⟩

Gray, C.: Paul H.T. Thorlakson. CMAJ 128:1211, 1983 ⟨I-05056⟩

Gray, C.: Robert Bews Kerr. CMAJ 130:194, 1984 ⟨I-05380⟩

Gray, F.W.: Pioneer Geologists of Nova Scotia. Dalhousie Review 26:10-25, 1946-47 ⟨I-02023⟩

Gray, J.H.: Bacchanalia Revisited. Western Canada's Boozy Skid to Social Disaster. Saskatoon, Western Producer Prairie Books, 1982. 206 p. ⟨II-05015⟩

Gray, W.A.: Early Years in our Medical School [U.W.O.]. University of Western Ontario Medical Journal 22:106-112, 1952 ⟨II-04183⟩

Green, D.: Dr. William John Knox, 1878-1967: Beloved Doctor of the Okanagan. Okanagan Historical Society Annual Report 33:8-18, 1969 ⟨I-05068⟩

Greenaway, R: Banting and Medical News. In: The News Game. Toronto/Vancouver, Clarke, Irwin and Co. Ltd., 1966, pp 59-71 ⟨I-03880⟩

Greenfield, K.: William Craigie. DCB 9:165-166, 1976 ⟨I-00930⟩

Greenhous, B.: Paupers and Poorhouses: the development of Poor Relief in early New Brunswick. Histoire Sociale/Social History 1:103-128, 1968 ⟨II-03306⟩

Greenland, C.: Ernest Jones in Toronto 1908-13: A Fragment of Biography. Canadian Psychiatric Association Journal 6:132-139, 1961 ⟨II-02319⟩

Greenland, C.: L'Affaire Shortis and the Valleyfield Murders. Canadian Psychiatric Association Journal 7:261-271, 1962 ⟨II-00588⟩

Greenland, C: Services for the Mentally Retarded in Ontario 1870-1930. Ontario History 54:267-274, 1962 ⟨II-04191⟩

Greenland, C.: Work as Therapy in the Treatment of Chronic Mental Illness. Canadian Psychiatric Association Journal 7:11-15, 1962 ⟨II-00525⟩

Greenland, C.: Richard Maurice Bucke, M.D. Canada's Mental Health 11:6, 1963 ⟨I-04388⟩

Greenland, C.: The Treatment of the Mentally Retarded in Ontario -- an Historical Note. Canadian Psychiatric Association Journal 8:328-336, 1963 ⟨II-00847⟩

Greenland, C.: Richard Maurice Bucke, M.D., 1837-1902 (A Pioneer of Scientific Psychiatry). CMAJ 91:385-391, 1964 ⟨I-01709⟩

Geenland, C.: Richard Maurice Bucke, 1837-1902. CMAJ 92:1136, 1965 ⟨I-01710⟩

Greenland, C.: The Life and Death of Louis Riel -- Part II -- Surrender, Trial, Appeal and Execution. Canadian Psychiatric Association Journal 10:253-259, 1965 ⟨II-04788⟩

Greenland, C.: C.K. Clarke: A Founder of Canadian Psychiatry. CMAJ 95:155-160, 1966 ⟨I-00901⟩

Greenland, C.: Charles Kirk Clarke, A Pioneer of Canadian Psychiatry. Toronto, Clarke Institute of Psychiatry, 1966. 31 p. ⟨II-00592⟩

Greenland, C.: Ernest Jones in Toronto 1908-13, part II. Canadian Psychiatric Association Journal 11:512-519, 1966 ⟨II-02320⟩

Greenland, C.: Richard Maurice Bucke, M.D. 1837-1902: The Evolution of a Mystic. Canadian Psychiatric Association Journal 11:146-154, 1966 ⟨I-01712⟩

Greenland, C.: Three Pioneers of Canadian psychiatry. JAMA 200:833-842, 1967 ⟨I-00008⟩

Greenland, C: Canadian Pioneers in Mental Retardation. Rehabilation in Canada 17:3-6, 1967-68 ⟨II-04189⟩

Greenland, C.: The Compleat Psychiatrist: Dr. R.M. Bucke's Twenty-Five Years as Medical Superinten-

dent, Asylum for the Insane, London, Ontario 1877-1902. Canadian Psychiatric Association Journal 17:71-77, 1972 ⟨I-03566⟩

Greenland, C.: Mary Edwards Merrill, 1858-1880: "The Psychic". Ontario History 68:81-92, 1976 ⟨II-00575⟩

Greenland, C., Griffin, J.D.: William Henry Jackson (1861-1952): Reil's secretary (another case of involuntary commitment). Canadian Psychiatric Association Journal 23:469-477, 1978 ⟨II-00591⟩

Greenland, C., Griffin, J.D.: The Honorable Mary MacDonald: a lesson in attitude. CMAJ 25:305-308, 1981 ⟨II-04221⟩

Greenland, C.: William George Metcalf. DCB 11:590-91, 1982 ⟨I-04852⟩

Greenland, C (edit): Ontario Neuro-Psychiatric Association: Recollections from the First Fifty Years. Ontario Psychiatric Association, 1970. ⟨II-04188⟩

Greenwald, I.: The History and Character of Goitre in Canada. CMAJ 84:379-388, 1961 ⟨II-00108⟩

Gregoire, J.: The Ministry of Health of the Province of Quebec. Canadian Journal of Public Health 50:411-420, 1959 ⟨II-00574⟩

Grenfell, W.T.: A Labrador Doctor (The Autobiography of Wilfred Thomason Grenfell). Boston/New York, Houghton Mifflin Co., 1919. 441 p. ⟨II-00490⟩

Grenfell, W.T.: Forty Years for Labrador. London, Hodder and Stoughton Ltd., 1934, 365 p. ⟨I-04421⟩

Greve, A.: Dr. McLoughlin's house. The Beaver 272(2):32-35, 1941 ⟨I-03240⟩

Gridgeman, N.T.: Biological Sciences at the National Research Council of Canada: The Early Years to 1952. Waterloo, Wilfrid Laurier University Press, 1979. 153 p. ⟨II-00448⟩

Griffin, J.D.: Planning Psychiatric Services. Medical Services Journal of Canada 23:1245-1260, 1967 ⟨II-04187⟩

Griffin, J.D., Greenland, C.: Manifestations of Madness in New France. In International Congress for the History of Medicine, 25th, Quebec, 1976. Proceedings, Volume II, 1976. p. 727-745 ⟨II-00112⟩

Griffin, J.D.: Trepanation Among Early Canadian Indians. Canadian Psychiatric Association Journal 21:123-125, 1976 ⟨II-04180⟩

Griffin, J.D.: Psychiatry in Ontario in 1880: Some Personalities and Problems. Ontario Medical Review 47:271-274, 1980 ⟨II-00154⟩

Griffin, J.D.: The Asylum at Lower Fort Garry. The Beaver, Spring 1980 pp 18-23 ⟨II-00153⟩

Griffin, J.D., Greenland, C.: Institutional Care of the Mentally Disordered in Canada - A 17th Century Record. Canadian Journal of Psychiatry 26:274-278, 1981 ⟨II-04215⟩

Griffith, H.R.: Cyclopropane: A Revolutionary Anesthetic Agent. CMAJ 36:496-500, 1937 ⟨II-04175⟩

Griffith, H.R.: The Evolution of the Use of Curare in Anesthesiology. Annals of the New York Academy of Science 54:493-497, 1951 ⟨II-04177⟩

Griffith, H.R.: Fifty Years of Progress in Surgery and Anesthesia. Canadian Nurse 54:540-542, 1958 ⟨II-04173⟩

Griffith, H.R.: The Early Clinical Use of Cyclopropane. Anesthesia and Analgesia....Current Researches 40;28-31, 1961 ⟨II-04176⟩

Griffith, H.R.: Some Canadian Pioneers in Anesthesia. Canadian Anesthetists' Society Journal 11:557-566, 1964 ⟨II-04172⟩

Griffith, H.R.: Dr. Wesley Bourne, an appreciation. CMAJ 92:895-896, 1965 ⟨I-02052⟩

Griffith, H.R.: Wesley Bourne (1886-1965). Canadian Anaesthetists' Society Journal 12:315-317, 1965 ⟨I-02053⟩

Griffith, H.R.: An Anesthetist's Valediction. Canadian Anesthetists' Society Journal 14:373-381, 1967 ⟨II-04178⟩

Griffith, H.R.: Anesthesia in Canada, 1847-1967: II. the Development of Anesthesia in Canada. Canadian Anesthetists' Society Journal 14:510-518, 1967 ⟨II-04174⟩

Grisdale, L.: Walter MacKenzie: a gift for friendship. CMAJ 120:985, 988, 1979 ⟨I-01414⟩

Groen, J.J.: Discovery of Insulin Told as a Human Story. Israel Journal of Medical Sciences 8:476-83, 1972 ⟨II-05335⟩

Groves, A.: All in a day's work. (Leaves from a doctor's case-book). Toronto, Macmillan Co. of Canada Ltd., 1934. 181 p. ⟨II-00423⟩

Gryfe, A.: Dr. John Rolph -- physician, lawyer and rebel. CMAJ 113:971-974, 1975 ⟨I-01133⟩

Guerra, F.: Les Medecins Patriotes. In International Congress for the History of Medicine, 25th, Quebec, 1976. Proceedings, Volume II, 1976. p. 746-754 ⟨II-00692⟩

Guest, R.G.: The Development of Patent Medicine Legislation. Applied Therapeutics 8:786-789, 1966 ⟨II-04169⟩

Guiou, N.M.: Haemorrhage at the Outposts. CMAJ 23:679-681, 1930 and 30:449, 1934 ⟨II-00363⟩

Gullen, A.S.: A Brief History of the Ontario Medical College for Women, 1906. Canadian Journal of Medicine and Surgery 65:82-88, 1929 ⟨II-02339⟩

Gullett, D.W.: Notes on the Development of the Canadian Dental Association. Journal of the Canadian Dental Association 18:303-309, 1952 ⟨II-05205⟩

Gullett, D.W.: A History of Dentistry in Canada. Toronto, University of Toronto Press, 1971. 308 p. ⟨II-00068⟩

Gundy, H.P.: Growing Pains: The Early History of Queen's Medical Faculty. Transactions of the Kingston Historical Society 4;14-25, 1954-55 ⟨II-04170⟩

Gunn, J.A.: Dr. Edward William Montgomery. CMAJ 59:494-5, 1948 ⟨I-04481⟩

Gunn, J.N.: Harry Goodsir Mackid, M.D., LRCP and S.(Edin), FACS. CMAJ 22:700-701, 1930 ⟨I-02180⟩

Gunn, S.W.A.: A Complete Guide to the Totem Poles in Stanley Park, Vancouver, B.C. Vancouver, W.E.G. MacDonald, Publisher, 1965. 24p. ⟨II-04179⟩

Gunn, S.W.A.: (Wallace Wilson). British Columbia Medical Journal 8:236, 1966 ⟨I-03398⟩

Gunn, S.W.A.: Kwatkiutl House and Totem Poles. British Columbia, Whiterocks Publications, 1966. 24 p. ⟨II-00612⟩

Gunn, S.W.A.: George Elias Darby: 1889-1962. Canadian Journal of Surgery 10:275-280, 1967 ⟨I-04227⟩

Gunn, S.W.A.: Medicine in primitive Indian and Eskimo Art. CMAJ 14:513-514, 1970 ⟨II-04168⟩

Gunn, S.W.A.: Medecine Totemique et Chamanisme Chez Les Indiens du Nord-Quest Americain. Bull d'abonnement a la revue 5:97-105, 1978 ⟨II-02470⟩

Gunn, S.W.A.: Traditional Medicine among Native Indians of Western Canada. Dialogue 68:6-7, 1979 ⟨II-00611⟩

Gunson, H.H.: Blood Transfusions in 1875. CMAJ 80:130-131, 1959 ⟨II-02333⟩

Gunter, J.U.: Burial of a Heart (R.T. McKenzie). Hospital Tribune, September 25, 1967, page 11 ⟨I-03216⟩

Guyot, M.: A brief history of the smallpox epidemic in Montreal from 1871 to 1880 and the late outbreak of 1885. Montreal, s.n. 1886 ⟨II-01530⟩

Gwyn, N.B.: Osler, student of the Toronto School of Medicine: a detail of the personal side of teaching. Annals of Medical History 5:305-308, 1923 ⟨I-02532⟩

Gwyn, N.B.: Dr. William Lockwood T. Addison. CMAJ 23:727, 1930 ⟨I-03025⟩

Gwyn, N.B.: The Chapter from the Life of John Rolph. Bulletin of the Academy of Medicine, Toronto 9:137-144, 1936 ⟨I-04965⟩

Gwyn, N.B.: The letters of a devoted Father to an Unresponsive Son. BHM 7:335-351, 1939 ⟨I-03877⟩

Gwyn, N.B.: Šir William Osler's Contributions to the Library of the Academy of Medicine, Toronto. Bulletin of the Academy of Medicine, Toronto 20:266-271, 1946-47 ⟨II-00145⟩

Gwyn, N.B.: A Short History of the Toronto Medical Historical Club. CMAJ 56:218-220, 1947 ⟨II-04167⟩

Gwyn, N.B.: The Medical Arena in the Toronto of Osler's Early Days in the Study of Medicine. Archives of Internal Medicine 84:2-6, 1949 ⟨II-00276⟩

Gwynn, N.B.: Some Details of Osler's Early Life as Collected by a Near Relation. North Carolina Medical Journal 10:491-496, 1949 ⟨I-01124⟩

H

H., G.: Dr. David A. Henderson, an appreciation. CMAJ 96:171-172, 1967 ⟨I-02490⟩

H., J.L.: Douglas Edward Cannell, M.C. LL.D., University of Toronto, Honoris Causa - B.Sc., (Med.) F.R.C.S.(C), F.A.C.O.G., F.R.S.M. (Hon.), F.R.C.O.G. Bull of the Academy of Med, Toronto 53:53-54, 1980 ⟨I-00892⟩

H., L.W.: Salute to a Centenarian (William McClure). CMAJ 74:654-655, 1956 ⟨I-03175⟩

H., R.: The Experiences of a Klondike Nurse. CMAJ 71:129-137, 1932 ⟨II-04166⟩

H., W.H.: Dr. Craik. Montreal Medical Journal 35:539-543, 1906 ⟨I-02015⟩

H., W.H.: Early Adventures with Chloroform in Nova Scotia. CMAJ 14:254-255, 1924 ⟨II-03098⟩

H., W.H.: Dr. J.B. Black. CMAJ 15:104-105, 1925 ⟨I-01591⟩

H., W.H.P.: Dr. F. Arthur H. Wilkinson. CMAJ 80:921-922, 1959 ⟨I-02728⟩

H., W.P.: Dr. Peter McKellar Spence. CMAJ 78:811, 1958 ⟨I-04749⟩

Hacker, C.: Jennie Trout: An Indomitable Lady Doctor Whose History Was lost for a Half-Century. CMAJ 110:841-3, 1974 ⟨I-05370⟩

Hacker, C.: The Indomitable Lady Doctors. Toronto, Clarke, Irwin and Co. Ltd., 1974. 259 p. ⟨II-00384⟩

Haffey, H.: Six Cots and a Prayer that became a Famous Children's Hospital. York Pioneer 71:15-25, 1975 ⟨II-03287⟩

Haig, K.M.: Dr. A.E. Medd. CMAJ 56:115-6, 1947 ⟨I-04405⟩

Haist, R.E.: Charles Herbert Best 1899-1978. PTRSC series 4, 16:45-47, 1978 ⟨I-04953⟩

Hall, A.: On the Past, Present, and Future of the Faculty of Medicine of McGill University. Canadian Medical Journal and Monthly Record of Medical and Surgical Science 3:289-302, 1866-1867 ⟨II-00314⟩

Hall, G.E.: Dr. John MacAlpine -- Physician and Surgeon. Canada Lancet and Practitioner 77:47-52, 1931 ⟨I-02839⟩

Hall, G.E.: James Bertram Collip:1892-1965. CMAJ 93:673, 1965 ⟨I-02010⟩

Hall, R., German, T.: Dental Pathology, Attrition, and Occlusal Surface Form in a Prehistoric Sample from British Columbia. Syesis 8:275-89, 1975 ⟨II-05456⟩

Hallowell, A.I.: The Passing of the Midewiwin in the Lake Winnipeg Region. American Anthropologist 38:33-51, 1936 ⟨II-00640⟩

Hallowell, A.I.: The social function of anxiety in a primitive society. American Sociological Review 6:869-881, 1941 ⟨II-00641⟩

Hallowell, A.I.: The role of conjuring in Saulteaux Society, Vol. 2. New York, Octagon Books, 1971. 96 p. ⟨II-00642⟩

Hallowell, G.A.: Prohibition in Ontario. Ontario Historical Society, 1972. 180 p. ⟨II-00078⟩

Halpenny, J.: George Turner Orton (1837-1901). In Kelly HW, Burrage WL; Dictionary of American Medical Biography. New York and London, D. Appleton and Co., 1928. p. 921. ⟨I-01268⟩

Halpenny, J.: Sir John Christian Schultz (1840-1896). In Kelly HW, Burrage WL: Dictionary of American Medical Biography, New York and London, D. Appleton and Co., 1928. pp. 1083-1084. ⟨I-01104⟩

Halpenny, J.: William Johnston Neilson (1854-1903). In Kelly HW, Burrage WL: Dictionary of American Medical Biography. New York and London, D. Appleton and Co., 1928. pp. 899-900 ⟨I-01272⟩

Hamel, P.: Evolution de la dentisterie dans Quebec et la region, de 1902 a nos jours. Journal of the Canadian Dental Association 18:372-378, 1952 ⟨II-05200⟩

Hamilton, H.D.: Dr. David James Evans. CMAJ 19:501, 1928 ⟨I-03495⟩

Hamilton, J.: George Lyman Duff, 1904-1956. PTRSC Series 3, 51:89-93, 1957 ⟨I-04776⟩

Hamilton, J.: Dr. Joseph Arthur MacFarlane; an appreciation. CMAJ 94:1069-1070, 1966 ⟨I-01732⟩

Hamilton, J.D.: Tributes presented at the memorial service for Professor R.F. Farquharson. CMAJ 93:234-235, 1965 ⟨I-02813⟩

Hamilton, W.F.: Dr. William Grant Stewart. CMAJ 18:630, 1928 ⟨I-01623⟩

Hamilton, Z.W.: Admiralty Documents concerning Dr. John Rae. CACHB 9(1):32-35, 1944 ⟨II-00394⟩

Hamilton, Z.W.: Admiralty documents concerning Dr. John Rae. CACHB 9:32-35, 1944 ⟨I-02769⟩

Hanaway, J: The Coats-of-Arms of McGill University and the Faculty of Medicine. McGill Medical Journal 29:78-87, 1960 ⟨II-04165⟩

Handcock, W.G.: John Waldron. DCB 5:837-839, 1983 ⟨I-05301⟩

Hanna, J.A.: A Century of Red Blankets: A History of Ambulance Service in Ontario. Ontario, Boston Mills Press, 1982. 100 p. ⟨II-05260⟩

Hannah, J.A.: The Development of Associated Medical Services Inc. CMAJ 54:606-610, 1946 ⟨II-00247⟩

Hanson, L.H. Jr.: The Excavation of the Engineer's Latrine at Louisbourg. Manuscript Report Number 55, National Historic Sites Service, 1968. pp. 63 ⟨II-00472⟩

Hardisty, R.H.M.: Dr. Alison Cumming. CMAJ 16:859, 1926 ⟨I-01619⟩

Hardwick, E., Jameson, E., Treguillus, E.: The Science, the Art and the Spirit: Hospitals, Medicine and Nursing in Calgary. Calgary, Century Calgary Publications, 1975, 160 p. ⟨II-04469⟩

Hareven, T.K.: An ambiguous alliance: some aspects of American influences on Canadian Social Welfare. Histoire Sociale/Social History #:82-98, 1969 ⟨II-03305⟩

Harris, C.W.: Abraham Groves of Fergus: The First Elective Appendectomy?. Canadian Journal of Surgery 4:405-410, 1961 ⟨II-00424⟩

Harris, C.W.: William Thomas Aikins, M.D., LL.D.,. Canadian Journal of Surgery 5:131-137, 1962 ⟨I-04243⟩

Harris, C.W.: Irving Heward Cameron (1855-1933): Professor of Surgery, University of Toronto, 1897-1920. Canadian Journal of Surgery 8:131-136, 1965 ⟨I-01565⟩

Harris, C.W.: Dr. Wilbur James Cryderman. CMAJ 95:1271, 1966 ⟨I-02028⟩

Harris, R.I.: As I remember him: William Edward Gallie, Surgeon, Seeker, Teacher, Friend. Canadian Journal of Surgery 10:135-150, 1967 ⟨I-02803⟩

Harris, R.I.: Osteological Evidence of Disease Amongst the Huron Indians. University of Toronto Medical Journal 27(1):71-75, 1949 ⟨II-00754⟩

Harris, R.I.: Alexander Primrose, 1861-1944. Canadian Journal of Surgery 1:183-8, 1957-8 ⟨I-04241⟩

Harris, R.I.: William Edward Gallie, 1882-1959: an appreciation. CMAJ 81:766-770, 1959 ⟨I-02143⟩

Harris, R.I.: Almon Fletcher. CMAJ 92:198, 1965 ⟨I-02789⟩

Harris, R.I.: Christopher Widmer, 1780-1858 and the Toronto General Hospital. York Pioneer 61:3-11, 1965 ⟨II-03610⟩

Harris, S.: Banting's Miracle: The Story of the Discoverer of Insulin. Toronto/Vancouver, J.M. Dent and Sons (Canada) Ltd., 1946. 245 p. ⟨II-00234⟩

Harrison, H.M.: The End of an Era. CMAJ 82:1166-1167, 1960 ⟨II-00248⟩

Harrison, R.C.: Canadian Contributions towards the Comprehension of Hyperinsulinism: the First Successful Excision of an Insulinoma. Canadian Journal of Surgery 23:401-403, 1980 ⟨II-02983⟩

Harshman, J.P.: Robert Tait McKenzie: Another Canadian Centennial. Ontario Medical Review 34:443-448, 452, 1967 ⟨II-01781⟩

Harshman, J.P.: Dr. Horace Bascom (1863-1956) Country Doctor, Court Officer. Ontario Medical Review 47(1):12-17, 1980 ⟨I-00934⟩

Hart, G.D.: The Confederation Worm Token. CMAJ 97:39-40, 1967 ⟨II-04161⟩

Hart, G.D.: George Wesley Miller. CMAJ 123:940, 1980 ⟨I-02507⟩

Hart, G.E.: The Halifax Poor Man's Friend Society, 1820-27, An Early Social Experiment. CHR 34:109-123, 1953 ⟨II-01861⟩

Harvey, A.G.: Meredith Gairdner: Doctor of Medicine. British Columbia Historical Quarterly 9:89-111, 1945 ⟨I-02802⟩

Harvey, F: Preliminaires a une Sociologie Historique des Maladies Mentales au Quebec. Recherches Sociographiques 16:113-118, 1975 ⟨II-04687⟩

Hattie, W.H.: The Early Story of Vaccination on this Continent. CMAJ 14:255, 1924 ⟨II-03097⟩

Hattie, W.H.: Pioneers of Medicine in Canada. CMAJ 14:324, 1925 ⟨II-04156⟩

Hattie, W.H.: Early Acadian Hospitals. CMAJ 16:707-708, 1926 ⟨II-01802⟩

Hattie, W.H.: Dr. John Harris, 1739-1802. CMAJ 18:214-215, 1928 ⟨I-01628⟩

Hattie, W.H.: Historical Sketch of the Dalhousie Medical School. CMAJ 15:539-541, 1925 ⟨II-01801⟩

Hattie, W.H.: A note on the founding of Dalhousie University. CMAJ 20:192-193, 1929 ⟨II-03666⟩

Hattie, W.H.: Note on a Medical Family [Almon]. CMAJ 20:306, 1929 ⟨II-04158⟩

Hattie, W.H.: The First Minute Book [Medical Society of Nova Scotia]. Nova Scotia Medical Bulletin 8:155-161, 1929 ⟨II-04159⟩

Hattie, W.H.: Canada's First Apothecary. Dalhousie Review 10:376-381, 1930-31 ⟨I-02017⟩

Hattie, W.H.: Dr. Murdoch Chisholm. CMAJ 22:295-96, 1930 ⟨I-03010⟩

Hattie, W.H.: On Apothecaries, Including Louis Hebert. CMAJ 24:120-123, 1931 ⟨I-01009⟩

Hayes, J.: Nova Scotia Medical Services in the Great War. In: Hunt, M.S.: Nova Scotia's Part in the Great War. Halifax, Nova Scotia Veteran Publishing Co., Ltd., 1920. pp 177-225 ⟨II-00813⟩

Hayes, J.: The Death of the Duke of Richmond from Hydrophobia in 1820. CMAJ 16:319, 1926 ⟨II-04163⟩

Hayward, P.: Surgeon Henry's Trifles: Events of a Military Life. London, Chatto and Windus, 1970. 281 p. ⟨I-01364⟩

Hazlett, J.W.: The Canadian Orthopaedic Association: A Historical Review. Canadian Journal of Surgery 13:1-4, 1970 ⟨II-04301⟩

Heagerty, J.J.: Mal de Siam. CMAJ 15:1243-1245, 1925 ⟨II-04155⟩

Heagerty, J.J.: Centenary of first Canadian medical journal. CMAj 16:59-60, 1926 ⟨II-01535⟩

Heagerty, J.J.: Plague in Canada. CMAJ 16:452-454, 1926 ⟨II-01803⟩

Heagerty, J.J.: Four Centuries of Medical History in Canada; and a Sketch of the Medical History of Newfoundland. Toronto, Macmillan Co. of Canada Ltd., 1928. 374 p. Vol. II ⟨II-00852⟩

Heagerty, J.J.: The retirement of Lt.-Col. John Andrew Amyot, CMG, MB, Deputy Minister of Pensions and National Health, Canada. CMAJ 27:544-545, 1933 ⟨I-03909⟩

Heagerty, J.J.: Medical Practice in Canada Under the British Regime. In: Tory, H.M. (edit): A History of Science in Canada. Toronto, The Ryerson Press, 1939, pp. 69-86. ⟨II-04915⟩

Heagerty, J.J.: The Romance of Medicine in Canada. Toronto, Ryerson Press, 1940. 113 p. ⟨II-00851⟩

Heal, F.C.: Dr. Harvey Gordon Young. CMAJ 96:1544, 1967 ⟨I-02715⟩

Heaney, N.S.: John Clarence Webster 1863-1950. Proceedings of the Institute of Medicine of Chicago 18:174-176, 1950- 51. ⟨I-01175⟩

Heizer, R.T.: The Use of the Enema Among the Aboriginal American Indians. Ciba Symposia 5:1686-1693, 1944 ⟨II-04153⟩

Hellstedt, L. McG.(edit): Agnes K. Moffat. In: Women Physicians of the World: Autobiographies of Medical Pioneers New York, Mcgraw-Hill Book Co, 1978. pp 220-223 ⟨I-03920⟩

Hellstedt, L.McG. (edit): E. Elizabeth Cass. In: Women Physicians of the World: Autobiographies of Medical Pioneers New York, McGraw-Hill Book Co., 1978. pp 306-12 ⟨I-03921⟩

Hellstedt, L.McG. (edit): Elizabeth Catherine Bagshaw. In: Women Physicians of the World: Autobiographies of Medical Pioneers New York, McGraw-Hill Book Co., 1978. pp 8-9 ⟨I-03942⟩

Hellstedt, L. McG (edit): Ellen C. Blatchford. In: Women Physicians of the World: Autobiographies of Medical Pioneers New York, McGraw Hill Book Co., 1978. pp 223-225 ⟨I-03919⟩

Hellstedt, L.McG. (edit): Enid MacLeod. In: Women Physicians of the World: Autobiographies of Medical Pioneers New York, McGraw-Hill Book Co., 1978. pp 383-85 ⟨I-03923⟩

Hellstedt, L.McG (edit): Florence McConney. In: Women Physicians of the World: Autobiographies of Medical Pioneers. New York, McGraw-Hill Book Co., 1978. pp 120-22 ⟨I-03944⟩

Hellstedt, L. McG (edit): Gladys Story Cunningham. In: Women Physicians of the World: Autobiographies of Medical Pioneers New York, McGray-Hill Book Co., 1978. pp 123-7 ⟨I-03918⟩

Hellstedt, L.McG. (edit): Jeannie Smillie Robertson. In: Women Physicians of the World: Autobiographies of Medical Pioneers New York, McGraw-Hill Book Co., 1978. pp 1-4 ⟨I-03941⟩

Hellstedt, L. McG (edit): Margaret Owens. In: Women Physicians of the World: Autobiographies of Medical Pioneers New York, McGraw-Hill Book Co., 1978. pp 79-84 ⟨I-03943⟩

Hellstedt, L.McG. (edit): Rebe Willits Schoenfeld. In: Women Physicians of the World: Autobiographies of Medical Pioneers New York, McGraw-Hill Book Co., 1978. pp 326-32 ⟨I-03922⟩

Helm, J.: Female infanticide, European diseases, and population levels among the Mackenzie Dene. American Ethnologist 7:259-285, 1980 ⟨II-04203⟩

Helmcken, J.S.: Some experiences in pioneer days. Western Canada Medical Journal 1:440-444, 1907 ⟨II-00531⟩

H.E.M.: Dr. James Brodie Ross. CMAJ 46:399-400, 1942 ⟨I-04273⟩

Henderson, A.F.: Resuscitation Experiments and Breathing Apparatus of Alexander Graham Bell. Chest 62:311-316, 1972 ⟨II-03867⟩

Henderson, J.L.H.: The Founding of Trinity College, Toronto. Ontario History 44:7-14, 1952 ⟨II-01828⟩

Henderson, R.D.: Dr. Jessie Gray (1910-1978). Canadian Journal of Surgery 23:220, 1980 ⟨I-02878⟩

Henderson, V.E.: The Search for an Ideal Anaesthetic. PTRSC, Ser.3, 32:1-19, 1938 ⟨II-00043⟩

Henderson, V.E.: Sir Frederick Grant Banting. CMAJ 44:429-430, 1941 ⟨I-03348⟩

Hendrie, H.C., Varsamis, J.: The Winnipeg Psychopathic Hospital 1919-1969: an Experiment in Community Psychiatry. Canadian Psychiatric Association Journal 16:185-186, 1971 ⟨II-04784⟩

Henripin, J.: From Acceptance of Nature to Control: The Demography of the French Canadians Since the Seventeenth Century. Canadian Journal of Economics and Political Science 23(1):10-19, 1957 ⟨II-02984⟩

Henry, S.: Mississauga Hospital: Largest Evacuation in Canada's History. CMAJ 122:582-585, 1980 ⟨II-00170⟩

Henry, W.: Trifles from my port-folio. Quebec, William Neilson (Printers), 1839. Vol 1, 251 p. Vol 2. 252 p. ⟨I-01363⟩

Henry, W.: Statistics of Delirium Tremens amongst the Troops in Canada for the last thirty years, with some observations on the Disease. Medical Chronicle 1:321-327, 1854 ⟨II-00076⟩

Hensman, B.: The Kilborn Family: A Record of a Canadian Family's Service to Medical Work and Education in China and Hong Kong. CMAJ 97:471-483, 1967 ⟨II-02316⟩

Hepburn, H.H.: Dr. F. Hastings Mewburn. CMAJ, 71:633, 1954 ⟨I-04570⟩

Hepburn, H.H.: The Evolution of Medical Practice During one Man's Lifetime. Alberta Medical Bulletin 24(3):127-132, 1959 ⟨II-00475⟩

Herald, J: History of Medical Education in Kingston,. Queen's Medical Quarterly 8:5-15, 1903 ⟨II-04152⟩

Herrernan, M., McLaughlin, R.S.: A Short History of the Oshawa General Hospital. N.P., 1935, 61 p. ⟨II-04604⟩

Hershfield, C.S.: Medical Memories. Winnipeg, [n.p.] 1973, 85 p. ⟨II-05083⟩

Hertzman, L.: Anthony von Iffland. DCB 10:375-376, 1972 ⟨I-01336⟩

Hewitt, R.M., Eckman, J.R., Miller, R.D.: The Mayo Clinic and the Canadians. CMAJ 91:1161-1172, 1964 ⟨II-04151⟩

Hewson, J.: What does Vaccination mean?. Newfoundland Quarterly 75(3):15-16, 1979 ⟨II-05122⟩

Hiebert, M: Manitoba's Rural Hospitals. Canadian Nurse 53:294-296, 1957 ⟨II-04150⟩

Hildes, J.A.: Recollections of Joseph Doupe. CMAJ 96:63, 1967 ⟨I-01500⟩

Hildes, J.A., Schaefer, O.: The Changing Picture of Neoplastic Disease in the Western and Central Canadian Arctic (1950-1980). CMAJ 130:25-32, 1984 ⟨II-05321⟩

Hill, H.P.: The Bytown Gazette: A Pioneer Newspaper. Ontario Historical Society Papers and Records 27:407-423, 1931 ⟨II-00529⟩

[Hill, P.]: A Brief History of the Hamilton Civic Hospitals. Link II, January, February, March, April, 1982. ⟨II-05006⟩

Hiller, J.K.: John Joseph Dearin. DCB 11:239-40, 1982 ⟨I-04865⟩

Hillsman, J.B.: Eleven Men and a Scalpel. Winnipeg, Columbia Press Ltd., 1948. 144p. ⟨II-04934⟩

Hiltz, J.E.: Dr. Arthur Frederick Miller, an appreciation. CMAJ 93:1374, 1965 ⟨I-03180⟩

Hincks, C.M.: Dr. A. Grant Fleming. CMAJ 48:548, 550, 1943 ⟨I-02787⟩

Hingston, W.H.: The climate of Canada and its relations to life and health. Montreal, Dawson Brothers, Publishers, 1884. 266 p. ⟨II-00065⟩

Hitsman, J.M.: A Medical Officer's Winter Journey in Canada. Canadian Army Journal 12:46-64, 1958 ⟨II-04149⟩

Hodder, E.M.: Transfusion of Milk in Cholera. Practitioner 10:14-16, 1873 ⟨II-04148⟩

Hogarth, W.P.: Dr. Albert E. Allin. CMAJ 96:61-62, 1967 ⟨I-03910⟩

Hogarth, W.P.: Dr. John Hoyle Dennison. CMAJ 96:120-121, 1967 ⟨I-01506⟩

Hoig, D.S.: Reminiscences and Recollections. Oshawa, Mundy-Goodfellow Printing Co. Ltd., 1933, 227 p. ⟨I-04816⟩

Holbrook, J.H.: The Story of the Hamilton Health Association. Canadian Journal of Public Health 15:158-164, 219-221, 1924 ⟨II-00564⟩

Holbrook, J.H.: A Century of Medical Achievement. In: Wingfield, A.H.(ed): The Hamilton Centennial, 1846-1946. The Hamilton Centennial Committee, 1946 ⟨II-03262⟩

Holbrook, J.H.: Forty Years of Advance. Progress and evolution in the care of tuberculosis as exemplified in the story of the mountain Sanatorium at Hamilton. The Canadian Hospital 23:29-33, 92-93, 1946 ⟨II-00127⟩

Holland, C.W.: An Historical Sketch of the Dalhousie Unit. Nova Scotia Medical Bulletin 8:105-108, 1929 ⟨II-04146⟩

Hollander, J.L.: Dr. Wallace Graham: an appreciation. CMAJ 88:168-169, 1963 ⟨I-02138⟩

Holling, S.A., Senior, J., Clarkson, B., Smith, D.A.: Medicine for Heroes: a Neglected Part of Pioneer Life. Mississauga, Mississauga South Historical Society, 1981. 93 p. ⟨II-04783⟩

Holman, W.L.: Oskar Klotz, 1878-1936. Archives of Pathology 22:840-845, 1936 ⟨I-02588⟩

Holman, W.L.: Prof. Oskar Klotz. CMAJ 36:97-98, 1937 ⟨I-01734⟩

Honigmann, J.J.: Witchcraft Among Kaska Indians. In: Walker, D.E.(edit): Systems of North American Witchcraft and Sorcery. Moscow, Idaho, Univ. of Idaho, 1970. pp 221-238 ⟨II-05361⟩

Hood, D.: Davidson Black: A Biography. Toronto, University of Toronto Press, 1964. 145 p. ⟨II-00226⟩

Hopwood, V.: William Fraser Tolmie: Natural Scientist and Patriot. British Columbia Studies, 5:45-51, 1970. ⟨I-03167⟩

Horne, J.: R.M. Bucke: Pioneer Psychiatrist, Practical Mystic. Ontario History 59:197-208, 1967 ⟨I-01662⟩

Horowics, J.H.: The Development of Health Services in Canada During the Last Twenty Years. Canadian Journal of Public Health, 57:123-125, 1966 ⟨II-04145⟩

Horsey, A.J.: Some medical and surgical cases in late campaign -- North-West Rebellion. The Canada Lancet 18:223-227, 1885-6 ⟨II-00814⟩

Horsfall, F.L.: Dr. Jonathan Campbell Meakins: an appreciation. CMAJ 81:956, 1959 ⟨I-03457⟩

Houston, C.J.: James Franklin Irving. CMAJ 44:640-641, 1941 ⟨I-03355⟩

Houston, C.J., Houston, C.S.: Pioneer of vision: The Medical and political memoirs of T.A. Patrick, M.D. CMAJ 119:964-967, 1978 ⟨I-01232⟩

Houston, C.J., Houston, C.S.: Pioneer of Vision: The Reminiscences of T.A. Patrick, M.D. Saskatoon, Western Producer Prairie Books, 1980. 149 p. ⟨II-00493⟩

Houston, C.S.: The early years of the Saskatchewan Medical Quarterly. CMAJ 118:1122,1127-1128, 1978 ⟨II-00717⟩

Houston, P.J.F.: Early Ophthalmology in Toronto. CMAJ 24:708-710, 1931 ⟨II-00357⟩

Howard, C.A.: Dr. Richard William Garrett. CMAJ 15:329, 1925 ⟨I-02829⟩

Howard, R.P.: A Sketch of the Life of the Late G.W. Campbell A.M.,M.D.,LL. D., Late Dean of the Medical Faculty, and a Summary of the History of the Faculty; Being the Introductory Address of the Fiftieth Session of the Medical Faculty of McGill University. Montreal Gazette, 1882 ⟨I-00910⟩

Howard, R.P.: William Osler: " A Potent Ferment" at McGill. Archives of Internal Medicine 84:12-15, 1949 ⟨I-02533⟩

Howard-Jones, N.: What was WHO -- Thirty Years Ago?. Dialogue 59:28-34, 1979 ⟨II-00447⟩

Howe, J.: Dr. and Mrs. H. McGregor. Okanagan Historical Society Annual Report 41:114-125, 1977 ⟨I-05065⟩

Howell, C.D.: Reform and the Monopolistic Impulse: the Professionalization of Medicine in the Maritimes. Acadiensis 9:3-22, 1981 ⟨II-04913⟩

Howell, C.D.: Elite Doctors and the Development of Scientific Medicine: The Halifax Medical Establishment and 19th Century Medical Professionalism. In: Roland, C.G.(ed.): Health, Disease and Medicine: Essays in Canadian History. Toronto, Hannah Institute for the History of Medicine, 1984, 105-122 ⟨II-05396⟩

Howell, G.R.: Dr. Arnold Bernstein. CMAJ 68:299, 1953 ⟨I-04532⟩

Howell, J.M.: Gillespie, J. CMAJ 126:205, 1982 ⟨I-04718⟩

Howell, W.B.: Medicine in Canada. New York, Paul B. Hoeber Inc., 1933. 137 p. ⟨II-00853⟩

Howell, W.B.: F.J. Shepherd: His Life and Times. Toronto and Vancouver, J.M. Dent and Sons Ltd., 1934. 251 p. ⟨I-01639⟩

Howell, W.B.: L'Hotel Dieu de Quebec. Annals of Medical History 6:396-409, 1934 ⟨II-04143⟩

Howell, W.B.: Walter Henry, Army Surgeon. CMAJ 36:302-310, 1937 ⟨I-02764⟩

Howell, W.B.: Colonel F.A.C. Scrimger, V.C. CMAJ 38:279-281, 1938 ⟨I-03372⟩

Howell, W.B.: Dr. Edward Archibald. CMAJ 54:317, 1946 ⟨I-04349⟩

Hoyt, J.: Great Grandmother's Medicine Ball. New Brunswick Historical Society Collections 17:41-43, 1961 ⟨II-04010⟩

Hrdlicka, A.: Disease, Medicine and Surgery Among the American Aborigines. JAMA 99:1661-1666, 1932 ⟨II-02960⟩

Huckell, R.G.: John Keith Munroe Fife. CMAJ 56:585, 1947 ⟨I-02816⟩

Humphrey, B.M.: A Medical Sphinx [James Barry]. CACHB 10:107-114. 1945 ⟨I-03926⟩

Hundahl, S.: Acupuncture and Osler. JAMA 240:737, 1978 ⟨II-05253⟩

Hunstman, A.G.: The Jubilee Reunion of the Class of 1905: The Varsity Tree. Toronto, 1955, University of Toronto ⟨II-00316⟩

Hunter, C.: Dr. Julius Edward Lehmann. CMAJ 31:227, 1934 ⟨I-03528⟩

Hunter, G.: Sir Frederick Banting. CMAJ 44:431, 1941 ⟨I-03349⟩

Hunter, J.: Dr. J.H. Richardson, (an appreciation). Canadian Practitioner and Review 35:121-122, 1910 ⟨I-01131⟩

Hunter, J.: An appreciation of Dr. Wm. Britton. Canadian Journal of Medicine and Surgery 37:165-167, 1915 ⟨I-01554⟩

Hunter, J: Half a Century in Medicine -- 1875-1925. Canadian Journal of Medicine and Surgery 64:71-74, 1928 ⟨II-04142⟩

Hunter, K.A., Andrew, J.E.: The R.C.A.M.C. in the Korean War. Canadian Services Medical Journal 10:5-15, 1954 ⟨II-00795⟩

Hurd, H.M.;Drewry, W.F., Dewey, R.;Pilgrim, C.W., Blumer, G.A., Burgess, T.J.W.: The Institutional Care of the Insane in the United States and Canada. Baltimore, Johns Hopkins Press, 1917, vol. 4. 352 pp. ⟨II-00155⟩

Hussey, C.: Tait McKenzie, A Sculptor of Youth. Philadelphia, J.B. Lippincott Co., 1930. 107 p. ⟨I-01287⟩

Hutchens, A.R.: Indian Herbalogy of North America. Windsor, Merco, 1969. 382 p. ⟨II-05258⟩

Hutcheson, M.M.: Pierre Romieux. DCB 1:578-579, 1966 ⟨I-01004⟩

Hutchison, H.S.: Dr. George Stewart Strathy. CMAJ 15:1172-1173, 1925 ⟨I-02300⟩

Hutchison, H.S.: Dr. Frederick Adam Cleland. CMAJ 30:107-108, 1934 ⟨I-03542⟩

I

Ingersoll, L.K.: A Man and a Museum. Museum Memo 4:2-5, 1972 ⟨II-04141⟩

Ingham, G.H.: Dr. Frederick Joseph Richardson Forster. CMAJ 98:63-64, 1968 ⟨I-02172⟩

Innis, M.Q.: The Record of an Epidemic. Dalhousie Review 16:371-375, 1936-7 ⟨II-02108⟩

Israels, L.G.: 1930-1980: From the Minutes of Early Years [Cancer Relief and Research Institute]. University of Manitoba Medical Journal 52:37-39, 1982 ⟨II-05004⟩

J

Jack, D.: Rogues, Rebels, And Geniuses: The story of Canadian Medicine. Toronto, Doubleday, 1981, 662p. ⟨II-04328⟩

Jackson, A.Y.: Banting As an Artist. Toronto, Ryerson Press, 1943. 37 p. ⟨I-00965⟩

Jackson, A.Y.: Memories of a Fellow Artist, Frederick Grant Banting. CMAJ 92:1077-1084, 1965 ⟨I-04951⟩

Jackson, M.P.: On the Last Frontier: Pioneering in the Peace River Block. Letters of Mary Percy Jackson. London, The Sheldon Press, 1933. 118 p. ⟨II-00476⟩

Jackson, M.P.: My Life at Keg River. Journal of the Medical Women's Federation 38:40-55, 1956 ⟨I-01327⟩

Jackson, P.: People's Doctor: Norman Bethune 1890-1939. Montreal, Red Flag Publications, 1979. 43 p. ⟨I-00955⟩

Jackson, S.W.: The First Pharmacy Act of Ontario. Ontario College of Pharmacy [1971?] ⟨II-05089⟩

Jackson, W.S.T.: Medicine among the North American Indians. CACHB 20(2):39-44, 1955 ⟨II-00613⟩

Jacques, A.: The Hotel-Dieu de Quebec, 1639-1964, 325th Anniversary: Anesthesia, Past and Present. Anesthesia and Analgesia -- Current Researches 45:15-20, 1966 ⟨II-04695⟩

Jacques, A: Anaesthesia in Canada, 1847-1967: The Beginnings of Anaesthesia in Canada. Canadian Anaesthetists' Society Journal 14:500-509, 1967 ⟨II-03984⟩

Jacques, A.: How it all began. CMAJ 97:934-937, 1967 ⟨II-00459⟩

James, J.F.: Pharmacy in Newfoundland. Canadian Pharmaceutical Journal 91:630-631, 1958 ⟨II-00711⟩

Jameson, M.A.: Richard Maurice Bucke: A catalogue based upon the collections of the University of Western Ontario libraries. London, The Libraries, University of Western Ontario, 1978. 126 pp. ⟨I-00003⟩

Jamieson, H.C.: Medical Teaching in Canada in 1824 and 1834. CMAJ 17:360-361, 1927 ⟨II-03983⟩

Jamieson, H.C.: A short sketch of medical progress in Alberta. CMAJ 20:188-190, 1929 ⟨II-03665⟩

Jamieson, H.C.: Frank Hamilton Mewburn. CMAJ 20:328, 1929 ⟨I-03433⟩

Jamieson, H.C.: The early medical history of Edmonton. CMAJ 29:431-437, 1933 ⟨II-03144⟩

Jamieson, H.C.: The Pioneer Doctor of Alberta: William Morrison MacKay. CMAJ 37:388-393, 1937 ⟨I-02843⟩

Jamieson, H.C.: The Early Doctors of Southern Alberta. CMAJ 38:391-397, 1938 ⟨II-03596⟩

Jamieson, H.C.: Southern Alberta Medicine in the Eighties. CMAJ 54:391-396, 1946 ⟨II-04377⟩

Jamieson, H.C.: Early Medicine in Alberta: The First Seventy-Five Years. Alberta, Canadian Medical Association, 1947. 214 p. ⟨II-00862⟩

Jamieson, H.C.: Milestones in Canadian Medicine. CMAJ 59:279-281, 1948 ⟨II-04622⟩

Jamieson, J.E.: Okanagan's First Amputation. Okanagan Historical Society Annual Report 36:139-140, 1972 ⟨II-05115⟩

Janes, [R.M.?]: The History of the Toronto General Hospital and Medical School. Middlesex Hospital Journal 57:74-76, 1957 ⟨II-03982⟩

Janes, R.M.: Dr. Clarence Leslie Starr. Canadian Journal of Surgery 3:109-111, 1959-60 ⟨I-04237⟩

Janson, G.: Charles Blake. DCB 5:88-89, 1983 ⟨I-05316⟩

Janson, G.: Dominique Mondelet. DCB 5:599-600, 1983 ⟨I-05309⟩

Janson, G.: Pierre-Joseph Compain. DCB 5:201-202, 1983 ⟨I-05313⟩

Jaques, L.B.: Reminiscences on completing twenty-five years of research in the blood coagulation field. University of Saskatchewan Medical Journal 3:4-6, 1960 ⟨II-00216⟩

Jaques. L.B.: The Department of Physiology, University of Saskatchewan. The Physiologist 2 (5): 12-14, 1978 ⟨II-04315⟩

J[archo], S.: Drugs Used at Hudson Bay in 1730. Bulletin of the New York Academy of Medicine 47:838-42, 1971 ⟨II-02626⟩

Jarvis, E.: Municipal Compensation Cases: Toronto in the 1860's. Urban History Review 3:14-22, 1976 ⟨II-04210⟩

Jenkins, E.: Neill Cream, Poisoner. In: Reader's Digest, 1978. pp 67-156 ⟨II-00362⟩

Jennings, F.C.: The New Brunswick Medical Society. CMAJ 81:400-402, 1959 ⟨II-03980⟩

Jilek, W.G.: Indian Healing: Shamanic Ceremonialism in the Pacific Northwest Today. Hancock House, 1982. ⟨II-05412⟩

Jobin, P.: La Faculte de Medecine de l'Universite Laval Depuis sa Fondation Jusqu'a 1875. L'UMC 75:1305-1313, 1946 ⟨II-02441⟩

Johansen, D.O.: William Fraser Tolmie of the Hudson's Bay Company 1833-1870. The Beaver 268(2):29-32, 1937 ⟨I-03230⟩

John, (Sister): Vancouver Hospital Oldest in Northwest Area. Hospitals 18:36-38, 1945 ⟨II-03981⟩

Johns, E.: The Winnipeg General Hospital School of Nursing, 1887-1953. Np/Nd ⟨II-00776⟩

Johnson, A.L.: John McCrae of Poppy Day: an overdue revelation. London, The British Legion, 1968 ⟨I-01289⟩

Johnson, G.: Dr. Hugh Malcolmson. CMAJ 91:92, 1964 ⟨I-03425⟩

Johnson, G.R.: Sir John Richardson (1787-1865). CACHB 7(1):1-10, 1942 ⟨II-00395⟩

Johnson, G.R.: Abraham Gesner - 1797-1864: A Forgotten Physician-Inventor. CACHB 13(2):30-34, 1948 ⟨II-00471⟩

Johnson, G.R., Oborne, H.V.: Abraham Gesner - 1797-1864: A Forgotten Physician-Inventor. CACHB 13:30-34, 1948 ⟨I-01393⟩

Johnson, G.R.: McGill University -- Medical Faculty, Part 1. CACHB 14:41-47, 1949 ⟨II-00317⟩

Johnson, G.R.: McGill University -- Medical Faculty, Part 11. CACHB 15:1-7, 1950 ⟨II-00277⟩

Johnson, G.R.: Ground Medicine. CACHB 17(2):37-39, 1952 ⟨II-00614⟩

Johnson, G.R.: Place Names Up to 1930 Commemorating Medical Men Who Have Practised Their Profession in Alberta. Alberta Medical Bulletin 18:53-54, 1953 ⟨II-03976⟩

Johnson, J.H.: The History of Dental Research in Canada. Journal of the Canadian Dental Association 18:315-320, 1952 ⟨II-05203⟩

Johnson, J.K.: The Chelsea Pensioners in Upper Canada. Ontario History 53:272-289, 1961 ⟨II-00464⟩

Johnson, R.E.: Sir John Richardson. DCB 9:658-661, 1976 ⟨I-01222⟩

Johnston, A.: Uses of Native Plants by the Blackfoot Indians. Alberta Historical Review 8(4):8-13, 1960 ⟨II-02971⟩

Johnston, J.L.: Pharmacy 100: The Centenary of Pharmacy in Manitoba. The Alumni Journal [University of Manitoba] 38:7-10, 1978 ⟨II-03978⟩

Johnston, S: The Growth of the Specialty of Anesthesia in Canada. CMAJ 17:163-165, 1927 ⟨II-03979⟩

Johnston, W.V.: John Hutchison Garnier a Canadian naturalist and physician. CMAJ 29:314-316, 1933 ⟨I-03008⟩

Johnston, W.V.: John Hutchison Garnier of Lucknow, Ont.: A Canadian Naturalist and Physician. Bulletin of the Academy of Medicine, Toronto 7:11-20, 1933 ⟨I-04964⟩

Jones, A., Rutman, L.: In the Children's Aid: J.J. Kelso and Child Welfare in Ontario. Toronto, University of Toronto Press, 1981. 210 p. ⟨II-04989⟩

Jones, D.: Mount Sinai Hospital Began in an old Yorkville House. Ontario Medical Review 47:340, 1980 ⟨II-01840⟩

Jones, E., McCalla, D.: Toronto Waterworks, 1840-77: Continuity and Change in Nineteenth- Century Toronto Politics. CHR 60(3):300-323, 1979 ⟨II-00358⟩

Jones, F.: John Clinch. DCB 5:189-190, 1983 ⟨I-05314⟩

Jones, G.C.: The knights of the order of St. John of Jerusalem in Canada under the French regime. CMAJ 31:431-432, 1934 ⟨II-03664⟩

Jones, O.M.: John Ash (1821-1886) [sic]. In Kelly HW, Burrage WL: Dictionary of American Medical Biography. New York and London, D. Appleton and Co., 1928. pp. 38-39. ⟨I-00030⟩

Jones, O.M.: William Fraser Tolmie (1812-1886). In Kelly HW, Burrage WL: Dictionary of American Medical Biography. New York and London, D. Appleton and Co., 1928. p. 1216. ⟨I-01153⟩

Jones, W.A.: Gordon Earle Richards -- a little about his life and times. Journal of the Canadian Association of Radiologists 6:1-7, 1955 ⟨I-02497⟩

Jones, W.A.: Lorimer John Austin, MA, MB, M.Ch, FRCS(C), FACS, 1880-1945. Canadian Journal of Surgery 5:1-5, 1962 ⟨II-03948⟩

Joslin, E.P.: A Personal Impression. Diabetes 5:67-68, 1956 ⟨II-02907⟩

Jost, A.C.: Jacques Bourgeois, Chirurgien 1621-1701. CMAJ 16:190-191, 1926 ⟨I-01603⟩

Jost, A.C.: Notes on Some Old Time Practitioners. Nova Scotia Medical Bulletin 6:3-10, 1927 ⟨II-03975⟩

Jury, E.M.: Carigouan. DCB 1:164-165, 1966 ⟨II-00648⟩

Jury, E.M.: Tehorenhaegnon. DCB 1:634-635, 1966 ⟨II-00647⟩

Jutras, A.: Dr. Leo Erol Pariseau, an appreciation. CMAJ 50:187-188, 1944 ⟨I-01697⟩

Jutras, A.: La Medecine Francaise au Canada. Le Journal de l'Hotel-Dieu de Montreal 15:85-105, 1947 ⟨II-04694⟩

K

K., J.D.: Dr. Hugh Alexander MacMillan, CMAJ 92:641-642, 1965 ⟨I-02838⟩

Kaiser, T.E.: A history of the medical profession of the County of Ontario. Ontario County Medical Association, 1934 ⟨II-03106⟩

Kajander, R.E.: 26 Years of Psychiatric Practice in Thunder Bay. Ontario Medical Review 50(1):13-16, 1983 ⟨II-05048⟩

Kalisch, P.A.: Tracadie and Penikese Leprosaria: a Comparative Analysis of Societal Response to Leprosy in New Brunswick, 1844-1880, and Massachusetts, 1904-1921. BHM 47:480-512, 1973 ⟨II-04887⟩

Kalsner, J.: The Unique Stress Library of Dr. Hans Selye. CMAJ 129:288-289, 1983 ⟨II-05208⟩

Kato, L, Marchand, J: Leprosy: "Loathsome Disease in Tracadie, New Brunswick" -- a glimpse into the past century. CMAJ 114:440-442, 1976 ⟨II-03993⟩

Katz, S.: A new, informal glimpse of Dr. Frederick Banting. CMAJ 129:1229-1232, 1983 ⟨I-05300⟩

Kaufman, A.R.: History of Birth Control Activities in Canada. International Planned Parenthood Federation 4th Report of the Proceedings, August 1953, pp 17-22 ⟨II-05031⟩

Kautz, S.: Trephining. Snaug. 3(2):16-19, 1975 ⟨II-03992⟩

Kay, D.: A Tribute from Scotland [W.C. MacKenzie]. Canadian Journal of Surgery 22:309, 1979 ⟨I-04286⟩

Kay, K.: Development of Industrial Hygiene in Canada. Industrial Safety Survey 22(1):1-11, 1946 ⟨II-00762⟩

Keddy, G.W.A.: Experiences in a 600 Bed Hospital in Normandy. Nova Scotia Medical Bulletin 25:131-135, 1947 ⟨II-03972⟩

Keel, O., Keating, P.: Author du Journal de Medecine de Quebec/Quebec Medical Journal (1826-1827): Programme Scientifique et Programme de Medicalisation. In: Jarrell, R.A.; Roos, A.E. (edit): Critical Issues in the History of Canadian Science, Technology and Medicine. Thornhill and Ottawa, HSTC Publications, 1983. pp 101-134. ⟨II-05190⟩

Keenan, C.G.: Notes of a Regimental Doctor in a Mounted Infantry Corps. Montreal Medical Journal 31:389-400, 1902 ⟨II-02317⟩

Keith, W.D.: John Mawer Pearson Lecture. Bulletin of the Vancouver Medical Association 25:60-64, 1949 ⟨I-02560⟩

Keith, W.D.: Some Early Canadian Ships' Surgeons. B.C. Medical Journal 1:103-116, 1959 ⟨I-04199⟩

Keith, W.S.: Dr. George F. Boyer. CMAJ 96:505-506, 1967 ⟨I-02055⟩

Keith, W.S.: Dr. Arthur B. LeMesurier. CMAJ 126:1353, 1982 ⟨I-04835⟩

Kelley, T.P., Jr.: The fabulous Kelley: Canada's King of the Medicine Men. Don Mills, Paper Jacks, 1975. 149 p. ⟨II-00115⟩

Kellgren, J.J.: Dr. Wallace Graham: an appreciation. CMAJ 88:168, 1963 ⟨I-02160⟩

K[elly], A.D.: W.O. and F.B.B. CMAJ 103:231-232 ⟨I-02883⟩

Kelly, A.D.: The Swift Current Experiment. CMAJ 58:506-511, 1948 ⟨II-03962⟩

Kelly, A.D.: Health Insurance in New France: A Footnote to the History of Medical Economics. BHM 28:535-541, 1954 ⟨II-00258⟩

K[elly], A.D.: Dr. George Frederick Strong. CMAJ 76:517, 1957 ⟨I-04731⟩

K[elly], A.D.: Dr. J. Harold Shaw. CMAJ 77:276, 1957 ⟨I-04752⟩

Kelly, A.D.: The Secretarial Succession in the Canadian Medical Association. CMAJ 81:583-86, 1959 ⟨II-03964⟩

Kelly, A.D.: Health Insurance in New France. CMAJ 82:1284-1286, 1960 ⟨II-00259⟩

Kelly, A.D.: The Crest and Seal of the Canadian Medical Association. CMAJ 85:1016, 1961 ⟨II-01790⟩

K(elly), A.D.: Herbert Alexander Bruce, M.D., FACS, LRCP, (Eng.). CMAJ 89:232-233, 1963 ⟨I-01483⟩

K(elly), A.D.: Thomas Clarence Routley: an appreciation. CMAJ 88:860, 1963 ⟨I-01695⟩

K[elly], A.D.: Dr. George Walton. CMAJ 90:704, 1964 ⟨I-05222⟩

Kelly, A.D.: Richard Maurice Bucke. CMAJ 91:769, 1964 ⟨I-01550⟩

K(elly), A.D.: Dr. William James Deadman. CMAJ 92:1138, 1965 ⟨I-01507⟩

Kelly, A.D.: (Wallace Wilson). British Columbia Medical Journal 8:229, 1966 ⟨I-03405⟩

Kelly, A.D.: Dr. Ernest Clifford Janes, an appreciation. CMAJ 95:1163-1164, 1966 ⟨I-02552⟩

Kelly, A.D.: Dr. Joseph Arthur MacFarlane: an appreciation. CMAJ 94:1070, 1966 ⟨I-01757⟩

K(elly), A.D.: Dr. Wallace Wilson: an appreciation. CMAJ 94:1021, 1966 ⟨I-02726⟩

Kelly, A.D.: China Hands. CMAJ 97:1363-64, 1967 ⟨I-03917⟩

K(elly), A.D.: Dr. C.W. Burns, an appreciation. CMAJ 96:1542-1543, 1967 ⟨I-01493⟩

Kelly, A.D.: Dr. Kelly Takes Over. Ontario Medical Review 34:532-33, 536, 1967 ⟨II-03764⟩

Kelly, A.D.: Effort to Control Cancer. Ontario Medical Review 34:585-86, 609, 1967 ⟨II-03758⟩

Kelly, A.D.: Hands Across the Sea. CMAJ 97:1494, 1967 ⟨II-03968⟩

Kelly, A.D.: Ontario-1867: The Common Health. Ontario Medical Review 34:435-442, 1967 ⟨II-00318⟩

Kelly, A.D.: Our Forgotten Man. CMAJ 96:1485-86, 1967 ⟨I-03916⟩

Kelly, A.D.: Publish or Perish. CMAJ 97:348, 1967 ⟨II-03965⟩

Kelly, A.D.: The Mace [Canadian Medical Association]. CMAJ 96:1540-41, 1967 ⟨II-03974⟩

Kelly, A.D.: Unclean no More. CMAJ 97:1298, 1967 ⟨II-03967⟩

Kelly, A.D.: Dr. Dunham Appointed. Ontario Medical Review 35:86-88, 1968 ⟨II-03768⟩

Kelly, A.D.: Our Oldest Affiliate [Canadian Medical Protective Association]. CMAJ 98:369-370, 1968 ⟨II-03966⟩

Kelly, A.D.: The Great Medical Prepayment Debates. Ontario Medical Review 35:28-30, 1968 ⟨II-03805⟩

Kelly, A.D.: Variable Veracity. Ontario Medical Review 35:256-258, 1968 ⟨II-03970⟩

K[elly], A.D.: Donald Hugh Paterson, M.D. CMAJ 100:466, 1969 ⟨I-05042⟩

K[elly], A.D.: John H. MacDermot, M.D. CMAJ 100:922, 1969 ⟨I-05039⟩

Kelly, A.D.: Origin and Organization of the CMA. CMA 107:559-561, 1972 ⟨II-03971⟩

Kelly, C.M.: An Account of Canadian Leprosy. Montreal Medical Journal 38:387-392, 1909 ⟨II-03969⟩

Kelly, H.A.: George Edgeworth Fenwick (1825-1894). In Kelly HW, Burrage WL: Dictionary of American Medical Biography. New York and London, D. Appleton and Co., 1928. p. 403. ⟨I-01214⟩

Kelly, H.A.: John Fulton (1837-1887). In Kelly HW, Burrage WL: Dictionary of American Medical Biography, New York and London, D. Appleton and Co., 1928. pp. 442-443. ⟨I-01212⟩

Kelly, H.A.: John McCrae (1872-1918). In Kelly HW, Burrage WL: Dictionary of American Medical Biography. New York and London, D. Appleton and Co., 1928. pp. 777-778 ⟨I-01291⟩

Kelly, H.A.: Michael Joseph Ahern (1844-1914). In Kelly HW, Burrage WL: Dictionary of American Medical Biography. New York, London, D. Appleton and Co., 1928. p. 10. ⟨I-00027⟩

Kelly, H.A.: Michel S. Sarrazin (1659-1734). In Kelly HW, Burrage WL: Dictionary of American Medical Biography. New York and London, D. Appleton and Co., 1928. pp. 1077-1078 ⟨I-01117⟩

Kelly, H.A.: Sir William Osler (1849-1919). In Kelly HW, Burrage WL: Dictionary of American Medical Biography. New York and London, D. Appleton and Co., 1928. pp. 921-923. ⟨I-01254⟩

Kelly, H.A.: William Dunlop (1791-1848). In Kelly HW, Burrage WL: Dictionary of American Medical Biography. New York and London, D. Appleton and Co., 1928. pp 358-359 ⟨I-00887⟩

Kelly, K: Medicine...The Distaff Side. Canadian Doctor, May 1961. pp 24-39 ⟨II-03961⟩

Kelsey, H.: Jean-Baptiste Chapoton. DCB 3:102-103, 1974 ⟨I-00925⟩

Kendall, A.S.: Cape Breton Medical Society. Nova Scotia Medical Bulletin 8:109-113, 1929 ⟨II-03973⟩

Kennedy, D.R.: One Hundred Years of Pharmacy Legislation. In One Hundred Years of Pharmacy in Canada 1867 - 1967. Toronto, Canadian Academy of the History of Pharmacy, 1969. pp. 25-37. ⟨II-00704⟩

Kennedy, E.: Immigrants, Cholera and the Saint John Sisters of Charity. Canadian Catholic Historical Association, Study Sessions 44, 1977. pp 25-44 ⟨II-00088⟩

Kennedy, J.E.: Jane Soley Hamilton, Midwife. Nova Scotia Historical Review 2:6-30, 1982 ⟨I-05070⟩

Kergin, F.G.: Robert Meredith Janes: an appreciation. CMAJ 95:1399-1400, 1966 ⟨I-02550⟩

Kergin, F.G.: Robert Meredith Janes 1894-1966. Canadian Journal of Surgery 10:1-2, 1967 ⟨I-02549⟩

Kernaghan, L.K.: John Philipps. DCB 5:670, 1983 ⟨I-05307⟩

Kernaghan, L.K.: William James Almon. DCB 5:23-24, 1983 ⟨I-05318⟩

Kerr, J.L.: Wilfred Grenfell: His Life and Work. New York, Dodd, Mead and Company, 1959, 270 p. ⟨I-04479⟩

Kerr, R.B.: (Wallace Wilson). British Columbia Medical Journal 8:232, 1966 ⟨I-03402⟩

Kerr, R.B.: History of the Medical Council of Canada. Ottawa, The Medical Council of Canada, 1979. 131 p. ⟨II-00131⟩

Kett, J.F.: American and Canadian Medical Institutions, 1800-1870. JHMAS 22:343-356, 1967 ⟨II-00319⟩

Keys, D.A.: Andre Joseph Cipriani, 1908-1956. Proceedings and Transactions of the Royal Society of Canada Series 3, 50:65-9, 1956 ⟨I-04775⟩

Keys, D.A.: Dr. Andre Joseph Cipriani. CMAJ 74:590, 1956 ⟨I-04743⟩

Keys, D.A.: James Bertram Collip, C.B.E., M.D., Ph.D., D.Sc., F.R.S. CMAJ 93:774-775, 1965 ⟨I-02004⟩

Keys, T.: Canada's Contribution to the Medical Library Association. Bulletin of the Medical Library Association 47:419-423, 1959 ⟨II-00146⟩

Keywan, Z.: Mary Percy Jackson: pioneer doctor. The Beaver, pp. 41-48, Winter 1977 ⟨II-00477⟩

Kidd, G.A.: Smallpox in Vancouver. Vancouver Medical Association Bulletin 23:86-88, 1946-47 ⟨II-03959⟩

Kidd, G.E.: Trepanation Among the Early Indians of British Columbia. CMAJ 55:513-516, 1946 ⟨II-03951⟩

Kidd, G.E.: History of the Vancouver Medical Association. Bulletin of the History of Medicine 19:50-52, 1945; 23:5-8, 1946-47; 23:101-102, 1946-47; 23:148-150; 195-196; 233-235; 264-67; 290-96, 1946-47; 24:7-10, 1947-48 ⟨II-03963⟩

Kidd, H.M.: The William Osler Medal Essay: Pioneer Doctor John Sebastian Helmcken. BHM 21:419-461, 1947 ⟨I-02487⟩

Kidd, H.M.: John Antle. CMAJ 65:484-489, 1951 ⟨I-03875⟩

Kidd, K.E.: A Note on the Palaeopathology of Ontario. American Journal of Physical Anthropology 12:610-615, 1954 ⟨II-03960⟩

Kidston, J.: Harry Wishart Keith, M.D. 1873-1933. Okanagan Historical Society Annual Report 30L145-147, 1966 ⟨I-05069⟩

Kiely, E.B.: Dr. M.W. Locke Heals with his Hands. 1937. n.p., no pagination (first published as a series of articles in the Montreal Daily Herald). ⟨I-01519⟩

King, F.E.: The Past and the Future of Canadian Voluntary Tuberculosis Associations. Canadian Journal of Public Health 59:123-125, 1968 ⟨II-03957⟩

King, M.K.: The development of university nursing education. In; Innis, M.Q.: Nursing Education in a Changing Society. Toronto, University of Toronto Press, 1970. pp 67-85 ⟨II-03652⟩

Kingsmill, D.P.: The International Grenfell Association. McGill Medical Journal 25:121-127, 1956 ⟨II-03958⟩

Kinietz, W.V.: Indians of the Great Lakes -- Huron: Shamans and Medical Practice. Michigan University Museum of Anthropology Occasional Contributions, 10:131-160, 1940 ⟨II-00615⟩

Kippen, D: [Reminiscences]. Winnipeg Clinic Quarterly 23:94-96, 1970 ⟨II-03956⟩

Kirkland, A.S.: Dr. Alban Frederick Emery. CMAJ 30:108-109, 1934 ⟨I-03544⟩

Kirkland, A.S.: Dr. Stephen Henry McDonald, an appreciation. CMAJ 34:358-359, 1936 ⟨I-03447⟩

Kirkland, A.S.: Dr. Frederick Henry Wetmore. CMAJ 39:510, 1938 ⟨I-03330⟩

Kirkland, A.S.: Dr. George Clowes VanWart. CMAJ 39:510, 1938 ⟨I-03329⟩

Kirkland, A.S.: Hon. Dr. W.F. Roberts. CMAJ 38:303, 1938 ⟨I-03371⟩

Kirkland, A.S.: Dr. H.I. Taylor. CMAJ 48:464-465, 1943 ⟨I-02698⟩

Kirkland, A.S.: Dr. William Warwick. CMAJ 49:68, 1943 ⟨I-04267⟩

Kirkland, A.S.: Dr. George Arthur Beldon Addy. CMAJ, 52:312, 1945 ⟨I-04368⟩

Kirkland, A.S.: Dr. John Clarence Webster, M.D.C.M., C.M.G., D. Sc., LL.D., F.R.C.P., F.A.C.S., F.R.S.,. CMAJ 62:521-2, 1950 ⟨I-04486⟩

Kirkland, A.S.: Dr. Hugh A. Farris. CMAJ 68:625-6, 1953 ⟨I-04528⟩

Klass, A.: Dr. Joseph Doupe, an appreciation. CMAJ 95:1329-1331, 1966 ⟨I-01472⟩

Klassen, H.C.: John Bunn. DCB 9:102-103, 1976 ⟨I-00991⟩

Klinck, C.F.: William "Tiger" Dunlop. "Blackwoodian Backwoodsman". Toronto, Ryerson Press, 1958. 185 p. ⟨II-00841⟩

Klotz, O.: The Library. Bulletin of the Academy of Medicine, Toronto, May 1932, pp 49-52 ⟨II-00147⟩

Knox, O.: The Question of Louis Riel's Insanity. Historical and Scientific Society of Manitoba. Papers, Series 3, No. 6:20-34, 1951 ⟨II-02102⟩

Kourllsky, R.: La medecine canadienne-francaise et la France. La Vie Medicale au Canada Francais 1:696-704, 1972 ⟨II-02401⟩

Kozar, A.J.: R. Tait McKenzie, The Sculptor of Athletes. Knoxville, University of Tennessee Press, 1975. 118 p. ⟨I-01286⟩

Krasnick, C.L.: "In Charge of the Loons" A Portrait of the London, Ontario Asylum for the Insane in the Nineteenth Century. Ontario History 74:138-184, 1982 ⟨II-05011⟩

Krumbhaar, E.B.: Memoir of R. Tait McKenzie, M.D. Transactions and Studies of the College of Physicians of Philadelphia 6:260-270, 1938 ⟨I-03218⟩

Kutcher, S.P.: Toronto's Metaphysicians: the social gospel and medical professionalization in Victorian Toronto. Journal of the History of Canadian Science, Technology and Medicine 5(1):41-51, 1981 ⟨II-03261⟩

L

L., A.: Dr. Thomas Lowell Butters. CMAJ 31:452-453, 1934 ⟨I-03513⟩

L., E.K.: Dr. Murray Scott Douglas. CMAJ 85:761-762, 1961 ⟨I-01496⟩

L., E.K.: Dr. C. Carman White, an appreciation. CMAJ 89:99-100, 1963 ⟨I-02707⟩

L., G.: Honourable William E. Egbert. CMAJ 36:210, 1937 ⟨I-03437⟩

L., G.E.: Lieutenant-Colonel John Nisbet Gunn, DSO, MB. CMAJ 37:510-511, 1937 ⟨I-02882⟩

L., J.: Dr. George Wilbur Graham. CMAJ 17:128, 1927 ⟨I-02148⟩

Lacey, L.: Micmac Indian Medicine: A Traditional Way of Health. Antigonish, N.S., Formac Limited, 1977. 74 p. ⟨II-00635⟩

Lacourciere, L.: A Survey of Folk Medicine in French Canada from Early Times to the Present. In: Hand, W.D.: American Folk Medicine a Symposium. Berkeley, University of California Press, 1976. pp 203-214 ⟨II-02334⟩

Ladell, M.: 'The Tiger': A Giant of a Man. The Medical Post, October 1983. p. 2 ⟨I-05217⟩

Laflamme, M.L.: I -- Michel Sarrazin: Materiaux pour servir a l'histoire de la science en Canada. PTRSC 5:1-23, 1887 ⟨I-01969⟩

Lafleche, G.: Le chamanisme des Amerindiens et des missionnaires de la Nouvelle-France. Studies in Religion/Sciences Religieuses 9:137-160, 1980 ⟨II-04219⟩

Lahaise, R.: L'Hotel-Dieu de Vieux-Montreal, 1642-1861. Montreal, Hurtubise HMH, 1973 ⟨II-05150⟩

Laird, D.H.: Prisoner Five-One-Eleven. Toronto, Ontario Press, Ltd. (1917?), 115 p. ⟨II-04217⟩

Lajoie, G.: A la Memoire de Sir Frederick Banting. L'UMC 71:1331-1332, 1942 ⟨I-00960⟩

Lamb, W.K.: William Fraser Tolmie. DCB 11:885-888, 1982 ⟨I-04856⟩

Landes, R.: Ojibwa religion and the Midewiwin. Madison/Milwaukee/London, University of Wisconsin Press, 1968. 250 p. ⟨II-00643⟩

Landon, F.: The Duncombe Uprising of 1837 and Some of its Consequences. PTRSC series 3, vol. 25:83-98, 1931 ⟨I-03367⟩

Landry, Y.: Mortalite, nuptialite et canadianisation des troupes francaises de la guerre de Sept Ans. Histoire Social/Social History 12:299-315, 1979 ⟨II-04663⟩

Langdon, E.: Medicines Out of the Earth. Canadian [Antique] Collector 13:28-31, 1978 ⟨II-00222⟩

Langley, R.: Bethune. Vancouver, Talonbooks, 1975. 119 p. ⟨I-05185⟩

Langmuir, J.W.: Asylums, Prisons and Public Charities of Ontario and their Systems of Management. Can. Mon. 5:239-47, 1880 ⟨II-05160⟩

Langstaff, J.R.: Dr. Lillian: A Memoir. Ontario, The Langstaff Medical Heritage Committee, 1979, 44 p. ⟨I-04432⟩

Lapierre, G.: Dr. Raoul Masson. CMAJ 19:739, 1928 ⟨I-03493⟩

Lapointe, M.: Hotel-Dieu Saint-Vallier de Chicoutimi. L'UMC 97:703-04, 1968 ⟨II-05422⟩

Laramee, A.: Georges Grenier, M.D. L'UMC 5:286-88, 1876 ⟨I-04829⟩

Large, R.G.: Drums and Scalpel. From Native Healers to Physicians on the North Pacific Coast. Vancouver, Mitchell Press Limited, 1968. 145 p. ⟨II-00532⟩

Large, R.G.: History of the Prince Rupert General Hospital. Vancouver, Mitchell Press Ltd., [1972?] 28 p. ⟨II-04610⟩

Laterriere, P. de S.: Memoires de Pierre de Sales Laterriere et de ses Traverses. Quebec, L'Imprimerie de L'Evenement, 1873. pp 271 ⟨I-02257⟩

Lauder, B.: Two Radicals: Richard Maurice Bucke and Lawren Harris. Dalhousie Review 56:307-318, 1976-77 ⟨I-02580⟩

Laugier, H.: Banting et la Decouverte de L'Insuline. L'UMC 70:347-351, 1941 ⟨II-02407⟩

Lauriston, V.: A Centennial Chronicle of Kent Doctors. Chatham, Shepherd Printing Co. Ltd. 1967. p. 248 ⟨II-04382⟩

Lauze, S: Louis-Charles Simard, 1900-1970. L'UMC 1314-1315, 1970 ⟨I-01077⟩

Lavell, A.E.: The Beginning of Ontario Mental Hospitals. Queen's Quarterly 49:59-67, 1942 ⟨II-01842⟩

Laver, A.B.: The Historiography of Psychology in Canada. Journal of the History of the Behavorial Sciences 13(3):243-41, 1977 ⟨II-05328⟩

Lawrence, D.G.: "Resurrection" and legislation or body-snatching in relation to the anatomy act in the Province of Quebec. BHM 32:408-424, 1958 ⟨II-00035⟩

Lawrence, J.W.: The Medical Men of St. John. New Brunswick Historical Society Collections 1:273-305, 1894-97 ⟨II-05157⟩

Layton, M.: Magico-Religious Elements in the Traditional Beliefs of Maillardville, B.C. British Columbia Studies 27:50-61, 1975 ⟨II-03255⟩

Lea, R.G.: History of the Practice of Medicine in Prince Edward Island. P.E.I., Prince Edward Island Medical Society. III p. ⟨II-00854⟩

Lea, R.G.: Dr. John MacKieson (1795-1885): Strangulated Hernia in the Early 19th Century. Canadian Journal of Surgery 8:1-9, 1965 ⟨I-04232⟩

Lea, R.G.: History of Medicine in Prince Edward Island. Nova Scotia Medical Bulletin 52:212-4, 1973 ⟨II-05438⟩

Leacock, S.: The Death of John McCrae. University Monthly [Toronto], April 1918, pp 245-248 ⟨I-03165⟩

Leacock, S.: Andrew Macphail. Queen's Quarterly 45:445-463, 1938 ⟨I-02129⟩

Learmonth, G.E.: Dr. Leverett George De Veber. CMAJ 15:868, 1925 ⟨I-01503⟩

Learmonth, G.E.: Dr. Thomas Henry Crawford. CMAJ 15:1281-1282, 1925 ⟨I-01593⟩

Learmonth, G.E.: Dr. Neville James Lindsay. CMAJ 16:204, 1926 ⟨I-01601⟩

Learmonth, G.E.: Dr. Daniel Rolston Dunlop. CMAJ 18:356, 1928 ⟨I-01627⟩

Learmonth, G.E.: The Hon. Dr. R.G. Brett. CMAJ 21:621, 1929 ⟨I-02045⟩

Learmonth, G.E.: Dr. John Collison. CMAJ 23:116, 1930 ⟨I-03022⟩

Learmonth, G.E.: Dr. Thomas Henry Blow. CMAJ 28:227. 1933 ⟨I-03081⟩

Learmonth, G.E.: Dr. Joseph Gamache. CMAJ 30:226, 1934 ⟨I-03551⟩

Learmonth, G.E.: The Fiftieth Anniversary of the Alberta Medical Association. Alberta Medical Bulletin 20:50-57, 1955 ⟨II-03738⟩

LeBlond, S.: Le Docteur P.C. Dagneau. CMAJ 43:193-194, 1940 ⟨I-03340⟩

LeBlond, S.: Dr. Paul Garneau. CMAJ 45:89, 1941 ⟨I-03534⟩

LeBlond, S.: Le Medecin Autrefois, au Canada (1534-1847). Laval Medicale 12:695-709, 1947 ⟨II-04667⟩

LeBlond, S.: History of the Hotel-Dieu de Quebec. CMAJ 60:75-80, 1949 ⟨II-04678⟩

LeBlond, S.: La France et la medecine canadienne. La Revue de L'Universite Laval 4:571-587, 1950 ⟨II-04666⟩

LeBlond, S.: L'Hopital de la Marine de Quebec. L'UMC 80:616-626, 1951 ⟨II-02370⟩

LeBlond, S.: L'Hotel-Dieu de Quebec. Laval Medical 16:5-17, 1951 ⟨II-04679⟩

LeBlond, S.: James Douglas, M.D. (1800-1886). CMAJ 66:283-287, 1952 ⟨I-01201⟩

LeBlond, S.: Joseph Painchaud. L'UMC 82:1-6, 1953 ⟨II-00454⟩

LeBlond, S.: Cholera in Quebec in 1849. CMAJ, 71:288-292, 1954 ⟨II-04647⟩

LeBlond, S.: Le Cholera A Quebec En 1849. CMAJ, 71:292-296 1954 ⟨II-04710⟩

LeBlond, S.: Le Meurtre de Pierre Dion. Laval Medical 21:3-10, 1956 ⟨II-01895⟩

LeBlond, S.: The Marine Hospital of Quebec. CACHB 21:33-46, 1956 ⟨II-00191⟩

LeBlond, S.: Le Dr. Dill. CMAJ 79:55-57, 1958 ⟨I-01502⟩

LeBlond, S.: Pierre-Martial Bardy. Laval Medical 27(4):3-10, 1959 ⟨I-03876⟩

LeBlond, S.: Le Docteur Cyrille-Hector-Octave Cote et le Mouvement Baptiste Francais au Canada. Lavale Medicale 30(5):634-641, 1960 ⟨II-02474⟩

LeBlond, S.: Michel Sarrazin: un document inedit. Laval Medical 31(3):1-8, 1961 ⟨I-01981⟩

LeBlond, S.: Alexis St-Martin: Sa Vie et Son Temps. Laval Medical 33:578-585, 1962 ⟨I-01970⟩

LeBlond, S.: Pioneers of Medical Teaching in the Province of Quebec. JAMA 200:843-848, 1967 ⟨II-02429⟩

LeBlond, S.: Quebec en 1832. Laval Medical 38:183-191, 1967 ⟨II-02408⟩

LeBlond, S.: Le docteur Alfred Gauvreau Belleau (1842-1905). Laval Medical 39:870-73, 1968 ⟨I-05296⟩

LeBlond, S.: Une Conference Inedite du Docteur Joseph Painchaud. Laval Medical 39:355-360, 1968 ⟨II-04661⟩

LeBlond, S.: Histoire de la Medecine au Canada Francais. Cahiers Med Lyonnais 45:2389-2396, 1969 ⟨II-02402⟩

LeBlond, S.: La Legislation Medicale a la Periode Francaise. Bulletin du College des Medecins et Chirurgiens da la Province de Quebec 9(3):50-53, 1969 ⟨II-02433⟩

LeBlond, S.: Le Docteur George Douglas (1804-1864). Cahier des Dix 34:144-164, 1969 ⟨I-00881⟩

LeBlond, S.: La Legislation Medicale a la Periode Anglaise. Bulletin du College des Medecins et Chirurgiens da la Province de Quebec 10(3):71-77, 1970 ⟨II-02414⟩

LeBlond, S.: La Medecine dan la Province de Quebec anant 1847. Cahier des Dix 35:69-95, 1970 ⟨II-00137⟩

LeBlond, S.: William Marsden (1807-1885): Essai Biographique. Laval Medical 41:639-658, 1970 ⟨II-00321⟩

LeBlond, S.: Le docteur Joseph Painchaud (1787-1871) conferencier populaire. Cahier des Dix 36:120-138, 1971 ⟨II-00320⟩

LeBlond, S.: La Medecine et les Medecins a Quebec en 1872. L'UMC 101:2720-2725, 1972 ⟨II-04665⟩

LeBlond, S.: Le drame de Kamouraska: d'apres les documents de l'epoque. Cahier des Dix 37:239-273, 1972 ⟨II-02412⟩

LeBlond, S.: Docteur Cyrille Hector Octave Cote (1809-1850). L'UMC 102:1572-1574, 1973 ⟨I-00928⟩

LeBlond, S.: Le profession medicale sous l'Union (1840-1867). Cahier des Dix 38:165-203, 1973 ⟨II-02430⟩

LeBlond, S.: Au Quebec, on volait aussi des cadavres. La Vie medicale au Canada francais 3:1210-1213, 1974 ⟨II-04669⟩

LeBlond, S.: La Societe Canadienne D'Histoire de la Medecine. Cahier des Dix 39:1-32, 1974 ⟨II-02423⟩

LeBlond, S.: Le testament de Michel Sarrazin. La Vie medicale au Canada francais 3:510-513, 1974 ⟨I-04655⟩

LeBlond, S.: Le vol des cadavres dans la legende au Quebec. La Vie medicale au Canada francais 3:67-68, 1974 ⟨II-02413⟩

LeBlond, S.: Ne a La Grosse-Ile. Cahier des Dix 40:113-139, 1975 ⟨I-00882⟩

LeBlond, S.: George Mellis Douglas. DCB 9:217-218, 1976 ⟨I-00880⟩

LeBlond, S.: Le genou malade de Madame d'Youville. Cahier des Dix 41:43-49, 1976 ⟨II-00109⟩

LeBlond, S.: Le Mal De La Baie Etait-Il La Syphilis?. In International Congress for the History of Medicine, 25th, Quebec, 1976. Proceedings, Volume II, 1976. p. 866-872 ⟨II-00120⟩

LeBlond, S.: La mal de la Baie: etait-ce la syphilis?. CMAJ 116:1284-88, 1977 ⟨II-00354⟩

LeBlond, S.: Homeopathie. Le Vie medicale au Canada Francais 7:1055-1061, 1978 ⟨II-04674⟩

LeBlond, S.: Le Dr. James Douglas, de Quebec, remonte le Nil en 1860-61. Les Cahiers Des Dix 42:101-123, 1979 ⟨I-01665⟩

LeBlond, S.: Arthur Vallee, M.D. Newsletter, Canadian Society for the History of Medicine, 6:15-16, 1981 ⟨I-04767⟩

LeBlond, S.: Medecins et Chirurgiens en France et en Houvelle-France. Canadian Society for the History of Medicine Newsletter, 5:3-12, 1981 ⟨II-04672⟩

LeBlond, S.: James Douglas. DCB 11:271-272. 1982 ⟨I-04866⟩

LeBlond, S.: Le Service de Sante des Anciens Combattants a Quebec en 1947. CSHM Newsletter, Spring 1982, pp 7-10 ⟨II-04944⟩

LeBlond, S.: Dr. Charles Auguste Gauthier. CMAJ 129:771-772, 1983 ⟨I-05163⟩

LeBlond, S.: L'enseignement de la medecine a l'Universite Laval de 1923 a 1928. Canadian Society for the History of Medicine Newsletter, 1983. pp 1-5 ⟨II-05278⟩

LeBlond, S.: Margaret Charlton. CSHM Newsletter, Spring 1983, pp 15-16 ⟨I-05063⟩

LeClair, M.: Leopold Morisette (1911-1970). L'UMC 100:770-2, 1971 ⟨I-02262⟩

Lecours, A.: La Medecine Francaise D'Hier et D'Aujourd'Hui au Canada. L'UMC 79:792-796, 1950 ⟨II-02355⟩

Leduc, J.: La vie et l'ouevre de Jean-Pierre Cordeau, 1922-1971. L'UMC 101:2641-5, 1972 ⟨I-05294⟩

Lee, D.: Jean Legere de la Grange. DCB 2:387-388, 1969 ⟨I-01021⟩

Lee, E.J.: History of the Osler Society of McGill. McGill Medical Journal 34:146-148, 1965 ⟨II-03737⟩

Lee, H.K.: Honoring the Founder in His Country: Conception and Struggle for Canada's Memorial College. Chiropractic History 1:43-46, 1981 ⟨II-04888⟩

Leechman, D.: Trephined Skulls from British Columbia. PTRSC 38:99-102, 1944 ⟨II-03869⟩

Leeder, F.: Dr. Melbourne Raynor. CMAJ 16:100, 1926 ⟨I-01605⟩

Leeder, F.: Dr. R.L. Fraser. CMAJ 16:99, 1926 ⟨I-01606⟩

Lefebvre, E.: Judith Moreau de Bresoles. DCB 1:512, 1966 ⟨I-01459⟩

Lefebvre, J.J., Desjardins, E.: Le Docteur George Selby, Medecin de L'Hotel-Dieu de 1807 a 1829, et sa Famille. L'UMC 100:1592-1594, 1971 ⟨I-02244⟩

Lefebvre, J.J., Desjardins, E.: Les medecins canadiens diplomes des universites etrangeres au XIX siecle. L'UMC 101:935-51, 1972 ⟨II-05334⟩

Leger, J.: L'association des medecins de langue francaise du Canada et L'Union Medicale du Canada. L'UMC 101:2376-2377, 1972 ⟨II-02460⟩

Legett, L.: History of Medicine in Guelph. Guelph, Westmount Medical Building, 1980 ⟨II-02101⟩

Lehmann, P.O.: Louis Riel -- patriot or zealot?. B.C. Medical Journal 5:154-171, 1963 ⟨II-02619⟩

Lem, C.: Bethune Memorial House. Ontario Museum Association Quarterly 7(2):5-6, 1978 ⟨I-00966⟩

Lenoch, F.: Dr. Wallace Graham: an appreciation. CMAJ 88:167-168, 1963 ⟨I-02139⟩

LeSage, A.: L'epidemie de grippe a Montreal en 1918. L'UMC 48:1-10, 1919 ⟨II-02388⟩

LeSage, A.: Bulletin 1872-1922: Le Cinquantenaire de LUnion Medicale du Canada. L'UMC 51:1-10, 1922 ⟨II-02448⟩

LeSage, A.: Le Programme de L'Union Medicale du Canada 1872-1932. L'UMC 61:553-562, 1932 ⟨II-02445⟩

LeSage, A.: Les Debuts de L'Union Medicale Durant L'Annee 1872. Le Dr. Rottot. L'UMC 61:78-95, 1932 ⟨I-02226⟩

LeSage, A.: Le Decanat a la Faculte de Medecine de L'Universite de Montreal: Trois Doyens (1880-1934) -- Rottot, Lachapelle, Harwood. L'UMC 68:166-178, 1939 ⟨I-02264⟩

LeSage, A.: Le Tricentenaire de la Fondation de L'Hotel-Dieu de Quebec 1639-1939. L'UMC 68:329-336, 1939 ⟨II-02368⟩

LeSage, A.: Le Tricentenaire de L'Hotel-Dieu et de Saint-Sulpice. L'UMC 70:1268-1270, 1941 ⟨II-02362⟩

LeSage, A.: Docteur Charles-Paul Gaboury, Colonel R.C.A.M.C. L'UMC 71:447-449, 1942 ⟨I-01767⟩

LeSage, A.: Jacques de Lorimier Bourgeois. L'UMC 72:1-4, 1943 ⟨I-02001⟩

LeSage, A.: 75e Anniversaire de la Fondation de "L'Union Medicale du Canada" 1872-1947. L'UMC 75:1265-1304, 1946; 76:300-327, 1947 ⟨II-02452⟩

Lessard, R.: Un De Nos Illustres Devanciers: Jean-Francois Gaultier. L'UMC 95:676-678, 1966 ⟨I-02237⟩

Lessard, R.: Les Debuts de la Cardiologie a Quebec. CSHM Newsletter, Spring 1982, pp 17-18 ⟨II-04943⟩

Lessard, R.: Alexandre Serres. DCB 5:752, 1983 ⟨I-05304⟩

Lessard, R.: Francois-Michel Suzor. DCB 5:788-89, 1983 ⟨I-05302⟩

Letondal, P.: Introduction a L'Histoire de la Pediatrie au Canada Francais. In International Congress for the History of Medicine, 25th, Quebec, 1976. Proceedings, Volume II, 1976. p. 885-894 ⟨II-00742⟩

Letondal, P.: Raoul Masson (1875-1928): Pionnier de la pediatrie au Canada francais. L'UMC 108:1-4, 1979 ⟨I-01422⟩

Levine, I.E.: The discoverer of insulin: Dr. Frederick G. Banting. Toronto, The Copp Clark Publishing Co. Ltd., 1959. pp 192 ⟨I-00962⟩

Lewis, D.S.: The Royal College of Physicians and Surgeons of Canada 1920-1960. Montreal, McGill University Press, 1962. 241 p. ⟨II-00441⟩

Lewis, D.S.: Royal Victoria Hospital 1887-1947. Montreal, McGill University Press, 1969, 327 p. ⟨II-00175⟩

Lewis, D.S.: Campbell B. Keenan, D.S.O., M.D., C.M., F.R.C.S. [C], 1867 to 1953. Canadian Journal of Surgery 15:287-294, 1972 ⟨I-04225⟩

Lewis, J.: Something Hidden: A Biography of Wilder Penfield. Toronto, Doubleday Canada Ltd., 1981, 311 p. ⟨I-04765⟩

Leys, J.F.: A physical fitness shrine in Canada. CMAJ 82:1330-1332, 1960 ⟨II-03736⟩

Leys, J.F.: Theirs Be The Glory. In: Davidson, S.A.; Blackstock, P. (Edit.) the R. Tait McKenzie Memorial Addresses. Canadian Association for Health, Physical Education and Recreation, 1980. 7-14 ⟨II-00376⟩

Libman, E.: Louis Gross, May 5, 1895 - October 17, 1937. Journal of the Mount Sinai Hospital Hospital 4, 1938 ⟨I-02120⟩

Linell, E.A.: The Academy of Medicine of Toronto 1907-1957. CMAJ 76:437-442, 1957 ⟨II-03735⟩

Linell, E.A.: A Cairn to the memory of Osler. CMAJ 85:1347-1350, 1961 ⟨I-02290⟩

Link, E.P.: Vermont physicians and the Canadian Rebellion of 1837. Vermont History 37(3), 1969 ⟨II-00677⟩

Linton, R.: The Collip Medical Research Laboratory. University of Western Ontario Medical Journal 28:39-45, 1958 ⟨II-03852⟩

Lipinski, J.K.: Original Publications in Diagnostic Radiology by Canadian Physicians 1896-1920. CSHM Newsletter, Spring 1983. pp 8-12 ⟨II-05112⟩

Lipinski, J.K.: Some Observations on Early Diagnostic Radiology in Canada. CMAJ 129:766, 768, 1983. ⟨II-05270⟩

Liptzin, B.: The Effects of National Health Insurance on Canadian Psychiatry: The Ontario Experience. American Journal of Psychiatry 134:248-252, 1977 ⟨II-00578⟩

Liston, A.: To Cure the Sick and Protect the Healthy. In International Congress for the History of Medicine, 25th, Quebec, 1976. Proceedings, Volume 1, 1976. p. 217-228 ⟨II-00437⟩

Little, H.M.: Dr. Frederick Albert Lawton Lockhart. CMAJ 15:220, 1925 ⟨I-03083⟩

Little, S.W.: Physicians to the Company of Adventurers. CAMSI Journal 17:7, 9-10,13-14, 1958 (Apr) ⟨II-00405⟩

Littmann, S.K.: A Pathography of Louis Riel. Canadian Psychiatric Association Journal 23:449-62, 1978 ⟨II-05257⟩

Littmann, S.K.: History and the Psychiatrist. Canadian Psychiatric Association Journal 23:430-31, 1978 ⟨II-05358⟩

Livermore, J.D.: The Personal Agonies of Edward Blake. CHR 56:45-58, 1975 ⟨II-04876⟩

Lloyd, S.: The Ottawa Typhoid Epidemics of 1911 and 1912: A Case Study of Disease as a Catalyst for Urban Reform. Urban History Review 8:66-89, 1979 ⟨II-04209⟩

Lockwood, A.L.: Dr. Robert Hugh Arthur. CMAJ 46:198-9, 1942 ⟨I-04252⟩

Lockwood, A.L.: Founder's Philosophy Still Pervades Toronto's Earliest Medical Clinic. Canadian Doctor 29(3):34-37, 1963 ⟨II-03760⟩

Lockwood, T.M.: A History of Medical Practice in and Around Port Credit (1789-1963). Ontario Medical Review 30:653-658, 1963 ⟨II-03745⟩

Loeb, L.J.: The Cholera Epidemics in Upper Canada 1832-1834. Western Ontario Historical Notes 11:44-54, 1953 ⟨II-04988⟩

Loew, F.M.: Veterinary Surgeons in the North West Mounted Police: Incident at Lethbridge, 1890. Canadian Veterinary Journal 18:233-40, 1977 ⟨II-05426⟩

Long, C.N.H.: Dr. Jonathan Campbell Meakins: an appreciation. CMAJ 81:955-956, 1959 ⟨I-03456⟩

Longley, J.W.: Sir Charles Tupper. Toronto, Makers of Canada (Morang) Ltd., 1916. 304 p. ⟨I-05051⟩

Lonjias, H.T.: Physicians as Explorers in the New World. Ciba Symposia 2:643-652, 1940 ⟨II-03955⟩

Lord, J.: The Song of Alopeix, and Other Poems [Terry Fox]. Hamilton, Epic Publishing Co., 1983. pp viii + 109 ⟨II-05283⟩

Lortie, L.: Jean-Baptiste Meilleur. DCB 10:504-509, 1972 ⟨I-01440⟩

Lortie, L.: Francois-Alexandre-Hubert La Rue. DCB 11:495-97, 1982 ⟨I-04849⟩

Lortie, L.: Joseph-Alexandre Crevier. DCB 11:217-18, 1982 ⟨I-04863⟩

Lougheed, P.: Inspiration and a source of pride. CMAJ 120:988, 1979 ⟨I-01413⟩

Louw, J.: A Tribute from South Africa [W.C. MacKenzie]. Canadian Journal of Surgery 22:310, 1979 ⟨I-04285⟩

Lovejoy, E.P.: Canada. In: Women Doctors of the World. New York, The MacMillan Company, 1957. pp 111-118 ⟨II-05014⟩

Low, D.M.: Robert Meredith Janes: The Man (an appreciation). CMAJ 95:1400, 1966 ⟨I-02278⟩

Low, J.: Dr. Charles Frederick Newcombe. The Beaver, Spring 1982, pp 32-39 ⟨I-04833⟩

Lowy, F.H.: Clarence B. Farrar 1874-1970 and the History of Psychiatry in Canada. Canadian Psychiatric Association Journal 20:1-2, 1975 ⟨II-05322⟩

Lozynsky, A.: Richard Maurice Bucke, Medical Mystic. Detroit, Wayne State University Press, 1977. 203 p. ⟨I-00001⟩

Lucas, D.M.: H. Ward Smith. CMAJ 97:363-364, 1967 ⟨I-01684⟩

Lucas, G.H.W.: The Discovery and Pharmacology of Cyclopropane. Canadian Anesthetists' Society Journal 7:237-256, 1960 ⟨II-03746⟩

Lucas, G.H.W.: The discovery of cyclopropane. Anesthesia and Analgesia...Current Researches, 40:15-27, 1961 ⟨II-03851⟩

Luke, J.C.: Dr. George Gavin Miller, an appreciation. CMAJ 92:247, 1965 ⟨I-03198⟩

Lusignan, C.A.: Dr. Robert Nelson. Canada Medical Record 1:213-14, 1872-3 ⟨I-04826⟩

Luxton, E.G.: Stony Indian Medicine. In: Foster, J.E. (edit): The Developing West, Alberta, Univ. of Alberta Press, 1983. pp 101-121. ⟨II-05050⟩

Lynch, D.O.: A century of psychiatric teaching at Rockwood Hospital, Kingston. CMAJ 70:283-87, 1954 ⟨II-03744⟩

Lynch, M.J., Raphael, S.S.: Medicine and the State. Illinois, Charles C. Thomas, Publisher, 1963. 449 p. ⟨II-00430⟩

Lynn, R.B.: James Cameron Connell:1863-1947. Canadian Journal of Surgery 2:336-339, 1968 ⟨I-02013⟩

Lyon, E.K.: Dr. Norman Arnold McCormick. CMAJ 98:64-65, 1968 ⟨I-01761⟩

Lysaght, A.M.: Joseph Banks in Newfoundland and Labrador, 1766: His Diary, Manuscripts and Collections. Berkeley, University of California Press [1971], 512 p. ⟨II-05355⟩

M

M., A.S.: Dr. Alison Cumming. CMAJ 16:990-991, 1926 ⟨I-01618⟩

M., G.W.: Dr. W. Stuart Stanbury. CMAJ 87:1208, 1962 ⟨I-01633⟩

M, H.E.: Dr. Lawrence J. Rhea. CMAJ 51:184-5, 1944 ⟨I-04258⟩

M., H.E.: William W. Francis. CMAJ 81:516, 1959 ⟨I-02821⟩

M., J.A.: Dr. W.J.P. MacMillan. CMAJ 78:71, 1958 ⟨I-02836⟩

M, J.H.: Robert E. McKechnie, C.B.E., M.D., C.M. (McGill), LL.D. (McGill and U.B.C.), F.A.C.S., F.R.C.S. (C). CMAJ 51:81-90, 1944 ⟨I-04246⟩

M., J.H.: Dr. A.W. Bagnall. CMAJ 52:313, 1945 ⟨I-04369⟩

M., J.H.: Morris W. Thomas, M.D., C.M. CMAJ 52:112, 1945 ⟨I-04361⟩

M., J.H.: Dr. Charles S. McKee: an appreciation. CMAJ 86:141, 1962 ⟨I-03204⟩

M., R.: Dr. Wesley Herbert Secord. CMAJ 35:105, 1936 ⟨I-02870⟩

M., R.: Dr. Alexander Gibson. CMAJ 74:852, 1956 ⟨I-02776⟩

M., R.: Dr. Frederick Todd Cadham. CMAJ 84:673, 1961 ⟨I-01482⟩

M., R.I.: Wilfred Parsons Warner, DSC, CBE, MB, FRCP(c), LL.D.(Tor). CMAJ 74:167-168, 1956 ⟨I-04741⟩

M., W.B.: Dr. George Ray Johnson. CMAJ 74:590-591, 1956 ⟨I-02274⟩

Macallum, A.B.: Robert Fulford Ruttan. CMAJ 22:596-97, 1930 ⟨I-03029⟩

Macallum, A.B.: Alexander Dougall Blackader. CMAJ 26:519-524, 1932 ⟨I-02988⟩

MacBeath, G.: Gernard Marot. DCB 1:490, 1966 ⟨I-01458⟩

Macbeth, R.A.: Alexander Russell Munroe: 1879-1965. Canadian Journal of Surgery 10:3-10, 1967 ⟨I-03184⟩

Macbeth, R.A.: Dr. Thomas John Speakman: an appreciation. CMAJ 100:782-783, 1969 ⟨I-05045⟩

Macbeth, R.A.: Medicine in French Canada from 1608 to 1763. In International Congress for the History of Medicine, 25th Quebec, 1976. Proceedings, Volume III, 1976. p. 931-943 ⟨II-00870⟩

Macbeth, R.A.: Canadian Surgery During the French Regime, 1608 to 1763." Canadian Journal of Surgery 20:71-82, 1977 ⟨II-04332⟩

Macbeth, R.A.: Walter C. MacKenzie, OC, BSc, MD, CM. MS, FACS, FRCS C, Hon FRCS, Hon FRCS (Edin), Hon FRCS (Ire), Hon FRCS (Glas), LLD (McGill), LLD (Dalhousie), LLD (Manitoba), 1909-1978. Canadian Journal of Surgery 22:303-307, 1979 ⟨I-04290⟩

MacCallum, G.A.: History of the hospital for the insane (formerly the Military and Naval Depot), Penetanguishene, Ont. Ontario Historical Society Papers and Records 12:121-127, 1914 ⟨II-00156⟩

MacCharles, M.R.: Dr. Patrick H. McNulty. CMAJ 98:328-329, 1968 ⟨I-02303⟩

MacD, J.H.: Dr. Charles F. Covernton. CMAJ 79:1026-1027, 1958 ⟨I-02033⟩

MacD., J.H.: Dr. Charles F. Covernton. CMAJ 90:1478, 1964 ⟨I-05228⟩

MacDermot, H.E.: The earliest clinical applications of the X-rays. CMAJ 28:321-22, 1933 ⟨II-03143⟩

MacDermot, H.E.: A Bibliography of Canadian Medical Periodicals. Montreal, Renouf Publishing Co., 1934. 21 pp ⟨II-01533⟩

MacDermot, H.E.: The Early Days of the Montreal General Hospital. Surgery, Gynecology, and Obstetrics 59:120-125, 1934 ⟨II-05018⟩

MacDermot, H.E.: The early admission books of the Montreal General Hospital. CMAJ 36:524-529, 1937 ⟨II-03638⟩

MacDermot, H.E.: Sir Thomas Roddick. His Work in Medicine and Public Life. Toronto, Macmillan Co. of Canada Ltd., 1938. 160 p. ⟨I-01120⟩

MacDermot, H.E.: John McCrae's Autopsy Book. CMAJ 40:495, 1939 ⟨II-03594⟩

MacDermot, H.E.: Dr. Walter H. Smyth. CMAJ 45:287-288, 1941 ⟨I-03521⟩

MacDermot, H.E.: Maude Abbott: A Memoir. Toronto, Macmillan Co. of Canada Ltd., 1941. 264 p. ⟨I-00024⟩

MacDermot, H.E.: Seventy-Five Years of the Association. CMAJ 47:69-72, 1942 ⟨II-03853⟩

M[acDermot], H.E.: Dr. George A. Fleet. CMAJ 49:149, 1943 ⟨I-02175⟩

MacDermot, H.E.: A Short History of Health Insurance in Canada. CMAJ 50:447-454, 1944 ⟨II-00253⟩

MacDermot, H.E.: Dr. Edward Archibald, 1872-1945. McGill News, Spring 1946, 4p. ⟨I-04389⟩

MacDermot, H.E.: The Annual Meeting at Banff, in 1889. CMAJ, 54:496-498, 1946 ⟨II-04378⟩

M[acDermot], H.E.: Dr. Fred Holland Mackay. CMAJ 57:408-9, 1947 ⟨I-04402⟩

M[acDermot], H.E.: Dr. Harold Beveridge Cushing. CMAJ 57:606-7, 1947 ⟨I-04400⟩

M[acDermot], H.E.: Dr. William Boyman Howell. CMAJ 57:177-8, 1947 ⟨I-04411⟩

MacDermot, H.E.: Jeanne Mance. CMAJ 57:67-73, 1947 ⟨I-03426⟩

MacDermot, H.E.: A History of the Montreal General Hospital. Montreal, Montreal General Hospital, 1950. 135 p. ⟨II-00192⟩

MacDermot, H.E.: Dr. Cecil C. Birchard. CMAJ 65:393, 1951 ⟨I-04545⟩

M[acDermot], H.E.: Dr. H.P. Wright. CMAJ 66:295, 1952 ⟨I-04543⟩

M[acDermot], H.E.: Dr. Norman Gwyn. CMAJ 66:402-3, 1952 ⟨I-04541⟩

MacDermot, H.E.: Early Medical Education in North America. CMAJ 67:370-375, 1952 ⟨II-03678⟩

M[acDermot], H.E.: Dr. Alvah Hovey Gordon. CMAJ 68:300, 1953 ⟨I-04531⟩

M[acDermot], H.E.: Dr. Archibald Malloch. CMAJ 69:543-4, 1953 ⟨I-04523⟩

M[acDermot], H.E.: Dr. Frank S. Patch. CMAJ 69:79-80, 1953 ⟨I-04526⟩

M[acDermot], H.E.: J. Frederick Burgess. CMAJ 68:625, 1953 ⟨I-04530⟩

MacDermot, H.E.: Early Medical Journalism in Canada. CMAJ 72:536-539, 1955 ⟨II-01532⟩

MacDermot, H.E.: Notes on Canadian Medical History. British Medical Journal 1:925-930, 1955 ⟨II-03691⟩

MacDermot, H.E.: The Medical Faculties of Canadian Universities. CMAJ 73:101-103, 1955 ⟨II-03670⟩

MacDermot, H.E.: Dr. Mackenzie Forbes and his hospital. McGill News 37:35, 62, 1956 ⟨I-02792⟩

M[acDermot], H.E.: Professor Horst Oertel. CMAJ 74:485, 1956 ⟨I-04742⟩

MacDermot, H.E.: The Osler Library, Montreal. CMAJ 76:1077, 1957 ⟨II-03679⟩

MacDermot, H.E.: The papers of Dr. Thomas Simpson (1833-1918). CMAJ 77:266-267, 1957 ⟨I-01687⟩

MacDermot, H.E.: Francis J. Shepherd, M.D. LL.D. (Harvard, McGill, Queen's), Hon. F.R.C.S. Engl, Hon. F.A.C.S. Canadian Journal of Surgery 1:5-7, 1957-8 ⟨I-04242⟩

MacDermot, H.E.: History of the Canadian Medical Association, Vol. II. Toronto, Murray Printing and Gravure Ltd., 1958. 153 p. ⟨II-00449⟩

MacDermot, H.E.: Nora Livingston and Maude Abbott. CACHB 22:228-235, 1958 ⟨I-00023⟩

MacDermot, H.E.: The Calgary Associate Clinic Historical Bulletin. CMAJ 78:792, 1958 ⟨II-01540⟩

MacDermot, H.E.: Dr. William W. Francis 1878-1959. McGill News 61:16-17, 1959 ⟨I-02796⟩

MacDermot, H.E.: The Scottish Influence in Canadian Medicine. The Practitioner 183:84-91, 1959 ⟨II-03690⟩

MacDermot, H.E.: History of the School of Nursing of the Montreal General Hospital. Montreal, The Southam Printing Co. Ltd., 1961, 152 p. ⟨II-04471⟩

MacDermot, H.E.: The Fiftieth Anniversary of the Association Journal. CMAJ 84:1-5, 1961 ⟨II-01854⟩

MacDermot, H.E.: Thomas George Roddick (1846-1923). Canadian Journal of Surgery 4:1-3, 1960-61 ⟨I-04238⟩

MacDermot, H.E.: Dr. T. Clarence Routley, an appreciation. CMAJ 88:1046, 1963 ⟨I-01672⟩

MacDermot, H.E.: One Hundred Years of Medicine in Canada, 1867-1967. Toronto, McClelland and Stewart Ltd., 1967. 224 p ⟨II-00863⟩

MacDermot, H.E.: George Edgeworth Fenwick (1825-1894). Canadian Journal of Surgery 11:1-4, 1968 ⟨I-04229⟩

MacDermot, H.E.: Pioneering in Public Health. CMAJ 99:267-273, 1968 ⟨II-03686⟩

MacDermot, H.E.: The Years of Change (1945-70) [Montreal General Hospital]. Montreal General Hospital, [1970], 44 p. ⟨II-04615⟩

MacDermot, J.H.: J.S. Helmcken, MRCP(Lond.), LSA. CMAJ 55:166-171, 1946 ⟨I-02486⟩

MacDermot, J.H.: Food and Medicinal Plants used by the Indians of British Columbia. CMAJ 61:177-183, 1949 ⟨II-00616⟩

MacDermot, J.H.: Medical Men and Place Names of British Columbia. CMAJ 61:533-536, 1949 ⟨II-03677⟩

MacD(ermot), J.H.: Dr. William Brenton Burnett, an appreciation. CMAJ 90:1478, 1964 ⟨I-01549⟩

MacDermot, J.H.: Dr. Robert Lynn Gunn: an appreciation. CMAJ 92:897, 1965 ⟨I-02178⟩

MacDermot, J.H.: Dr. Thomas R.B. Nelles, an appreciation. CMAJ 98:180, 1968 ⟨I-01766⟩

MacDonald, A.E.: William Herbert Lowry, M.D., C.M., M.R.C.S., F.R.C.S. (C),. CMAJ 47:384, 1942 ⟨I-04277⟩

MacDonald, E.: Indian Medicine in New Brunswick. CMAJ 80:220-224, 1959 ⟨II-00618⟩

MacDonald, E.: Outport Medicine in Newfoundland. Canadian Pharmaceutical Journal 92(11):40-41, 1959 ⟨II-03689⟩

MacDonald, J.: Dr. Locke, Healer of Men. Toronto, Maclean Publishing Co., 1933. 83 p. ⟨I-01520⟩

MacDonald, J.A.: The Daffydil Story. University of Toronto Medical Journal 31:64-67, 1953 ⟨II-03642⟩

MacDonald, R.I.: Canadian Milestones in Clinical Medicine. Bulletin of the Medical Librarians Association 48:27-32, 1960 ⟨II-03671⟩

MacDonald, R.I.: Dr. Joseph Arthur MacFarlane, an appreciation. CMAJ 94:1067-1069, 1966 ⟨I-01054⟩

MacDonnell, R.: The Oldest Medical Journal in Canada. Canada Medical and Surgical Journal 13:1-7, 1884 ⟨II-00732⟩

MacDougall, D.S.: This Nova Scotia Pharmacy. Modern Pharmacy 63(2):12-13, 1948 ⟨II-03755⟩

MacDougall, H.: Researching Public Health Services in Ontario, 1882-1930. Archivaria 10:157-172, 1980 ⟨II-00565⟩

MacDougall, H.: Public Health in Toronto's Municipal Politics: The Canniff Years, 1883-1890. BHM 55:186-202, 1981 ⟨II-04638⟩

MacDougall, H.: Epidemics and the Environment: The Early Development of Public Health Activity in Toronto, 1832-1872. In: Jarrell, R.A.; Roos, A.E. (edit): Critical Issues in the History of Canadian Science, Technology and Medicine. Thornhill and Ottawa, HSTC Publications, 1983. pp 135-151 ⟨II-05194⟩

MacDougall, H.: "Enlightening the Public": The Views and Values of the Association of Executive Health Officers of Ontario, 1886-1903. In: Roland, C.G.(ed.): Health, Disease and Medicine: Essays in Canadian History. Toronto, Hannah Institute for the History of Medicine, 1984, 436-464 ⟨II-05411⟩

MacFarlane, J.A.: Dieppe in Retrospect. Lancet 1:498-500, 1943 ⟨II-04327⟩

MacFarlane, J.A.: Medical Education in Canada. Ottawa, Queen's Printer, 1965. 373 p. ⟨II-00238⟩

MacG., J.W.: Dr. John James Ower, an appreciation. CMAJ 86:796-797, 1962 ⟨I-02530⟩

Mackenzie, A.J.: A Canadian Naturalist; John Hutchison Garnier of Lucknow. CMAJ 17:355-356, 1927 ⟨I-02805⟩

Mackenzie, D.J.: The origin and development of a medical laboratory service in Halifax. Nova Scotia Medical Bulletin 43:179-184, 1964 ⟨II-03673⟩

Mackenzie, J.J.: Number 4 Canadian Hospital. The Letters of Professor Mackenzie, K.C. from the Salonika Front. Toronto, Macmillan Co. of Canada Ltd., 1933. 247 p. ⟨II-00816⟩

MacKenzie, K.A.: Abraham Gesner, M.D., Surgeon Geologist, 1797-1864. CMAJ 59:384-387, 1948 ⟨I-04480⟩

MacKenzie, K.A.: A Century of Medicine in Nova Scotia. Nova Scotia Medical Bulletin 32:290-295, 1953 ⟨II-03697⟩

MacKenzie, K.A.: Founders of the Medical Society of Nova Scotia. Nova Scotia Medical Bulletin 32:240-245, 1953 ⟨II-03688⟩

MacKenzie, K.A.: The First Physicians in Nova Scotia. CMAJ 68:610-612, 1953 ⟨II-03696⟩

MacKenzie, K.A.: Doctor John Fox: 1793-1866. Nova Scotia Medical Bulletin 33:302-303, 1954 ⟨I-02820⟩

MacKenzie, K.A.: Dr. Isaac Webster, 1766-1851. Nova Scotia Medical Bulletin 33:215-219, 1954 ⟨I-02734⟩

MacKenzie, K.A., Stewart, C.B.: Dalhousie University. CAMSI Journal 15:15-20, 1956 ⟨II-03676⟩

MacKenzie, K.A., Kirk, T.E., Lemoine, R.E.: Camp Hill Hospital: Its History and Development. Nova Scotia Medical Bulletin 36:369-74, 1957 ⟨II-03672⟩

MacKenzie, K.A.: In Retrospect. Dalhousie Medical Journal II:18-20, 1958 ⟨I-01410⟩

MacKenzie, K.A.: The beginnings of Dalhousie Medical School. Dalhousie Med J 11(1):7-11, 1958 ⟨II-00324⟩

MacKenzie, L., Johnston, S.R.: Dr. Robert Evatt Mathers. CMAJ 76:592, 1957 ⟨I-04732⟩

Mackenzie, N.: (Wallace Wilson). British Columbia Medical Journal 8:228, 1966 ⟨I-03320⟩

Mackie, H.G.: The Polio Epidemic of 1927. Okanagan Historical Society Annual Report 29:43-48, 1965 ⟨II-05116⟩

MacKinnon, C.: Sewell Foster. DCB 9:276-277, 1976 ⟨I-01213⟩

Macklin, C.C.: James Playfair McMurrich. CMAJ 40:409-410, 1939 ⟨I-02841⟩

Macklin, C.C.: Paul Stilwell McKibben 1886-1941. PTRSC 37:79-85, 1943 ⟨I-03571⟩

MacKnight, J.J.: George Arnold Burbidge, Dean of Pharmacy in the Maritimes and a Founder of Canadian Pharmacy; A Biography. Toronto, Canadian Academy of the History of Pharmacy, 1976. ⟨II-05234⟩

MacLaren, M.: Dr. George Eli Armstrong. CMAJ 29:103, 1933 ⟨I-03074⟩

MacLaren, M.: Col. F.G. Finley. CMAJ 43:193, 1940 ⟨I-03339⟩

MacLean, H.: A Pioneer Prairie Doctor. Saskatchewan History 15:58-66, 1962 ⟨II-00494⟩

MacLean, J.: The Medicine Stone. The Beaver 258:116-7, 1927 ⟨II-03251⟩

MacLean, J.: Blackfoot Medical Priesthood. Alberta Historical Review 9(2):1-7, 1961 ⟨II-02970⟩

MacLean, J.A.: Dr. Samuel Willis Prowse. CMAJ 25:366, 1931 ⟨I-03158⟩

MacLeod, W., Park, L., Ryerson, S.: Bethune: The Montreal Years. Toronto, James Lorimer and Company, 1978, 167 p. ⟨II-04930⟩

MacMillan, C.L.: Memoirs of a Cape Breton Doctor. Toronto, Montreal, New York, McGraw-Hill Ryerson Limited, 1975. 177 p. ⟨I-01411⟩

MacMillan, J.A.: Notes on the history of ophthalmology in Canada. American Journal of Ophthalmology 31:199-206, 1948 ⟨II-03674⟩

MacMillan, W.J.: Alexander MacNeill, MD, CM, FACS. CMAJ 16:707, 1926 ⟨I-01598⟩

MacMillan, W.J.P.: Dr. Harry Dawson Johnson. CMAJ 51:186-7, 1944 ⟨I-04256⟩

MacNab, E.: A Legal History of Health Professions in Ontario. Toronto, Queen's Printer, 1970. 152 p. ⟨II-00139⟩

Macphail, A.: Francis Wayland Campbell (1837-1905). In Kelly HW, Burrage WL: Dictionary of American Medical Biography. New York and London, D. Appleton and Co., 1928. pp. 195-196 ⟨I-00911⟩

Macphail, A.: Francis Buller (1844-1905). In Kelly HW, Burrage WL: Dictionary of American Medical Biography. New York and London, D. Appleton and Co., 1928. pp. 170-171 ⟨I-00978⟩

Macphail, A.: George Ross (1834-1892). In Kelly HW, Burrage WL: Dictionary of American Medical Biography. New York and London, D. Appleton and Co., 1928. p. 1058 ⟨I-01140⟩

Macphail, A.: James Stewart (1846-1906). In Kelly HW, Burrage WL: Dictionary of American Medical Biography New York and London, D. Appleton and Co., 1928. p 1166-1167 ⟨I-01097⟩

Macphail, A.: John Stephenson (1797-1842). In Kelly HW, Burrage WL: Dictionary of American Medical Biography. New York and London, D. Appleton and Co., 1928. p. 1157 ⟨I-01108⟩

Macphail, A.: Robert Craik (1829-1907). In Kelly HW, Burrage WL: Dictionary of American Medical Biography. New York and London, D. Appleton and Co., 1928. p. 265. ⟨I-00914⟩

Macphail, A.: Robert Palmer Howard (1823-1889). In Kelly HW, Burrage WL: Dictionary of American Medical Biography. New York and London, D. Appleton and Co., 1928. p. 606. ⟨I-01351⟩

Macphail, A.: William Hales Hingston (1829-1907). In Kelly, HW, Burrage WL: Dictionary of American Medical Biography. New York and London, D. Appleton and Co., 1928. pp. 569-570. ⟨I-01349⟩

Macphail, A.: Wyatt Galt Johnston (1859-1902). In Kelly HW, Burrage WL: Dictionary of American Medical Biography. New York and London, D. Appleton and Co., 1928. p. 670. ⟨I-01329⟩

Macphail, A.: Howell's "Shepherd". CMAJ 669-672, 1934 ⟨I-01676⟩

Macphail, A.: The Master's Wife. Toronto, McClelland and Stewart Limited, 1977. 173 p. ⟨I-01424⟩

MacPherson, C.: Medical History in Newfoundland. Nova Scotia Medical Bulletin 28:61-67, 1949 ⟨II-03682⟩

MacPherson, C.: The First Recognition of Beri-beri in Canada?. CMAJ 95:278-279, 1966 ⟨II-03687⟩

Macrae, H.M.: Dr. Walter Walker Wright. CMAJ 98:1158, 1968 ⟨I-01724⟩

MacTaggart, K.: The First Decade. Ottawa, Canadian Medical Association, 1973. 132 p. ⟨II-00432⟩

Maddison, G.E.: Dr. J. Arthur Melanson. CMAJ 100:543-544, 1969 ⟨I-05044⟩

Magner, L.N.: Ernest Lyman Scott's work with insulin: a reappraisal. Pharmacy in History 19:103-108, 1977 ⟨II-03620⟩

Magner, W.: Dr. P.W. McKeown, CBE, BA, MD, CM, MRCS. CMAJ 15:1281, 1925 ⟨I-01594⟩

Maheux, A.A.: Centenary of the Faculty of Medicine of Laval University. CMAJ 67:64-67, 1952 ⟨II-04629⟩

Major, E.J.S.: Les Medecins et les Troubles de 1837-1838. L'UMC 95:1429-131, 1966 ⟨II-02453⟩

Malloch, A.: Dr. George Alexander MacCallum: an appreciation. CMAJ 37:200-202, 1937 ⟨I-03050⟩

Malloch, A.: Dr. Ingersoll Olmsted, an appreciation. CMAJ 37:93-94, 1937 ⟨I-03445⟩

Malloch, A.: Short Years: The Life and Letters of John Bruce MacCallum, M.D., 1876-1906. Chicago, Normandie House, 1938. 343 p. ⟨I-01435⟩

Malloch, A.: Medical Interchange Between the British Isles and America Before 1801. London, Royal College of Physicians, 1946, pp ix, 143 ⟨II-03681⟩

Maltais, R.: Le Centre Medical De L'Universite de Sherbrooke: Une esquisse de son histoire (1961-1979). Sherbrooke, de L'Universite de Sherbrooke, 1980. ⟨II-04664⟩

Manion, R.J.: A Surgeon in Arms. New York, D. Appleton and Co., 1918. 310 p. ⟨I-03417⟩

Manion, R.J.: Life is an Adventure. Toronto, The Ryerson Press, 1936, 360 p. ⟨I-04780⟩

Mao Tse-Tung: In Memory of Norman Bethune. Chinese Medical Journal 84(11):699-700, 1965 ⟨I-00957⟩

Margetts, E.L.: Dr. Douglas Earle Alcorn. CMAJ 100:42, 1969 ⟨I-05040⟩

Margetts, E.L.: Indian and Eskimo medicine, with notes on the early history of psychiatry among French and British colonists. In Howells, John G.,ed. World History of Psychiatry. New York, Brunner/Mazel, Publisher, 1975. pp 400-431 ⟨II-00619⟩

Marion-Landais, G.: The first European hospital in the Western hemisphere. Transactions and Studies of the College of Physicians of Philadelphia 4th Ser. 43(3):136-141, 1976 ⟨II-00199⟩

Markson, E.R.: The Life and Death of Louis Riel: A Study in Forensic Psychiatry Part I. Canadian Psychiatric Association Journal 10:246-252, 1965 ⟨II-04789⟩

Marlow, F.W.: A Few Notes Referring to the Contributions to Medical Literature and the Writings of the late Dr. James F.W. Ross, Toronto. Canada Lancet 45:334-337, 1912 ⟨I-01144⟩

Marquis, A.S.: Dr. John McLoughlin (The Great White Eagle). Toronto, The Ryerson Press, 1929, 31 p. ⟨I-03172⟩

Marrie, T.: In Retrospect (Cluny Macpherson). Dalhousie Medical Journal 20:89 + 91, 1967 ⟨I-02301⟩

Marsden, W.: An Essay on the Contagion, Infection, Portability, and Communicability of the Asiatic Cholera in its Relations to Quarantine; with a brief History of its Origin and Course in Canada, from 1832. Canada Medical Journal and Monthly Record of Medical and Surgical Science. 4:529-543, 1868; 5:1-7, 49-53,101-108, 145-151, 195-203, 243-250, 1868-1869. ⟨II-00090⟩

Marshall, J.S.: Charles Smallwood. DCB 10:658-659, 1972 ⟨I-01096⟩

Marshall, J.T.: A Century of Population Growth in British Columbia. Canadian Journal of Public Health 50:64-70, 1959 ⟨II-03770⟩

Marshall, M.R.: Dr. Harold Orr. CMAJ 68:185, 1953 ⟨I-04550⟩

Martel, P.G.: Joliette: dix ans d'evolution psychiatrique. Laval Medical 42:1-3, 1971 ⟨II-05419⟩

Martell, J.S.: Nova Scotia's Contribution to the Canadian Relief Fund in the War of 1812. CHR 23:297-302, 1943 ⟨II-00466⟩

Martin, C.: The European Impact on the Culture of a Northeastern Algonquian Tribe: an ecological interpretation. William and Mary Quarterly 31:3-26, 1974 ⟨II-03259⟩

Martin, C.A.: Alexis le fistuleux. Vie Medicale au Canada Francais 2:378-83, 1973 ⟨II-05442⟩

Martin, C.F.: Dr. Gordon Stewart Mundie. CMAJ 16:608, 1926 ⟨I-01423⟩

Martin, C.F.: Dr. J.G. Adami. CMAJ 16:1281-1282, 1926 ⟨I-01616⟩

Martin, C.F.: Dr. William Grant Stewart, an appreciation. CMAJ 18:630-631, 1928 ⟨I-01652⟩

Martin, C.F.: The Mental Hygiene Movement in Canada. The Canadian Journal of Medicine and Surgery 63:167-173, 1928 ⟨II-03683⟩

Martin, C.F.: Sir Andrew Macphail. CMAJ 39:508-509, 1938 ⟨I-03373⟩

Martin, C.F.: William Harvey Smith, an appreciation. CMAJ :87, 1940 ⟨I-03357⟩

Martin, C.F.: Dean J.C. Simpson. McGill Medical Journal 13:257-260, 1944 ⟨I-01680⟩

Martin, C.F.: The Montreal General Hospital in Osler's Time. Montreal General Hospital Bulletin 2:11-15, 1955 ⟨II-03684⟩

M[artin], C.P.: Dr. George Lyman Duff. CMAJ 75:964, 1956 ⟨I-04738⟩

Martin, K.R.: Life and Death at Marble Island, 1864-73. The Beaver, Spring 1979, pp 48-56 ⟨II-00117⟩

Martin, R.: Medicine, Then and Now. Manitoba Medical Review 30:645-47, 1950 ⟨II-03771⟩

Massicotte, E.Z.: Les Chirurgiens de Montreal au XVIIe Siecle. L'UMC 46:310-315, 1917 ⟨II-02435⟩

Massicotte, E.Z.: Comptes de Chirurgiens Montrealais au 18eme Siecle. L'UMC 48:507-511, 1919 ⟨II-02360⟩

Massicotte, E.Z.: Documents pour L'Histoire de la Medecine au Canada. L'UMC 48:463-465, 1919 ⟨II-02387⟩

Massicotte, E.Z.: Document pour l'histoire de la medecine en Canada. L'UMC 49:375-376, 1920 ⟨II-02385⟩

Massicotte, E.Z.: L'Engagement d'un Chirurgien Pour L'Ouest au Dix-Huitieme Siecle. L'UMC 49:204-205, 1920 ⟨I-01774⟩

Massicotte, E.Z.: Un Document du Docteur Sarrazin. L'UMC 49:418-420, 1920 ⟨I-01770⟩

Massicotte, E.Z.: Le Sieur de la Houssaye. L'UMC 50:302-303, 1921 ⟨I-01771⟩

Massicotte, E.Z.: Les Medecins et Chirurgiens de la Region de Montreal. L'UMC 50:483-485, 1921 ⟨II-02382⟩

Massicotte, E.Z.: Medecins et Chirurgiens Sous le Regime Francais. L'UMC 50:156, 1921 ⟨II-02384⟩

Massicotte, E.Z.: Notes pour l'Histoire de la Medecine au Canada: Les Chirurgiens de Montreal au XVIIe Siecle. L'UMC 50:266-271, 1921 ⟨II-02383⟩

Matas, J.: The Story of Psychiatry in Manitoba. Manitoba Medical Review 41:360-364, 1961 ⟨II-00527⟩

Mather, J.M.: Myron McDonald Weaver, AB, MS, PhD, MD, DSc, FACP, FRCP(C). CMAJ 90:750, 1964 ⟨I-02704⟩

Mathers, A.T.: Dr. Julius Edward Lehmann. CMAJ 31:227, 1934 ⟨I-03527⟩

Matsuki, A., Zsigmond, E.K.: The first fatal case of chloroform anaesthesia in Canada. Canadian Anesthetists' Society Journal 20:395-397, 1973 ⟨II-00041⟩

Matsuki, A., Zsigmond, E.K.: A bibliography of the history of surgical anaesthesia in Canada (supplement to Dr. Roland's Checklist). Canadian Anesthetists' Society Journal 21:427-430. 1974 ⟨II-00040⟩

Matsuki, A.: A Chronology of the Very Early History of Inhalation Anaesthesia in Canada. Canadian Anaesthetists Society Journal 21:92-5, 1974 ⟨II-05439⟩

Matsuki, A., Zsigmond, E.K.: The Early Anesthesia Chart in Canada. Anaesthesist 23:268-9, 1974 ⟨II-05452⟩

Matthews, R.M.: Philosophy of the Fee Schedule. Ontario Medical Review 31:21-23, 1964 ⟨II-03685⟩

Matthews, R.M.: James Metcalfe MacCallum, BA, MD, CM (1860-1943). CMAJ 114:621-624, 1976 ⟨I-01426⟩

Matthews, R.M.: Permissiveness and Dr. Blatz: Where Did Society's Ideas on Child-Raising Go Wrong?. CMAJ 122:99-101, 1980 ⟨II-00739⟩

Maurault, O.: Gabriel Souart. DCB 1:612-613, 1966 ⟨I-01001⟩

Maus, J.H.: Dr. Norman Arnold McCormick. CMAJ 98: 65-66, 1968 ⟨I-01760⟩

Mazumdar, P.M.H.: History, science and the community. CMAJ 117:313-317, 1977 ⟨II-00205⟩

McArton, D.: 75 Years in Winnipeg's Social History. Canadian Welfare 25:11-19, 1949 ⟨II-03663⟩

McAuley, R.G., Moore, C.A.: Family Medicine in Hamilton 1965-1981: Change Over Time. Canadian Family Physician 28:556-558, 1982 ⟨II-04813⟩

McCabe, J.P.: The Birth of the Royal Canadian Army Medical Corps. U.S. Armed Forces Medical Journal 5:1016-1024, 1954 ⟨II-03832⟩

McCaffery, M.: Missionary Doctor -- In Deepest Toronto [Dr. Robert B. Salter]. Canadian Family Physician 25:487-490, 1979 ⟨I-01078⟩

McCardle, B.: Bibliography of the History of Canadian Indian and Inuit Health. Edmonton, Treaty and Aboriginal Rights Research of the Indian Association of Alberta, 1981 89 p. ⟨II-04641⟩

McCaughey, D.: Professional Militancy: The Medical Defence Association vs. the College of Physicians and Surgeons of Ontario, 1891-1902. In: Roland, C.G. (ed.): Health, Disease and Medicine: Essays in Canadian History. Toronto, Hannah Institute for the History of Medicine, 1984, 96-104 ⟨II-05395⟩

McConnachie, K.: A Note on Fertility Rates Among Married Women in Toronto, 1871. Ontario History 75:87-98, 1983 ⟨II-05087⟩

McConnachie, K.: Methodology in the Study of Women in History: A Case Study of Helen MacMurchy, M.D. Ontario History 75:61-70, 1983 ⟨I-05055⟩

McConnell, D.: A Study of the British Military Buildings at Niagara-on-the-Lake, 1838-71. Manuscript Report No. 226, Parks Canada, 1977 ⟨II-00193⟩

McConnell, F.: Highlights in the Early History of the Faculty of Medicine, the University of Toronto. CAMSI Journal 10:29, 1951 (Feb) ⟨II-00327⟩

McConnell, J.B.: Dr. James Perrigo. CMAJ 18:757-758, 1928 ⟨I-01620⟩

McConnell, V.: An early venture in heteroplasty. CMAJ 83:609, 1960 ⟨II-03775⟩

McCoy, E.C.: (Wallace Wilson). British Columbia Medical Journal 8:235, 1966 ⟨I-03399⟩

McCrae, J.: A Canadian Hospital of the 17th Century. Montreal Medical Journal 35:459-65, 1906 ⟨II-03774⟩

McCrae, J.: In Flanders Fields. New York/London, G.P. Putnam's Sons, 1919. 141 p. ⟨II-00877⟩

McCrae, T.: Some Medical Teachers of the Nineties. Canadian Journal of Medicine and Surgery 50:138-141, 1921 ⟨II-03773⟩

McCrae, T.: Dr. Angus MacKinnon. CMAJ 21:110, 1929 ⟨I-02848⟩

McCrae, T.: Mr. Irving Heward Cameron. CMAJ 30:225-226, 1934 ⟨I-03550⟩

McCrae, T.: Dr. Alexander McPhedran. CMAJ 32:222-223, 1935 ⟨I-01284⟩

McCreary, J.F.: (Wallace Wilson). British Columbia Medical Journal 8:230, 1966 ⟨I-03404⟩

McCuaig, K.: From Social Reform to Social Service. The Changing Role of Volunteers: the Anti-tuberculosis Campaign, 1900-30. CHR 71:480-501, 1980 ⟨II-02944⟩

McCuaig, K.: From "A Social Disease with a Medical Aspect" to "A Medical Disease with a Social Aspect": Fighting the White Plague in Canada, 1900-1940. In: Shephard, D.A.E.: Levesque, A.(edit): Norman Bethune: His Times and His Legacy, Ottawa, Canadian Public Health Assoc., 1982. pp 54-64 ⟨II-04925⟩

McCuaig, K.: Tuberculosis: The Changing Concepts of the Disease in Canada 1900-1950. In: Roland, C.G. (ed.): Health, Disease and Medicine: Essays in Canadian History. Toronto, Hannah Institute for the History of Medicine, 1984, 296-307 ⟨II-05404⟩

McCulloch, E.A.: That Reminds Me of N.A.P. Toronto, The Ryerson Press, 1942, 78 p. ⟨I-04517⟩

McCullough, J.W.S.: 1910-1920, A Review of Ten Years' Progress. The Provincial Board of Health, Ontario, [1920], pp. 1-48 ⟨II-03835⟩

McCullough, J.W.S.: Early History of Public Health in Upper and Lower Canada. National Hygiene and Public Welfare 58:17-31, 1922 ⟨II-00572⟩

McCullough, J.W.S.: Dr. Frederick Montizambert, CMG, ISO, FRCSE, DCL (an appreciation). CMAJ 21:747, 1929 ⟨I-01759⟩

McCutcheon, J.W.: The Second-War Years. Ontario Medical Review 34:755-57, 1967 ⟨II-03809⟩

McDonald, J.F.: William Henry Drummond. Toronto, The Ryerson Press, n.d., 132 p. ⟨I-02145⟩

McDonnell, C.E.: B.C. Medical History. British Columbia Medical Journal 19:348-9, 1977 ⟨II-03148⟩

McDonnell, C.E.: Contract medicine before the railway. British Columbia Medical Journal 19:418-19, 1977 ⟨II-03119⟩

McDonnell, C.E.: Medical care on Burrard Inlet 1877-1882. British Columbia Medical Journal 19:394-5, 1977 ⟨II-03149⟩

McDonnell, C.E.: Some early Practitioners. British Columbia Medical Journal 19:446-7, 1977 ⟨II-03257⟩

McDonnell, C.E.: CPR contract physicians and early hospital development in Vancouver. British Columbia Medical Journal 20:18-19, 1978 ⟨II-03118⟩

McDonnell, C.E.: Early medical legislation. British Columbia Medical Journal 20:44-5, 1978 ⟨II-03117⟩

McDonnell, C.E.: Early VMA activities -- The founding of the BCMA. British Columbia Medical Journal 20:182-4, 1978 ⟨II-03113⟩

McDonnell, C.E.: The founding of the VMA [Vancouver Medical Association]. British Columbia Medical Journal 20:144-6, 1978 ⟨II-03114⟩

McDonnell, C.E.: The founding of St. Paul's hospital. British Columbia Medical Journal 20:112-4, 1978 ⟨II-03115⟩

McDonnell, C.E.: The golden years and the founding of the Vancouver General Hospital. British Columbia Medical Journal 20:221-3, 1978 ⟨II-03112⟩

McDonnell, C.E.: The VMA and the government. British Columbia Medical Journal 20:246-8, 1978 ⟨II-03318⟩

McDonnell, C.E.: Vancouver's early years. British Columbia Medical Journal 20:78-9, 1978 ⟨II-03116⟩

McDougall, D.: The History of Pharmacy in Manitoba. Historical and Scientific Society of Manitoba. Papers. Series 3, No. 11:18-29, 1956 ⟨II-02105⟩

McEwan, C.: Dr. Wallace Graham: an appreciation. CMAJ 88:107, 1963 ⟨I-02162⟩

McEwen, D.: Robert Palmer Howard. McGill Medical Journal 34:141-145, 1965 ⟨I-02557⟩

McFadden, I.: The Indomitable Savage. Toronto, United Church of Canada, Board of Information and Stewardship, 1963. ⟨I-05060⟩

McFall, W.A.: The Life and Times of Dr. Christopher Widmer. Annals of Medical History, ser. 3, 4:324-334, 1942 ⟨I-04898⟩

McFarlane, C.J.: Manitoba's First Woman Doctor. University of Manitoba Medical Journal 53:11-14, 1983 ⟨I-05130⟩

McGahan, E.W.: John Thomson. DCM 11:878-888, 1982 ⟨I-04855⟩

McGahan, E.W.: Sylvester Zobieski Earle. DCB 11:295-96, 1982 ⟨I-04867⟩

McGhie, A.G.: Historical notes on medical personalities in the Hamilton area. McGregor Clinic Bulletin 23(2):1-9, 1962 ⟨II-00537⟩

McGhie, A.G.: The development of medical education in Canada. McGregor Clinic Bulletin 23(2):10-16, 1962 ⟨II-00328⟩

McGhie, A.G.: The development of group practice. McGregor Clinic Bulletin 23(2):17-23, 1962 ⟨II-00442⟩

McGhie, A.G.: The growth of medical practice and medical education in Canada. Wentworth Bygones 9:48-55, 1971 ⟨II-03108⟩

McGill, J.: Medals and Medallions of R. Tait McKenzie. Canadian Collector, July/August 1976. pages 21-23 ⟨II-04808⟩

McGill, J.: The Joy of Effort: A Biography of R. Tait McKenzie. Sewdley, Ontario, Clay Publishing Company Limited, 1980. 241 p. ⟨I-03002⟩

McGinnis, J.P.D.: "Unclean, Unclean": Canadian Reaction to Lepers and Leprosy. In: Roland, C.G.(ed.): Health, Disease and Medicine: Essays in Canadian History. Toronto, Hannah Institute for the History of Medicine, 1984, 250-275 ⟨II-05402⟩

McGinnis, J.P.D.: A City Faces an Epidemic. Alberta History 24(4):1-11, 1976 ⟨II-00819⟩

McGinnis, J.P.D.: The Impact of Epidemic Influenza: Canada, 1918-1919. Historical Papers, CHA, 1977. pp 120-140 ⟨II-00820⟩

McGinnis, J.P.D.: Records of Tuberculosis in Calgary. Archivaria 10:173-189, 1980 ⟨II-00369⟩

McGinnis, J.P.D.: The White Plague in Calgary; Sanatorium Care in Southern Alberta. Alberta History 28(4):1-15, 1980 ⟨II-02945⟩

McGinnis, J.P.D.: Whose Responsibility? Public Health in Canada, 1919-1945. In: Staum, M.S., Larsen, D.E. (edit.): Doctors, Patients, and Society. Power and Authority in Medical Care. Waterloo, Wilfrid Laurier Univ. Press, 1981. pp 205-229 ⟨II-05026⟩

McGovern, J.P., Roland, C.G.: William Osler: The Continuing Education. Springfield, Charles C. Thomas, Publisher, 1969 ⟨II-00279⟩

McGrath, J.: Dr. Cluny Macpherson. CMAJ 96:172-174, 1967 ⟨I-03421⟩

McGregor, M.: Le Troisieme Cinquantenaire de la Faculte de Medecine de McGill. L'UMC 100:435-437, 1971 ⟨II-02431⟩

McGugan, A.C.: Dr. W. Fulton Gillespie. CMAJ 62:208-9, 1950 ⟨I-04484⟩

McGugan, A.C.: Hospitals and Hospital Administration Then and Now. Alberta Medical Bulletin 25:99-106, 1960 ⟨II-03695⟩

McGugan, A.C.: The First Fifty Years. A History of the University of Alberta Hospital, 1914-1964. Edmonton, University of Alberta Hospital, 1964 ⟨II-05104⟩

McGuire, C.R.: The Canadian Connection with St. Helena. Stampex Canada Catalogue 1981, pp [6] - [13], [16] ⟨I-03873⟩

McInnis, R.: Sir Charles Tupper -- Nova Scotia's Father of Confederation. Dalhousie Medical Journal 20:99-106, 1967 ⟨I-03562⟩

McIntosh, A.W.: The Career of Sir Charles Tupper in Canada, 1864-1900. Thesis, University of Toronto, Ph.D., 1970, 598 pages ⟨I-04893⟩

McK, N.: Alexander Francis Mahaffy, CMG, BA, MB, DPH; an appreciation. CMAJ 88:906-907, 1963 ⟨I-03424⟩

McK., N.: David Bruce Wilson, BA, MB, DPH: an appreciation. CMAJ 88:639, 1963 ⟨I-02710⟩

McKechnie, R.E.: Strong Medicine. Vancouver, J.J. Douglas Ltd., 1972, 193 p. ⟨II-04466⟩

McKee, S.H.: Abstracts from the Early Records of the Montreal Medico-Chirurgical Society. CMAJ 16:839-844, 1926 ⟨II-01805⟩

McKelvie, B.A.: Lieutenant-Colonel Israel Wood Powell, M.D., C.M. British Columbia Historical Quarterly 11:33-54, 1947 ⟨I-05064⟩

McKendry, J.B.R.: Closed Chest Cardiac Massage: An Early Case Report. CMAJ 87:305-30, 1962 ⟨II-01788⟩

McKenna, C.A.: Toronto in 1896. Journal of the Canadian Dentistry Association 19:133-136, 1953 ⟨II-03776⟩

McKenzie, J.W.: Dr. Stephen Rice Jenkins, FACS. CMAJ 21:620, 1929 ⟨I-02276⟩

McKenzie, K.A.: The Dalhousie Medical School. CACHB 11:78-81, 1947 ⟨II-00280⟩

McKenzie, R.T.: Compensations at 70. Transactions and Studies of the College of Physicians of Philadelphia 6:271-281, 1838 ⟨II-03662⟩

McKerracher, D.G.: Dr. Allan A. Bailey. CMAJ 97:1428, 1967 ⟨I-01489⟩

McKervill, H.W.: Darby of Bella Bella. Toronto, Ryerson Press, 1964 ⟨I-02986⟩

McKillop, A.B.: Dr. Bovell's Quadrilateral Mind. In: A Disciplined Intelligence. Montreal, McGill-Queen's University Press, 1979, pp 73-91. ⟨I-03189⟩

McKim, L.H.: Fraser Baillie Gurd: an appreciation. CMAJ 58:394-395, 1948 ⟨I-02177⟩

McKinnon, N.E.: Mortality Reductions in Ontario, 1900-1942. Canadian Journal of Public Health 35:481-4, 1944 ⟨II-04456⟩

McKinnon, N.E.: Mortality Reductions in Ontario 1900-1942 IV. Tuberculosis. Canadian Journal of Public Health 36:423-9, 1945 ⟨II-04451⟩

McKinnon, N.E.: Mortality Reductions in Ontario 1900-1942 III. The Age Groups of 50 and Over. Canadian Journal of Public Health 36:368-73, 1945 ⟨II-04452⟩

McKinnon, N.E.: Mortality Reductions in Ontario, 1900-1942 II. Canadian Journal of Public Health 36:285-298, 1945 ⟨II-04453⟩

McKinnon, N.E.: Mortality Reductions in Ontario, 1900-42 VI. Scarlet Fever. Canadian Journal of Public Health 37:407-10, 1946 ⟨II-04454⟩

McKinnon, N.E.: Mortality Reductions in Ontario, 1900-1945 VIII. Respiratory Disease. Canadian Journal of Public Health 39:417-21, 1948 ⟨II-04457⟩

McKinnon, N.E.: Mortality Reductions in Ontario, 1900-45 VII. Measles and Whooping Cough. Canadian Journal of Public Health 39:95-8, 1948 ⟨II-04476⟩

McLaren, A.: Birth Control and Abortion in Canada, 1870-1920. CHR 59:319-340, 1978. ⟨II-00047⟩

McLaren, A.: What Has This to Do with Working Class Women?: Birth Control and the Canadian Left, 1900-1939. Histoire Sociale/Social History 14:435-454, 1981 ⟨II-04792⟩

McLeod, S.H.: Nova Scotia Farm Boy to Alberta M.D. np., 1970. 110 p. ⟨I-03411⟩

McM., J.P.: Prof. R. Ramsay Wright. Nature 132:631, 1933 ⟨I-02719⟩

McMaster, J.: Despite Tempest and Ague: an 1844 letter to the folks at home. York Pioneer 74:1-4, 1979 ⟨II-03285⟩

McMullin, S.E.: Walt Whitman's Influence in Canada. Dalhousie Review 49:361-368, 1969-70 ⟨I-02022⟩

McNally, L.B.: Dr. William Drummond: Poet - Physician to the "Habitant". CAMSI Journal 22:9-16, 1963 (Feb) ⟨II-00878⟩

McNally, W.J.: Herbert Stanley Birkett. CMAJ 47:280-283, 1942 ⟨I-02050⟩

McNaughton, F.L.: Colin Russel, a pioneer of Canadian neurology. CMAJ 77:719-723, 1957 ⟨I-02576⟩

McNeel, B.H., Lewis, C.H.: Care of the Mentally Ill in Ontario: History of Treatment. Canadian Hospital 37(2):34-36, 102, 1960. 37(3):45, 106-107, 1960 ⟨II-03772⟩

McNichol, V.E.: Smiling through Tears. Bloomingdale, Ont., One M Printing Co., 1970, 1:256p. Bridgeport, Ont., Union Print, 1971, 2:408 p., 3:489 p., 4:494 p. 5:379 p. ⟨I-04891⟩

Meakins, J.C.: Typhoid Fever in the 1890's and the 1930's. CMAJ 42:81-82, 1940 ⟨II-03462⟩

Meakins, J.C.: Edward William Archibald, B.A., M.D., C.M. (McGill); Hon. F.R.C.S. (Eng.); F.R.C.S. [C].; Hon. F.R.C.S. (Australasia); F.A.C.S. CMAJ 54:194-7, 1946 ⟨I-04346⟩

Meakins, J.C.: Charles Ferdinand Martin. CMAJ, 70:95-6, 1954 ⟨I-04562⟩

Mechling, W.H.: Medical Practices. Anthropologica 8:239-263, 1959 ⟨II-00620⟩

Medovy, H.: Pediatrics in Manitoba: Goals and Accomplishments. The Journal-Lancet 87:34-37, 1967 ⟨II-05019⟩

Medovy, H.: The Early Jewish Physicians in Manitoba. Historical and Scientific Society of Manitoba. Papers. Series 3, No. 29:23-39, 1972-3 ⟨II-02103⟩

Medovy, H.: The History of Western Encephalomyelitis in Manitoba. Canadian Journal of Public Health 67 Suppl. 1:13-4, 1976 ⟨II-05235⟩

Medovy, H.: Blue Babies and Well Water. Alumni Journal [University of Manitoba] 38:4-7, 18-19, 1978 ⟨I-04962⟩

Medovy, H.: A Vision Fulfilled. The Story of the Children's Hospital of Winnipeg 1909-1973. Winnipeg, Peguis Publishers Limited, 1979. 156 p. ⟨II-00176⟩

Medovy, H.: Seven Decades of Service at the Children's Hospital of Winnipeg. CMAJ 123:1259-1261, 1980 ⟨II-02981⟩

Meiklejohn, M.L.: The early hospital history of Canada 1535-1875. Montreal Medical Journal 39:397-320, 1910 ⟨II-03794⟩

Melanson, J.A.: The New Brunswick Department of Health and Social Services. Canadian Journal of Public Health 49:370-381, 1958 ⟨II-00573⟩

Melville, K.I.: A progress report on the Canadian Society of Chemotherapy. International Journal of Clinical Pharmacology 1:373-375, 1968 ⟨II-03109⟩

Menzies, A.M.: An unusual introduction to practice. CMAJ 80:985-987, 1959 ⟨II-03769⟩

Mercer, W.: William Edward Gallie. CMAJ 81:691-692, 1959 ⟨I-02171⟩

Mercer, W.: Edinburgh and Canadian Medicine: The First Alexander Gibson Memorial Lecture, part 1. CMAJ 84:1241-1257, 1313-1317, 1961 ⟨I-01573⟩

Mercier, O.: Medecins et Chirurgeins de L'Hotel-Dieu. L'UMC 70:1273-1276, 1941 ⟨II-02364⟩

Mercier, O.: Echo du Tricentenaire. L'UMC 71:608-609, 1942 ⟨II-02365⟩

Mercier, O.: Trois Siecles de Medecine au Canada Francais. L'UMC 71:801-806, 1942 ⟨II-02366⟩

Mercier, O.: Three Centuries of Medicine in French Canada. Nova Scotia Medical Bulletin 29:207-212, 1950 ⟨II-03747⟩

Mestern, P.M.: Clara: an Historical Novel of an Ontario Town 1879-1930 [Fiction]. Guelph, Ontario, Back Door Press, 1979. 187 p. ⟨I-01375⟩

Metcalfe, A.: The evolution of organized physical recreation in Montreal, 1840-1895. Histoire Sociale/Social History II(21):144-166, 1978 ⟨II-03090⟩

Metson, G.: The Halifax explosion, December 6, 1917. Toronto/Montreal/New York, McGraw-Hill Ryerson Limited, 1978. 173 p. ⟨II-00386⟩

Meyers, C: The historical development of the institutional care of the insane in Ontario. McMaster University, Hamilton, Ontario, 1978. 19 p. n.p. ⟨II-00165⟩

Middleton, F.C.: Evolution of Tuberculosis Control in Saskatchewan. Canadian Public Health Journal 24:505-513, 1933 ⟨II-00067⟩

Mignault, L.D.: Histoire de L'Ecole de Medecine et de Chirurgie de Montreal. L'Union Medicale du Canada 55:597-674, 1926 ⟨II-05110⟩

Mignault, L.D.: A Short History of the Medical Faculty of the University of Montreal. CMAJ 17:242-245, 1927 ⟨II-03645⟩

Miles, J.E.: The Psychiatric Aspects of the Traditional Medicine of the British Columbia Coast Indians. Canadian Psychiatric Association Journal 12:429-431, 1967 ⟨II-04786⟩

Miller, G. (Edit.): Historiography of the History of Medicine of the United States and Canada, 1939-1960. Baltimore, John Hopkins Press, 1964. 428 p. ⟨II-00200⟩

Miller, J.: Dr. Thomas Gibson. CMAJ 45:192-193, 1941 ⟨I-03519⟩

Miller, J.: The Late Dr. L.J. Austin. CMAJ 52:644-5, 1945 ⟨I-04334⟩

Miller, L.A.: The Newfoundland Department of Health. Canadian Journal of Public Health 50:228-239, 1959 ⟨II-00570⟩

Miller, L.A.: Dr. Walter Templeman, an appreciation. CMAJ 95:1219, 1966 ⟨I-02753⟩

Millman, T.: Impressions of the West in the Early 'Seventies, from the Diary of the Assistant Surgeon of the B.N.A. Boundary Survey,. Women's Canadian Historical Society of Toronto 26: 15-56, 1927-1928 ⟨II-04627⟩

Mills, J.A.: Dr. Francis John Shepherd. McGill Medical Journal 22:67-72, 1953 ⟨I-01678⟩

Mills, T.M.: Women's Lib in the 1890's: they didn't have to fight for it. Atlantic Advocate 63:51-52, 1972 ⟨II-03712⟩

Mills, T.M.: Gold Rush Nurse. North/Nord 3:10-13, 1973 ⟨II-04625⟩

Minhinnick, J.: Macaulay House, Picton. Ontario Museum Association Quarterly 7(2):17-21, 1978 ⟨II-00786⟩

Minuck, M.: Recent advances in anaesthesia in Manitoba. Manitoba Medical Review 47:146-148, 1967 ⟨II-03647⟩

Minuck, M.: [Dr. W. Webster]. Manitoba Medical Review 47:315-316, 1967 ⟨I-03561⟩

Minuck, M.: Pioneers of Canadian Anaesthesia -- Dr. William Webster. Canadian Anaesthetists Society Journal 19:322-6, 1972 ⟨I-05373⟩

Mitchell, C.A.: Walter Henry et l'Autopsie de l'Empereur Napoleon I. L'UMC 94:1651-1653, 1965 ⟨I-01521⟩ .

Mitchell, CA: Walter Henry and the Autopsy of Emperor Napoleon I. University of Ottawa Medical Journal 9:3-8. 1965 ⟨I-03927⟩

Mitchell, C.A.: Events Leading up to and the Establishment of the Grosse Ile Quarantine Station. Medical Services Journal, Canada 23:1436-1444, 1967 ⟨II-03644⟩

Mitchell, C.A.: Rabies in Quebec City: Case Report 1839. Medical Services Journal of Canada, 23:809-812, 1967 ⟨II-03643⟩

Mitchell, J.R.: Alexandra Park -- Johnston Park: "One Man's Fight to Save a Park" [Dr. Ross Mitchell]. University of Manitoba Medical Journal 51:61-69, 1981 ⟨I-04713⟩

Mitchell, J.R.: Elinor F.E. Black, an appreciation. University of Manitoba Medical Journal 52:6-7, 1982 ⟨I-04972⟩

Mitchell, R.: Dr. Harry D. Morse. Winnipeg Clinic Quarterly 19:105-109 ⟨I-02531⟩

Mitchell, R.: Medicine in Manitoba: The Story of Its Beginnings. Winnipeg, Stovel-Advocate Press, Ltd., 141 p. ⟨II-00855⟩

Mitchell, R.: Physician, fur trader and explorer. The Beaver 267(2):16-20 ⟨I-03227⟩

Mitchell, R.: James Wilford Good, M.B., L.R.C.P.(Edin), F.A.C.S. CMAJ 16:1283, 1926 ⟨I-02137⟩

Mitchell, R.: Dr. Frank L. McKinnon. CMAJ 21:350, 1929 ⟨I-02847⟩

Mitchell, R.: Dr. John Ernest Coulter. CMAJ 21:747-748, 1929 ⟨I-02034⟩

Mitchell, R.: Dr. John Orchard Todd. CMAJ 21:748, 1929 ⟨I-02746⟩

Mitchell, R.: H.M. Cameron, M.C., B.A., M.D., LL.B. CMAJ 20:329-330, 1929 ⟨I-01568⟩

Mitchell, R.: Dr. Edwin S. Popham. CMAJ 22:443, 1930 ⟨I-02581⟩

Mitchell, R.: Manitoba's medical school. CMAJ 706-708, 1930 Vol. 22 ⟨II-03111⟩

Mitchell, R.: Manitoba's Educational Institutions. CMAJ 22:705-708, 1930 ⟨II-03648⟩

Mitchell, R.: The 55 "Hospitals" and nursing missions of greater Winnipeg. CMAJ 22:861-866, 1930 ⟨II-03145⟩

Mitchell, R.: Dr. Jasper Halpenny. CMAJ 24:323-24, 1931 ⟨I-03045⟩

Mitchell, R.: Dr. R.E. Alleyn. CMAJ 24:474, 1931 ⟨I-03065⟩

Mitchell, R.: Dr. Norman Kitson McIvor. CMAJ 26:259, 1932 ⟨I-03060⟩

Mitchell, R.: Dr. John Rae, Arctic explorer, and his search for Franklin. CMAJ 28:85-90, 1933 ⟨I-03004⟩

Mitchell, R.: The Manitoba Medical College, 1883-1933. CMAJ 29:549-552, 1933 ⟨II-03087⟩

Mitchell, R.: Dr. John Alexander MacArthur. CMAJ 31:453, 1934 ⟨I-02846⟩

Mitchell, R.: Dr. William Webster. CMAJ 31:691, 1934 ⟨I-01668⟩

Mitchell, R.: The Development of Public Health in Manitoba. Canadian Public Health Journal 26:62-69, 1935 ⟨II-03693⟩

Mitchell, R.: The early doctors of Manitoba. CMAJ 33:89-94 ⟨II-03668⟩

Mitchell, R.: Dr. D.A. Stewart. CMAJ 36:435, 1937 ⟨I-03879⟩

Mitchell, R.: Alexander Jardine Hunter, MD, DD, MBE. CMAJ 43:396, 1940 ⟨I-03344⟩

Mitchell, R.: William Harvey Smith. CMAJ 43:86-87, 1940 ⟨I-03364⟩

Mitchell, R.: Doctor Alexander Rowand 1816(?)-1889. CACHB 7(4):1-5, 1943 ⟨I-01126⟩

Mitchell, R.: Dr. William Wesley Lorne Musgrove. CMAJ 56:349, 1947 ⟨I-04408⟩

Mitchell, R.: Early Doctors of Red River and Manitoba. Historical and Scientific Society of Manitoba. Papers. Series 3, No. 4:37 -47, 1947-8 ⟨II-02106⟩

Mitchell, R.: Dr. Alex. J. Douglas 1874-1940. Manitoba Medical Review 38:47-48, 1948 ⟨I-01467⟩

Mitchell, R.: Manitoba's Medical School. CACHB 12:66-69, 1948 ⟨II-03649⟩

Mitchell, R.: Medical Services in the North-West Rebellion of 1885. CMAJ 60:518-521, 1949 ⟨II-04623⟩

Mitchell, R.: Dr. H.M. Speechly. CMAJ 64:460, 1951 ⟨I-04546⟩

Mitchell, R.: Dr. Donald S. McEachern. CMAJ 66:82-3, 1952 ⟨I-04522⟩

Mitchell, R.: Sir James Hector. CMAJ 66:497-499, 1952 ⟨I-02485⟩

Mitchell, R.: Early northern surgeons. The Beaver 284(4):22-24, 1954 ⟨II-03309⟩

Mitchell, R.: Early Medical Journals in Manitoba. Manitoba Medical Review 35:39-40, 1955 ⟨II-01538⟩

Mitchell, R.: North American Indian Medicine. Manitoba Medical Review 36:242-244, 1956 ⟨II-00621⟩

Mitchell, R.: Samuel Willis Prowse, MD 1869-1931: Fourth Dean of Medicine. Manitoba Medical Review 38:551-553, 1958 ⟨I-02694⟩

Mitchell, R.: Dr. Gordon Bell 1863-1923. Manitoba Medical Review 39:521 + 523, 1959 ⟨I-05057⟩

Mitchell, R.: H.H. Chown, Third Dean of Manitoba Medical College 1859-1944. Manitoba Medical Review 39:189-191, 1959 ⟨I-01702⟩

Mitchell, R.: Dr. T. Glen Hamilton: The Founder of the Manitoba Medical Review. Manitoba Medical Review 40:219-221, 1960 ⟨I-02131⟩

Mitchell, R.: Manitoba Surgical Pioneers James Kerr (1849-1911) and H.H. Chown (1859-1944). Canadian Journal of Surgery 3:281-285, 1960 ⟨I-03555⟩

Mitchell, R.: Pioneer! Dr. Elizabeth Beckett Matheson, 1866-1958. Manitoba Medical Review 40:617 + 619, 1960 ⟨I-05058⟩

Mitchell, R.: Iceland's Gift to Canadian Medicine. CMAJ 4:145-151, 1961 ⟨II-01792⟩

Mitchell, R.: Samuel Willis Prowse. Manitoba Medical Review 41:455-459, 1961 ⟨I-02695⟩

M[itchell], R.: Dr. B.J. Ginsburg. CMAJ 86:796, 1962 ⟨I-02808⟩

Mitchell, R., Ferguson, C.C.: Alexander Hugh Ferguson 1853-1911. Canadian Journal of Surgery 6:1-4, 1963 ⟨I-02785⟩

Mitchell, R.: Dr. John Clarence Webster (1863-1950) Man of Two Careers. Canadian Journal of Surgery 6:407-413, 1963 ⟨I-04234⟩

Mitchell, R.: Dr. F.W.E. Burnham 1872-1957: A Life of Strange Adventure. Manitoba Medical Review 46:569-570, 1966 ⟨I-02130⟩

Mitchell, R.: Dr. F.W.E. Burnham 1872-1957. Manitoba Medical Review 46:549-550, 1966 ⟨II-03864⟩

Mitchell, R., Thorlakson, T.K.: James Kerr, 1849-1911 and Harry Hyland Kerr, 1881-1963: Pioneer Canadian-American Surgeons. Canadian Journal of Surgery 9:213-220, 1966 ⟨I-02569⟩

Mitchell, R.: The Progress of an idea: the story of the Winnipeg Clinic Research Institute. CMAJ 94:132-137, 1966 ⟨II-03650⟩

Mitchell, R.: A Centennial Medical Calendar (Manitoba) 1867-1967. Winnipeg Clinic Quarterly 20:72-88, 1967 ⟨II-03692⟩

Mitchell, R.: Dr. Patrick H. McNulty. CMAJ 97:1429-1430, 1967 ⟨I-01764⟩

Mitchell, R.: Dr. Wilfred Abram Bigelow, an appreciation. CMAJ 97:874, 877, 1967 ⟨I-01492⟩

Mitchell, R.: Dr. Wilfred A. Bigelow. Manitoba Medical Review 47:421-422, 1967 ⟨I-01964⟩

Mitchell, R.: John Harrison O'Donnell, M.D. (1838-1912). Canadian Journal of Surgery 10:399-402, 1967 ⟨I-02535⟩

Mitchell, R.: Manitoba Medical Journals. Winnipeg Clinical Quarterly. 20:9-19, 1967 ⟨II-01537⟩

Mitchell, R.: Acorus Calamus. The Beaver 298(4):24-26, 1968 ⟨II-03313⟩

Mitchell, R.: Dr. Donald I. Bowie. CMAJ 99:509, 1968 ⟨I-01961⟩

Mitchell, R.: Manitoba Anatomists. Canadian Journal of Surgery 11:123-134, 1968 ⟨II-04304⟩

Mitchell, R.: How Winnipeg Waged War on Typhoid. Manitoba Medical Review 49:166-67, 1969 ⟨II-05144⟩

Mitchell, R.: An Abortive Attempt. How a Meeting of Medical Men Met in 1883 Hoping to Establish a Medical Association in Winnipeg. Manitoba Medical Review 50:17, 1970 ⟨II-05423⟩

M[itchell], R.M.: Dr. Owen C. Trainor,. CMAJ 76:165, 1957 ⟨I-04756⟩

M [itchell] R.: Dr. Digby Wheeler. CMAJ, 73:920, 1955 ⟨I-04582⟩

Mitchinson, W.: Historical Attitudes Toward Women and Childbirth. Atlantis 4(2)13:34, 1979, Part II ⟨II-00770⟩

Mitchinson, W.: Medical Attitudes Towards Female Sexuality in Late Nineteenth Century English Canada. Department of History, University of Windsor, 1979. 32 p. n.p. ⟨II-00470⟩

Mitchinson, W.: Gynecological Operations on the Insane. Archivaria 10:125-144, 1980 ⟨II-00595⟩

Mitchinson, W.: R.M. Bucke: A Victorian Asylum Superintendent. Ontario History 63:239-254, 1981 ⟨I-04715⟩

Mitchinson, W.: Causes of Disease in Women: The Case of Late 19th Century English Canada. In: Roland, C.G.(ed.): Health, Disease and Medicine: Essays in Canadian History. Toronto, Hannah Institute for the History of Medicine, 1984, 381-395 ⟨II-05408⟩

Monet, J.: Etienne Pigarouich. DCB 1-548-549, 1966 ⟨II-00649⟩

Monet, J.: Edmund Bailey O'Callaghan. DCB 10:554-556,1972 ⟨I-01262⟩

Monro, A.S.: The Medical History of British Columbia. CMAJ 25:336-42, 470-77; 26:88-93, 225-230, 345-348, 601-607, 725-732, 27:187-193, 1931-32 ⟨II-03288⟩

Montagnes, J.: Emily Howard Stowe, physician and social reformer. Canadian Doctor 47(2):27, 1981 ⟨I-04195⟩

Montagnes, J.: McGill Grad Honored by U.S. [C.R. Drew]. Canadian Doctor 48(7):33, 1982 ⟨I-04952⟩

Montague, J., Montague, S.: Impressions of Some Canadian Medical Institutions in 1837. Extracts from the Diary of Dr. James MacDonald. Canadian Psychiatric Association Journal 21:181-2, 1976 ⟨II-05323⟩

Montgomery, E.W.: Dr. William Webster, an appreciation. CMAJ 31:691, 1934 ⟨I-01669⟩

Montgomery, E.W.: Dr. Brandur Jonsson Brandson. CMAJ 51:185-6, 1944 ⟨I-04257⟩

Montgomery, E.W.: Dr. Neil John Maclean. CMAJ 56:115, 1947 ⟨I-03408⟩

Montgomery, E.W.: J.W. Good - The Most Unforgettable Character I Have Known. University of Manitoba Medical Journal 21:27-34, 1949 ⟨I-01582⟩

Montgomery, M.I.R.: The Legislative Healthscape of Canada: 1867-1975. In: LaSor, B.; Elliott, M.R.: Issues in Canadian Nursing. Scarborough, Prentice-Hall of Canada, Ltd., 1977. pp 128-153 ⟨II-03291⟩

Montgomery, W.D.: Dr. J.H. Richardson. Canada Lancet and Practitioner 66:18-21, 1926 ⟨I-02765⟩

Montizambert, F.: The Story of Fifty-Four Years' Quarantine Service from 1866-1920. CMAJ 16:314-319, 1926 ⟨II-01804⟩

Montizambert, L: An Account of the origin, rise and progress of the Montreal General Hospital. Canadian Magazine and Literary Repository 4:100-126, 1825 ⟨II-04002⟩

Montpetit, E.: Albert Prevost. L'Union Medicale du Canada 55:675-680, 1926 ⟨I-05062⟩

Moody, J.P., de Grott van Embden, W.: Arctic Doctor. New York, Dodd, Mead and Company, 1955, 274 p. ⟨I-04433⟩

Moogk, P.N.: Antoine-Bertrand Forestier. DCB 3:220-221, 1974 ⟨I-01016⟩

Moogk, P.N.: Jean-Fernand Spagniolini. DCB 3:597-598, 1974 ⟨I-01107⟩

Moogk, P.N.: Jordain Lajus. DCB 3:344-345, 1974 ⟨I-01010⟩

Moogk, P.N.: Simon Soupiran. DCB 3:595-596, 1974 ⟨I-01106⟩

Moore, D.F.: Dr. Allan A. Bailey, an appreciation. CMAJ 97:1429, 1967 ⟨I-01490⟩

Moore, K.L.: The Discovery of the Sex Chromatin. IN: the Sex Chromatin, Philadelphia, W.B. Saunders Co., 1966 ⟨II-03750⟩

Moore, K.L.: Dr. Ian MacLaren Thompson. University of Manitoba Medical Journal 52:9, 1982 ⟨I-04971⟩

Moore, P.E.: No Longer Captain: A History of Tuberculosis and its Control Amongst Canadian Indians. CMAJ 84:1012-1015, 1961 ⟨II-03290⟩

Moore, P.E.: George Donald [Don] Cameron. CMAJ 129:771, 1983 ⟨I-05162⟩

Moore, S.E.: Dr. F.J. Ball. CMAJ 19:628-629, 1928 ⟨I-03489⟩

Moore, S.E.: David Low, MD. CMAJ 44:534, 1941 ⟨I-03351⟩

Moore, T.: Wilfred Grenfell. Toronto, Fitzhenry and Whiteside Limited, 1950, p.64. ⟨I-04519⟩

Moorhead, E.S.: The Late Dr. Gordon Bell. CMAJ 14:895-896, 1924 ⟨I-02992⟩

Moorhead, E.S.: A Page in Medical History Prepared by Request. Manitoba Medical Review 38:250 + 251, 1958 ⟨II-05088⟩

Moorman, L.J.: Bill Stewart as Student, Patient and Friend. CMAJ 63: 618-9, 1950 ⟨I-04514⟩

Morgan, H.V.: David Alexander Stewart (1874-1937). CACHB 6(2):1-5, 1941 ⟨II-00124⟩

Morgan, M.V.: Indian Medicine. The Beaver 264(2):38, 1933 ⟨II-03307⟩

Morgan, R.J.: William Smith. DCB 5:766-67, 1983 ⟨I-05303⟩

Morin, J.: Liveright Piuze. DCB 5:676, 1983 ⟨I-05306⟩

Morin, V: Superstitions et Croyances Populaires. PTRSC 31 [1]:51:60, 1937 ⟨II-03985⟩

Morin, V.: L'evolution de la medecine au Canada francais. Cahier Des Dix 25:65-83, 1960 ⟨II-04690⟩

Morison, D.: The Doctor's Secret Journal. Mackinac Island, Mackinac Island State Park Commission, 1960. 48 p. ⟨II-00380⟩

Morisset, A.: Le Langage Populaire de la Medecine du Debut du Siecle au Canada Francais. La Vie Medicale 6:276-281, 1977 ⟨II-04945⟩

Morley, W.F.E.: William Henry Smith. DCB 10:660-661, 1972 ⟨I-01101⟩

Morphy, A.G.: Thomas J.W. Burgess, M.D., F.R.C.S. CMAJ 16:203, 1926 ⟨I-01569⟩

Morphy, A.G.: Old Times in Medicine. CMAJ 63:507-511, 1950 ⟨II-03749⟩

Morrell, C.A.: Government Control of Food and Drugs. Canadian Pharmacy Journal 90:342-344, 1957 ⟨II-00438⟩

Morrison, D.N.: The Eagle and The Fort: The Story of John McLoughlin. New York, Atheneum, 1979. 119 p. ⟨I-01586⟩

Morrow, P.A.: James Elliott Graham (1847-1899). In Kelly HW, Burrage WL: Dictionary of American Medical Biography. New York and London, D. Appleton and Co., 1928. pp. 486-487. ⟨I-01386⟩

Morse, F.W.: A Country Doctor's Life, 1855-1898. Nova Scotia Medical Bulletin 46:169-175, 1967 ⟨I-03183⟩

Morton, C.S.: John George MacDougall, MD, CM(McGill), FACS, FRCS(Can), 1897-1947. Nova Scotia Medical Bulletin 26:105-110, 1947 ⟨I-03233⟩

Morton, C.S.: Doctor Herbert Smith. Nova Scotia Medical Bulletin 28:122-124, 1949 ⟨I-01997⟩

Morton, C.S.: John George MacDougall, MD, CM (McGill), FACS, FRCS(C). Nova Scotia Medical Bulletin 29:185-194, 1950 ⟨I-03221⟩

Morton, C.S.: John George MacDougall, MD, CM(McGill), FACS, FRCS(C). Nova Scotia Medical Bulletin 29:185-194, 1950 ⟨II-03293⟩

Morton, D.: "Noblest and Best": Retraining Canada's War Disabled 1915-23. Journal of Canadian Studies 16:75-85, 1981 ⟨II-04881⟩

Mott, F.W.: Charles Kirk Clarke, M.D., LL.D. British Medical Journal 1:219, 1924 ⟨I-02006⟩

Mullally, E.J.: Dr. Ronald Hugh MacDonald. CMAJ 61:641-2, 1949 ⟨I-04492⟩

Mullin, J.H.: Dr. John Gerald FitzGerald. CMAJ 43:192, 1940 ⟨I-01218⟩

Mundie, G.S.: The Need of Psychopathic Hospitals in Canada. CMAJ 10:537-542, 1920 ⟨II-00157⟩

Mundie, G.S.: The Problem of the Mentally Defective in the Province of Quebec. CMAJ 10:63-69, 1920 ⟨II-00597⟩

Murphy, A.L.: The Anti-Scurvy Club, 1606 AD. CMAJ 82:541-43, 1960 ⟨II-03753⟩

Murphy, D.A.: Osler, Now a Veterinarian!. CMAJ 83:32-35, 1960 ⟨II-02331⟩

Murphy, D.A.: James Bell's Appendicitis. Canadian Journal of Surgery 15:335-338, 1972 ⟨I-04224⟩

Murphy, G.H.: John Stewart. CMAJ 30:222-223, 1934 ⟨I-03549⟩

Murphy, G.H.: Dr. William F. MacKinnon. CMAJ 67:379, 1952 ⟨I-04535⟩

Murphy, G.H.: Golden Jubilee Saint Joseph's Hospital 1955. Nova Scotia Medical Bullletin 35:109-15, 1956 ⟨II-03754⟩

Murphy, H.H.: Indian Medicine. CMAJ 17:725-27, 1927 ⟨II-03752⟩

Murphy, H.H.: Dr. M.S. Wade. CMAJ 20:682, 1929 ⟨I-02738⟩

Murphy, H.H.: Dr. Forrest B. Leeder. CMAJ 52:644, 1945 ⟨I-04371⟩

Murphy, H.H.: Dr. H. W. Hill. CMAJ 57:607, 1947 ⟨I-04417⟩

Murphy, H.H.: Dr. Harold Edward Ridewood. CMAJ 68:186, 1953 ⟨I-04534⟩

Murphy, H.H.: Dr. J.S. Burris 1875-1953. CMAJ, 70:479, 1954 ⟨I-04564⟩

Murphy, M: A Hundred Years in St. Boniface. Canadian Nurse 40:311-319, 1944 ⟨II-03988⟩

Murray, E.G.D.: Frederick Smith. McGill Medical Journal 18:155-157, 1949 ⟨I-01631⟩

Murray, F.E.: Memoir of LeBaron Botsford, M.D. New Brunswick, J. and A. McMillan, 1892. 285 p. ⟨I-00983⟩

Murray, F.J.: At the Foot of Dragon Hill. New York, E.P. Dutton and Co., 1975. 240 p. ⟨II-04115⟩

Murray, G.: Medicine in the Making. Toronto, Ryerson Press, 1960. 235 p. ⟨II-00415⟩

Murray, G.: Quest in Medicine. Toronto, Ryerson Press, 1963. 185 p. ⟨II-00416⟩

Murray, G.: In Funerals also -- Time Brings Changes. York Pioneer 73:10-17, 1978 ⟨II-03284⟩

Murray, J.R.: Pharmaceutical Education in Alberta. Canadian Pharmaceutical Journal 91:692-94, 1958 ⟨II-03748⟩

Musgrove, W.M.: The Progress of Mental Hygiene in Manitoba. CMAJ 14:377-378, 1924 ⟨II-00158⟩

Myers, C.R.: Notes on the History of Psychology in Canada. Canadian Psychologist 6:4-19, 1965 ⟨II-03751⟩

N

N., A.G.: Dr. A.D. Blackader and the Journal. CMAJ 21:367, 1929 ⟨I-00947⟩

N., J.E., W., J.C., W., P.: Dr. John Ridge: an appreciation. CMAJ 97:1496, 1967 ⟨I-02504⟩

N, R.: Dr. Jane L. Heartz Bell. CMAJ 90:946, 1964 ⟨I-02046⟩

N., R.: Dr. Jane L. Heartz Bell. CMAJ 90:946, 1964 ⟨II-02077⟩

Nadeau, G.: A T.B.'s Progress: The Story of Norman Bethune. BHM 8:1135-1171, 1940 ⟨II-00125⟩

Nadeau, G.: Indian Scalping: Technique in Different Tribes. BHM 10:178-194, 1941 ⟨II-00385⟩

Nadeau, G.: Un Cas d'Adipocire a Berthier en 1844. L'UMC 72:180-184, 1943 ⟨II-02344⟩

Nadeau, G.: Le Plus Illustre de Nos Poitrinaires: Sir Wilfred Laurier. L'UMC 73:404-433, 1944 ⟨II-01867⟩

Nadeau, G.: Ledoyen and His Disinfectant: An Episode in the History of Typhus Fever in Quebec. CMAJ 50:471-476, 1944 ⟨II-04325⟩

Nadeau, G.: Un Episode de L'Histoire du Typhus a Quebec: Ledoyen et son Desinfectant. L'UMC 73:52-66, 1944 ⟨II-02450⟩

Nadeau, G.: Un Savant Anglais a Quebec a La Fin du XVIIIe Siecele le Docteur John-Mervin Nooth. L'UMC 74:49-74, 1945 ⟨I-02249⟩

Nadeau, G.: Les Vieux Remedes de la Nouvelle-France: l'huile de Petits Chiens. L'UMC 77:327-329, 1948 ⟨II-02349⟩

Nadeau, G.: Histoire de la Medecine Dans la Nouvelle-France: L'Alkermes et le Kermes Mineral. L'UMC 79:924-928, 1950 ⟨II-02354⟩

Nadeau, G.: Le dernier chirurgien du roi a Quebec, Antoine, Briault, 1742-1760. L'UMC 8:720, 1951 ⟨I-04938⟩

Nadeau, G.: Francois le Beau, Medecin du Roi. L'UMC 82:312-316, 1953 ⟨I-02242⟩

Nadeau, G.: Etienne Bouchard. DCB 1:108-109, 1966 ⟨I-00999⟩

Nadeau, G.: Francois Gendron. DCB 1:328, 1966 ⟨I-01402⟩

Nadeau, G.: Gervais Baudouin. DCB 1:80-81, 1966 ⟨I-00996⟩

Nadeau, G.: Jean de Bonamour. DCB 1:106-107, 1966 ⟨I-00997⟩

Nadeau, G.: Jean Madry. DCB 1:478-479, 1966 ⟨I-01455⟩

Nadeau, G.: Louis Pinard. DCB 1:550, 1966 ⟨I-01005⟩

Nadeau, G.: Timothee Roussel. DCB 1:583, 1966 ⟨I-01003⟩

Nadeau, G.: Vincent Basset du Tartre. DCB 1:79-80, 1966 ⟨I-00995⟩

Nadeau, G.: Le Docteur Paul Dufault (1895-1969). L'UMC 99:1672-1673, 1970 ⟨I-01052⟩

Nadeau, G.: Un Medecin de Roi a Quebec Qui Ne Vint Pas au Canada: Gandoger de Foigny. L'UMC 100:1990-1992, 1971 ⟨I-02233⟩

Naimark, A.: About Joe (Joseph Doupe). University of Manitoba Medical Journal 28:1, 1966 ⟨I-01474⟩

Nasmith, G.G.: On the Fringe of the Great Fight. Toronto, McClelland, Goodchild and Stewart Publishers, 1917. 263 p. ⟨II-00821⟩

Nation, E.F., Roland, C.G., McGovern, J.P.: An Annotated Checklist of Osleriana. Kent State University Press, 1970. 289 p. ⟨II-00212⟩

Naylor, C.D.: Canadian Doctors and State Health Insurance, 1911-1918. HSTC Bulletin 6:127-150, 1982 ⟨II-04991⟩

Neary, H.B.: William Renwick Riddell: Judge, Ontario Publicist and Man of Letters. Law Society of Upper Canada Gazette II:144-174, 1977 ⟨II-00213⟩

Neatby, H.: The Political Career of Adam Mabane. CHR 16:137-150, 1935 ⟨II-00693⟩

Neatby, H.: The political career of Adam Mabane. CHR 16:137-150, 1935 ⟨I-01454⟩

Neatby, H.: The Medical Profession in the North-West Territories. CACHB 14:61-77, 1950 ⟨II-03787⟩

Neatby, L.H.: Marien Tailhandler. DCB 2:617-618, 1969 ⟨I-01193⟩

Neatby, L.H.: Chronicle of a Pioneer Prairie Family. Saskatoon, Western Producer Prairie Books, 1979. 93 p. ⟨II-00495⟩

Neufeld, A.H.: Seventy-fifth birthday of Dr. Jonathan C. Meakins. CMAJ 77:58, 1957 ⟨I-03455⟩

Nevitt, J.: White Caps and Black Bands: Nursing in Newfoundland to 1934. Newfoundland, Jesperson Press Printing Limited, 1978 ⟨II-00771⟩

New, P.K., Cheung, Y.: Medical Missionary Work of a Canadian Protestant Mission in China, 1902-1937. CSHM Newsletter, Spring 1982, pages 11-16 ⟨II-04883⟩

Newerla, G.J.: Canadian Medical History: James Henry Tofield. M.D. September 1967, page 31 ⟨I-02745⟩

Newman, M.T.: Aboriginal New World Epidemiology and Medical Care, and the Impact of Old World Disease Imports. American Journal of Physical Anthropology 45:667-672, 1976 ⟨II-04996⟩

Nicholas, W.B.: Dr. W. Gordon Brown, an appreciation. CMAJ 98:795, 1968 ⟨I-01705⟩

Nicholls, A.G.: Dr. J.G. Adami. CMAJ 16:1282, 1926 ⟨I-01615⟩

Nicholls, A.G.: The Romance of Medicine in New France. Dalhousie Review 7:226-234, 1927-28 ⟨II-02109⟩

Nicholls, A.G.: The Late Louis de Lotbiniere Harwood. CMAJ 31:539-541, 1934 ⟨I-02136⟩

N(icholls), A.G.: Dr. A.D. Blackader and the Journal. CMAJ 21:367, 1939 ⟨II-00724⟩

Nicholls, A.G.: L'Hotel-Dieu. CMAJ 47:372-374, 1942 ⟨II-04677⟩

Nicholls, R.V.V.: McGill University and the Teaching of Chemistry in Canada. Chemistry and Industry, August 1958, pp 1106-1107 ⟨II-03788⟩

Nichols, R.B.: Early Women Doctors of Nova Scotia. Nova Scotia Medical Bulletin 29:14-21, 1950 ⟨II-03826⟩

Nicholson, G.W.: The White Cross in Canada; A History of St. John Ambulance. Montreal, Harvest House, 1967. 206 p. ⟨II-05451⟩

Nicholson, G.W.L.: Canada's Nursing Sisters. Toronto, A.M. Hakkert Ltd., 1975. 272 p. ⟨II-00778⟩

Noble, A.B.: Frederick Arthur Harvey Wilkinson. Canadian Anaesthetists Society Journal 6:292-293, 1959 ⟨I-02727⟩

Noble, R.L.: Memories of James Bertram Collip. CMAJ 93:1356-1364, 1965 ⟨I-02009⟩

Noble, R.L.: James Bertram Collip. Dictionary of Scientific Biography 3:351-354, 1971 ⟨I-02762⟩

Normandeau, L., Legare, J.: La Mortalite infantile des Inuit du Nouveau-Quebec. Canadian Review of Sociology and Anthropology 16:260-275, 1979 ⟨II-05117⟩

Norris, J: The Country Doctor in British Columbia: 1887-1975. An Historical Profile. B.C. Studies 49:15-39,1981 ⟨II-04070⟩

Norris, J.: Typhoid in the Rockies: Epidemiology in a Constrained Habitat, 1883-1939. In: Roland, C.G.(ed.): Health, Disease and Medicine: Essays in Canadian History. Toronto, Hannah Institute for the History of Medicine, 1984, 276-295 ⟨II-05403⟩

Northway, M.L.: William Emet Blatz. CMAJ 123:15-16, 1980 ⟨I-01066⟩

Nowell-Smith, F.M.: The History of Medicine Museum Academy of Medicine, Toronto 1907-1981. Thesis (Master of Museum Studies), Toronto, University of Toronto, 1981. 65 p. ⟨II-05285⟩

Noyes, F.W.: Stretcher-Bearers...at the Double. Toronto, The Hunter-Rose Company, Limited (printers), 311 p. ⟨II-00408⟩

Nyce, J.M.: The Gordon C. Eby Diaries, 1911-13: Chronicle of a Mennonite Farmer. Multicultural History Society of Ontario, 1982. 208 p. ⟨II-05268⟩

O

O., W.: Sir Charles Tupper, Bart. Lancet 2:1049-50, 1915 ⟨I-05177⟩

Oborne, H.G.: Samuel Tilley Gove 1813-1897: The Chronicle of a Canadian Doctor of a Century Ago. CACHB 12(2):31-38, 1947 ⟨II-00533⟩

Oborne, H.G.: Samuel Tilley Gove 1813-1897: The Chronicle of a Canadian Doctor of a Century Ago. CACHB 12:31-38, 1947 ⟨I-02113⟩

O'Donnell, J.H.: Manitoba as I saw it from 1869 to Date, with Flash-Lights on the First Riel Rebellion. Winnipeg, Clark Brothers and Co., 1909, 158 p. ⟨II-05084⟩

Oertel, H.: Dr. J.G. Adami. CMAJ 16:1282, 1926 ⟨I-01955⟩

Oertel, H.: Dr. D. D. MacTaggart. CMAJ 20:214-215, 1929 ⟨I-01754⟩

Oertel, H.: Louis Gross. McGill Medical Undergraduate Journal 7:8-10, 1937 ⟨I-02121⟩

Oertel, H.: Prof. Oskar Klotz. CMAJ 36:98-99, 1937 ⟨I-02863⟩

Oillie, J.A.: My experiences in medicine. CMAJ 91:855-860, 1964 ⟨I-02307⟩

Oko, A.J.: The Frontier art of R.B. Nevitt: Surgeon, North-West Mounted Police, 1874-78. Calgary, Glenbow-Alberta Institute, n.d.,n.p. ⟨II-00045⟩

Oliver, B.C.: Dr. Margaret MacKellar: The Story of Her Early Years. Canada, Women's Missionary Society of the Presbyterian Church in Canada, 1920. 42 p. ⟨I-01425⟩

Oliver, C.: Toronto's Medical Museum Packed with Items of Historical Significance. CMAJ 117:525-30, 1977 ⟨II-05248⟩

Oliver, E.B.: Department of Health. Thunder Bay Historical Society Annual 5:29-33, 1914 ⟨II-03828⟩

Oliver, E.B.: The Influenza Epidemic of 1918-19. Thunder Bay Historical Society Annual 10:9-10, 1919 ⟨II-03827⟩

Olmsted, A.I.: Ingersoll Olmsted (1864-1937). Canadian Journal of Surgery 3:1-4, 1959-60 ⟨I-04235⟩

O'Malley, M.: A Doctor's Dilemma. Saturday Night, May 1983, pp 19-29, 1983 ⟨I-05073⟩

Ong, E.G.: A Tribute from Hong Kong [W.C. MacKenzie]. Canadian Journal of Surgery 22:311-312, 1979 ⟨I-04284⟩

Oppenheimer, J.: Childbirth in Ontario: The Transition from Home to Hospital in the Early 20th Century. Ontario History 75:36-60, 1983 ⟨II-05092⟩

Ormsby, W.: William Rees. DCB 10:610-611, 1972 ⟨I-01128⟩

Orr, H.: Dr. William Charles Laidlaw. CMAJ 16:1285, 1926 ⟨I-01610⟩

Orr, R.B.: Practice of Medicine and Surgery by the Canadian tribes in Champlain's time. Annual Archaeological Report, 1915. pp. 35-37 ⟨II-00650⟩

Orr, W.J.: Dr. Ernest Janes: an appreciation. CMAJ 96:64, 1967 ⟨I-01742⟩

Osborne, B.S.: The Cemeteries of the Midland District of Upper Canada: A Note on Mortality in a Frontier Society. Pioneer America 6:46-55, 1974 ⟨II-05267⟩

[Osler, W.]: James Hamilton, L.R.C.S. Canada Medical and Surgical Journal 5:478-80, 1876-77 ⟨I-04959⟩

[Osler, W.]: Edward Mulberry Hodder, M.D. Canada Medical and Surgical Journal 6:428-31, 1877-88 ⟨I-04960⟩

[Osler, W.]: James Bovell, M.D. The Canada Lancet 12:249-51, 1880 ⟨I-01580⟩

Osler, W.: Obituary of Richard Zimmerman of the Toronto School of Medicine. Canada Medical and Surgical Journal 16:510-511, 1887-88 ⟨I-05183⟩

[Osler, W.]: Robert Palmer Howard, M.D. Medical News 54:419, 1889 ⟨I-05182⟩

[Osler, W.]: Richard Lea MacDonnell. New York Medical Journal 54:162, 1891 ⟨I-05181⟩

[Osler, W.]: John Bruce MacCallum, B.A., M.D. British Medical Journal 1:955-956, 1906 ⟨I-05180⟩

[Osler, W.]: Sir William Hales Hingston, M.D., LL.D., D.C.L., F.R.C.S., Eng. Lancet 1:770, 1907 ⟨I-05179⟩

O[sler], W.: The Right Hon. Sir Charles Tupper, Bart. M.D., Edin. The Lancet, 2:1049-50, 1915 ⟨I-05218⟩

[Osler, W.]: Thomas Wesley Mills. Lancet 1:466, 1915 ⟨I-05178⟩

Owen, M.: Annual Reports -- By-Laws and other Printed Documents of the Montreal General Hospital 1823-1971 Accession No. 1501/9 and 1501/75. Montreal, University Archives McGill University, January 1973, 62 p. ⟨II-04608⟩

Ower, J.J.: Dr. Harold Main Vango. CMAJ 26:377, 1932 ⟨I-03061⟩

Ower, J.J.: Pictures on Memory's Walls. CACHB 19:1-22, 1954 ⟨I-01245⟩

Ower, J.J.: Pictures on Memory's Walls, Part II (Army Days). CACHB 19:35-62, 1954 ⟨I-01246⟩

Oxorn, H.: Harold Benge Atlee, M.D.: A Biography. Hantsport, N.S., Lancelot Press, 1983. pp 352. ⟨I-05164⟩

P

P., G.R.: Jason A. Hannah: Pathologist, Economist, Historian. CMAJ 117:193, 1977 ⟨II-02212⟩

P., R.W.: Henry P. Wright, M.D. Montreal Medical Journal 27:879-880, 1898 ⟨I-02718⟩

P., V.H.T.: Dr. John C. Ballem. CMAJ 90:1138, 1964 ⟨I-05225⟩

Painchaud, R.: Theogene Fafard. DCB 11:306-307, 1982 ⟨I-04836⟩

Paine, A.L.: Manitoba Perspective on Tuberculosis. University of Manitoba Medical Journal 52:21-37, 1982 ⟨II-05005⟩

Pannekoek, F.: "Corruption" at Moose. Beaver, Spring 1979, pp. 4-11 ⟨II-00074⟩

Panneton, P.: Les Notes Medicales dan les Ecrits d'Americ Vespuce. L'UMC 74:1388-1397, 1945 ⟨II-02345⟩

Panneton, P.: Comment le premier Chirurgien a pratiquer en Quebec faillit contracter une maladie cordiere et definitive. L'UMC 76:41-45, 1947 ⟨II-02434⟩

Paper, J.: From shaman to mystic in Ojibwa religion. Studies in Religion/Sciences Religieuses 9:185-199, 1980 ⟨II-04201⟩

Paquin, M.: Gervais Baudoin. DCB 3:35, 1974 ⟨I-00994⟩

Paquin, M.: Rene Gaschet. DCB 3:236-237, 1974 ⟨I-02258⟩

Parfitt, C.D.: Dr. Jabez Henry Elliott. CMAJ 48:181-2, 1943 ⟨I-04250⟩

Pariseau, L.: Le Centenaire de la Fondation du "Journal de Medecine de Quebec". L'UMC 55:1-7, 1926 ⟨II-02478⟩

Pariseau, L.E.: Canadian Medicine and Biology During the French Regime. In: Tory, H.M. (edit): A History of Science in Canada. Toronto, The Ryerson Press, 1939, pp. 58-68. ⟨II-04914⟩

Park, L.: The Bethune Health Group. In: Shephard, D.A.E.; Levesque, A.(edit): Norman Bethune: His Times and His Legacy. Ottawa, Ontario, Canadian Public Health Association, 1982. pp 138-144. ⟨II-04920⟩

Parker, A.C.: Indian Medicine and Medicine Men. Thirty-Sixth Annual Archaeological Report (Toronto), 1928. pp 9-17 ⟨II-04820⟩

Parker, S.: Eskimo Psychopathology in the Context of Eskimo Personality and Culture. American Anthropologist, 64:76-96, 1962 ⟨II-03783⟩

Parker, W.F.: Daniel McNeill Parker, M.D.: His ancestry and a memoir of his life. Toronto, William Briggs, 1910. pp. 604 ⟨I-01032⟩

Parks, A.E.: The evolution of Canadian Medical practice during the last century. Modern Medicine of Canada 32:41-90, 1967 ⟨II-00864⟩

Parsons, W.B.: The day sulfanilamide came to town. Canadian Doctor 45:61-62,65, 1979 ⟨I-00262⟩

Parsons, W.B.: Medicine in the Thirties. Canadian Doctor 46:69-73, 1980 ⟨II-02326⟩

Parsons, W.D.: A brief history of medicine in Newfoundland. Newfoundland Medical Association Newsletter 13:5-7, 1971 ⟨II-03785⟩

Paterson, A.O.: Dr. Daniel S. McMillan. CMAJ 27:109, 1933 ⟨I-02542⟩

Paterson, G.R., Moisley, P.T.: 50 Years of the Canadian Pharmaceutical Association. Journal of American Pharmaceutical Association 18(8):481-485, 1957 ⟨II-00707⟩

Paterson, G.R.: A Year of Pharmaceutical Legislation -- 1908. Canadian Pharmaceutical Journal 91:385, 1958 ⟨II-00705⟩

Paterson, G.R.: The Canadian Conference of Pharmaceutical Faculties. American Journal of Pharmaceutical Education 22:201-209, 1958 ⟨II-05086⟩

Paterson, G.R.: The Canadian Formulary. American Journal of Hospital Pharmacy 17:427-437, 1960 ⟨II-00706⟩

Paterson, G.R.: Canadian Pharmacy in Preconfederation Medical Legislation. JAMA 200:89-852, 1967 ⟨II-00350⟩

Paterson, G.R.: The History of Pharmacy in Ontario. Canadian Pharmaceutical Journal 100:3-8, 1967 ⟨II-05094⟩

Paterson, G.R.: A Non-Active Practice: An Active Museum. Bulletin of the Ontario College of Pharmacy pp 49-51, 1971 ⟨II-05081⟩

Paterson, G.R.: Jason A. Hannah: Pathologist, Economist, Historian. CMAJ 117:193, 1977 ⟨I-02133⟩

Paterson, G.R.: The Hannah Institute: Promoting Canadian History of Medicine. CMAJ 128:1325-1328, 1983 ⟨II-05078⟩

Patterson, H.S.: Sir James Hector, M.D. 1834-1906. CACHB 6(3):2-10, 1941 ⟨I-01353⟩

Patterson, M.A.: The Cholera Epidemic of 1832 in York, Upper Canada. Bulletin of the Medical Library Association 46:165-184, 1958 ⟨II-00091⟩

Patton, W.W.: Hopital du Roy, Louisbourg. Nova Scotia Medical Bulletin 31:193-203, 1952 ⟨II-03786⟩

Peacock, F.W.: Some Eskimo Remedies and Experiences of an Amateur Doctor among the Labrador Eskimo. CMAJ 56:328-330, 1947 ⟨II-00622⟩

Pearson, A.A.: John and William Hunter: Patrons of the Arts. In International Congress for the History of Medicine, 25th, Quebec, 1976. Proceedings, Volume III, 1976. p. 1053-1062 ⟨II-00645⟩

Peart, A.F.W.: The Medical Viewpoint. Journal of Public Health 53:724-728, 1963 ⟨II-03821⟩

Pedley, F.D.: Grant Fleming. CMAJ 48:464, 1943 ⟨I-02788⟩

Peer, E.T.: A Nineteenth Century Physician of Upper Canada and His Library. Bulletin of the Cleveland Medical Library 19:78-85, 1972 ⟨I-04908⟩

Peikoff, S.S.: Dr. Sydney Caminetsky. CMAJ 97:1495, 1967 ⟨I-01562⟩

Peikoff, S.S.: Yesterday's Doctor: An Autobiography. Winnipeg, The Prairie Publishing Co., 1980. 145 p. ⟨II-00480⟩

Pelrine, E.W.: Morgentaler: The Doctor who couldn't turn away. Canada, Gage Publishing Ltd., 1975. 210 p. ⟨I-01299⟩

Penfield, W.: The significance of the Montreal Neurological Institute. In: Neurological Biographies and Addresses. London, Oxford University Press, 1936. pp 36-54 ⟨II-03823⟩

Penfield, W., Francis, W.W., Russell, C.: Tributes to Colin Kerr Russel 1877-1956. CMAJ 77:715-723, 1957 ⟨I-02590⟩

Penfield, W.: Edward Archibald :1872-1945. Canadian Journal of Surgery 1:167-174, 1958 ⟨I-01576⟩

Penfield, W.: Edward Archibald: 1872-1945. CMAJ I:167-174, 1958 ⟨II-01785⟩

Penfield, W.: China Mission Accomplished. CMAJ 97:468-470, 1967 ⟨II-03822⟩

Penfield, W.: No Man Alone. Boston/Toronto, Little, Brown and Co., 1977. 398 p. ⟨II-00782⟩

Penfield, W.: Penfield Remembered. The Review [Imperial Oil Ltd.] 66(2):26-29, 1982 ⟨I-04771⟩

Pennefather, J.D.: Thirteen Years on the Prairies: From Winnipeg to Cold Lake, Fifteen Hundred Miles. London, Kegan Paul, Trench, Trubner and Co. Ltd, 1892. 127 p. ⟨II-05085⟩

Pennefather, J.P.: A Surgeon with the Alberta Field Force. Alberta History 26(4):1-14, 1978 ⟨II-02979⟩

Percival, E.: Women in Medicine. CMAJ 23:436-438, 1930 ⟨II-03146⟩

Perlin, A.B.: History and Health in Newfoundland. Canadian Journal of Public Health 61:313-316, n.d. ⟨II-03784⟩

Persaud, T.V.N.: A Brief History of Anatomy at the University of Manitoba. Anatomischer Anzeiger 153:3-31, 1983 ⟨II-05121⟩

Peterkin, A., Shaw, M.: Mrs. Doctor: reminiscences of Manitoba doctors' wives. Winnipeg, Manitoba, The Prairie Publishing Company, 1978. 168 p. ⟨II-00496⟩

Peters, C.A.: Henri Amedee LaFleur. CMAJ 62:607-8, 1950 ⟨I-04936⟩

Peters, H.: A History of the Education of Selected Health Professions in Manitoba, Thesis (Master of Education). Department of Educational Foundation, University of Manitoba, January 1979 ⟨II-00281⟩

Pettigrew, E.: The Healing Archives: Exploring our Medical Past. The Review [Imperial Oil Ltd.] 66(4): 10-13, 1982 ⟨II-05007⟩

Pettigrew, E.: The Silent Enemy: Canada and the Deadly Flu of 1918. Saskatoon, Western Producer Prairie Books, 1983. pp 156 ⟨II-05368⟩

Phair, J.T., McKinnon, N.E.: Mortality Reductions in Ontario 1900-1942 V. Diptheria. Canadian Journal of Public Health 37:69-73, 1946 ⟨II-04455⟩

Phair, J.T., Defries, R.D.: The Ontario Department of Health. Canadian Journal of Public Health 50:183-196, 1959 ⟨II-03819⟩

Phelan, J.: A Duel on the Island. Ontario History 69:235-238, 1977 ⟨I-01666⟩

Phelps, M.L.: Moses French Colby. DCB 9:144-145, 1976 ⟨I-00927⟩

Philippe, P., Gomila, J.: Inbreeding Effects in a French Canadian Isolate. Evolution of Inbreeding. Zeitschrift Fur Morphologie und Anthropologie 64:54-9, 1972 ⟨II-05333⟩

Philpott, N.W.: Dr. Walter William Chipman. CMAJ 62:519-20, 1950 ⟨I-04485⟩

Pierce, L.: Albert Durrant Watson (1859-1926). Toronto, 1924. 30 p. n.p. ⟨I-03420⟩

Pierce, L.: Some Unpublished Letters of John Strachan, First Bishop of Toronto. Proceedings and Transactions of the Royal Society of Canada, series 3, vol. 23:25-35, 1929 ⟨I-03338⟩

Pierre-Deschenes, C.: La tuberculose au Quebec au debut au XXe Siecle: Probleme social et reponse reformiste. Thesis (M.A.) Quebec a Montreal, 1980 ⟨II-05146⟩

Pierson, R.R.: The double bind of the double standard: V.D. control and the Canadian women's army corps in WWII. Presented at annual meeting of Can Hist Assoc, Saskatoon, 1979. Memorial Univ of Newfoundland, 1979. 41 p. n.p. ⟨II-00122⟩

Pilon, H.: Edward Mulberry Hodder. DCB 10:350-351, 1972 ⟨I-01354⟩

Piva, M.J.: The Workmen's Compensation Movement in Ontario. Ontario History 67:39-56, 1975 ⟨II-04875⟩

Plamondon, L.: Marie-Catherine Payen de Noyan. DCB 5:661-662, 1983 ⟨I-05308⟩

Plewes, B.: William Edward Gallie: A Tribute by a Gallie Slave. CMAJ 81:692, 1959 ⟨I-02123⟩

Plewes, B.: Dr. James Young Ferguson: an appreciation. CMAJ 92:896, 1965 ⟨I-02819⟩

Pocius, G.L.: Eighteenth and Nineteenth Century Newfoundland Gravestones: Self-Sufficiency, Economic Specialization, and the Creation of Artifacts. Material History Bulletin 12:1-16, 1981 ⟨II-05390⟩

Pollock, S.J.: Social Policy for Mental Health in Ontario 1930-1967. Thesis (Ph.D.), Toronto, University of Toronto, 1978. unpublished ⟨II-05034⟩

"Pooch" [Corrigan, C.E.]: Tales of a Forgotten Theatre. Winnipeg, D Day Publishers, 1969. 223 p. ⟨II-00799⟩

Poole, M.E.M.: The Library of the Academy of Medicine, Toronto. Canadian Journal of Medicine and Surgery 76:144-146, 1934 ⟨II-03820⟩

Pope, E.: The profession in Winnipeg. Western Canada Medical Journal 2:121-128, 1908 ⟨II-00455⟩

Porritt, A.: A Tribute from England [W.C. MacKenzie]. Canadian Journal of Surgery 22:312-313, 1979 ⟨I-04283⟩

Porteous, C.A.: Some notes on the formation of the Canadian National Committee for Mental Hygiene. CMAJ 8:634-639, 1918 ⟨II-03789⟩

Porter, D.: Dr. Joseph Arthur MacFarlane, an appreciation. CMAJ 94:1070, 1966 ⟨I-01406⟩

Porter, G.D.: Pioneers in Tuberculosis Work in Canada. Canadian Public Health Journal 31:367-69, 1940 ⟨II-03790⟩

Porter, G.D.: Pioneers in Public Health. Canadian Journal of Public Health 40:84-86, 1949 ⟨II-00566⟩

Porter, J.R.: L'Hopital-General de Quebec et le soin des alienes (1717-1845). La Societe Canadienne d'Histoire de l'Eglise Catholique, Study Session 44, pp 23-55, 1977 ⟨II-02416⟩

Porter, McK.: To All Men. The Story of the Canadian Red Cross. Toronto, McClelland and Stewart Ltd., 1960. 146 p. ⟨II-00548⟩

Pos, R., Walters, J.A., Sommers, F.G.: D. Campbell Meyers, M.D., L.R.C.P., M.R.C.S. (Eng.): 1863-1927 Pioneer of Canadian General Hospital Psychiatry. Canadian Psychiatric Association Journal 20:393-403, 1975 ⟨I-05290⟩

Poulet, J.: L'Implanation Medicale en Nouvelle France. In International Congress for the History of Medicine, 25th, Quebec, 1976. Proceedings, Volume III, 1976. p. 1081-1093 ⟨II-00871⟩

Pouliot, L.: Rene Goupil. DCB 1:343-344, 1966 ⟨I-02260⟩

Powell, M.: Public Health Litigation in Ontario, 1884-1920. In: Roland, C.G.(ed.): Health, Disease and Medicine: Essays in Canadian History. Toronto, Hannah Institute for the History of Medicine, 1984, 412-435 ⟨II-05410⟩

Powell, N.A.: In Memoriam of Dr. J.F.W. Ross. Canada Lancet 45:327-329, 1912 ⟨I-01143⟩

Powell, N.A.: Christopher Widmer (1780-1858). In Kelly HW, Burrage WL: Dictionary of American Medical Biography. New York and London, D. Appleton and Co., 1928. pp. 1299-1300. ⟨I-01160⟩

Powell, N.A.: James Frederick William Ross (1857-1911). In Kelly HW, Burrage L: Dictionary of American Medical Biography. New York and London, D. Appleton and Co., 1928. pp. 1058-1059. ⟨I-01141⟩

Powell, R.W.: Dr. Grant Powell. CMAJ 18:213-214, 1928 ⟨I-02299⟩

Power, D'Arcy: John George Adami. In: Plarr's Lives of the Fellows of the Royal College of Surgeons of England. Bristol and London, The Royal College of Surgeons, 1930. Vol. I, pp 2-3 ⟨I-02760⟩

Power, D'Arcy: Sir Thomas George Roddick. In: Plarr's Lives of the Fellows of the Royal College of Surgeons of England. Bristol and London, The Royal College of Surgeons, 1930. Vol 2:236-37 ⟨I-02763⟩

Power, D'Arcy: The Hon. Sir William Hales Hingston. In : Plarr's Lives of the Fellows of the Royal College of Surgeons of England. Bristol and London, The Royal College of Surgeons, 1930. Vol. 1:545-6 ⟨I-02758⟩

Power, D'Arcy: William John Ogilvie Malloch. In: Plarr's Lives of the Fellows of the Royal College of Surgeons of England. Bristol and London, The Royal College of Surgeons, 1930. Vol. 2:18-19 ⟨I-02757⟩

Power, D'Arcy: William Rawlins Beaumont. In: Plarr's Lives of the Fellows of the Royal College of Surgeons of England. Bristol and London, The Royal College of Surgeons 1930. Vol. 1:73-75 ⟨I-02759⟩

Poynter, F.N.L.: James Yonge. DCB 2:670-672, 1969 ⟨I-01013⟩

Poynter, F.N.L.(edit): The Journal of James Yonge (1647-1721). Hamden, Connecticut, Archon Books, 1963 ⟨II-02905⟩

Pratt, J.H.: A reappraisal of researches leading to the discovery of Insulin. JHMAS 9:281-289, 1954 ⟨II-00105⟩

Prescott, J.F.: The Extensive Medical Writings of Soldier-Poet John McCrae. CMAJ 122-110, 113-114, 1980 ⟨II-00876⟩

Preston, J.W.: The Canadian Pharmaceutical Association, 1907-1957. Canadian Pharmaceutical Association, 1957 ⟨II-05090⟩

Preston, R.A.: A Field Hospital in the American Civil War. CACHB 17:10-13, 1952 ⟨II-00195⟩

Price, G.A.: A History of the Ontario Hospital, Toronto. Thesis (M.S.W.), Toronto, University of Toronto, 1950 ⟨II-05161⟩

Price, G.C.: A History of the Ontario Hospital. Thesis (Ph.D.). University of Toronto, 1974. ⟨II-05032⟩

Price, H.W.: A Jubilee Survey of Alberta Hospitals. CACHB 20:62-67, 1955 ⟨II-00177⟩

Price, M.J.: The Professionalization of Medicine in Ontario During the 19th Century. Thesis (M.A.), Hamilton, McMaster University, 1977 ⟨II-05155⟩

Priest, F.O.: Dr. John Clarence Webster. CMAJ 64:351-353, 1951 ⟨I-01070⟩

Prieur, G.O.: Rene Goupil, Surgeon: The First of the Jesuit Martyrs. CACHB 12:25-31, 1947 ⟨I-02112⟩

Prieur, G.O.: Francois Gendron: the First Physician of Old Huronia. CACHB 21:1-7, 1956 ⟨I-01403⟩

Primrose, A.: The Faculty of Medicine. In: The University of Toronto and its Colleges, 1827-1906. Toronto, University Library, 1906. pp 168-179 ⟨II-02329⟩

Primrose, A.: C.K. Clarke, M.D., LL.D.: A Man of Many Parts. University of Toronto Monthly 24:223-224, 1924 ⟨I-01515⟩

Primrose, A.: Dr. Clarence L. Starr. CMAJ 20:212, 1929 ⟨I-01634⟩

Primrose, A.: Dr. Francis J. Shepherd, an appreciation. CMAJ 20:211-212, 1929 ⟨I-01691⟩

Primrose, A.: The Canadian Medical Association. CMAJ 27:194-199, 1932 ⟨II-03086⟩

Primrose, A.: Irving Heward Cameron. CMAJ 30:224-225, 1934 ⟨I-03480⟩

Proctor, H.A.: Historical Sketches of the Defence Medical Association of Canada and of the Canadian Forces Medical Services. Medical Services Journal pp 305-309, 1965 ⟨II-03818⟩

Provost, H.: Robert Giffard de Moncel. DCB 1:330-331, 1966 ⟨I-01399⟩

Prud'Homme, L-A: Forts en Medicine et Jongleurs. PTRSC 30[1]:7-10, 1936 ⟨II-04696⟩

Pugsley, L.I.: The Administration and Development of Federal Statutes on Foods and Drugs in Canada. Medical Services Journal, Canada 23:387-449, 1967 ⟨II-03817⟩

Purdon, A.L.: Early Medical Practice in the Niagara Peninsula. In: Villages in the Niagara Peninsula. Proceeding, Second Annual Niagara Peninsula History Conference, Brock University, April 1980, pp. 103-112. ⟨II-04916⟩

Q

Quaggin, A.: Prisoner and Doctor: Practice in a POW Camp. Canadian Family Physician 28:1431-1432, 1434, 1982 ⟨II-04982⟩

Quaggin, A.: 'For the Public Good': Early Birth control Clinics in Canada. Canadian Family Physician 28:1868-1869, 1982 ⟨II-05024⟩

Quastel, J.H.: Fifty Years of Biochemistry. A Personal Account. Canadian Journal of Biochemistry 52:71-82, 1974 ⟨II-05450⟩

Quinn, R.W.: The Four Founders. McGill Medical Undergraduate Journal 5:5-11, 1936 ⟨II-00330⟩

Quintin, T.J.: Dr. Murray Stalker, an appreciation. CMAJ 92:437, 1965 ⟨I-01632⟩

R

R., A.C.: Professor J. Olszewski, M.D., Ph.D. CMAJ 90:1379, 1964 ⟨I-05227⟩

R., A.N.: James Barnston, M.D. Medical Chronicle 6:90-92, 1859 ⟨I-00987⟩

R., H.R.: David Sclater Lewis: student and maker of history. CMAJ 116:314, 1977 ⟨I-03883⟩

R., I.: Dr. Hartley Frederic Patterson Grafton: an appreciation. CMAJ 86:995-996, 1962 ⟨I-02150⟩

R., J.C.: Herbert Hylton Hyland. Canadian Journal of Neurological Science 5:51, 1978 ⟨I-01337⟩

Rae, H. [pseud]: Maple Leaves in Flanders Fields. Toronto, William Briggs, n.d. 268 p. ⟨II-02328⟩

Rae, I.: The strange story of Dr. James Barry. London, Longmans, Green and Co., 1958. pp 124 ⟨I-00992⟩

Rafter, G.W.: Banting and Best and the Sources of Useful Knowledge. Perspectives in Biology and Medicine 26:281-286, 1983 ⟨II-05049⟩

Ramsay, G.: Towards Hudson Bay. CMAJ 58:614-616, 1948 ⟨II-03816⟩

Rankin, A.C.: Dr. Frank Hamilton Mewburn. CMAJ 20:328-329, 1929 ⟨I-03506⟩

Rankin, L.: A Many Sided Man [T.G.Hamilton]. The Alumni Journal [University of Manitoba] 41:4-7, 1981 ⟨II-04114⟩

Ranta, L.E.: The Medical School of British Columbia. CACHB 16:1-9, 1951 ⟨II-00243⟩

Rasporich, A.W., Clarke, I.H.: John Palmer Litchfield. DCB 9:470-471, 1976 ⟨I-01313⟩

Rasporich, A.W., Clarke, I.H.: John Scott. DCB 9:706-707, 1976 ⟨I-01114⟩

Rasporich, A.W., Getty, I.A.L.: George Verey. DCB 11:900-901, 1982 ⟨I-04858⟩

Rawlinson, H.E.: Frank Hamilton Mewburn, OBE, MD, CM, LLD, LT.-COL., CAMC, Professor of Surgery, University of Alberta, Pioneer Surgeon. Canadian Journal of Surgery 2:1-5, 1958 ⟨I-03432⟩

Rawson, N.B.: Dr. Herbert P. Byers. CMAJ 30:108-109, 1934 ⟨I-03543⟩

Ray, A.J.: Smallpox: the epidemic of 1837-38. The Beaver, Autumn 1975, pp 8-13 ⟨II-00118⟩

Ray, A. J.: Diffusion of Disease in the Western Interior of Canada, 1830-1850. Geographical Review 66:139-157, 1976 ⟨II-00230⟩

Ray, A.J.: Opportunity and Challenge: The Hundson's Bay Company Archives and Canadian Science and Technology. In: Jarrell, R.A. Ball, N.R.: Science, Technology and Canadian History. Kingston, Wilfrid Laurier Univ. Press, 1980. pp 45-59 ⟨II-00374⟩

Ray, J.: Emily Stowe. Fitzhenry and Whiteside Ltd., 1978. 63 p. ⟨II-03641⟩

Raymond, R.: Hopital General de Montreal, Registre de lentree des pauvres (1691- 1741). Memories de la Societe Genealogique Canadienne-Francaise 20:238-42, 1969 ⟨II-05151⟩

Read, C.: The Duncombe rising, its aftermath, anti-Americanism, and sectarianism. Histoire Sociale/Social History 9(17):47-69, 1976 ⟨I-03003⟩

Read, C.F.: The Rising in Western Upper Canada, 1837-38. Thesis (Ph.D.), University of Toronto, 1976. Microfiche #2795 ⟨II-00681⟩

Reddy, H.L.: J. Bradford McConnell, MD, DCL. CMAJ 22:893, 1930 ⟨I-03017⟩

Redford, J.B.: Some pioneers in the medical history of British Columbia. CAMSI Journal 11:24-26, 1952 ⟨II-03814⟩

Reed, T.A.: "The Toronto General". CACHB 9(1):13-18, 1944 ⟨II-00196⟩

Rehwinkel, B.L.: Dr. Bessie. The Life Story and Romance of a Pioneer Lady Doctor on our Western and the Canadian Frontier. St. Louis, Mo., Concordia Pub. House, 1963 ⟨I-05059⟩

Reid, A.G.: The first poor-relief system of Canada. CHR 27:424-431, 1946 ⟨II-00467⟩

Reid, D.: De la medecine traditionnelle a la medecine preventive: analyse des reformes de sante au Quebec. L'UMC 109:774-777, 1980 ⟨II-04682⟩

Reid, E.G.: The Great Physician. (A Short LIfe of Sir William Osler). London/New York/Toronto, Oxford University Press, 1931. 299 p. ⟨I-01253⟩

Reid, J.W.: Presidential Address. CMAJ 70:335-338, 1954 ⟨II-03815⟩

Reimber, M.: Cornelius W. Wiebe: A Beloved Physician. Winnipeg, Hyperion Press Limited, 1983 ⟨I-05054⟩

Rene, S.M.-C.: Soeurs Grises Nicoletaines; Mere Youville, Ses Auxiliaries, Son Oeuvre. Editions du Bien Public, Trois-Rivieres 1948. 355 p. ⟨II-04671⟩

Repka, W.: Howard Lowrie M.D.: Physician Humanitarian. Toronto, Progress Books, 1977 104p. ⟨I-04240⟩

Revell, D.G.: The Medical Faculty -- University of Alberta. CACHB 13:65-75, 1949 ⟨II-00284⟩

Rheaume, P.Z.: Notes sur l'hopital general Canadien No. 6. L'UMC 49-345-348, 1920 ⟨II-02371⟩

Rheaume, P.Z.: Dr. Eugene Latreille. CMAJ 19:738, 1928 ⟨I-03492⟩

Rheaume, P.Z.: Latreille, 1879-1928. L'UMC 57:699-702, 1928 ⟨I-01769⟩

Rich, E.E.: The Fur Traders: Their Diet and Drugs. The Beaver, Summer 1976. pp 43-53 ⟨II-00220⟩

Rich, E.E. (edit): The Letters of John McLoughlin from Fort Vancouver to the Governor and Committee, first series, 1825-38; second series 1839-44; third series 1844-46. Toronto, The Champlain Society 1941; 1943; 1944 ⟨I-05173⟩

Richard, L.: La Famille Loedel. Le Bulletin des Recherches Historiques 56:78-89, 1950 ⟨II-00331⟩

Richards, G.E.: William Howard Dickson, MD. CMAJ 29:690-91, 1933 ⟨I-03049⟩

Richards, R.L.: Rae of the Arctic. Medical History 19(2):176-193, 1975 ⟨II-00400⟩

Richardson, G.: Mrs. Letitia (Lecitia) Munson. DCB 11:629-30, 1982 ⟨I-04853⟩

Richardson, J.H.: The mystery of the medals. University of Toronto Monthly 2:130-135, 1902 ⟨II-02625⟩

Richardson, R.A.: Archibald Byron Macallum. In: Dictionary of Scientific Biography 8:583-4, 1973 ⟨I-05293⟩

Richmond, G.: Prison Doctor. Surrey, Nunaga Publishing, 1975. 186 p. ⟨I-04197⟩

Riddell, D.G.: Nursing and the law: The History of Legislation in Ontario. In: Innis, M.Q.: Nursing Education in a Changing Society. Toronto, University of Toronto Press, 1970. pp 16-45 ⟨II-03653⟩

Riddell, [W.R.]: The Court of King's Bench in Upper Canada, 1824-1827. N.P./n.d. pp. 1-28 ⟨I-01136⟩

Riddell, W.R.: The First Medical Case in the Province. N.p. / n.d. ⟨II-00255⟩

Riddell, W.R.: Was the handsome "Doctor" of Carleton Place a faker?. Offprint, (n.p., n.d.) pp. 3. ⟨II-00555⟩

Riddell, W.R.: The medical profession in Ontario. A legal and historical sketch. Canadian Journal of Medicine and Surgery 30:131-153, 1911 ⟨II-03792⟩

Riddell, W.R.: A medical slander case in Upper Canada, 85 years ago. Canada Lancet 46:330-332, 1913 ⟨II-03834⟩

Riddell, W.R.: Examination for license to practise sixty years ago. Canada Lancet 46:735-741, 1913 ⟨II-03833⟩

Riddell, W.R.: Some Early Legislation and Legislators in Upper Canada. Toronto, The Carswell Co., Limited, 1913. 39 p. ⟨II-00140⟩

Riddell, W.R.: A Medical Slander Case in 1831. Canada Lancet 48:501-3, 1915 ⟨II-04475⟩

Riddell, W.R.: An Eighteenth Century Quack in French Canada. New York Medical Journal 102:881-882, 1915 ⟨II-04474⟩

Riddell, W.R.: The Mosquito in Upper Canada. Ontario Historical Society Papers and Records 17:85-89, 1919 ⟨II-00111⟩

Riddell, W.R.: La Maladie de la Baie de St. Paul. Public Health Journal 15:145-157, 1924 ⟨II-04473⟩

Riddell, W.R.: Popular medicine in Upper Canada a century ago. Ontario Historical Society Papers and Records, 25:1-8, 1929 ⟨II-03791⟩

Riddell, W.R.: A Case of 'Ship Fever' in French Canada. Canada Lancet and Practitioner 74:132-1934, 1930 ⟨II-00347⟩

Riddell, W.R.: Sidelights on disease in French Canada before the conquest. Canadian Journal of Medicine and Surgery 69:5-12, 1931 ⟨II-03793⟩

Riddell, W.R.: The First College of Surgeons in Canada. Canadian Journal of Medicine and Surgery 70:25-30, 1931 ⟨II-04001⟩

Ridge, J.M.: The Impact of a Great Discovery [TB Bacillus]. University of Manitoba Medical Journal 28:75, 77-78, 1957 ⟨II-05263⟩

Rioux, C.: L'hopital militaire a Quebec: 1759-1871. Canadian Society for the History of Medicine Newsletter, 5:16-19, 1981 ⟨II-04673⟩

Risk, M.Mc.: A Study of the Origins and Development of Public Health Nursing in Toronto, 1890-1918. Thesis (M.Sc.), Toronto, University of Toronto, 1973 ⟨II-05143⟩

Ritchie, J.B.: Early Surgeons of the North West Mounted Police. CACHB 21(4):93-101, 1957 ⟨II-00825⟩

Ritchie, J.B.: Early Surgeons of the North West Mounted Police. III Doctor George Alexander Kennedy, Part 2. CACHB 22:201-218, 1957 ⟨I-01322⟩

Ritchie, J.B.: Early Surgeons of the North West Mounted Police. III Doctor George Alexander Kennedy. CACHB 22:171-181, 1957 ⟨I-01323⟩

Ritchie, J.B.: Early Surgeons of the North West Mounted Police, II: Doctor John George Kittson: First Surgeon. CACHB 22:130-143, 1957 ⟨I-02589⟩

Ritchie, J.B.: Early Surgeons of the North West Mounted Police: V. Doctor Richard Barrington Nevitt. CACHB 22:249-265, 1958 ⟨I-02540⟩

Ritchie, J.B.: Early Surgeons of the North-West Mounted Police (R.B. Nevitt. RCMP Quarterly 24:61-65, 1958 ⟨I-02541⟩

Ritchie, J.B.: George Alexander Kennedy, M.D. 1858-1913. CMAJ 1:279-286, 1958 ⟨I-01575⟩

Ritzenthaler, R.E.: Chippewa Preoccupation with Health; Change in a Traditional Attitude Resulting from Modern Health Problems. Bulletin of the Public Museum of the City of Milwaukee 19:175-258, 1953 ⟨II-02691⟩

Roach, M.R.: Alan Chadburn Burton 1904-1979. PTRSC series 4, 18: 57-59, 1980 ⟨I-04955⟩

Robert, G.: L'Aide a la Famille Dans la Province de Bourgogne et son Extension au Royaume de France ainsi Qu'au Canada. International Congress for the History of Medicine, Paris, 1982. Proceedings, vol. 1:56-59, 1982. ⟨II-05274⟩

Roberts, C.A.: Thirty-five years of psychiatry in Canada, 1943-1978. Psychiatric Journal of the University of Ottawa 4(1):35-38, 1979 ⟨II-00579⟩

Roberts, K.B.: Smallpox: an Historic Disease. St. John's, Nfld.,Memorial University of Newfoundland, 1979. 49 p. ⟨II-00353⟩

Roberts, W.: Six New Women: A Guide to the Mental Map of Women Reformers in Toronto. Atlantis 3:145-164, 1977-8 ⟨I-01975⟩

Roberts, W.F.: Dr. H.L. Abramson. CMAJ 30:696, 1934 ⟨I-03541⟩

Robertson, H.R.: Edward Archibald, the "New Medical Science" and Norman Bethune. In: Shephard, D.A.E.; Levesque, A. (edit): Norman Bethune; His Times and His Legacy. Ottawa, Canadian Public Health Assoc., 1982 pp 71-78 ⟨I-04895⟩

Robertson, J.K.: An experiment in medical education. The British Journal of Radiology 27:593-603, 1954 ⟨II-03797⟩

Robertson, J.S.: The Nova Scotia Department of Public Health. Canadian Journal of Public Health 50:270-283, 1959 ⟨II-03796⟩

Robertson, P.: The All-Penetrating "X". Archivaria 10-258-260, 1980 ⟨II-00551⟩

Robillard, D.: Armand Frappier. CMAJ 123:807, 1980 ⟨I-02020⟩

Robillard, D.: L'Hopital Notre-Dame de Montreal celebre avec dynamisme 100 ans de progres. CMAJ 122:837-389, 1980 ⟨II-02417⟩

Robillard, D.: Profil: Renaud Lemieux. CMAJ 125:383, 1981 ⟨I-04556⟩

Robinson, D.: Early CPR Doctors of Alberta and the West. Alberta Medical Bulletin 18: August 1953 ⟨II-03798⟩

Robinson, M.O.: Give my Heart. (The Dr. Marion Hilliard Story). New York, Doubleday and Co., Inc., 1964. 348 p. ⟨II-00768⟩

Robinson, R.R.: Bates of the Health League: An Insider's Reminiscence. Ontario Medical Review 49:305-308, 1982 ⟨I-04871⟩

Robson, R.B.: Windsor Medical Services Incorporated. CMAJ 82:604-607, 1960 ⟨II-00249⟩

Roby, Y.: Pierre-Claude Boucher de la Bruere. DCB 10:76-77, 1972 ⟨I-00013⟩

Roche, W.J.: Reminiscences. University of Western Ontario Medical Journal 1:8-10, 1930 ⟨I-04761⟩

Rodin, A.E.: John McCrae, Poet-Pathologist. CMAJ 88:204-205, 1963 ⟨II-00753⟩

Rodin, A.E.: Osler's Museum Specimens of Heart Disease. Chest 60:587-594, 1971 ⟨II-03866⟩

Rodin, A.E.: Canada's Foremost Pathologist of the Nineteenth Century -- William Osler. CMAJ 107:890-896, 1972 ⟨II-00752⟩

Rodin, A.E.: Osler's Autopsies: Their Nature and Utilization. Medical History 17:37-48, 1973 ⟨I-01247⟩

Rodin, A.E.: Oslerian Pathology: an Assessment and Annotated Atlas of Museum Specimens. Kansas, Coronado Press, 1981. 250 p. ⟨II-03761⟩

Roemer, M.I.: The Saskatchewan Air Ambulance Service: Medical and Public Health Aspects. CMAJ 75:529-533, 1956 ⟨II-00407⟩

Roger, I.L.: John Mackieson. DCB 11:565-66, 1982 ⟨I-04851⟩

Roland, C.G.: Priority of Clinical X-Ray Reports: A Classic Dethroned?. Canadian Journal of Surgery 5: 247-251, 1962 ⟨II-04626⟩

[Roland, C.G.]: Canada's Psychiatrists and their History. CMAJ 89:520-521, 1963 ⟨II-00576⟩

[Roland, C.G.]: The First Operation for Cleft Palate. CMAJ 89:825-826, 1963 ⟨II-00095⟩

Roland, C.G.: James Bovell (1817-1880): The Toronto Years. CMAJ 91:812-814, 1964 ⟨I-00010⟩

Roland, C.G.: Some Addena to Abbott's Classified Bibliography of Sir William Osler. BHM 38:78-79, 1964 ⟨II-01860⟩

Roland, C.G.: Teaching Medical History in Canadian Universities. CMAJ 90:887, 1964 ⟨II-05282⟩

Roland, C.G.: The First Death From Chloroform at the Toronto General Hospital. Canadian Anesthetists' Society Journal 11:437-439, 1964 ⟨II-03799⟩

Roland, C.G.: Dr. Clarence Meredith Hincks. CMAJ 92:305, 1965 ⟨I-01663⟩

Roland, C.G.: Clarence Hincks in Manitoba, 1918. Manitoba Medical Review 46:107-113, 1966 ⟨I-03415⟩

Roland, C.G.: James Neish and the Canadian Medical Times. McGill Medical Journal 36:107-125, 1967 ⟨II-00727⟩

Roland, C.G.: The Osler Library. JAMA 200:161-166, 1967 ⟨II-05021⟩

Roland, C.G.: Bibliography of the History of Anesthesia in Canada: Preliminary Checklist. Canadian Anesthetists' Society Journal 15:202-214, 1968 ⟨II-04884⟩

Roland, C.G.: Doctors Afield: Walter Henry -- a Very Lilyputian Hero. New England Journal of Medicine 280:31-33, 1969 ⟨I-04870⟩

Roland, C.G.: Maude Abbott and J.B. MacCallum: Canadian Cardiac Pioneers. Chest 57:371-77, 1970 ⟨I-03564⟩

Roland, C.G.: Diary of a Canadian Country Physician: Jonathan Woolverton (1811-1883). Medical History 14:168-180, 1971 ⟨I-04872⟩

Roland, C.G.: Dr. James Bowman vs Canada: A Struggle to Obtain Payment for Government Service. In: International Congress for the History of Medicine, 25th, Quebec, 1976. Proceedings, Volume III, 1976. p. 1158-1170 ⟨II-00439⟩

Roland, C.G.: Gerald O'Reilly. DCB 9:611-612, 1976 ⟨I-01267⟩

Roland, C.G.: James Barry. DCB 9:33-34, 1976 ⟨I-00985⟩

Roland, C.G., Potter, P.: An Annotated Bibliography of Canadian Medical Periodicals 1826-1975. Toronto, The Hannah Institute for the History of Medicine, 1979. 77 p. ⟨II-05027⟩

Roland, C.G.: Dr. Earle Scarlett: melding tradition and beauty in historical writing. Canadian Medical Association Journal 122:822-826, 1980 ⟨II-00206⟩

Roland, C.G.: Dr. Earle Scarlett: melding tradition and beauty in historical writing. CMAJ 122:822-826, 1980 ⟨I-01074⟩

Roland, C.G.: Ontario Medical Periodicals as Mirrors of Change. Ontario History 72:5-15, 1980 ⟨II-00735⟩

Roland, C.G.: The Possible Consequences of a Bibliography of Canadian Medical Periodicals. In: Jarrell, R.A., Ball, N.R.: Science, Technology and Canadian History. Kingston, Wilfrid Laurier Univ. Press, 1980. pp 208-211 ⟨II-00375⟩

Roland, C.G.: War Amputations in Upper Canada. Archivaria 10:73-84, 1980 ⟨II-00842⟩

Roland, C.G.: Battlefield Surgery and the Stretcher-bearers' Experience. In: Shephard, D.A.E.: Levesque, A.(edit): Norman Bethune: His Time and His Legacy. Ottawa, Canadian Public Health Assoc., 1982. pp 44-53 ⟨II-04926⟩

Roland, C.G.: George William Campbell. DCB 11:148-149, 1982 ⟨I-04868⟩

Roland, C.G.: John Fulton. DCB 11:328-29, 1982 ⟨I-04838⟩

Roland, C.G.: The Natural History of 19th Century Canadian Medical Periodicals. In: International Congress for the History of Medicine, 28th, Paris, 1982. Proceedings, vol. 1:219-223, 1982 ⟨II-05279⟩

Roland, C.G.: When Did John Rolph First Practice Medicine in Upper Canada?. Canadian Society for the History of Medicine Newsletter, Autumn, 1982. pp 24-25 ⟨I-04975⟩

Roland, C.G.: "Sunk under the Taxation of Nature": Malaria in Upper Canada. In: Roland, C.G. (ed.): Health, Disease and Medicine: Essays in Canadian History. Toronto, Hannah Institute for the History of Medicine, 1984, 154-170 ⟨II-05397⟩

Roland, C.G. (edit): Health, Disease and Medicine: Essays in Canadian History. Toronto, Hannah Institute for the History of Medicine, 1984. 464 pp. ⟨II-05391⟩

Roman, C.L.: Dr. E.M. Eberts. CMAJ 53:412, 1945 ⟨I-04343⟩

Roman, C.R.: Dr. Benjamin Franklin Macnaughton. CMAJ 45:468-469, 1941 ⟨I-03523⟩

Romaniuk, A.: Increase in Natural Fertility During the Early Stages of Modernization: Canadian Indians Case Study. Demography 18:157-172, 1981 ⟨II-04912⟩

Romanov, A.: Dr. Ernest Clifford Janes: an appreciation. CMAJ 96:64, 1967 ⟨I-01741⟩

Romkey, R.: Johann Burghard Erad. DCB 3:212, 1974 ⟨I-01015⟩

Ronaghan, A.: The Hospital on the Hill, 1912-1962. Islay, Municipal Hospital Board Historical Committee, 1962 ⟨II-05105⟩

Rooke, R.P., Schnell, R.L.: Childhood and Charity in Nineteenth-Century British North America. Social History 15:157-179, 1982 ⟨II-04928⟩

Roper, G.: Robertson Davies' Fifth Business and "That Old Fantastical Duke of Dark Corners, C.G. Jung". Journal of Canadian Fiction 1:33-39, 1972 ⟨II-05387⟩

Rose, J.: The Perfect Gentleman. [Dr. James Barry]. London, England, Hutchinson and Co. (Publishers) Ltd., 1977. 160 p. ⟨II-00837⟩

Rose, T.F.: From Shaman to Modern Medicine. A Century of the Healing Arts in British Columbia. Vancouver, Mitchell Press Ltd., 1972. 187 p. ⟨II-00856⟩

Rosen, G.: The Idea of Social Medicine in America. CMAJ 61:316-323, 1949 ⟨II-04621⟩

Ross, A.: Dr. A. Stanley Kirkland: an appreciation. CMAJ 89:733-734, 1963 ⟨I-01746⟩

Ross, A.M.: Recollections and Experiences of an Abolitionist; from 1885 to 1865. Toronto, Rowsell and Hutchison, 1875. 224 p. ⟨I-01641⟩

Ross, A.M.: Memoirs of a Reformer (1832-1892). Toronto, Hunter Rose and Co., 1893. 271 p. ⟨I-01643⟩

Ross, E.F.: Wilfred Alan Curry, ba, MD, FRCS(Eng.), FRCS(C), FACS. CMAJ 96:62-63, 1967 ⟨I-02026⟩

Ross, H.E.: A Glimpse of 1885. Saskatchewan History 21:24-29, 1968 ⟨II-03800⟩

Ross, J.F.W.: The Indian and the Indian Medicine Man. Canadian Practitioner and Review, May 1903 ⟨II-00623⟩

Ross, J.W.: A Half-Century in Medicine. Bulletin of the Academy of Medicine, Toronto 25:28-32, 1951 ⟨I-01050⟩

Ross, M.A.: Typhoid Fever Mortality in Ontario, 1880-1931. Canadian Public Health Journal 26:73-84, 1935 ⟨II-04878⟩

Ross, S.G.: Dr. Lionel Mitcheson Lindsay: an appreciation. CMAJ 95:738-739, 1966 ⟨I-03085⟩

Roth, F.B., Defries, R.D.: The Saskatchewan Department of Public Health. Canadian Journal of Public Health 49:276-285, 1958 ⟨II-03801⟩

Rothwell, A.: Love and Good Sense -- The First Half-Century of the Salvation Army Grace Hospital, Calgary 1926-1976. n.p., n.d. [ca. 1976] ⟨II-05016⟩

Rottot, J.P.: Retrospective; L'Union Medicale du Canada. L'UMC 101:952, 1972 ⟨II-05332⟩

Roulston, T.M.: Elinor F.E. Black. University of Manitoba Medical Journal 52:5-6, 1982 ⟨I-04973⟩

Rousseau, F.: L'Hospitalisation en Nouvelle-France, l'Hotel-Dieu de Quebec, 1689-1698. Thesis (M.A.), Laval University, 1975 ⟨II-05153⟩

Rousseau, F.: Hopital et Societe en Nouvelle-France: L'Hotel-Dieu de Quebec a la Fin du XVIIe Siecle. Revue d'Histoire de l'Amerique Francaise 31:29-47, 1977-78 ⟨II-04692⟩

Rousseau, F.: Marie-Venerande Melancon. DCB 5:587-588, 1983 ⟨I-05310⟩

Rousseau, J.: Diereville. DCB 2:188-189, 1969 ⟨I-01018⟩

Routley, T.C.: Canadian Experiments in Medical Economics. CMAJ 40:599-605, 1939 ⟨II-03778⟩

Routley, T.C.: Dr. John Ferguson. CMAJ 42:94, 1940 ⟨I-01219⟩

Routley, T.C.: Canadian Medical Association Journal. CACHB 10:10-16, 1945 ⟨II-03803⟩

Routley, T.C.: Volume one -- Number one of the Canadian Medical Association Journal. CACHB 10:10-16, 1945 ⟨II-00726⟩

Routley, T.C.: John Sinclair McEachern. CMAJ 58:290, 1948 ⟨I-03178⟩

Routley, T.C.: Dr. Charles Martin. CMAJ, 70:96-7, 1954 ⟨I-04563⟩

Routley, T.C.: Harry Goudge Grant. Nova Scotia Medical Bulletin 33:165, 1954 ⟨I-02158⟩

Routley, T.C.: The Founding of the Royal College of Physicians and Surgeons of Canada. CMAJ, 73:104-106, 1955 ⟨II-04648⟩

Routley, T.C.: The Murray Brothers. CMAJ 78:449-450, 1958 ⟨II-01791⟩

Routley, T.C.: Dr. Leon Gerin-Lajoie. CMAJ 80:397-398, 1959 ⟨I-02247⟩

Routley, T.C.: Affiliation with CMA. Ontario Medical Review 30:785-787, 801, 1963 ⟨II-03763⟩

Routley, T.C.: Introduction (Routley's History of the OMA). Ontario Medical Review 30:593-94, 1963 ⟨II-03762⟩

Routley, T.C.: Some Early Achievements. Ontario Medical Review 30:725-729, 1963 ⟨II-03811⟩

Routley, T.C.: The Formative Years. Ontario Medical Review 30:659-662, 1963 ⟨II-03812⟩

Routley, T.C.: Adopting an Offical Journal. Ontario Medical Review 31:349-354, 1964 ⟨II-03766⟩

Routley, T.C.: Membership Becomes Continuous. Ontario Medical Review 31:208-211, 231, 1964 ⟨II-03765⟩

Routley, T.C.: Setting up the districts. Ontario Medical Review 31:95-99, 1964 ⟨II-03810⟩

Routley, T.C.: The Bid to Rout Routley. Ontario Medical Review 31:285-287, 290, 1964 ⟨II-03767⟩

Routley, T.C.: The War Years. Ontario Medical Review 31:27-30, 1964 ⟨II-03759⟩

Routley, T.C.: Medical Welfare plan is born. Ontario Medical Review 33:864-68, 1966 ⟨II-03807⟩

Routley, T.C.: A Breach of Contract. Ontario Medical Review 34:165-68, 176, 1967 ⟨II-03802⟩

Routley, T.C.: Dr. Kelly Joins the Staff. Ontario Medical Review 34:237-241, 1967 ⟨II-03779⟩

Routley, T.C.: Dr. Routley Resigns. Ontario Medical Review 34:387-392, 1967 ⟨II-03780⟩

Routley, T.C.: Managing Medical Relief. Ontario Medical Review 34:30-34, 1967 ⟨II-03806⟩

Routley, T.C.: Routley's History of the O.M.A. : Conclusion. Ontario Medical Review 34:453-456, 1967 ⟨II-01797⟩

Routley, T.C.: The Reluctant Contractors. Ontario Medical Review 34:91-98, 1967 ⟨II-03781⟩

Routley, T.C.: Trial Plans in Health Insurance. Ontario Medical Review 34:315-319, 1967 ⟨II-03804⟩

Rowles, E.: Bannock, Beans and Bacon: An Investigation of Pioneer Diet. Saskatchewan History 5:1-15, 1952 ⟨II-00360⟩

Rowntree, L.G.: Banting's "Miracle". In: Amid Masters of Twentieth Century Medicine. Springfield, Charles C. Thomas Publisher, 1958. pp 339-354 ⟨I-02593⟩

Roy, J.E.: Medicine and the Law. In Histoire due Notariat au Canada, Vol 1, 1889. pp 8-23 ⟨II-00341⟩

Roy, J.E.: Licensure and Control of the Profession. In:Histoire du Notariat au Canada, Vol. II, 1900. pp 498-516 ⟨II-00141⟩

Roy, P-G.: A Travers l'histoire de l'Hotel-Dieu de Quebec. Levis, 1939 ⟨II-05152⟩

Royer, B.F.: Dr. William Harop Hattie, (an appreciation). CMAJ 26:121-122, 1932 ⟨I-01341⟩

Rudkin, D.W.: Henry Boys. DCB 9:79-80, 1976 ⟨I-00009⟩

Rudowski, W.: A tribute from Poland [W.C. MacKenzie]. Canadian Journal of Sugery 22:313-314, 1979 ⟨I-04282⟩

Runnalls, J.L.: A Century with the St.Catharines General Hospital. St. Catharines, St. Catharines General Hospital, 1974. 150 p. ⟨I-01526⟩

Russel, C.K.: Dr. James Douglas, 1800-1886, Adventurer. Transactions of the American Neurological Association, pp 2-6, 1935 ⟨I-04834⟩

Russel, C.M.: The Origin, Organization and Scope of the Canadian National Committee for Mental Hygiene. CMAJ 8:538-546, 1918 ⟨II-03714⟩

Russell, G.: Phrenological Sketch of the Character of Dr. Wm. Dunlop, Late Member of Parliament for the County of Huron. British American Journal of Medical and Physical Science 4:153-154, 1848-9 ⟨I-01497⟩

Russell, L.S.: Abraham Gesner. DCB 9:308-312, 1976 ⟨I-01394⟩

Russell, R.: The Spanish Civil War: Reminiscences of a Veteran of the Mackenzie- Papineau Battalion. In: Shephard, D.A.E. Levesque, A.(edit): Norman Bethune: His Times and His Legacy. Ottawa, Canadian Public Health Association, 1982. pp 170-76 ⟨II-04921⟩

Rutman, L.: In the Children's Aid: J.J. Kelso and Child Welfare in Ontario. Toronto, University of Toronto Press, 1982. 356 p. ⟨II-04918⟩

Ruttan, H.R.: The Leprosy Problem in Canada with Report of a Case. CMAJ 78:19-21, 1958 ⟨II-03713⟩

Ruttan, R.F.: William Robertson (1784-1844). In Kelly HW, Burrage WL: Dictionary of American Medical Biography. New York and London, D. Appleton and Co., 1928. p. 1044 ⟨I-01224⟩

Ryan, G: [Reminiscences]. Winnipeg Clinic Quarterly 23:97-99, 1970 ⟨II-04121⟩

Ryerson, E.S.: Frederick LeMaitre Grasett. CMAJ 22:594-95, 1930 ⟨I-03028⟩

Ryerson, E.S.: Events Leading to the Formation of an Academy. Bulletin of the Academy of Medicine [Toronto] 5:26-33, 1932 ⟨II-00457⟩

Ryerson, G.S.: Medical Notes from the North West Field Force. The Canada Lancet 17:295-297, 1884-5 ⟨II-00826⟩

Ryerson, G.S.: Looking backward. Toronto, The Ryerson Press, 1924. 264 p. ⟨II-00387⟩

S

S., A.B.: Clarence B. Farrar. CMAJ 103:307, 1970 ⟨I-02783⟩

S., C.B.: Dr. Harry Dodge Morse, an appreciation. CMAJ 95:885, 1966 ⟨I-03194⟩

S., E.: Le docteur Francois Roy. CMAJ 111:569, 1974 ⟨I-05170⟩

S., E.H.: Torono Insane Asylum. Canadian Journal of Medicine and Surgery 3:164-166, 1898 ⟨II-03704⟩

S, F.J.: Rev. Prof. Wm. Wright, M.D. Died, April 15th, 1908, Aet. 81. Montreal Medical Journal 37:366-368, 1908 ⟨I-01169⟩

S, F.J.: Robert A. Stevenson, M.D. CMAJ 10:207-208, 1920 ⟨I-01651⟩

S., G.D.: Edward Hector Rouleau. CACHB 5:4-10, 1940 ⟨II-03813⟩

S., G.D.: Unforgettable Incidents. CACHB 7:12-14, 1942 ⟨II-03717⟩

S, H.L.: Dr. Roberta Bond Nichols. CMAJ 96:234, 1967 ⟨I-02537⟩

S., L.J.: Dr. E.R. Tiffin. CMAJ 90:1139, 1964 ⟨I-05226⟩

S., M.J.: Dr. George T. Zumstein, an appreciation. CMAJ 85:1215, 1961 ⟨I-02714⟩

S., O.A.: Elinor Frances Elizabeth Black. The Lancet 1:694, 1982 ⟨I-04963⟩

Sabia, M.J.: Dr. Joseph F. Vogl, an appreciation. CMAJ 89:834, 1963 ⟨I-02739⟩

Salisbury, S.: The Montreal Children's Hospital. McGill Medical Journal 26:154-156, 1957 ⟨II-03727⟩

Salter, R.B.: Scientific Contributions to Orthopaedic Surgery by the Staff of the Hospital for Sick Children, Toronto 1875 to 1975. In International Congress for the History of Medicine, 25th, Quebec, 1976. Proceedings, Volume III, 1976. p. 1225-1243 ⟨II-00756⟩

Sanders, E.M. (Edit.): The Life and Letters of the Rt. Hon. Sir Charles Tupper, Bart., K.C.M.G., Vol. 1 and Vol. 2. New York, Frederick A. Stokes Co., 1916. 319 p. -- Vol. II 298 p. ⟨I-01155⟩

Sandomirsky, J.R.: Toronto's Public Health Photography. Archivaria 10:145-155, 1980 ⟨II-00567⟩

Sapir, E.: A Girl's Puberty Ceremony among the Nootka Indians. PTRSC, section II:67-80, 1913 ⟨II-00644⟩

Sarwer-Foner, G.J.: In Memoriam: Professor Aldwyn Brockway Stokes, CBE, MA, BM, BCH (Oxon), DCH, DPM, FRCP (Lond), FRCP (C), February 23, 1906 - May 3, 1978. Psychiatric Journal of the University of Ottawa 3:235-236, 1978 ⟨I-01080⟩

Sarwer-Foner, G.J.: Hyman Caplan, M.D., C.M., F.R.C.P.(C). Psychiatric Journal of the University of Ottawa 5:145-146, 1980 ⟨I-01585⟩

Saucier, J.: Petite Histoire du Journalisme Medical au Canada Francais. L'UMC 65:1039-1049, 1936 ⟨II-02376⟩

Saucier, J.: Quand nos Peres Lisaient "L'Union Medicale". L'UMC 75:1341-1346, 1946 ⟨II-01856⟩

Saucier, J.: Montreal Neurology. CMAJ 82:892-894, 1960 ⟨II-03726⟩

Sauerland, E.K.: Dr. J.C. Boileau Grant, Anatomist Extraordinaire. JAMA 232:1347-1348, 1975 ⟨I-01373⟩

Saunders, E.M. (Edit.): The Life and Letters of the Rt. Hon. Sir Charles Tupper, Bart., K.C.M.G., Vol. 1 and Vol. 2. New York, Frederick A. Stokes Co., 1916. 319 p. -- Vol II 298 p. ⟨II-00663⟩

Saunders, L.Z.: Some Pioneers in Comparative Medicine. Canadian Veterinary Journal 14:27-35, 1973 ⟨II-00388⟩

Saunders, W.: Pharmacy in Canada before 1871. Canadian Pharmaceutical Journal 75:10-11, 70, 1942 ⟨II-00712⟩

Saunderson, H.H.: Class of '28 -- 50 Years Later. University of Manitoba Medical Journal 48:95-105, 1978 ⟨II-00244⟩

Savard, P.: Pierre-Martial Bardy. DCB 9:32-33, 1976 ⟨I-00977⟩

S[awyer], G.: Thomas Clarence Routley, MD, FRCP(C), LLD, DSc, CBE. Ontario Medical Review 30:202-203, 1963. ⟨I-02601⟩

Sawyer, G.: The First 100 Years: A History of the Ontario Medical Association. Toronto, Ontario Medical Association, 1980. 337 p. ⟨II-01810⟩

Scammell, H.L.: Dr. Murdock Daniel Morrison. CMAJ 55:88, 1946 ⟨I-03193⟩

Scammell, H.L.: The Old Lady Steps Back. Nova Scotia Medical Bulletin 26:266-269, 1947 ⟨II-03708⟩

Scammell, H.L.: Medicine Hat. Nova Scotia Medical Bulletin 28:146-148, 1949 ⟨I-03553⟩

Scammell, H.L.: John George MacDougall, M.D.C.M., F.A.C.S., F.R.C.S. [C.]. CMAJ 63:314-5, 1950 ⟨I-04512⟩

Scammell, H.L.: Dr. Louis Morton Silver. Nova Scotia Medical Bulletin 30:165-167, 1951 ⟨I-01689⟩

Scammell, H.L.: The Halifax Bridewell. CMAJ 64:163-15, 1951 ⟨II-01841⟩

Scammell, H.L.: A Century in Retrospect. CMAJ 69:349-352, 1953 ⟨II-03722⟩

Scammell, H.L.: Remember "Pa" Kenney?. Nova Scotia Medical Bulletin 32:260-265, 1953 ⟨I-02570⟩

Scammell, H.L.: Harry Goudge Grant. Nova Scotia Medical Bulletin 33:167-168, 1954 ⟨I-02156⟩

Scammell, H.L.: The Halifax Medical College. Dalhousie Medical Journal 11(1):12-17, 1958 ⟨II-00285⟩

Scammell, H.L.: John Stewart. Canadian Journal of Surgery 4:263-237, 1960-61 ⟨I-04239⟩

Scammmell. H.L.: A brief history of medicine in Nova Scotia. Dalhousie Medical Journal 19:33-36, 79-83, 91-96, 1965-66 ⟨II-03723⟩

Scarlett, E.P.: Reginald Burton Deane 1870-1941. CACHB 6(3):9-16, 1941 ⟨I-02489⟩

Scarlett, E.P.: Sir John Christian Schultz (1840-1896). CACHB 8(2):1-7, 1943 ⟨II-00664⟩

Scarlett, E.P.: Tenth Anniversary of the Bulletin. CACHB 10:1-4, 1945 ⟨II-01541⟩

Scarlett, E.P.: Delta: A Problem in Authorship. CMAJ 55:299-304, 1946 ⟨I-04363⟩

Scarlett, E.P.: "The Macnab". CACHB 16:21-24, 1951 〈I-01417〉

Scarlett, E.P.: Salutation to an elder. CACHB 17:59-60, 1952 〈I-01083〉

Scarlett, E.P.: And...at the last. No Marble, No Conventional Phrase. CACHB 19:32-34, 1954 〈I-01087〉

Scarlett, E.P.: Ave Atque Vale: Albert Earl Aikenhead 1882-1954. CACHB 19:84-85, 1954 〈I-00021〉

S[carlett], E.P.: Frederick Pilcher 1906-1954. CACHB 19:63-4, 1954 〈I-04387〉

Scarlett, E.P.: Medical Sources of Alberta Place-Names. CACHB 20:70-72, 1955 〈II-03709〉

Scarlett, E.P.: A Walled Stead. Alberta Medical Bulletin 21:3-9, 1956 〈II-03710〉

Scarlett, E.P.: Eastern Gate and Western Cavalcade. Canadian Services Medical Journal 12:851-870, 1956 〈II-03711〉

Scarlett, E.P.: A Doctor of the Frontier. Group Practice 16:659-664, 1967 〈I-03554〉

Scarlett, E.P.: A Forgotten Figure. Group Practice, pp 24, 26, 1970 〈I-03412〉

Scatliff, H.K.: A Doctor Specializes -- in Crime. Chicago Medicine 69(16):691-698, 1966 〈I-00908〉

Schaeffer, C.E.: Blackfoot shaking tent. Calgary, Glenbow-Alberta Inst 1969. 39 p. 〈II-00624〉

Schmidt, A.: An Rh Retrospective. The Alumni Journal [U. Manitoba] 43:6-7, 1983 〈II-05209〉

Schoenfeld, R.: Dr. B.F. Boyce. Okanagan Historical Society Annual Report 37:52-55, 1973 〈I-05067〉

Schrire, C., Steiger, W.L.: Arctic Infanticide Revisited. Etudes/Inuit/Studies 5:111-117, 1981 〈II-05414〉

Schwitalla, A.M.: The Tercentenary of the Hotel-Dieu of Montreal 1642-1942. Hospital Progress 23:159-63, 235-44, 1942 〈II-04697〉

Scott, G.D.: Inmate: The Casebook Revelations of a Canadian Penitentiary Psychiatrist. Montreal, Optimum Publishing International Inc., 1982. 226 pages 〈II-04818〉

Scott, J.W.: Faculty of Medicine, University of Alberta. Alberta Medical Bulletin 20:58-61, 1955 〈II-03706〉

Scott, J.W.: The History of the Faculty of Medicine of the University of Alberta 1913-1963. Alberta, The University of Alberta, 1963. 43 p. 〈II-00286〉

Scott, J.W.: Osler and the Science of Medicine. In: International Congress for the History of Medicine, 25th, Quebec, 1976. Proceedings, Volume III, 1976. p. 1244-1252 〈I-01269〉

Scott, J.W.: Preconfederation Medical Instruments. Canadian (Antique) Collector 13:42-45, 1978 〈II-00150〉

Scott, J.W.: Medical Education Sites in Toronto Commemorated. Ontario Medical Review 47:452-454, 1980 〈II-01951〉

Scott, J.W.: Rolph's Medical School. Ontario Medical Review 47:454-455, 1980 〈II-01952〉

Scott, J.W.: The History of Medicine Museum. In: Jarrell, R.A.; Ball, N.R.: Science, Technology, and Canadian History. Waterloo, Wilfrid Laurier Univ. Press, 1980. pp 206-207 〈II-00787〉

Scott, M.: McClure: The China Years of Dr. Bob McClure. Toronto, Canec Publishing and Supply House, 1977. 409 p. 〈I-01278〉

Scott, M.: McClure: Years of Challenge. Toronto, Canec Publishing and Supply House, 1979, 295 pp. 〈I-04439〉

Scratch, G.W.: John Tait 1878-1944. PTRSC 39:119-122, 1945 〈I-03570〉

Scrivener, L.: Terry Fox: His Story. Toronto, McClelland and Stewart, 1981, pp 176 〈II-05284〉

Scriver, J.B.: McGill's First Women Medical Students. McGill Medical Journal 16:237-43, 1947 〈II-02327〉

Scriver, J.B.: The Montreal Children's Hospital: Years of Growth. Montreal, McGill-Queen's University Press, 1979, 179 p. 〈II-04614〉

Scriver, J.B.: The Royal Victoria Hospital, Montreal: Common Diseases in the 1920's and 1930's. In: Shephard, D.A.E.; Levesque, A.(edit): Norman Bethune: His Times and His Legacy. Ottawa, Canadian Public Health Assoc., 1982. pp 79-84 〈II-04927〉

Scriver, W de M.: Nothing new under the sun [Montreal Medico-Chirurgical Society]. CMAJ 80:299-303, 1959 〈II-03724〉

Seaborn, E.: The Asiatic Cholera in 1832 in the London District. PTRSC 31:153-169, 1931 〈II-03871〉

Seaborn, E.: The March of Medicine in Western Ontario. Toronto, Ryerson Press, 1944. 386 p. 〈II-00857〉

Seaborn, E.: Doctor Thomas Patrick: A Pioneer Saskatchewan Doctor. CACHB 10:83-88, 1945 〈I-02561〉

Secord, E.R.: Thomas Henry Bier. CMAJ 29:575, 1933 〈I-03077〉

Segal, R.L.: The Pharmacy and its Pharmacists. Bulletin of the Ontario College of Pharmacy 20:36-39, 1971 〈II-03730〉

Segall, H.N.: Dr. Louis Gross. CMAJ 37:609, 1937 〈I-02142〉

Segall, H.N.: Histoire de la Societe Canadienne de Cardiologie. L'UMC 89:82-85, 1960 〈II-04681〉

Segall, H.N.: History of the Canadian Heart Association. Mantioba Medical Review 40:94-96, 1960 〈II-03265〉

Segall, H.N.: Introduction of the Stethoscope and Clinical Auscultation in Canada. JHMAS 22:414-417, 1967 〈II-00149〉

Segall, H.N.: L'Introduction du Stethoscope et de L'Auscultation Clinique au Canada. L'UMC 97:1115-1117, 1968 〈II-02346〉

Segall, H.N.: William Stairs Morrow, Canada's First Physiologist-cardiologist. CMAJ 114:543-545, 1976 〈I-03182〉

Segall, H.N.: Stories of and about Goldbloom, Goldblatt, Greenspon and Gross, "The Four G's" of the Class of the McGill Medicine Class of 1916. Journal of the Canadian Jewish Historical Society 6:17-32, 1982 〈II-05193〉

Segsworth, W.E.: Retraining Canada's Disabled Soldiers. Ottawa, J. de Labroquerie Tache, 1920. 193 p. 〈II-00698〉

Seguin, R-L.: Le docteur Valois, un patriote ignore. Le Bulletin des Recherches Historiques 60:85-91, 1954 ⟨I-01024⟩

Seguin, R-L: "L'Apprentissage" de la Chirurgie en Nouvelle-France. Revue d'Histoire de l'Amerique Francaise 20:593-599, 1966-67 ⟨II-04940⟩

Seidelman, W.: Pages from the past: B.C's first medical journal. B.C. Medical Journal 18:7-9, 1976 ⟨II-01855⟩

Selye, H.: The story of the adaptation syndrome. Montreal, ACTA, Inc., Medical Publishers, 1952. 225 p. ⟨I-01076⟩

Selye, H.: From dream to discovery: on being a scientist. New York/Toronto, McGraw-Hill Book Co., 1964. 419 p. ⟨II-00072⟩

Selye, H: The Stress of My Life: A Scientist's Memories. Toronto, McClelland and Stewart, 1977/ 272 p. ⟨I-03938⟩

Senex (N. Howard-Jones): Fifteen Words that Saved Humanity. WHO Dialogue 73:7-8, 1979 ⟨II-00580⟩

Senior, J.E.: Feeding the 19th Century Baby. Canadian Collector, May/June 1978, pages 37-41 ⟨II-04804⟩

Senior, J.E.: A Different Museum. Ontario Museum Association Quarterly 8(2):16-17, 1979 ⟨II-00788⟩

Sersha, T.M.: The Use of Plant Medicines by the Dakota Indians. Thesis (M.A.) Manitoba, University of Manitoba, 1973. ⟨II-05022⟩

Sexton, A.M.: Wyatt Galt Johnston and the Founding of the Laboratory Section. American Journal of Public Health 40:160-164, 1950 ⟨I-02572⟩

Seymour, M.M.: Public Health Work in Saskatchewan. CMAJ 15:271-278, 1925 ⟨II-03731⟩

Shane, S.J.: Dr. Alfred Turner Bazin, appreciation. CMAJ 79:600-601, 1958 ⟨I-03893⟩

Shastid, T.H.: Henry Howard (1815-1889). In Kelly HW, Burrage WL: Dictionary of American Medical Biography. New York and London, D. Appleton and Co., 1928. pp. 604-605. ⟨I-01350⟩

Shastid, T.H.: W. Franklin Coleman (1838-1917). In Kelly HW,Burrage WL: Dictionary of American Medical Biography. New York and London, D. Appleton and Co., 1928. p. 247. ⟨I-00922⟩

Shaw, E.C.: Make the Attempt. (This doctor-historian out-flanked the bureaucrats and enriched his area's heritage by doing it.). Canadian Doctor 45:30-32, 34-35, 1978 ⟨II-00789⟩

Shaw, M.M.: He Conquered Death: The Story of Frederick Grant Banting. Toronto, Macmillan Co. of Canada Ltd., 1946. III p. ⟨II-00235⟩

Shaw, M.M.: Frederick Banting. Toronto, Fitzhenry and Whiteside Limited, 1976, p.62 ⟨I-04521⟩

Shephard, D.A.E.: Alexander Graham Bell, Doctor of Medicine. New England Journal of Medicine 288:166-69, 1973 ⟨II-03868⟩

Shephard, D.A.E.: The Contributions of Alexander Graham Bell and Thomas Alva Edison to Medicine. BHM 51:610-616, 1977 ⟨II-03707⟩

Shephard, D.A.E.: First in Fear and Dread -- Cancer Control in Saskatchewan: A History of the Saskatchewan Cancer Commission, 1929-1979. [Saskatchewan Cancer Commission, 1982] pp 354 + [75] ⟨II-05009⟩

Shepherd, F.J.: Origin and History of the Montreal General Hospital. N.p., n.d. 47 p. ⟨II-04613⟩

Shepherd, F.J.: Reminiscences of Student Days and Dissecting Room. Montreal, 1919. Printed for private circulation only. 28 p. ⟨I-01640⟩

Shepherd, F.J.: Sir Thomas George Roddick, M.D., LL.D., F.R.C.S.(Eng.). CMAJ 13:283-284, 1923 ⟨I-03001⟩

Shepherd, F.J.: The First Medical School in Canada. CMAJ 15:418-525, 1925 ⟨II-03702⟩

Shepherd, F.J.: William Gardner, M.D. CMAJ 16:1284-1285, 1926 ⟨I-01611⟩

Sherman, L.R.: Manitoba's Response to a Major Epidemic of Poliomyelitis and the Consequences for Rehabilitation Services. University of Manitoba Medical Journal 50:80-83, 1980 ⟨II-03734⟩

S[herrington] A.: Seventy Years of Editorial Excellence. CMAJ 125:85-83, 1981 ⟨II-04640⟩

Shields, H.J.: The History of Anaesthesia in Canada. Canadian Anesthetists' Society Journal 2:301-307, 1955 ⟨II-03700⟩

Shields, H.J.: Pioneers of Canadian Anaesthesia: Dr. Samuel Johnston: A Biography. Canadian Anaesthetist's Society Journal 19:589-593, 1972 ⟨I-02574⟩

Shillington, C. H.: The Road to Medicare in Canada. Toronto, Del Graphics Pub. Dept., 1972, 208 p. ⟨II-04443⟩

Shimony, A.: Iroquois Witchcraft at ix Nations. In: Walker, D.E.(edit): Systems of North American Witchcraft and Sorcery. Moscow, Idaho, Univ. of Idaho, 1970. pp 239-265 ⟨II-05362⟩

Shipton, C.K.: Peter de Sales Laterriere. Sibley's Harvard Graduates 16(1764-67):492-9, 1972 ⟨I-05378⟩

Shortliffe, E.C.: Dr. Charles H. Lawford. Alberta Medical Bulletin 18:50-51, 1953 ⟨I-03225⟩

Shortt, E.S.: Historical Sketch of Medical Education of Women in Kingston, Canada. N.p., Kingston, September, 1916, 24 p. ⟨II-03701⟩

Shortt, S.E.D. (edit.): Medicine in Canadian Society: Historical Perspectives. Montreal, McGill-Queen's University Press, 1981.

Shortt, S.E.D.: Andrew Macphail: The Ideal in Nature. In: The Search for an Ideal: Six Canadian Intellectuals and Their Convictions in an Age of Transition 1890-1930. Toronto/Buffalo, Univ. of Toronto Press, 1976. pp 13-38 ⟨II-00879⟩

Shortt, S.E.D.: Sir Andrew Macphail: Physician, Philosopher, Founding Editor of CMAJ. CMAJ 118.323-325, 1978 ⟨I-01516⟩

Shortt, S.E.D.: R.M. Bucke: Vital Force, Evolution and Somatic Psychiatry, 1862-1902. In: 27th International Congress of the History of Medicine, p.149-153, 1980 ⟨II-04207⟩

Shortt, S.E.D.: The New Social History of Medicine: Some Implications for Research. Archivaria 10:5-22, 1980 ⟨II-00201⟩

Shortt, S.E.D.: Antiquarians and Amateurs: Reflections on the Writing of Medical History in Canada. In: Medicine in Canadian Society: Historical Perspectives. Montreal, McGill-Queen's University Press, 1981. pp 1-17 ⟨II-04880⟩

Shortt, S.E.D.: Banting, Insulin and the Question of Simultaneous Discovery. Queen's Quarterly 89:260-273, 1982 ⟨II-04981⟩

Shortt, S.E.D.: The Influence of French Biomedical Theory on Nineteenth-Century Canadian Neuropsychiatry: Bichat and Comte in the Work of R.M. Bucke. International Congress for the History of Medicine, Paris, 1982. Proceedings, vol. 1:309-312, 1982 ⟨I-05219⟩

Shortt, S.E.D.: "Before the Age of Miracles": The Rise, Fall, and Rebirth of General Practice in Canada, 1890-1940. In: Roland, C.G.(ed.): Health, Disease and Medicine: Essays in Canadian History. Toronto, Hannah Institute for the History of Medicine, 1984, 123-152 ⟨II-05398⟩

Shortt S.E.D.: Medical Professionalization: Pitfalls and Promise in the Historiography. Journal of the History of Canadian Science, Technology and Medicine 5: 210-219, 1981 ⟨II-04637⟩

Shulman, M.: Coroner. Toronto/Montreal/Winnipeg/Vancouver, Fitzhenry and Whiteside, 1975. 154 p. ⟨II-00744⟩

Shulman, M.: Member of the legislature. Toronto/Montreal/Winnipeg/Vancouver, Fitzhenry and Whiteside, 1979. 226 p. ⟨II-00653⟩

Siegel, L.S.: Child Health and Development in English Canada, 1790-1850. In: Roland, C.G.(ed.): Health, Disease and Medicine: Essays in Canadian History. Toronto, Hannah Institute for the History of Medicine, 1984, 360-380 ⟨II-05407⟩

Sigerist, H.E.: Saskatchewan Health Services Survey Commission. In: Roemer, M.I. (edit). Henry E. Sigerist on the Sociology of Medicine. New York, M.D. Publications, Inc. pp 209-228. ⟨II-00435⟩

Sigurdson, L.A.: Dr. Ian MacLaren Thompson. University of Manitoba Medical Journal 52:8-9, 1982 ⟨I-04970⟩

Silverman, B.: The Early Development of Child Psychiatry in Canada. Canadian Psychiatric Association Journal 6:239-240, 1961 ⟨II-04819⟩

Silverman, B.: Dr. E. Ewan Cameron. CMAJ 97:985-986, 1967 ⟨I-01700⟩

Simard, L.C.: Le Docteur Eugene Latreille. L'UMC 58:55-56, 1929 ⟨I-01768⟩

Simard, L.C.: Le Professeur Pierre Masson a L'Academie de Medecine de Paris. L'UMC 64:1401-1404, 1935 ⟨I-02228⟩

Simard, L.C.: Le Professeur Pierre Masson, Medecin Honoraire a L'Hospital Notre-Dame (de Montreal). L'UMC 83:194-195, 1954 ⟨I-02229⟩

Simpson, E.E.: William Willoughby Francis. Placerville, California, Blackwood Press, 1981, 7 p. ⟨I-04362⟩

Simpson, J.H.L.: The life of Sir Charles Tupper. CMAJ 40:606-610, 1939 ⟨I-03375⟩

Sims, C.A.: An Institutional History of Rockwood Asylum at Kingston, 1856-1905. Thesis (M.A.), Kingston, Queen's University, 1981 ⟨II-04979⟩

Sinnot, J.C.: A History of the Charlottetown Clinic. Charlottetown, 1975 ⟨II-05145⟩

Sirluck, E.: Dr. Ian MacLaren Thompson. University of Manitoba Medical Journal 52:7-8, 1982 ⟨I-04969⟩

Sismey, E.D.: Quil'-Sten Okanagan Steam Bath. The Beaver 297(1):41-43, 1966 ⟨II-03317⟩

Sissons, C.B.: Dr. John Rolph's own account of the Flag of Truce incident in the Rebellion of 1837. CHR 19:56-59, 1938 ⟨II-00685⟩

Skinner, M.: The Seafort Burial Site (FcPr100), Rocky Mountain House (1835-1861): Life and Death During the Fur Trade. Western Canadian Journal of Anthropology 3:126-145, 1972-73 ⟨II-04204⟩

Small, B.: Medical Memoirs of Bytown. Montreal Medical Journal 34:549-560, 1905 ⟨II-03732⟩

Small, H.B.: John Franklin Kidd, CMG, MD, LLD. CMAJ 29:452-53, 1933 ⟨I-03073⟩

Smellie, T.S.T.: The origin and history of the Fort William Relief Society. Thunder Bay Historical Society Annual 3:17-19, 1912-13 ⟨II-03728⟩

Smith, A.S.: Thomas Dryburgh's Dream; A Story of the Sick Children's Hospital. Toronto, Briggs, 1889 ⟨II-00178⟩

Smith, D.B.: Robert William Weir Carrall. DCB 10:138-140, 1972 ⟨I-00924⟩

Smith, D.B. (Edit.): The Reminiscences of Doctor John Sebastian Helmcken. British Columbia, University of British Columbia Press, 1975. 373 p. ⟨I-01359⟩

Smith, F.E.: Dr. Mary Whittaker. CMAJ 67:378-9, 1952 ⟨I-04536⟩

Smith, J.F.: Life's Waking Part. Toronto, Thomas Nelson and Sons, Ltd., 1937. 345 p. ⟨I-02306⟩

Smith, J.W.: Fifty Years of General Practice. Nova Scotia Medical Bulletin 27:93-96, 1948 ⟨II-03729⟩

Smith, K.: Dr. Augusta Stowe-Gullen: A Pioneer of Social Conscience. CMAJ 126:1465-1467, 1982 ⟨I-04900⟩

Smith, K.: Maude Abbott: Pathologist and Historian. CMAJ 127:774-776, 1982 ⟨I-04976⟩

Smith, K.M.: Dr. James Barry: military man -- or woman?. CMAJ 126:854-857, 1982 ⟨I-04770⟩

Smith, P.H.: Pharmacy in British Columbia. Canadian Pharmaceutical Journal 91:690-692, 1958 ⟨II-00714⟩

Smith, W.D.: Curtis James Bird. DCB 10:67-68, 1972 ⟨I-00984⟩

Smith, W.E.: A Canadian Doctor in West China: Forty Years under Three Flags. Toronto, Ryerson Press, 1939. 2768 p. ⟨II-00545⟩

Smith, W.G.: Immigration, Past and Future. Canadian Journal of Mental Hygiene, 1:47-57,130-140, 1919-20. ⟨II-04799⟩

Smith, W.H.: Dr. Samuel Willis Prowse. CMAJ 25:366-67, 1931 ⟨I-03157⟩

Snell, A.E.: The C.A.M.C. with the Canadian Corps during the Last Hundred Days of the Great War. Ottawa, F.A. Acland, 1924. 292 p. ⟨II-00828⟩

Snidal, D.P.: Garfield M. Moffatt. CMAJ 124:516, 1981 ⟨I-03163⟩

Somerville, A.: Dr. William Alexander Campbell. CMAJ 31:573, 1934 ⟨I-03516⟩

Somerville, A.: The Alberta Department of Public Health. Canadian Journal of Public Health 50:6-19, 1959 ⟨II-00568⟩

Sonnedecker, G.: Pharmaceutical Education, 1867 and 1967. In One Hundred Years of Pharmacy in Canada 1867 - 1967. Toronto, Canadian Academy of the History of Pharmacy, 1969. pp. 1-10. ⟨II-00708⟩

Sourkes, T.L.: Twenty-Five Years of Biochemical Psychiatry. Canadian Psychiatric Association Journal 15:625-29, 1970 ⟨II-05337⟩

Spack, V.M.: The story of a pioneer doctor -- Harmaunus Smith. Wentworth Bygones 5:40-43, 1964 ⟨I-01630⟩

Spalding, J.W.: Sunrise to Sunset. Scarborough, Centennial College Press, 1978. 174 p. ⟨II-00381⟩

Spaulding, W.B.: Smallpox Control in the Ontario Wilderness, 1880-1910. In: Roland, C.G.(ed.): Health, Disease and Medicine: Essays in Canadian History. Toronto, Hannah Institute for the History of Medicine, 1984, 194-214 ⟨II-05400⟩

Spence, E.: Hugh A. McCallum, M.D., FRCP, LL.D. CMAJ 15:1173, 1925 ⟨I-02298⟩

Splane, R.B.: Social Welfare in Ontario 1791-1893: A Study of Public Welfare Administration. Toronto, University of Toronto Press, 1965. 305 p. ⟨II-02692⟩

Spragge, G.W.: The Trinity Medical College. Ontario Historical Society Journal 58:63-98, 1966 ⟨II-00333⟩

Sprague, J.D.: Medical Ethics and Cognate subjects. Toronto, Chas. P. Sparling and Co., Publishers, 1902. 248 p. ⟨II-00227⟩

Spray, W.A.: John Waddell. DCB 10:695-696, 1972 ⟨I-01190⟩

Spurr, J.W.: Edward John Barker, M.D. Editor and Citizen. Historic Kingston 27:113-126, 1979 ⟨I-00016⟩

Spurr, J.W.: Edward John Barker. DCB 11:47-49, 1982 ⟨I-04841⟩

Squair, J.: Admission of Women to the University of Toronto. Part 1. University of Toronto Monthly 24:209-212, 1924 ⟨II-03640⟩

Stanley, G.D.: A Brief Summary of Medical Beginnings. CACHB 2(3):9-12, 1937 ⟨II-00504⟩

Stanley, G.D.: Dr. Henry George. CACHB 2(2):8-10, 1937 ⟨I-01381⟩

Stanley, G.D.: Hon. L.G. DeVeber. CACHB 2(1):11-12, 1937 ⟨I-01208⟩

Stanley, G.D.: Medical Pioneering in Alberta (Dr. E.A. Braithwaite). CACHB 1(4):7-8, 1937 ⟨I-00975⟩

Stanley, G.D.: A Medical Pilgrim's Progress. CACHB 3(2):5-9, 1938 ⟨I-01084⟩

Stanley, G.D.: Dr. W.B. Cheadle. CACHB 3(1):307, 1938 ⟨I-00916⟩

Stanley, G.D.: Doctor William Morrison MacKay. CACHB 4(3):13-15, 1939 ⟨I-01447⟩

Stanley, G.D.: Dr. Neville James Lindsay. CACHB 4(2):6-9, 1939 ⟨I-01308⟩

Stanley, G.D.: Dr. Robert George Brett (1851-1929). CACHB 4(1):5-12, 1939 ⟨II-00506⟩

Stanley, G.D.: Andrew Henderson. CACHB 5(3):5-7, 1940 ⟨I-01344⟩

Stanley, G.D.: Edward Hector Rouleau. CACHB 5(1):4-10, 1940 ⟨I-01221⟩

Stanley, G.D.: Andrew Everett Porter (1855-1940). CACHB 6(2):5-11, 1941 ⟨I-01236⟩

Stanley, G.D.: Herbert Rimington Mead (? - 1898). CACHB 6(3):10-14, 1941 ⟨I-01448⟩

Stanley, G.D.: Irving Heward Cameron: The Philosophical Surgeon. CACHB 6:1-11, 1941 ⟨I-01564⟩

Stanley, G.D.: James Delamere Lafferty. CACHB 5(4):12-16, 1941 ⟨I-01307⟩

Stanley, G.D.: Further notes on Irving Heward Cameron. CACHB 7:8-10, 1942 ⟨I-01566⟩

Stanley, G.D.: Sir Charles Tupper 1812-1915. CACHB 6(4):1-9, 1942 ⟨I-01157⟩

Stanley, G.D.: Unforgettable incidents in pioneer practice. CACHB 7:8-10, 1942 ⟨II-00518⟩

Stanley, G.D.: Dr. Michael Clark. CMAJ 48:449453, 1943 ⟨I-01525⟩

Stanley, G.D.: Early days at High River, Alberta. CACHB 8(3):13-14, 1943 ⟨II-00512⟩

Stanley, G.D.: Medical Pioneering in Alberta: Unforgettable Incidents in Pioneer Practice. CACHB 7(4):9-10, 1943 ⟨II-00511⟩

Stanley, G.D.: Dr. John Rolph: Medicine and Rebellion in Upper Canada. CACHB 9:1-13, 1944 ⟨I-01137⟩

Stanley, G.D.: The medical annals of Alberta. CACHB 8(4):17-22, 1944 ⟨II-00538⟩

Stanley, G.D.: Unforgettable Incidents. CACHB 9:54-56, 1944 ⟨II-03718⟩

Stanley, G.D.: How to make a successful start. CACHB 9(4):76-78, 1945 ⟨II-00513⟩

Stanley, G.D.: Medical Pioneering in Alberta. CACHB 10(1):74-78, 1945 ⟨II-00514⟩

Stanley, G.D.: Unforgettable incidents in private practice. CACHB 10(3):147-148, 1945 ⟨II-00508⟩

Stanley, G.D.: A Pioneer Funeral. CACHB 11(1):13-15, 1946 ⟨II-00793⟩

Stanley, G.D.: A pioneer funeral. CACHB 11:13-15, 1946 ⟨I-01088⟩

Stanley, G.D.: Dr. Edward M. Sharpe. CACHB 11:57-63, 1946 ⟨I-02169⟩

Stanley, G.D.: One physician's honeymoon. CACHB 11:47-48, 1946 ⟨I-01090⟩

Stanley, G.D.: 'Bob' Edwards again and his Eye-Opener!. CACHB 12:38-40, 1947 ⟨II-00224⟩

Stanley, G.D.: Campbell of Lethbridge. CACHB 12:56-62, 1947 ⟨I-01563⟩

Stanley, G.D.: Dr. G.M. Atkin. CACHB 12(1):18-20, 1947 ⟨I-00019⟩

Stanley, G.D.: The pioneer doctor and a famous newspaper editor. CACHB II:82-84, 1947 ⟨II-00225⟩

Stanley, G.D.: Dr. Abraham Groves 1847-1935: A Great Crusader of Canadian Medicine. CACHB 13:4-10, 1948 ⟨I-01376⟩

Stanley, G.d.: Dr. Alfred Hamman of Taber, Alberta. CACHB 13:39-40, 1948 ⟨I-01339⟩

Stanley, G.D.: Dr. Charles Ernest Smyth: pioneer doctor of Medicine Hat. CMAJ 58:200-204, 1948 ⟨I-01660⟩

Stanley, G.D.: Surgeon-General A.H. Fraser. CACHB 12:83-84, 1948 ⟨I-01210⟩

Stanley, G.D.: Dr. Daniel Graisberry Revell: Medical teacher, scholar and gentleman. CACHB 14:48-54, 1949 ⟨I-01119⟩

Stanley, G.D.: Dr. Walter S. Galbraith of Lethbridge. CACHB 13:79-82, 1949 ⟨I-01380⟩

Stanley, G.D.: Dr. George Malcolmson. CACHB 14:78-85, 1950 ⟨I-01430⟩

Stanley, G.D.: Dr. Richard Parsons of Red Deer. CACHB 15:41-51, 1950 ⟨I-02562⟩

Stanley, G.D.: Medical Archives and their Relation to the Profession. CACHB 15:28-35, 1950 ⟨II-00202⟩

Stanley, G.D.: Unforgettable Incidents. CACHB 15:13-14, 1950 ⟨II-03721⟩

Stanley, G.D.: Daniel Stewart Macnab, October 28, 1879 - February 2, 1951. CACHB 16(1):10-20, 1951 ⟨II-00445⟩

Stanley, G.D.: Dr. Hugh Lang of Granton: A Family Physician on the Old Ontario Strand. CACHB 16:82-87, 1951 ⟨I-01314⟩

Stanley, G.D.: Dr. Louis J. O'Brien. CACHB 15:72-80, 1951 ⟨I-01244⟩

Stanley, G.D.: The North-West Territories Medical Association. CACHB 16(2):38-39, 1951 ⟨II-00458⟩

Stanley, G.D.: Who was Stephen Ayres?. CACHB 17:54-56, 1952 ⟨II-00556⟩

Stanley, G.D.: Early Days at the Muskoka San. CACHB 18(1):17-20, 1953 ⟨II-00126⟩

Stanley, G.D.: Medical Pioneering in Alberta. CACHB 17(4):75-78, 1953 ⟨II-00503⟩

Stanley, G.D.: Dr. J.F. ("Windy") Ross. Medical Recollections of Toronto Varsity. CACHB 18:88-95, 1954 ⟨I-01142⟩

Stanley, G.D.: Medical Pioneers in Alberta. Alberta Medical Bulletin 19:40-43, 1954 ⟨II-03844⟩

Stanley, G.F.G.: John Clarence Webster the Laird of Shediac. Acadiensis 3:51-71, 1973-4. ⟨II-00207⟩

Stark, E.: The History of Medical Bacteriology in Manitoba. Canadian Journal of Public Health 39:168-170, 1948 ⟨II-03720⟩

Starna, W.A.: Mohawk Iroquois Populations: A Revision. Ethnohistory 27:371-382, 1980 ⟨II-05363⟩

Starr, F.N.G.: The passing of the surgeon in Toronto. Canadian Journal of Medicine and Surgery 10:313-335, 1901 ⟨II-03719⟩

Stearn, E.W., Stearn, A.E.: The Effect of Smallpox on the Destiny of the Amerindian. Boston, Bruce Humphries, Inc., 1945. 153 p. ⟨II-03618⟩

Stephenson, J.: Repair of Cleft Palate by Philibert Roux in 1819. Plastic and Reconstructive Surgery 47:277-283, 1971 ⟨II-00096⟩

Stevenson, G.H.: The Life and Work of Richard Maurice Bucke, (an appraisal). American Journal of Psychiatry 93:1127-1150, 1937 ⟨II-01930⟩

Stevenson, G.H.: The Life and Work of Richard Maurice Bucke. American Journal of Psychiatry 93:1127-50, 1937 ⟨I-02305⟩

Stevenson, G.H.: Bucke and Osler: a personality study. CMAJ 44:183-188, 1941 ⟨I-03337⟩

Stevenson, L.G.: Sir Frederick Banting. Toronto, The Ryerson Press, 1946. 446 p. ⟨II-00236⟩

Stevenson, L.G.: Canadian Medical Faculties through the years: University of Western Ontario. CAMSI Journal 13:17-21, 1954 ⟨II-03839⟩

Stevenson, L.G.: University of Western Ontario. CAMSI Journal 13:17-18, 21, 1954 (Dec) ⟨II-00289⟩

Stevenson, L.G.: Dr. William W. Francis 1878-1959. CMAJ 81:515-516, 1959 ⟨I-02797⟩

Stevenson, L.G.: W.W. Francis 1878-1959. BHM 34:373-378, 1960 ⟨I-02795⟩

Stevenson, L.G.: Frederick Grant Banting. Dictionary of Scientific Biography 1:440-443, 1970 ⟨I-02761⟩

Steward, D.J.: The Early History of Anaesthesia in Canada: The Introduction of Ether to Upper Canada, 1847. Canadian Anaesthesist Society Journal 24(2):153-61, 1977 ⟨II-05326⟩

Stewart, B.: [Reminiscences]. Winnipeg Clinic Quarterly 23:110-113, 1970 ⟨II-03986⟩

Stewart, B.: CMA's Dr. T. Clarence Routley: 34 Years of Devoted Service. CMAJ 129:642-643, 645, 1983 ⟨I-05171⟩

Stewart, C.B.: Canadian Research in Aviation Medicine. Nova Scotia Medical Bulletin 26:86-95, 1947 ⟨II-03838⟩

Stewart, C.B.: Highlights of the Past Anniversaries. Nova Scotia Medical Bulletin 32:246-252, 1953 ⟨II-03837⟩

Stewart, C.B.: Harry Goudge Grant. Nova Scotia Medical Bulletin 33:166-167, 1954 ⟨I-02154⟩

Stewart, C.B.: Ian MacKenzie, MBE, MB, ChB, FRCS(Edin), FRCS(C), FACS. CMAJ 95:1218-1219, 1966 ⟨I-03409⟩

Stewart, D.A.: An Obstetrician-Adventurer to the Hudson's Bay in 1812 -- Dr. Thomas McKeevor. CMAJ 18:738-740, 1928 ⟨II-01806⟩

Stewart, D.A.: Sir John Richardson: Surgeon, Physician, Sailor, Explorer, Naturalist, Scholar. CMAJ 24:292-297, 1931 ⟨II-00351⟩

Stewart, D.A.: Malaria in Canada. CMAJ 26:239:241, 1932 ⟨II-00364⟩

Stewart, I.: These were our yesterdays. A history of district nursing in Alberta. Calgary, Irene Stewart, 1979. ⟨II-05107⟩

Stewart, I.A.: The 1841 Election of Dr. William Dunlop as Member of Parliament for Huron County. Ontario Historical Society Papers and Records 39:51-62, 1947 ⟨I-02018⟩

Stewart, J.: Dr. Robert Johnstone Blanchard, an appreciation. CMAJ 19:500-501, 1928 ⟨I-03504⟩

Stewart, J.: Dr. Francis J. Shepherd, an appreciation. CMAJ 20:212, 1929 ⟨I-01692⟩

Stewart, J.: Alexander Dougall Blackader, MA, MD, LL.D, MRCS, FRCP(C). CMAJ 26:519-524, 1932 ⟨I-00948⟩

Stewart, R.: Norman Bethune. Don Mills, Fitzhenry and Whiteside Ltd., 1974. 60 p. ⟨I-00971⟩

Stewart, R.: Bethune. Toronto, New Press, 1973. 210 p. ⟨I-00972⟩

Stewart, R.: The Mind of Norman Bethune. Toronto/Montreal/Winnipeg/Vancouver, Fitzhenry and Whiteside, 1977. 150 p. ⟨I-00973⟩

Stewart, R.C.: Early Vaccinations in British North America. CMAJ 39:181-183, 1938 ⟨II-03840⟩

Stewart, R.C.: Hospital Care of Smallpox in Montreal. CMAJ 43:381-383, 1940 ⟨II-03598⟩

Stewart, R.C.: The Montreal General Hospital and the Care of Contagious Diseases 1822-1897. CMAJ 43:282-284, 1940 ⟨II-03597⟩

Stewart, R.J.: Dr. Bethune is a hero to the Chinese. The Medical Post, pp 32-33, Nov.16, 1971 ⟨I-03881⟩

Stewart, W.B.: Medicine in New Brunswick. New Brunswick, New Brunswick Medical Society, 1974. 413 p. ⟨II-00858⟩

Stewart, W.B.: Indian Medicine in New Brunswick. In International Congress for the History of Medicine, 25th Quebec, 1976. Proceedings, Volume III, 1976. p. 1320-1326 ⟨II-00625⟩

Stewart, W.B.: Early Medicine and Surgery in New Brunswick. Canadian Journal of Surgery 22:183-190, 1979 ⟨II-04330⟩

Stewart, W.G.: Dr. Alexander Esselmont Garrow. CMAJ 13:931, 1923 ⟨I-02998⟩

Stewart, W.G.: Personal reminiscences of Sir William Osler. Bulletin IX, International Association of Medical Museums, 1927, pp. 4381-j. ⟨I-02289⟩

Stich, K.P.: Eclampsia and the study of F.P. Grove's women. Canadian Notes and Queries, No. 22, December 1978. pp 7-8 ⟨II-00873⟩

Stieb, E.W.: One Hundred Years of Organized Pharmacy. In One Hundred Years of Pharmacy in Canada 1867 - 1967. Toronto, Canadian Academy of the History of Pharmacy, 1969. pp. 11-24. ⟨II-00709⟩

Stieb, E.W.: Tinctures, Salt-Mouths, and Carboys. Bulletin of the Ontario College of Pharmacy 20:42-43, 1971 ⟨II-03836⟩

Stieb, E.W., Quance, E.J.: Drug Adulteration: Detection and Control in Canada I: Beginnings: The Inland Revenue Act of 1875. Pharmacy in History 14:18-24, 1972 ⟨II-05433⟩

Stieb, E.W.: Pharmaceutical Education in Ontario. I: Prelude and Beginnings. Pharmacy in History 16:64-71, 1974 ⟨II-05449⟩

Stieb, E.W.: Drug Adulteration: Detection and Control in Canada. A Step Forward: The Adulteration Act of 1884. Pharmacy in History 18(1):17-24, 1976 ⟨II-05432⟩

Stieb, E.W.: Three centennials: a retrospective view of Canada's pure food and drug legislative. In International Congress for the History of Medicine, 25th, Quebec, 1976. Proceedings, Volume 111, 1976. p. 1327.1340 ⟨II-00440⟩

Stiver, W.B.: Flight of the White Mice: A World War II Flashback. Ontario Medical Review 47:629-632, 1980 ⟨II-02977⟩

St. Jacques, E.: Hon. Dr. L.P. Normand. CMAJ 19:260-261, 1928 ⟨I-03502⟩

St. Jacques, E.: Histoire Medicale de Montreal Depuis sa Fondation Jusqu'a la Fin du XIXe Siecle. L'UMC 61:256-259, 1932 ⟨II-02375⟩

Stokes, A.B.: The Toronto Psychiatric Hospital 1926-1966. Canadian Psychiatric Association Journal 12:521-523, 1967 ⟨II-03843⟩

Stokes, P.J.: The Restoration of the Niagara Apothecary. Bulletin of the Ontario College of Pharmacy 20:33-35, 1971 ⟨II-03841⟩

Stone, A.C.: The Life of James Douglas, M.D. McGill Medical Undergraduatre Journal 8:6-20, 1938 ⟨I-01469⟩

Stone, E.: Medicine Among the Iroquois. Annals of Medical History 6:529-539, 1934 ⟨II-03842⟩

Stortz, G.: Of Tactics and Prophylactics. Canadian Lawyer 6(2):4-6, 1982 ⟨II-05002⟩

Strachan, M.: "Dr. Stanley" 1876-1954. CACHB 19:23-26, 1954 ⟨I-01085⟩

Street, M.M.: Watch-Fires on the Mountains: The Life and Writings of Ethel Johns. Toronto, University of Toronto Press, 1973. 336 p. ⟨I-03939⟩

Street, M.M.: Watch-Fires on the Mountains: The Life and Writings of Ethel Jones. Toronto, University of Toronto Press, 1973. 336 p. ⟨II-04118⟩

Stringer, R.M., Catton, D.V.: The history of anaesthesia in Hamilton, Ontario, Canada. October 1977. 45p. n.p. ⟨II-00042⟩

Strong-Boag, V.: Canada's Women Doctors: Feminism Constrained. In: Kealey, L.(edit): A Not Unreasonable Claim. Toronto, The Women's Press, 1979. pp 109-129 ⟨II-03150⟩

Strong-Boag, V.: Intruders in the Nursery: Childcare Professionals Reshape the Years One to Five, 1920-1940. In: Parr, J(ed): Childhood and Family in Canadian History, Toronto, McClelland and Stewart, 1982. pp 160-178 ⟨II-04885⟩

Strong-Boag, V.(edit.): A Woman with a Purpose: The Diaries of Elizabeth Smith 1872-1884. Toronto/Buffalo/London, University of Toronto Press, 1980. 298 p. ⟨I-02592⟩

Struthers, E.B.: A Doctor Remembers: Days in China and Korea. 1976, 146 p. ⟨I-04435⟩

Stuart, H.A.: Sir Wilfred Thomason Grenfell, 1865-1940. CACHB 5(3):1-3, 1940 ⟨I-02182⟩

Stuart, H.A.: Sir Andrew Macphail (1864-1938). CACHB 9:61-67, 1945 ⟨I-01421⟩

Stubbs, R.S.: Dr. John Bunn. In: Four Recorders of Rupert's Land. Winnipeg, Peguis Publishers, 1967. pp 91-134 ⟨I-04779⟩

Styran, R., Watson, A.: Books of Materia Medica in Toronto Libraries: The Renaissance Publications of a Traditional Character. Renaissance Reformation 6:23-9, 1969/70 ⟨II-05331⟩

Sullivan, M.: Retrospect of Fifty Years of the Medical School of Kingston. Np, nd, pp. 35 ⟨II-03716⟩

Sulte, B.: Le Mal De La Baie Saint-Paul. Le Bulletin des Recherches Historiques 22:36-39, 1916 ⟨II-00121⟩

Surveyer, E.F.: The Honourable William Renwick Riddell 1852-1945. PTRSC 39:111-114, 1945 ⟨I-03576⟩

Sutherland, N.: To create a Strong and Healthy Race.: School Children in the Public Health Movement, 1880-1914. History of Education Quarterly, ser.3, 12:304-333, 1972. ⟨II-00059⟩

Sutherland, N.: To create a strong and health race: school children in the Public Health Movement, 1880-1914. In Katz, MIchael B., Mattingly, Paul H. (ed.) Education and social change: themes from Ontario's past. New York, New York University Press, 1975. pp. 133-166 ⟨II-00058⟩

Sutherland, N.: Social Policy, 'Deviant' Children, and the Public Health Apparatus in British Columbia Between the Wars. Journal of Educational Thought 14:80-91, 1980 ⟨II-04877⟩

Svartz, N.: Dr. Wallace Graham: an appreciation. CMAJ 88:222, 1963 ⟨I-02141⟩

Swainson, D.: William Henry Brouse. DCB 11:114, 1982 ⟨I-04862⟩

Swan, R.: The history of medicine in Canada. Medical History 12:42-51, 1968 ⟨II-03733⟩

Swartz, D.: Canadian Doctors Who Have Distinguished Themselves in Other Fields. Manitoba Medical Review 34:645-655, 1954 ⟨II-03845⟩

Swartz, D.: An appreciation of C.B. Stewart. Manitoba Medical Review 46:486-487, 1966 ⟨I-01647⟩

Swinton, W.E.: Physician contributions to nonmedical science: William "Tiger" Dunlop, soldier, editor, lecturer and warden of the forests. CMAJ 115:690-4, 1976 ⟨I-01480⟩

Swinton, W.E.: Physicians as Explorers: Richard King: Arugmentative Cassandra in the Search for Franklin. CMAJ 117:1330,1333,1336,1341, 1977 ⟨II-02671⟩

Swinton, W.E.: Physicians as Explorers: Robert McCormich: Travels by Open Boat in Arctic Canada. CMAJ 117:1205-1208, 1977 ⟨II-03266⟩

Swinton, W.E.: William Henry Drummond -- A Master of the Peasant Thought. CMAJ 114:265-6, 1976 ⟨I-01477⟩

Swinton, W.E.: John McCrae, physician, soldier, poet. CMAJ 113:900-2, 1975 ⟨I-04442⟩

Swinton, W.E.: Abraham Gesner, inventor of kerosene. CMAJ 115:1126-9, 1976 ⟨I-04429⟩

Swinton, W.E.: Davidson Black, our Peking man. CMAJ 115:251-3, 1976 ⟨I-04430⟩

Swinton, W.E.: Robert Bell, the great geologist. CMAJ 115:948-50, 1976 ⟨I-04428⟩

Swinton, W.E.: Physicians as explorers: the contribution of John Rae to Canada's development. CMAJ 117:531-6 and 541, 1977 ⟨I-04385⟩

Swinton, W.E.: Sir John Richardson: Immense journeys in Rupert's Land. CMAJ 117:1095-1100, 1977 ⟨II-04478⟩

Swinton, W.E.: George Mellis Douglas: typhus and tragedy. CMAJ 125:1284-6, 1981 ⟨I-04561⟩

Sylvain, P.: Jean-Etienne Landry. DCB 11:483-86, 1982 ⟨I-04848⟩

T

T., J.: Dr. R.A.H. MacKeen, an appreciation. CMAJ 77:522, 1957 ⟨I-04754⟩

T., M.W.: Roy Fraser, BSA, MA, FRMS, LLD, an appreciation. CMAJ 77:357-58, 1957 ⟨I-04753⟩

Tabel, H., Corner, A.H., Webster, W.A., Casey, C.A.: History and Epizootiology of Rabies in Canada. Canadian Veterinary Journal 15:271-81, 1974 ⟨II-05441⟩

Tablyn, W.F.: Faculties of Medicine and Public Health, 1924-1938. In: These Sixty Years. London, Univ. of Western Ontario, 1938. pp 111-116 ⟨II-05360⟩

Tache, J.C.: The late Dr. Blanchet. Medical Chronicle 5:165-169, 1857-58 ⟨I-00988⟩

Tache, J.C.: Memorandum On Cholera, Adopted at a Medical Conference held in the Bureau of Agriculture, in March, 1866. Bureau of Agriculture and Statistics, 1866. (Ottawa) ⟨II-00092⟩

Tait, D.H.: Dr. Charles Tupper: A Father of Confederation. Collections of the Nova Scotia Historical Society 36:279-300, 1968 ⟨I-01156⟩

Tait, R.: The First Western Canadian X-Ray Specialist. University of Manitoba Medical Journal 45:57-59, 1975 ⟨II-00552⟩

Tait, W.M.: The Evacuation from Greece. CMAJ 49:314-317, 1943 ⟨II-03757⟩

Taylor, H.L.: Henry Taylor (1790-1890). In Kelly H.W., Burrage W.L.: Dictionary of American Medical Biography. New York and London, D. Appleton and Co., 1928. p. 1188 ⟨I-01158⟩

Taylor, J.A.: Dr. Gregoire F. Amyot. CMAJ 98:795, 1968 ⟨I-03908⟩

Taylor, J.F.: Sociocultural Effects of Epidemics on the Northern Plains: 1734-1850. Western Canadian Journal of Anthropology 7(4):55-81, 1977 ⟨II-04205⟩

Taylor, J.G.: An Eskimo Abroad, 1880: His Diary and Death. Canadian Geographic 101(5):38-43, 1981 ⟨II-04980⟩

Taylor, J.H.: Fire, Disease and Water in Ottawa: an Introduction. Urban History Review 7(1):1-37, 1979 ⟨II-03289⟩

Taylor, Lord.: Saskatchewan adventure: a personal record. Part I, background to the story. CMAJ 110:720,723,725,727, 1974 ⟨II-00654⟩

Taylor, Lord.: Saskatchewan adventure: a personal record. Part II, making contact. CMAJ 110:829,831-836, 1974 ⟨II-00655⟩

Taylor, M.G.: The Role of the Medical Profession in the Formulation and Execution of Public Policy. Canadian Journal of Economics and Political Science 26:108-127, 1960 ⟨II-00694⟩

Taylor, R.B.: Dr. William Oliver Taylor. CMAJ 49:150, 152, 1943 ⟨I-02756⟩

Taylor, W.I.: Dr. Karl Edward Hollis. CMAJ 92:198-199, 1965 ⟨I-02282⟩

Teece, W.K.: John Ash. DCB 11:32-33, 1982 ⟨I-04839⟩

Telford, G.S.: The First Child Welfare Conferences in Saskatchewan. Saskatchewan History 4:57-61, 1951 ⟨II-00060⟩

Temple, J.A.: Dr. Ross as a Surgeon. Canada Lancet 45:329-330, 1912 ⟨I-01147⟩

Tetrault, M.: L'etat de sante des Montrealais, 1880-1914. Thesis (M.A.), Montreal, 1979 ⟨II-05142⟩

Tew, W.P.: Dr. Frank R. Clegg. CMAJ 95:1045, 1966 ⟨I-02044⟩

Texter, J.H.: Misfortune to Fame. The Story of William Beaumont, M.D. and his Famous Patient Alexis St. Martin. Virginia Medical Monthly 102(10):821-6, 1975 ⟨II-05430⟩

Thaler, A.F.: Dr. Hugh Ross. CMAJ 19:738, 1928 ⟨I-03491⟩

Thibault, M.: Histoire de la Radiotherapie a l'hotel de Quebec. Vie Medicale au Canada Francais 2:955-6, 1973 ⟨II-05434⟩

Thomas, D.: The Making of a Saint. Quest 11(8):21-30, 1982 ⟨II-04997⟩

Thomas, G.W.: Wilfred T. Grenfell, 1865-1941 [sic]. Founder of the International Grenfell Association. Canadian Journal of Surgery 9:125-130, 1966 ⟨I-02119⟩

Thomas, G.W.: Surgery in the Sub-Arctic: A Thoracic Surgeon's Odyssey. Journal of Thoracic and Cardiovascular Surgery 70:203-13, 1975 ⟨II-05324⟩

Thomas, G.W.: The International Grenfell Association: Its Role in Northern Newfoundland and Labrador: part I: The Early Days. CMAJ 118:308-310, 326, 1978 ⟨II-02340⟩

Thomas, L.B.: Some Manitoba Women who did First Things. Historical and Scientific Society of Manitoba. Papers. Series 3, No. 4:13-25, 1947-8 ⟨II-02107⟩

Thomas, L.H.: Early Territorial Hospitals. Saskatchewan History 2:16-20, 1949 ⟨II-00179⟩

Thomas, M.W.: Dr. R.L. Fraser. CMAJ 16:99, 1926 ⟨I-01608⟩

Thomas, T.A.: Dr. Melbourne Raynor. CMAJ 16:100, 1926 ⟨I-01604⟩

Thompson, I.M.: F.J. Shepherd as anatomist. CMAJ 39:287-290, 1938 ⟨I-01679⟩

Thompson, I.M.: A doctor of the old school. CMAJ 69:74-75, 1953 ⟨I-02749⟩

Thompson, I.M.: Charles Clifford Macklin. PTRSC 54:133-135, 1960, 3d series ⟨I-01407⟩

Thompson, I.M.: Dr. Adamson as a medical historian. Manitoba Medical Review 44:564-565, 1964 ⟨I-00018⟩

Thompson, I.M.: Robert Tait McKenzie. CMAJ 93:551-555, 1965 ⟨I-01281⟩

Thompson, I.M.: Sir Andrew MacPhail, 1864-1938. Winnipeg Clinic Quarterly 20(1and2):20-32, 1967 ⟨I-01420⟩

Thompson, I.M.: Sir Andrew Macphail, 1864-1938. CMAJ 98:40-44, 1968 ⟨I-02833⟩

Thompson, J.B.: Wolfred Nelson. DCB 9:593-597, 1976 ⟨I-01274⟩

Thompson, J.E.: The influence of Dr. Emily Howard Stowe on the woman suffrage movement in Canada. Ontario History 54:253-266, 1962 ⟨I-01638⟩

Thompson, J.H.: The Beginning of our Regeneration: The Great War and Western Canadian Reform Movements. Canadian Historical Association: Historical Papers, pp 227-245, 1972 ⟨II-00463⟩

Thompson, J.H.: The Voice of Moderation: The Defeat of Prohibition in Manitoba. Mercury Series, History Div. Paper No. 1, The Twenties in Western Canada, 1972. pp 170-190. ⟨II-00077⟩

Thomson, A.R.: James Walter Woodley. CMAJ 20:682, 1929 ⟨I-02722⟩

Thomson, C.A.: Doc Shadd. Saskatchewan History 30:41-55, 1977 ⟨II-00519⟩

Thomson, C.A.: Saskatchewan's black pioneer doctor [Alfred Schmitz Shadd]. Canadian Family Physician 23:1343-1351, 1977 ⟨I-01980⟩

Thomson, D.L.: Dr. James Bertram Collip. Canadian Journal of Biochemistry and Physiology 35:1-5, 1957 ⟨I-02011⟩

Thomson, St. C.: Dr. John Stewart. CMAJ 30:222, 1934 ⟨I-01718⟩

Thomson, W.: Press Coverage of the Medicare Dispute in Saskatchewan: II. Queen's Quarterly 70:362-371, 1963-64 ⟨II-02323⟩

Thomson, W.A.: Incidents in early practice in the west. CACHB 10(1):79-82, 1945 ⟨II-00520⟩

Thorington, J.M.: Four Physicians-Explorers of the Fur Trade Days. Annals of Medical History, ser. 3, 4:294-301, 1942 ⟨I-04904⟩

Thorlakson, P.H.T.: The Late Brandur Jonsson Brandson. Manitoba Medical Review 24:223, 1944 ⟨I-05029⟩

Thorlakson, P.H.T.: The History of Prepaid Hospital and Medical Care Plans in Manitoba. CMAJ 84:896-899, 1961 ⟨II-05082⟩

Thorlakson, P.H.T.: A Tribute to Dr. Ross B. Mitchell. Winnipeg Clinic Quarterly 23:65-68, 1970 ⟨I-03181⟩

Thorlakson, T.K.: A Patient and His Pioneer Doctors. Winnipeg Clinic Quarterly 20:33-47, n.d. ⟨II-05080⟩

Thornton, L.A.: Grandmother's Pharmacy. New Brunswick Historical Society Collections 18:58-63, 1963 ⟨II-04011⟩

Thornton, R.S.: Hon. J.W. Armstrong, an appreciation. CMAJ 18:475, 1928 ⟨I-03904⟩

Tidmarsh, C.J.: The History of the Osler Society. McGill Medical Journal 25:176-78, 1956 ⟨II-03870⟩

Timothy, H.B.: Rediscovering R.M. Bucke. Western Historical Notes 21(1):34-40, 1965 ⟨I-03187⟩

Toket, M.H.: Highlights of a Half Century. Journal Dentaire du Quebec Dental Journal 8:7, 13, 1971 ⟨II-03756⟩

Tollefson, E.A.: Bitter Medicine. The Saskatchewan Medicare Feud. Saskatoon, Modern Press. 236 p. ⟨II-00433⟩

Tolmie, S.F.: My Father: William Fraser Tolmie, 1812-1886. British Columbia Historical Quarterly 1:227-240, 1937 ⟨I-05066⟩

Tompkins, G.: A History of the Kitchener-Waterloo Hospital. Waterloo Historical Society 52:44-60, 1964 ⟨II-04821⟩

Tompkins, M.G.: Harry Goudge Grant. Nova Scotia Medical Bulletin 33:165-166, 1954 ⟨I-02155⟩

Tondreau, R.L.: Michel Sarrazin (1659-1734): the father of French Canadian science. Trans. and Studies of the College of Physicians of Philadelphia 31:124-127, 1963 ⟨I-01983⟩

Tondreau, R.L.: Michel Sarrazin (1659-1734): the Father of French Canadian Science. Trans. and Studies of the College of Physicians of Philadelphia 31:124-127, 1963 ⟨II-02074⟩

Tory, H.M.: Robert Fulford Ruttan. CMAJ 22:597, 1930 ⟨I-03013⟩

Tracy, M.: William Bennett Webster. DCB 9:824-825, 1976 ⟨I-01191⟩

[Travill, A.A.]: Queen's University at Kingston, Faculty of Medicine 1854-1979. One Hundred and Twenty-Five Years Dedicated to Education and Service. Kingston, Queen's University, 48 p. ⟨II-01852⟩

Trent, B.: Northwoods Doctor. Philadelphia/New York, J.B. Lippincott Co., 320 p. ⟨II-00474⟩

Trigger, B.G.: The Individual and Society: Theories About Illness. In: The Huron Farmers of the North. New York/Chicago, Holt, Rinehart and Winston, 1969. pp 113-120 ⟨II-02628⟩

Troy, M.T.: Early Medicine and Surgery in Calgary. Canadian Journal of Surgery 19:449-453, 1976 ⟨II-04329⟩

Truax, W.: Reminiscences of a Country Doctor. CMAJ 60:411-415, 1949 ⟨II-00521⟩

Trudel, J.J.: Quelques journaux medicaux de langue Francaise au Canada historique. Winnipeg Clinical Quarterly 20:5-8, 1967 ⟨II-02395⟩

Tse-Tung, M.: In Memory of Norman Bethune. China's Medicine 5:325-333, 1967 ⟨II-00658⟩

Tuke, D.H.: Chapter 5: The Insane in Canada. In The Insane in the United States and Canada. London, H.K. Lewis, 1885. pp. 189-259 ⟨II-00159⟩

Tunis, B., Bensley, E.H.: A La Recherche de William Leslie Logie, Premier Diplome de L'Universite McGill. L'UMC 100:536-538, 1971 ⟨I-02227⟩

Tunis, B.: Inoculation for Smallpox in the Province of Quebec, a Re-appraisal. In: Roland, C.G.(ed.): Health, Disease and Medicine: Essays in Canadian History. Toronto, Hannah Institute for the History of Medicine, 1984, 171-193 ⟨II-05399⟩

Tunis, B.R.: In Caps and Gowns. Montreal, McGill University Press, 1966. 154 p. ⟨II-03120⟩

Tunis, B.R., Bensley, E.H.: William Lesley Logie: McGill University's first graduate and Canada's first medical graduate. CMAJ 105:1259-1263, 1971 ⟨II-00336⟩

Tunis, B.R.: Medical Licensing in Lower Canada: The Dispute over Canada's First Medical Degree. CHR 55:489-504, 1974 ⟨II-00138⟩

Tunis, B.R.: Tribute to William Leslie Logie. CMAJ 122:273, 1980 ⟨I-01311⟩

Tunis, B.R.: Issues in the Professionalization of Medicine, Lower Canada, 1788-1847. Newsletter, Canadian Society for the History of Medicine, 6:17-20, 1981 ⟨II-04800⟩

Tunis, B.R.: Medical Education and Medical Licensing in Lower Canada: Demographic Factors, Conflict and Social Change. Histoire Sociale/Social History 14:67-91, 1981 ⟨II-04793⟩

Tunis, B.R.: Public Vaccination in Lower Canada, 1815-1823: Controversy and a Dilemma. Historical Reflections 9:264-278, 1982 ⟨II-04995⟩

Tunis, B.R.: George Longmore. DCB 5:501-503, 1983 ⟨I-05311⟩

Tunney, E.: Sisters of Service, Edson, Alberta, 1926-1976, 50 Years of Service. Edson, Sisters of Service, 1976 ⟨II-05108⟩

Tupper, C.: Recollections of Sixty Years. Cassell and Company, Ltd, London, New York, Toronto, and Melbourne, 1914, 414p. ⟨I-04553⟩

Turnbull, F.: (Wallace Wilson). British Columbia Medical Journal 8:226-227, 1966 ⟨I-03321⟩

Turnbull, F.: Neurosurgery in Canada. Surgical Neurology 2:81-4, 1974 ⟨II-05418⟩

Turnbull, F.A.: Kenneth George McKenzie as the Young Chief: Retrospect. CMAJ 92:146, 1965 ⟨I-03179⟩

Turner, R.E.: The life and death of Louis Riel: part III -- medico-legal issues. Canadian Psychiatric Association Journal 10:259-264, 1965 ⟨II-02623⟩

Tuttle, M.W.: Peter McGregor Campbell. CMAJ, 71:631, 1954 ⟨I-04568⟩

Tyre, R.: Saddlebag Surgeon The story of Murrough O'Brien M.D. Toronto, J.M. Dent and Sons (Canada) Limited, 1954, 261 p. ⟨I-04515⟩

Tyre, R.: Douglas in Saskatchewan: The Story of a Socialist Experiment. Vancouver, Mitchell Press, 1962. 212 p. ⟨II-00659⟩

V

V., K: Lady Henrietta Banting: a life of service. CMAJ 116:85, 1977 ⟨I-03882⟩

Vachon, C.: Joseph-Octave Beaubien. DCB 10:36-37, 1972 ⟨I-00015⟩

Valens, J.A.: Dr. Alexander MacGillvray Young. CMAJ 41:213, 1939 ⟨I-03395⟩

Valens, J.A.: Dr. Harold Egbert Alexander. CMAJ 47:599, 1942 ⟨I-04278⟩

Valens, J.A.: Dr. Alexander Howard Armitage. CMAJ 48:279, 1943 ⟨I-04270⟩

Valens, J.A.: Dr. Andrew William Argue. CMAJ 52:530-1, 1945 ⟨I-04370⟩

Vallee, A.: Feu Dr. Ahern. In: Annuaire de l'Universite Laval pour l'annee 1914-15. Quebec 1914 ⟨I-05214⟩

Vallee, A.: Dr. Georges Ahern. CMAJ 17:1233, 1927 ⟨I-03423⟩

Vallee, A.: Un Biologiste Canadien, Michel Sarrazin (1659-1739). Quebec, Archives de Quebec, 1927. 291 pp ⟨I-01968⟩

Vallee, A.: The Medical Faculty of Laval University, Quebec. Surgery, Gynecology, and Obstetrics 60:1149-1150, 1935 ⟨II-05017⟩

Vallee, A.: Michel Sarrazin (1659-1734). The Crest 5(5):9-10, 1962 ⟨I-01990⟩

Vandall, P.E.: History of the Canadian Medical Association's attitude toward health insurance. University of Western Ontario Medical Journal 20:42-53, 1950 ⟨II-00254⟩

Van Nostrand, F.H.: Three years of neuropsychiatry in the Canadian army (overseas). CMAJ 49:295-301, 367-373, 1943 ⟨II-03743⟩

Van Wart, A.F.: The Indians of the Maritime Provinces, their diseases and native cures. CMAJ 59:573-577, 1948 ⟨II-00626⟩

Vaux, R.L.: Some notes on the organization and working of a cavalry field ambulance. The Western Medical News 4(7):167-173, 191-201, 1912 ⟨II-00831⟩

Verge, W.: Mon Cinquantenaire de Pratique Medico-Chirurgicale. L'UMC 87:958-962, 1958 ⟨I-01057⟩

Vipond, M.: A Canadian Hero of the 1920's: Dr. Frederick G. Banting. Canadian Historical Review 58:461-486, 1982 ⟨I-05028⟩

Vogel, V.J.: American Indian Medicine. Norman, University of Oklahoma Press, 1970 ⟨II-00628⟩

W

W., A.S., P., I.E.: Dr. Roberta Bond Nichols, an appreciation. Canadian Anaesthetists Society Journal 14:152, 1967 ⟨I-02538⟩

W., J.D.: Dr. Donald F. Moore. CMAJ 111:171, 1974 ⟨I-05169⟩

W., J.D.: Dr. J. Beatty Wallace. CMAJ 111:171, 1974· ⟨I-05168⟩

W., S.L.: Arthur Edward Grant Forbes, MD, CM. Nova Scotia Medical Bulletin 6:29-31, 1927 ⟨I-02807⟩

W., S.L.: The Medical Society of Nova Scotia 1869 to 1916. Nova Scotia Medical Bulletin 8:423-427, 1929 ⟨II-04164⟩

Wagner, R.L.: Robert Hale. DCB 3:274-275, 1974 ⟨I-01365⟩

Wahl, P., Greenland, C.: Du Suicide: F.A.H. LaRue, M.D. (1833-1881). Canadian Psychiatric Association Journal 15:95-97, 1970 ⟨I-04717⟩

Wales, H.C.: Dr. Charles Hawkins Gilmour 1879-1933. CMAJ 27:689, 1933 ⟨I-02809⟩

Wales, W.F.: Dr. Robert Meredith Janes: an appreciation. CMAJ 95:1401, 1966 ⟨I-01744⟩

Walker, E.R.C.: Dr. T. Clarence Routley, an appreciation. CMAJ 88:1223, 1963 ⟨I-02597⟩

Walker, S.L.: Michael Thomas Sullivan, MD. CMAJ 19:739-740, 1928 ⟨I-03494⟩

Walker, S.L.: Philip Doane McLarren, MD, CM. CMAJ 19:124-125, 1928 ⟨I-03501⟩

Walker, S.L.: Andrew James Cowie, M.D. CMAJ 20:449-450, 1929 ⟨I-02031⟩

Walker, S.L.: Fitzgerald Uniacke Anderson. CMAJ 20:681, 1929 ⟨I-03500⟩

Walker, S.L.: Medical Society Rennaisance. Nova Scotia Medical Bulletin 8:570-79, 1929 ⟨II-03742⟩

Walker, S.L.: The Medical Society of Nova Scotia. Nova Scotia Medical Bulletin 8:191-96, 1929 ⟨II-03741⟩

Walker, S.L.: Evan Kennedy, MD. CMAJ 22:743, 1930 ⟨I-03015⟩

Walker, S.L.: James Norbert Lyons, MD, CM. CMAJ 22:743, 1930 ⟨I-03016⟩

Wallace, A.B.: Canadian-Franco-Scottish co-operation: A Cleft-Palate Story. British Journal of Plastic Surgery 19:1-14, 1966 ⟨II-00097⟩

Wallace, A.F.C.: Dreams and the Wishes of the Soul: A Type of Psychoanalytic Theory among the Seventeenth Century Iroquois. American Anthropologist 60:234-247, 1958 ⟨II-00651⟩

Wallace, A.W.: History of Family Practice in B.C. British Columbia Medical Journal 21:264-5, 1979 ⟨II-03248⟩

Wallace, W.S.: The Periodical Literature of Upper Canada. CHR 12:4-22, 1931 ⟨II-01853⟩

Wallace, W.S.: The Graduates of King's College, Toronto. Ontario History 42:163-4, 1950 ⟨II-03256⟩

Wallis, W.D.: Medicines used by the Micmac Indians. American Anthropologist 24:24-30, 1922 ⟨II-00639⟩

Walmsley, L.C.: Dr. Leslie Gifford Kilborn: an appreciation. CMAJ 97:490-491, 1967 ⟨I-02566⟩

Walters, A.: James Wallace Graham, M.D., F.R.C.P.(Lond), F.R.C.P.(C). CMAJ 88:104-106, 1963 ⟨I-02116⟩

Walton, C.: [Reminiscences]. Winnipeg Clinic Quarterly 23:103-110, 1970 ⟨II-03740⟩

Walton, C.H.A.: A Medical Odyssey. Winnipeg, The Winnipeg Clinic, 1980 ⟨I-05052⟩

Wangensteen, O.H.: Dr. Donald Church Balfour: Builder of the University Name. University of Minnesota, 1950 ⟨I-00933⟩

Wansbrough, E.M.: Royal Canadian Dental Corps. Journal of the Canadian Dental Association 18:322-27, 1952 ⟨II-05202⟩

Ward, P.W.: The Standard of Living in Montreal, Canada, 1850-1900. International Congress for the History of Medicine, Paris, 1982. Proceedings, vol. 1:71-74, 1982. ⟨II-05273⟩

Ward, W.P.: Unwed Motherhood in Nineteenth-Century English Canada. Historical Papers, Halifax, 1981. Canadian Historical Association, pages 34-56 ⟨II-04815⟩

Ward, W.P.: Family Papers and the New Social History. Archivaria 14:63-73, 1982 ⟨II-05265⟩

Warfe, C.: Search for Pure Water in Ottawa: 1910-1915. Urban History Review 8:90-112, 1979 ⟨II-04211⟩

Warren, F.C., Fabre-Surveyer, E.: From Surgeon's Mate to Chief Justice - Adam Mabane (1734-1792). PTRSC 3rd series, 24(II): 189-210, 1930 ⟨I-03038⟩

Warren, M.R.: Dr. Henry Munro -- An elusive Figure. CMAJ 92:377-378, 1965 ⟨I-03191⟩

Warwick, O.H.: James Bertram Collip -- 1892-1965. CMAJ 93:425-426, 1965 ⟨I-02005⟩

Wasteneys, H.: Velyien Ewart Henderson, 1877-1945. PTRSC 40:91-93, 1946 ⟨I-04386⟩

Watermann, R.A.: Medizinalwesen Kanadas: in der Zeit von Nouvelle France (1600 bis 1763). R.A. Waterman, 1978. 60p. ⟨II-04983⟩

Waterson, E.: William James Anderson. DCB 10:13-14, 1972 ⟨I-00026⟩

Watkins, D.: The Practice of Medicine Among the Indians. Okanagan Historical Society Report 34:30-32, 1970 ⟨II-03609⟩

Watson, E.H.A.: History Ontario Red Cross 1914-1946. Toronto, Ontario Division Headquarters, 91 p. ⟨II-04987⟩

Watson, E.M.: John Alexander Macgregor, MD. CMAJ 41:518, 1939 ⟨I-03397⟩

Watson, I.A.: Allan Cameron. In: Physicians and Surgeons of America. Concord, Republican Press Association, 1896. pp 277 ⟨I-02511⟩

Watson, I.A.: Andrew McDiarmid. In: Physicians and Surgeons of America. Concord, Republican Press Association, 1896. pp 585-6 ⟨I-02520⟩

Watson, I.A.: Auguste Achille Foucher. In: Physicians and Surgeons of America. Concord, Republican Press Association, 1896. pp 207-208 ⟨I-02515⟩

Watson, I.A.: Duncan Campbell MacCallum. In: Physicians and Surgeons of America. Concord, Republican Press Association, 1896. p 34 ⟨I-02521⟩

Watson, I.A.: Edward Attrill Spilsbury. In:Physicians and Surgeons of America. Concord, Republican Press Association, 1896. p 45 ⟨I-02525⟩

Watson, I.A.: Edward Playter. In: Physicians and Surgeons of America. Concord, Republican Press Association, 1896. p 199 ⟨I-02523⟩

Watson, I.A.: Emmanuel P. Lachapelle. In: Physicians and Surgeons of America. Concord, Republican Press Association, 1896. p 19 ⟨I-02519⟩

Watson, I.A.: Francis W. Campbell. In: Physicians and Surgeons of America. Concord, Republican Press Association, 1896. pp 675 ⟨I-02512⟩

Watson, I.A.: Francis L. Howland. In: Physicians and Surgeons of America. Concord, Republican Press Association, 1896. p 156 ⟨I-02517⟩

Watson, I.A.: Frederick Montizambert. In: Physicians and Surgeons of America. Concord, Republican Press Association 1896. pp 27-28 ⟨I-02508⟩

Watson, I.A.: George Lawson Milne. In: Physicians and Surgeons of America. Concord, Republican Press Association, 1896. p 649 ⟨I-02522⟩

Watson, I.A.: George Sterling Ryerson. In: Physicians and Surgeons of America. Concord, Republican Press Association, 1896. pp 545 ⟨I-02524⟩

Watson, I.A.: Henry Aubrey Husband. In: Physicians and Surgeons of America. Concord, Republican Press Association, 1896. p 329 ⟨I-02518⟩

Watson, I.A.: John J. Cassidy. In: Physicians and Surgeons of America. Concord, Republican Press Association, 1896. pp 86-87 ⟨I-02513⟩

Watson, I.A.: John Morrison O'Donnell. In: Physicians and Surgeons of America. Concord, Republican Press Association, 1896. pp 772-3 ⟨I-03246⟩

Watson, I.A.: Peter H. Bryce. In: Physicians and Surgeons of America. Concord, Republican Press Association, 1896. pp 268-69 ⟨I-02510⟩

Watson, I.A.: Robert George Brett. In: Physicians and Surgeons of America. Concord, Republican Press Association, 1896. pp 753. ⟨I-02509⟩

Watson, I.A.: Robert J. Darragh. In: Physicians and Surgeons of America. Concord, Republican Press Association, 1896. p. 66 ⟨I-02514⟩

Watson, I.A.: Sir James A. Grant. In: Physicians and Surgeons of America. Concord, Republican Press Association, 1896. pp 402-403 ⟨I-02516⟩

Watson, M.C.: An account of an obstetrical practice in Upper Canada. CMAJ 40:181-188, 1939 ⟨II-03591⟩

Watson, M.C.: Medical aspects of the Normandy invasion. CMAJ 53:99-111, 1945 ⟨II-03739⟩

Waugh, F.P.: Symposium on Manitoban Memories. Winnipeg Clinic Quarterly 22:116-120, 1970 ⟨II-02906⟩

Waxman, S.B.: Dr. Emily Stowe: Canada's First Female Practitioner. Canada West 10(i) 17:23, 1980 ⟨I-04764⟩

Way, B.W.: Versatile Doctors of Upper Canada. Canadian Doctor, April 1962, pp 33-37, 65 ⟨II-03987⟩

Weatherilt, J.L.: Morley Alphonse Ryerson Young. CMAJ 125:218, 1981 ⟨I-04194⟩

Weaver, S.M.: Medicine and politics among the Grand River Iroquois: A study of the Non-Conservatives. Publications in Ethnology 4:1-182, 1972 ⟨II-00636⟩

Webster, C.A.: Yarmouth Doctors of the 1870's. Nova Scotia Medical Bulletin 6:5-14, 1927 ⟨II-03675⟩

Webster, C.A.: History of the early medical men of Yarmouth and conditions in the early days. Nova Scotia Medical Bulletin 16:193-198, 1937 ⟨II-03989⟩

Webster, J.C.: Those Crowded Years 1863-1944: An Octogenarian's Record of Work. Shediac, New Brunswick. Privately printed for His Family 1944. 51 p. ⟨I-01172⟩

Webster, J.C. (edit.): Diary of John Thomas. In: Diary of John Thomas: Journal of Louis de Courville. Nova Scotia, Public Archives of Nova Scotia, 1937. pp. 10-39 ⟨II-00844⟩

Webster, W.: Notes on the development of anaesthesia in Western Canada. CMAJ 17:727-728, 1927 ⟨II-03583⟩

Webster, W.: Major George Willard Treleaven. CMAJ 24:475, 1931 ⟨I-03066⟩

Weil, P.: Norman Bethune and the Development of Blood Transfusion Services. In: Shephard, D.A.E.; Levesque. A.(edit): Norman Bethune: His Times and His Legacy. Ottawa, Canadian Public Health Association, 1982. pp 177-181 ⟨II-04923⟩

Weiner, M.A.: Earth Medicine -- Earth Food. Plant Remedies, Drugs, and Natural Foods of the North American Indians. New York, Collier Books, 1972. 230 p. ⟨II-05259⟩

Weiss, G.: Hyman Caplan: 1920-1980. Canadian Journal of Psychiatry 25:684, 1980 ⟨I-02879⟩

Welch, C.E.: History of Canadian Surgery: The M.G.H. Twins. Canadian Journal of Surgery 8:325-331, 1965 ⟨II-03461⟩

Wells, D.B.: Scurvy: The First Disease Found in North America. CAMSI Journal 20:30-31, 1961 (Feb) ⟨II-00116⟩

Wenzel, G.W.: Inuit Health and the Health Care System: Change and Status Quo. Etudes/Inuit/Studies, 5:7-15, 1981 ⟨II-05413⟩

Weslager, C.A.: Cures Among the Delawares in Canada. In: Magic Medicines of the Indians. Somerset, N.J., Middle Atlantic Press ⟨II-00629⟩

Wetherell, A.: Charles Daniel Parfitt. Ontario History 44:45-56, 1952 ⟨I-02564⟩

Whalen, J.M.: "Almost as bad as Ireland": Saint John, 1847. Archivaria 10:85-97, 1980 ⟨II-00355⟩

Whalen, J.M.: The nineteenth-century Almshouse System in Saint John County. Histoire Sociale/Social History #7:5-27, 1971 ⟨II-03089⟩

Whalen, J.M.: Edwin Arnold Vail. DCB 11:896-97, 1982 ⟨I-04857⟩

Whalley, G.(edit.): Death in the Barren Ground: Edgar Christian. Canada, Oberon Press, 1980 ⟨II-02618⟩

Wherrett, G.J.: The Diamond Jubilee of the Canadian Tuberculosis Association. CMAJ 84:99-101, 1961 ⟨II-03460⟩

Wherrett, G.J.: Dr. Robert G. Ferguson. CMAJ 90:995-996, 1964 ⟨I-05224⟩

Wherrett, G.J.: The Miracle of the Empty Beds: A History of Tuberculosis in Canada. Toronto/Buffalo, University of Toronto Press, 1977. 299 p. ⟨II-00383⟩

Wherrett, G.J.: Norman Bethune and Tuberculosis. In: Shephard, D.A.E.; Levesque, A.(edit): Norman Bethune: His Times and His Legacy. Ottawa, Canadian Public Health Association, 1982. pp 65-70. ⟨II-04924⟩

White, G.M.: The history of obstetrical and gynecological teaching in Canada. American Journal of Obstetrics and Gynecology 77:465-474, 1959 ⟨II-03582⟩

White, J.: Gordon Lamberd. University of Manitoba Medical Journal 52:66, 1982 ⟨I-04966⟩

White, J.J.: Edward Archibald and William Rienhoff, Jr.: Fathers of the Modern Pneumonectomy -- An Historical Footnote. Surgery 68:397-402, 970 ⟨II-05424⟩

White, P.D.: A Tribute to Louis Gross. CMAJ 37:609, 1937 ⟨I-02153⟩

White, W.: Paul Z. Hebert, M.D.: "The Last Leaf" of Oslers's McGill Class of 1872. The Bulletin of the Los Angeles County Medical Association 71:520-527, 1941 ⟨I-04654⟩

White, W.: Medical Education at McGill in the Seventies: Excerpts from the "Autobiographie" of the late Paul Zotique Hebert, MD. BHM 13:614-626, 1943 ⟨II-02606⟩

Whiteford, W.: Reminiscences of Dr. John Stephenson, one of the Founders of McGill Medical Faculty. Canada Medical and Surgical Journal 11:728-731, 1883 ⟨II-00338⟩

Whitehead, F.L.: Leprosy in New Brunswick: the end of an era. CMAJ 97:1299-1300, 1967 ⟨II-03589⟩

Whitelaw, T.H.: Dr. Henry Richard Smith. CMAJ 19:737-738, 1928 ⟨I-03490⟩

Whitelaw, T.H.: Dr. Edgar W. Allin. CMAJ 29:338, 1933 ⟨I-03070⟩

Whitelaw, W.H.: Lieutenant-Colonel W.D. Ferris, MB. CMAJ 17:1233, 1927 ⟨I-02815⟩

Whiteside, C.: The Nomadic Life of a Surgeon. Edmonton, Alberta, Douglas Printing Co., 1950. 89 p. ⟨I-01173⟩

Whyte, J.C.: Dr. John Francis Puddicombe. CMAJ 96:507, 1967 ⟨I-02771⟩

Wightman, K.J.R.: Tributes presented at the memorial service for Professor R.F. Farquharson. CMAJ 93:233-234, 1965 ⟨I-02781⟩

Wilkins, R.: L'Inegalite Sociale face a la Mortalite a Montreal, 1975-1977. Cahiers quebecois de demographie 9:157-184, 1980 ⟨II-04946⟩

Willer, B., Miller, G.: Classification, Cause and Symptoms of Mental Illness 1890-1900 in Ontario.

Canadian Psychiatric Association Journal 22:231-235, 1977 ⟨II-04794⟩

Willer, B., Miller, G: Prognosis and Outcome of Mental Illness 1890-1900 in Ontario. Canadian Psychiatric Association Journal 22:235-8, 1977 ⟨II-04795⟩

Williams, G.: Edward Thompson. DCB 3:624-625, 1974 ⟨I-01195⟩

Williams, G.: John Potts. DCB 3:533-534, 1974 ⟨I-01243⟩

Williams, J.R.: The "S.S. Frederick Banting". CMAJ 50:181, 1944 ⟨I-04260⟩

Williams, J.R.: The Most Important Dog in History. The Bulletin, volume 3, number 9, 1946 ⟨II-00106⟩

Williams, R.: Poor Relief and Medicine in Nova Scotia, 1749-1783. Collections of the Nova Scotia Historical Society, 24:33-56, 1938 ⟨II-03099⟩

Willinsky, A.I.: A Doctor's Memoirs. Toronto, Macmillan Co. of Canada Ltd., 1960. 183 p. ⟨II-00389⟩

Wilson, B.: To Teach This Art. The History of the Schools of Nursing at the University of Alberta, 1924-1974. Edmonton, Hallamshire Publishers, 1977 ⟨II-05109⟩

Wilson, C.: Colin W. Graham: a tribute. CMAJ 55:315, 1946 ⟨I-02149⟩

Wilson, D.L.: G. Malcolm Brown 1916-1977. PTRSC series 4, 16:59-60, 1978 ⟨I-04954⟩

Wilson, M.C.: The Canadians, Marion Hilliard. Toronto, Fitzhenry and Whiteside Limited, 1977, p. 64 ⟨I-04520⟩

Wilson, R.: A Retrospect. A Short Review of the Steps taken in Sanitation to transform the Town of Muddy York into the Queen City of the West. Department of Public Health, City of Toronto. 37 p. ⟨II-00473⟩

Wilson, W.A.: Health Insurance -- A Flash-back. British Columbia Medical Journal 2:795-808, 1960 ⟨II-00250⟩

Wilt, J.C.: The history of medical microbiology at the University of Manitoba. Manitoba Medical Review 50(3):16-21, 1970 ⟨II-03586⟩

Wilt, J.C.: The History of Medical Education in Manitoba. University of Manitoba Medical Journal 39:125-132, 1968 ⟨II-03585⟩

Wilton, M.H.: Dr. Frederick Wilbur Jackson, an appreciation. CMAJ 78:296-297, 1958 ⟨I-02555⟩

Wishart, J.G.: Canadian Oto-Laryngology. Canadian Journal of Medicine and Surgery 52:127-135, 1922 ⟨II-03587⟩

Witridge, M.E.: Some observations on the evolution of rehabilitation in Canada. Medical Services Journal, Canada 23:869-894, 1967 ⟨II-03584⟩

Wolfe, S.: The Saskatchewan Medical Care Insurance Act, 1961, and the Impasse with the medical profession. Journal of Public Health 53:731-735, 1963 ⟨II-03588⟩

Wolffe, J.B.: A Man Unique in History. In: Davidson, S.A.; Blackstock, P. (edit): The R. Tait McKenzie Memorial Addresses. Canadian Association for Health, Physical Education and Recreation, 1980. pp 15-23 ⟨II-00378⟩

Woods, D.: Canadian Council on Hospital Accreditation. I: History and Philosophy of the Council. CMAJ 110:851-2, 1974 〈II-05440〉

Woods, D.: The family doctor in Canada evolves. CMAJ 112:92-95, 1975 〈II-00218〉

Woods, D.: Strength in Study. Toronto, College of Physicians of Canada, 1979. 248 p. 〈II-00217〉

Woods, J.H.: Hon. Dr. Robert George Brett, an appreciation. CMAJ 21: 621-622, 1929 〈I-02003〉

Woodside, M.St.A.: Dr. Wallace Graham: an appreciation. CMAJ 88:223, 1963 〈I-02159〉

Woolcock, H.R.: Attitudes to Health and Disease in London, Canada, 1826-1854. Thesis (M.A.), London, University of Western Ontario, 1977 〈II-05141〉

Woolner, W.: Dr. Dan Buchanan. CMAJ 29:575-576, 1933 〈I-03078〉

Woolner, W.: Dr. Joseph Henry Radford. CMAJ 36:99, 1937 〈I-02876〉

Workman, J.: Cholera in Canada in 1832 and 1834. Canada Medical Journal and Monthly Record of Medical and Surgical Science 2:485-489, 1865-1866 〈II-00093〉

Workman, J.: Discourse on Education. York Pioneer 67:32-38, 1971 〈II-03286〉

Worthington, E.D.: Reminiscences of student life and practice. Sherbrooke, Quebec, 1897. 〈I-01644〉

Wrenshall, E.: Hotel Dieu of Montreal Celebrates Three Hundred Years of Service. Canadian Hospital 19:13-15, 1942 〈II-03464〉

Wrenshall, G.A., Hetenyi, G., Feasby, W.R.: The Story of Insulin. Canada, Max Reinhardt, 1962. 232 p. 〈II-00237〉

Wride, R.J.: 'Surgery in British Columbia'. American Surgeon 38:471-6, 1972 〈II-05425〉

Wright, A.H.: The Medical Schools of Toronto. CMAJ 18:616-620, 1928 〈II-01807〉

Wright, H.P.: Dr. Richard Henry Moore Hardisty, D.S.O., M.C. CMAJ 56:114. 1947 〈I-04403〉

Wright, J.S.: Dr. Alexander Gillespie. CMAJ 36:99, 1937 〈I-02875〉

Wylde, C.F.: A Short History of the Medical Library of McGill University. The Canadian Journal of Medicine and Surgery 76:146-153, 1934 〈II-03463〉

Wylie, W.N.T.: Poverty, Distress, and Disease: Labour and the Construction of the Rideau Canal, 1826-32. Journal of Canadian Labour Studies, Spring 1983. pp 7-30 〈II-05275〉

Y

Young, D.: Was there an unsuspected killer aboard "The Unicorn". The Beaver 304(3):9-15, 1973 〈II-03315〉

Young, E.M.: The Hospitals and Charities of Vancouver City. British Columbia Magazine 7:608-11, 1911 〈II-05154〉

Young, G.: Dr. Frank Jones Farley. CMAJ 22:742, 1930 〈I-03014〉

Young, G.S.: Dr. Alexander Primrose, C.B., LL.D.,. CMAJ 50:389-390, 1944 〈I-04247〉

Young, J.: Frontier Pharmacies of Flin Flon. Modern Pharmacy 38(3):18-20, 1953 〈II-00700〉

Young, M.A.R.: A.E. Archer, M.D. CMAJ 61:193-4, 1949 〈I-04488〉

Young, M.R.: Then and Now. Nova Scotia Medical Journal 16:560-565, 1937 〈II-03465〉

Young, T.K.: Sweat Baths and the Indians. CMAJ 119:406, 408-09, 1978 〈II-05254〉

Young, T.K.: Changing Patterns of Health and Sickness among the Cree-Ojibwa of Northwestern Ontario. Medical Anthropology 3:191-223, 1979 〈II-04212〉

Y[oung], W.A.:: The Death of Dr. James H. Richardson. Canadian Journal of Medicine and Surgery 27:111-113, 1910 〈I-02499〉

Youngken, H.W.: The drugs of the North American Indian. American Journal of Pharmacy 96:485-502, 1924 〈II-00630〉

Youngken, H.W.: The drugs of the North American Indian (II). American Journal of Pharmacy 97:257-271, 1925 〈II-00631〉

Z

Ziegler, H.R.: Dr. W.E. Gallie. CMAJ 81:854-855, 1959